Obesity

Genomics and Postgenomics

Obesity
Genomics and Postgenomics

Edited by
Karine Clément
Pitié-Salpêtrière Hospital
Paris, France

Thorkild I.A. Sørensen
Institute of Preventive Medicine
Copenhagen University Hospitals
Copenhagen, Denmark

informa
healthcare

New York London

Informa Healthcare USA, Inc.
52 Vanderbilt Avenue
New York, NY 10017

© 2008 by Informa Healthcare USA, Inc.
Informa Healthcare is an Informa business

No claim to original U.S. Government works
Printed in the United States of America on acid-free paper
10 9 8 7 6 5 4 3 2 1

International Standard Book Number-10: 0-8493-8089-8 (Hardcover)
International Standard Book Number-13: 978-0-8493-8089-1 (Hardcover)

Library of Congress Cataloging-in-Publication Data

Library of Congress Cataloging-in-Publication Data
  Obesity: genomics and postgenomics / edited by Karine Clément,
Thorkild I.A. Sørensen.
    p. ; cm.
  Includes bibliographical references and index.
  ISBN-13: 978-0-8493-8089-1 (hardcover : alk. paper)
  ISBN-10: 0-8493-8089-8 (hardcover : alk. paper) 1. Obesity–Genetic aspects.
I. Clément, Karine, 1966- II. Sørensen, Thorkild I. A.
  [DNLM: 1. Obesity–genetics. WD 210 G3281 2007]

  RC628.G47 2007
  616.3'98042–dc22   2007015263

Visit the Informa web site at
www.informa.com

and the Informa Healthcare Web site at
www.informahealthcare.com

For Professor Albert J. Strunkard
—T.I.A. Sørensen

For Professor Daniel Ricquier
—K. Clément

Preface

The understanding of how genes influence the development and maintenance of obesity and its complications, such as type 2 diabetes and cardiovascular disease, has increased dramatically in recent decades, not in the least due to the development of tools for investigating genes and gene functions (i.e., large-scale genome screening). However, there is still much to learn. During this period several books on this topic have been published, but advances have been so rapid that a new one offering an updated overview of where we are now, the current front line questions, the technology that may help answer the questions, as well as future challenges and opportunities, is justified.

For some years, an annually updated comprehensive catalogue of findings on the genetics of obesity, defined as the role of interindividual genetic variation, has been published under the name, "The Obesity Gene Map," and the information it contains has been compiled in a useful website (www.obesitygene.pbrc.edu). However, for researchers and teachers approaching this field, there is a need to combine this source with an overview of the genomics of obesity, by which we mean the study of gene functions, the regulation of gene functions, and downstream relationships, including the interaction with environmental exposures in the broadest sense. Insight into possibilities and limitations is also needed to achieve a reasonable understanding of the current status and progress in the field. We have attempted to cover all the relevant main topics in the study of the genomics of human obesity, which clearly must also include rodent and nonvertebrate research. We have included both phenotypic quantitative genetics and molecular genetics, and we have added epigenetics and postgenomic processes, in addition to genotype-phenotype relationships.

On the other hand, the book does not intend to provide a completely up-to-date and comprehensive picture of the field. In view of the time it takes to produce a book and the amount of information emerging almost daily from many different laboratories, this would not be feasible. Since we began working on the book, several new discoveries have been made, and new technologies have come to prevailing use. A good example is the recent discovery, in a genome-wide search for genes associated with type 2 diabetes, of a very strong statistical association between a common, single nucleotide polymorphism in the *FTO* gene and the level of body mass index in the general population, published just before the final typesetting (www.scienceexpress.org 12 April, 2007). Aiming to incorporate each new important finding and technological development would make the writing of the book a never-ending story.

Our intention is rather to present a series of chapters in which competent and experienced experts, still actively involved in research in the field, give their current view on the topic of the chapter they were assigned to write. We have given contributors the freedom to set their own priorities in what and how they want to present their material within each chapter, with no editorial interference. This has a number of important implications for the reader. First, each chapter may be read as if it is an independent review article; second, there may well be repetition and even discordance among chapters, reflecting the diversity of opinions on the same issues; third, the selection of references in each chapter is based on what the contributors feel represents the core literature on the particular topic; fourth, the editors may not always share the opinions of the authors on various issues. The terminology and abbreviations used also reflect current customs in a particular area, except that we have used gene and gene product names and abbreviations in accordance with international standards.

ACKNOWLEDGMENT

The authors would also like to thank Ms. Catherine Couton for her excellent technical work in formatting the chapters.

Karine Clément
Thorkild I.A. Sørensen

Contents

Section 5: Syndromic and Monogenic Human Obesity

Section 6: Polygenic Human Obesity

Section 7: Gene-Environment Interaction in Human Obesity

Section 8: Epigenetics in Obesity

Contributors

Michael Affolter   Functional Genomics Group, Bioanalytical Science Department, Nestlé Research Center, Lausanne, Switzerland

David B. Allison   Section on Statistical Genetics, Department of Biostatistics, University of Alabama at Birmingham, Birmingham, Alabama, U.S.A.

Peter Arner   Karolinska Institutet, Department of Medicine, Karolinska University Hospital-Huddinge, Stockholm, Sweden

Paola Artioli   Department of Psychiatry, San Raffaele Institute, Milan, Italy

Gregory S. Barsh   Department of Genetics, Stanford University School of Medicine, Stanford, California, U.S.A.

Arnaud Basdevant   INSERM, U872, Nutriomique, Centre de Recherche des Cordeliers, Université Pierre et Marie Curie-Paris6, UMRS 872, Université Paris Descartes, Assistance Publique Hôspitaux de Paris, AP-HP, and Department of Endocrinology and Nutrition, Pitié-Salpêtrière Hospital, Paris, France

Philip Beales   Molecular Medicine Unit, UCL Institute of Child Health, London, U.K.

Monica Bertolini   Cattedra e Servizio di Endocrinologia e malattie del metabolismo, University degli Studi di Modena e Reggio Emilia, Modena, Italy

Yves Boirie   INRA, UMR 1019, Université de Clermont-Ferrand, Auvergne and Unité de Nutrition Humaine, Clermont-Ferrand, France

Claude Bouchard   Human Genomics Laboratory, Pennington Biomedical Research Center, Baton Rouge, Louisiana, U.S.A.

Jérémie Boucher   INSERM, U858, Institut de Médecine Moléculaire de Rangueil and Institut Louis Bugnard, Université Paul Sabatier, Toulouse, France

Andrew A. Butler   Pennington Biomedical Research Center, Louisiana State University System, Baton Rouge, Louisiana, U.S.A.

Frédéric Capel   INSERM, U858, Laboratoire de Recherches sur les Obésités, Institut de Médecine Moléculaire de Rangueil, Institut Louis Bugnard IFR 31, Université Paul Sabatier, and Centre Hospitalier, Universitaire de Toulouse, Toulouse, France

Isabelle Castan-Laurell   INSERM, U858, Institut de Médecine Moléculaire de Rangueil and Institut Louis Bugnard, Université Paul Sabatier, Toulouse, France

Yvon C. Chagnon   Psychiatric Genetic Unit, Laval University Research Center Robert-Giffard, Beauport, Quebec, Canada

Wendy K. Chung   Division of Molecular Genetics and The Naomi Berrie Diabetes Center, Columbia University Medical College, New York, New York, U.S.A.

Karine Clément   INSERM, U872, Nutriomique, Centre de Recherche des Cordeliers, Université Pierre et Marie Curie-Paris6, UMRS 872, Université Paris Descartes, Assistance Publique Hôpitaux de Paris, AP-HP, and Department of Endocrinology and Nutrition, Pitié-Salpêtrière Hospital, Paris, France

R. Keira Curtis Department of Clinical Biochemistry, University of Cambridge, Cambridge, U.K.

Ingrid Dahlman Karolinska Institutet, Department of Medicine, Karolinska University Hospital-Huddinge, Stockholm, Sweden

Jasmin Divers Section on Statistical Genetics, Department of Biostatistics, University of Alabama at Birmingham, Birmingham, Alabama, U.S.A.

Vernon Dolinsky Department of Molecular and Integrative Physiology, University of Michigan Medical Center, Ann Arbor, Michigan, U.S.A.

Hélène Dollfus Laboratoire EA 3949, Faculté de Médecine de Strasbourg, Centre de Référence pour les Affections Genetiques Ophtalmologiques, Hôpitaux Universitaires de Strasbourg, Strasbourg, France

Cédric Dray INSERM, U858, Institut de Médecine Moléculaire de Rangueil and Institut Louis Bugnard, Université Paul Sabatier, Toulouse, France

Oenone Dudley Institut de Biologie du Développement de Marseille Luminy, Marseille, France

Sven Enerbäck Medical Genetics, Department of Medical Biochemistry, Göteborg University, Göteborg, Sweden

I. Sadaf Farooqi Departments of Medicine and Clinical Biochemistry, Addenbrooke's Hospital, Cambridge University Hospitals NHS Foundation Trust, Cambridge, U.K.

C. Gallou-Kabani INSERM, AP-HP, Université Paris Descartes and Faculté de Médecine, INSERM Unit 781, Clinique Maurice Lamy, Hôpital Necker-Enfants Malades, Paris, France

M.S. Gross INSERM, AP-HP, Université Paris Descartes and Faculté de Médecine, INSERM Unit 781, Clinique Maurice Lamy, Hôpital Necker-Enfants Malades, Paris, France

Jorg Hager IntegraGen SA, Evry, France

Jennifer R. Harris Department of Genes and Environment, Division of Epidemiology, Norwegian Institute of Public Health, Oslo, Norway

Johannes Hebebrand Department of Child and Adolescent Psychiatry, University of Duisburg-Essen, Essen, Germany

Anke Hinney Department of Child and Adolescent Psychiatry, University of Duisburg-Essen, Essen, Germany

Jens Juul Holst Faculty of Health Sciences, Institute of Biomedicine, The Panum Institute, University of Copenhagen, Copenhagen, Denmark

C. Junien INSERM, AP-HP, Université Paris Descartes and Faculté de Médecine, INSERM Unit 781, Clinique Maurice Lamy, Hôpital Necker-Enfants Malades, Paris, France

Sona Kang Department of Molecular and Integrative Physiology, University of Michigan Medical Center, Ann Arbor, Michigan, U.S.A.

Jaakko Kaprio Department of Public Health, University of Helsinki and Department of Mental Health and Alcohol Research, National Public Health Institute, Helsinki, Finland

Nicholas Katsanis McKusick-Nathans Institute of Genetic Medicine, Johns Hopkins University, Baltimore, Maryland, U.S.A.

Irina Kratchmarova   Center for Experimental Bioinformatics, Department of Biochemistry and Molecular Biology, University of Southern Denmark, Odense, Denmark

Karsten Kristiansen   Eukaryotic Gene Expression and Differentiation Group, Department of Biochemistry and Molecular Biology, University of Southern Denmark, Odense, Denmark

Martin Kussmann   Functional Genomics Group, Bioanalytical Science Department, Nestlé Research Center, Lausanne, Switzerland

Dominique Langin   INSERM, U858, Laboratoire de Recherches sur les Obésités, Institut de Médecine Moléculaire de Rangueil, Institut Louis Bugnard IFR 31, Université Paul Sabatier, and Centre Hospitalier, Universitaire de Toulouse, Toulouse, France

Philip Just Larsen   Rheoscience, Rødovre, Denmark

Martine Laville   Human Nutrition Research Center, Rhône-Alpes, University Lyon-I and Department of Endocrinology-Nutrition, E. Herriot Hospital, Lyon, France

Rudolph L. Leibel   Division of Molecular Genetics and The Naomi Berrie Diabetes Center, Columbia University Medical College, New York, New York, U.S.A.

Ruth J.F. Loos   Medical Research Council (MRC) Epidemiology Unit, Cambridge, U.K.

Cécile Lubrano-Berthelier   INSERM, U872, Nutriomique, Centre de Recherche des Cordeliers, Université Pierre et Marie Curie-Paris6, Paris, France

Ormond A. MacDougald   Department of Molecular and Integrative Physiology, University of Michigan Medical Center, Ann Arbor, Michigan, U.S.A.

Lise Madsen   Eukaryotic Gene Expression and Differentiation Group, Department of Biochemistry and Molecular Biology, University of Southern Denmark, Odense, Denmark

Patrik K.E. Magnusson   Department of Medical Epidemiology and Biostatistics, Karolinska Institute, Stockholm, Sweden

Ariane Minet   Eukaryotic Gene Expression and Differentiation Group, Department of Biochemistry and Molecular Biology, University of Southern Denmark, Odense, Denmark

Béatrice Morio   INRA, UMR 1019, Unité de Nutrition Humaine, Clermont-Ferrand, France

Solomon Musani   Section on Statistical Genetics, Department of Biostatistics, University of Alabama at Birmingham, Birmingham, Alabama, U.S.A.

Françoise Muscatelli   Institut de Biologie du Développement de Marseille Luminy, Marseille, France

David Mutch   INSERM, U872, Nutriomique, Centre de Recherche des Cordeliers, Université Pierre et Marie Curie-Paris6, Paris, France

Jean-Michel Oppert   Department of Nutrition, Pitié-Salpétrière Hospital, AP-HP, Université Pierre et Marie Curie-Paris6, and Human Nutrition Research Center Ile-de-France, Paris, France

Stephen O'Rahilly   Departments of Medicine and Clinical Biochemistry, Addenbrooke's Hospital, Cambridge University Hospitals NHS Foundation Trust, Cambridge, U.K.

Matej Orešič   VTT Technical Research Centre of Finland, Espoo, Finland

Miguel Padilla Section on Statistical Genetics, Department of Biostatistics, University of Alabama at Birmingham, Birmingham, Alabama, U.S.A.

Rasmus Koefoed Petersen, Eukaryotic Gene Expression and Differentiation Group, Department of Biochemistry and Molecular Biology, University of Southern Denmark, Odense, Denmark

Daniel Pomp Departments of Nutrition and Cell and Molecular Physiology, The University of North Carolina at Chapel Hill, Chapel Hill, North Carolina, U.S.A.

Tuomo Rankinen Human Genomics Laboratory, Pennington Biomedical Research Center, Baton Rouge, Louisiana, U.S.A.

Finn Rasmussen Child and Adolescent Public Health Epidemiology Group, Department of Public Health Sciences, Karolinska Institute, Stockholm, Sweden

Frédéric Raymond Functional Genomics Group, Bioanalytical Science Department, Nestlé Research Center, Lausanne, Switzerland

David T. Redden Section on Statistical Genetics, Department of Biostatistics, University of Alabama at Birmingham, Birmingham, Alabama, U.S.A.

Treva Rice Division of Biostatistics and Department of Psychiatry, Washington University in St. Louis School of Medicine, St. Louis, Missouri, U.S.A.

Elke Roschman IntegraGen SA, Evry, France

Roland Rosmond Partille, Sweden

Alessandro Serretti Institute of Psychiatry, University of Bologna, Bologna, Italy

Thorkild I.A. Sørensen Institute of Preventive Medicine, Copenhagen University Hospitals, Centre for Health and Society, Copenhagen, Denmark

Gregory M. Sutton Pennington Biomedical Research Center, Louisiana State University System, Baton Rouge, Louisiana, U.S.A.

Antonio Tataranni Sanofi-Aventis, Bridgewater, New Jersey, U.S.A.

Hemant K. Tiwari Section on Statistical Genetics, Department of Biostatistics, University of Alabama at Birmingham, Birmingham, Alabama, U.S.A.

James L. Trevaskis Pennington Biomedical Research Center, Louisiana State University System, Baton Rouge, Louisiana, U.S.A.

Christian Vaisse Diabetes Center and Department of Medicine, University of California, San Francisco, San Francisco, California, U.S.A.

Philippe Valet INSERM, U858, Institut de Médecine Moléculaire de Rangueil and Institut Louis Bugnard, Université Paul Sabatier, Toulouse, France

Laura K. Vaughan Section on Statistical Genetics, Department of Biostatistics, University of Alabama at Birmingham, Birmingham, Alabama, U.S.A.

Hubert Vidal INSERM UMR870, INRA U-1235, and Human Nutrition Research Centre, Laennec Medical Faculty, Lyon 1 University, Lyon, France

Antonio Vidal-Puig Department of Clinical Biochemistry, University of Cambridge, Cambridge, U.K.

A.Vigé INSERM, AP-HP, Université Paris Descartes and Faculté de Médecine, INSERM Unit 781, Clinique Maurice Lamy, Hôpital Necker-Enfants Malades, Paris, France

Karani S. Vimaleswaran Medical Research Council (MRC) Epidemiology Unit, Cambridge, U.K.

Stéphane Walrand   INRA, UMR 1019, Unité de Nutrition Humaine, Clermont-Ferrand, France

Nicholas J. Wareham   Medical Research Council (MRC) Epidemiology Unit, Cambridge, U.K.

Allison W. Xu   Diabetes Center and Department of Anatomy, University of California, San Francisco, San Francisco, California, U.S.A.

Introduction

According to the World Health Organization, there are an estimated one billion overweight adults (BMI $\geq$ 25 kg/m^2); 300 million of these are considered clinically obese (BMI $\geq$ 30 kg/m^2), and the number is steadily increasing. Such staggering statistics clearly suggest that despite overt recognition of the taxing effects of obesity on both individual health and well-being and medical and social programs, we are still succumbing to this global epidemic, and it shows no sign of abating. Developing countries also face a transition in the alarming progression of obesity and its related comorbidities, especially diabetes, which has inspired a combination of the two words in the "diabesity." All the ancient authors, including one of the most ancient, Hippocrates, having an observant clinical eye, recognized that health risks were more common among obese subjects than lean ones. In 1956, Jean Vague pointed out the extraordinary variation in obese phenotypes, and, notably, that fat accumulation on the trunk and especially in the abdominal part of the body compared to the peripheral deposition, might be associated with this increased disease risk.

This overwhelming public health problem needs to be addressed in several ways. In spite of the parallel development of the obesity epidemic and the presumed obesogenic features of societies, it is clear that, in order to be able to find new ways of combating the epidemic, we need a better understanding of molecular mechanisms that lead to the accumulation of fat. While technological progress over the last twenty years has yielded the tools to comprehensively explore the perturbed biochemistry underlying the obese state, it is clear that both the individual's genetic makeup and the environment he or she is exposed to are critical for the regulation of adipose mass function. But discovering whether and how specific genes and specific environmental factors interact is still a great research challenge in this field. Finding the most efficient way of interfering with this process will obviously require much more progress in the identification of the diverse environmental factors that may interact with a given biological susceptibility to favor fat mass accumulation in different areas of the body. Medical and nutritional recommendations based on genetically undefined and/or environmentally heterogeneous population-based studies have had minimal success. Tremendous efforts have been invested in identifying new drug targets, so far with limited success, but the search is ongoing.

It is this relative lack of success that is now paving the way for the widely discussed concepts of personalized medicine and nutrition, which take into account genetic, environmental, and biological complexity at the population level. It is hoped that an important component of this complexity is the admixture of many different elements that, when disentangled, may lead to more straightforward and specific interventions that can be successfully administered at the individual level.

However, before realizing either of these ambitious ideas, the genetic components underlying obesity must be elucidated.

The idea that genetic susceptibility may contribute to the development of overweight and obesity is not new. In an 1872 medical treatise, Hufeland, a

German physician, in his definition of obesity noted, "In general, a congenital disposition has a big influence; so some people remain skinny in spite of the richest food, and others become obese whereas they are submitted to restriction." Even if this statement was a bit of a caricature, more than one century later, experiments with humans aimed at modifying an individual's environment revealed extraordinary individual variations in weight gain or weight loss in response to changes in food intake and/or physical activity.

At the beginning of the 20th century, works by Davenport (1923) mention that obesity tends to run in families. The development of genetic epidemiology using accurate statistical tools for data analysis of large populations of families, especially families with adopted children and twins, showed that various measures of obesity or fatness, such as body mass index, are influenced by genes throughout the range. On the other hand, the environmental influences are as obvious and clearly proven. The rapidly developing obesity epidemic in almost all world populations not subject to famine, is in itself a clear demonstration of the role of the environment, although it remains to be unraveled which environmental factors are crucial.

In spite of the diversity of environmental conditions, the familial correlation appears to be present everywhere, and twin and adoption studies indicate that among adults living separately, the familial correlation is due to the genetic relationships. While family members live in the same household, there is some contribution from the shared environment, especially in the children, but this fades away when the family member leaves the home. How heritable the different obesity traits are is less clear at this stage, but it is necessary to distinguish between the various obesity phenotypes in future research of both the genetic and environmental influences. The genetic epidemiology shows that the common forms of obesity must be multifactorial conditions influenced by many genes and many different environmental factors, and this has set the stage for the ongoing and future research that tries to elucidate the origins of obesity in general and the epidemic in particular.

In the past ten to fifteen years, the study of complex diseases has benefited greatly from the extraordinary advances made in molecular biology. While each form of obvious familial obesity was first thought to be a disease obeying Mendelian traits of inheritance for single major genes, the application of new technologies has painted a far more complex picture and led to unsuspected and fascinating new developments.

An illustrative example is provided by such syndromic forms of obesity as the Bardet-Biedl or Prader-Willi syndromes, among others. Although very rare, these cases have been well defined in the clinical context for years. Analysis of the genetic components of these conditions now suggests that multiple genes within a biological pathway may produce identical or close phenotypes. New fields of research have been opened by the molecular investigation of the Bardet-Biedl syndrome, for example, into the potential and mysterious role of ciliary cells in controlling some mechanisms of body-weight regulation. This means that pursuing the molecular exploration of rare but well-defined human phenotypes or syndromes is valuable for opening up fascinating new tracks, although the relevance for common obesity is still to be elucidated. Obesity stemming from a single, naturally occurring, dysfunctional gene (i.e., monogenic obesity) is both severe and rare when compared to the more common form of obesity, in which numerous genes make minor contributions to the phenotype (i.e., polygenic obesity).

Although some genetic candidates underlying monogenic obesities in the mouse have been defined, transferring this knowledge to man has produced more questions than answers. Indeed, the molecular approach has revealed novel candidate genes for the various "types" of human obesities, but it has also suggested that several cases previously defined as monogenic are genetically more complex than previously thought. This has made gene-gene and gene-environment interactions fundamentally important processes for the understanding of the mechanisms involved in fat mass expansion.

In view of these interactions, it is a great challenge to provide foolproof guidelines for the identification of a novel candidate gene that is important in determining a complex trait. Features such as expected-effect size, context-dependency, multiple testing, sample size, and replication must continue to be addressed on an experiment-by-experiment basis. Progress in the knowledge of the human genome, development of comprehensive technologies, and, notably, new analytical strategies will permit both the genetic and environmental aspects of complex traits to be addressed simultaneously.

The task is so great that success will ultimately lie with the creation of international consortia working toward a common goal, bringing together the expertise and resources needed to define and functionally annotate the genetic factors underlying the various forms of obesity. Our ability to identify promising candidates is progressing rapidly in the postgenomic era. This era is characterized by immense progress in the development of the tools of molecular biology (e.g., microarrays, mass spectrometry, bioinformatics, and so forth). Whether the consortia aim to sequence genomes, develop classification terminologies, create publicly accessible databases (such as HapMap), or provide scientific and ethical guidelines for emerging fields, the effect of collaboration is the same: Pooling together resources and knowledge from laboratories around the world achieves ambitious goals far more quickly and accurately than can be done by an individual research group working alone.

Programs comprising academic and industrial partners aim to study gene-environment interactions and identify the genomic processes susceptible to environmental stimuli. Within such programs the use of comprehensive platforms (i.e., genetics, transcriptomics, proteomics, peptidomics, lipidomics, and metabolomics) coupled with clinical data will probably play an important role in elucidating the perturbed functions leading to obesity.

In this rapidly changing context, we should not underestimate the necessity of adequately defining the human obesity phenotype, which is characterized by great diversity in subphenotypes and by natural evolution within the individual passing through different stages, which are probably associated with different molecular mechanisms. Bioclinical resources and individual characterizations created in accordance with this complexity are warranted. In this context, modern tools of exploration precisely aimed at dissecting the individual's obesity subphenotypes in population-based studies are needed. Indeed, individual complexity in humans relates to the influence of common disease alleles in different genetic backgrounds. Various genetic combinations, possibly influenced by different epigenetic factors—including the role of in utero environmental determinants—or environmental factors during an individual's lifetime are what face us in the task of deepening our understanding of the origin of obesity. Evaluation of perturbed functions at the multi-tissue level (for example, innovative imaging coupled with metabolic investigation) and environmental profiles are needed. Until now, the precise degree to which particular genes contribute to obesity has been poorly defined, and the importance of subtle, diverse environmental factors may not have been appreciated.

The future will tell us whether the current mix of the classical, hypothesis-driven approach and the hypothesis-generating approach using exploratory "omics" will succeed. While the latter approach is rapidly fed by extraordinary technological development (enabling the study of thousands of genes and gene products, thanks notably to progress in miniaturization) that will become accessible to many laboratories, bioinformatics, necessary for analysis and interpretation of the produced data, is itself a vast interdisciplinary field (involving computer science, physics, mathematics, and the contribution of biologic knowledge). Obesity as an environmentally-dependent disease is an exemplary model of an area where scientific experts from different fields need to exchange information and interact. In this context, new bioinformatics tools can be developed for a vast array of tasks, including integrating information from diverse sources and scales (environmental, clinical, genetics, genomics, and other "omics") obtained in humans and animal models; predicting and detecting genes and functional regulatory networks in key tissues of body weight regulation; and examining the kinetic influence of environmental changes in these networks of interaction including at the cell, tissue, organ, and whole-body levels, limited of course by the accessibility of tissues and organs.

The modeling of these effects can also be envisaged. Evaluating the pertinence of "omics"-derived results obtained in cells and in animal models in human physiopathology will probably become a prevailing activity the future. One pragmatic expectation is that through these technologies, we will be able to identify master candidate genes that will reveal novel biological pathways capable of affecting energy status, thereby enhancing our understanding of the multiple evolutionary stages in cellular adaptation during the development of human obesity. Some pivotal pathways could also be involved in other common diseases associated with obesity, e.g., diabetes and atherosclerosis. However, the success of these challenging cross-disciplinary approaches will probably be in translating the acquired scientific knowledge and predicting with confidence what can be used as treatment tailored to individual profiles.

USEFUL WEB SITES

Obesity gene map data base: www.obesitygene.pbrc.edu/
Nomenclature for genes and approved gene names (HUGO guidelines):
    www.gene.ucl.ac.uk/nomenclature/
Informations on genes:
    smd-www.stanford.edu/cgi-bin/source/sourceSearch
Mouse models and tools:
    jaxmice.jax.org/models/ www.genome.gov/10005834
Basis on molecular biology: www.web-books.com/MoBio/

1.1 Human Phenotypes

Jean-Michel Oppert
Department of Nutrition, Pitié-Salpétrière Hospital, AP-HP, Université Pierre et Marie Curie-Paris6, and Human Nutrition Research Center Ile-de-France, Paris, France

Martine Laville
Human Nutrition Research Center, Rhône-Alpes, University Lyon-I and Department of Endocrinology-Nutrition, E. Herriot Hospital, Lyon, France

Arnaud Basdevant
INSERM, U872, Nutriomique, Centre de Recherche des Cordeliers, Université Pierre et Marie Curie-Paris6, UMRS 872, Université Paris Descartes, Assistance Publique Hôpitaux de Paris, AP-HP, and Department of Endocrinology and Nutrition, Pitié-Salpêtrière Hospital, Paris, France

DEFINITION AND NATURAL HISTORY OF OBESITY

According to the World Health Organization, obesity is defined as "a condition of abnormal or excessive fat accumulation in adipose tissue, to the extent that health may be impaired" (1). Body composition, more specifically body fat content, and its relation to ill health are therefore central to the definition of obesity.

Obesity is a chronic disease characterized by the fact it is multifactorial in origin and heterogeneous, both in terms of determinants and phenotypes (1). With a temporal perspective, obesity can be viewed as a set of phenotypes that develop over time with a succession of stages that need to be differentiated (Fig. 1) (2). Schematically, it is possible to distinguish a *preobese static phase* when the individual at risk of obesity is weight stable and in energy balance, a *dynamic weight gain phase* during which weight is gained as a result of positive energy balance with intakes exceeding expenditures, and an *obese static phase* when the individual is weight stable again, but at a higher level, and energy balance regained (1). This phase is however rarely static as weight fluctuations are very frequent, usually as a result of efforts to lose weight and return to initial weight (Fig. 1).

Frequent weight fluctuations correspond to the notion of weight cycling (or "yoyo syndrome") and in many cases result in further increase in weight. Indeed, once the obese phase is established, the new weight appears to be defended both by biological and psychological regulatory mechanisms. It has been hypothesized that at the initial phase, behavioral and environmental factors would play a key role in the constitution of adipose-tissue excess on a genetically predisposed background. Then, progressively biological alterations of adipose-tissue metabolism would lead to some degree of irreversibility of the disease and contribute to the development of its metabolic and cardiovascular complications (2).

During the initial phase of obesity development, it has been suggested that even minor energy imbalance will lead to gradual but persistent weight (and fat) gain over time. For example, it has been recently calculated that an increase in

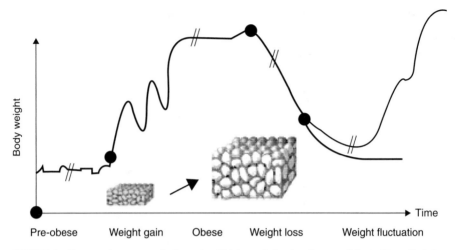

FIGURE 1   Temporal sequence in the natural history of obesity. *Source*: Adapted from Ref. 2.

energy intake or a decrease in energy expenditure through physical activity, on the order of only 100 kcal/day would theoretically be sufficient to explain the average rate of weight gain in the past decade in the United States (3). Such a small imbalance is, however, difficult to assess when using instruments currently available for measuring energy expenditure, and especially energy intake.

Given the natural history of obesity, as briefly outlined above, and the multiple determinants and consequences of this condition, the emphasis in this chapter is on the "obesities" rather than simply "obesity." Our aim is to delineate the most important of the numerous phenotypes that geneticists will have to deal with when exploring inherited factors contributing to obesity (Table 1).

PRIMARY PHENOTYPES: TOTAL AND REGIONAL BODY FAT
Overall Corpulence: the Body Mass Index
Body Mass Index Cutoffs in Adults and Children
There is an international consensus to use the body mass index (BMI), defined as the ratio of weight (in kg) over height squared (in m^2), to assess weight status and define obesity (Table 2) (1). In adults of both genders, obesity is currently defined as a BMI ≥ 30 kg/m^2. BMI is used for two main reasons. First, on a group basis, the BMI has been shown to be reasonably correlated with body fat content (r around 0.70–0.80) (4). Second, in a number of studies, a J- or U-shaped relationship was demonstrated between BMI and relative risk of mortality (all causes or cardiovascular) (5). Based on this type of relationship, current BMI cutoffs were defined, as shown in Table 2. In subjects of Asian origin, lower cutoffs have been proposed (overweight: ≥ 23 kg/m^2, obesity: ≥ 25 kg/m^2) (6) because a substantial proportion of Asian people was found at high risk of type 2 diabetes and cardiovascular disease at BMIs lower than 25 kg/m^2 (7).

In children, obesity is defined based on growth curves that describe, by sex, the development of BMI according to age (8). During childhood, BMI changes substantially over time (Fig. 2). After an initial increase in the first year of life, BMI declines and reaches a nadir around five to six years of age. The subsequent

TABLE 1 Overview of Obesity Phenotypes of Potential Interest in Genetic Studies[a]

Domain	Phenotype
Body fat	Overall corpulence (BMI)
	Total body fat
	Body fat distribution, abdominal visceral fat
	Weight changes over time
Energy expenditure	Total (24-hr) EE and components (resting EE, physical activity EE)
	Respiratory quotient, nutrient oxidation (lipid vs. carbohydrate)
	Physical activity level (TEE/REE)
	Nonexercise activity thermogenesis
Food intake	Energy intake, macronutrient intake
	Eating patterns (meal frequency, snacking), eating disorders (binge eating, cognitive restraint)
Physical activity	"Dose" (frequency, intensity, duration), type; sedentary behavior
Hormones, metabolites	Insulin, insulin sensitivity, ghrelin, inflammatory markers
	Adipocyte secretory products (leptin, adiponectin, angiotensinogen, PAI-1, IL-6, etc.)
Adipose tissue morphology	Adipocyte number and size, nonadipocyte components (stroma vascular fraction)
	Vascularization, innervation
Comorbidities	Metabolic and endocrine disorders: insulin resistance/metabolic syndrome, type 2 diabetes, dyslipidemia, hyperuricemia, nonalcoholic steatohepatitis, polycystic ovary syndrome, hypogonadism
	Cardiovascular: hypertension, ischemic heart disease, left ventricular hypertrophy, cardiac insufficiency, arrhythmia
	Respiratory: sleep apnea syndrome, obesity hypoventilation syndrome, asthma
	Joint diseases: knee, hip arthritis
	Cancers (colon, prostate, breast, uterus)
	Depression

[a]A variety of clinical features are related to syndromic forms of obesity, such as developmental abnormalities (short stature, abnormal growth, sensorial defects, polydactyly, and mental retardation/learning disability). Further details are found in Section 5.
Abbreviations: BMI, body mass index; EE, energy expenditure; REE, resting energy expenditure; TEE, total energy expenditure.

increase in BMI has been termed "adiposity rebound" (9). There is evidence that children with an early adiposity rebound have an increased BMI as adults (Fig. 2) (9,10). An international definition of childhood obesity has been proposed by the International Obesity Task Force (8). The definition relies on the BMI centile curves that pass through the cutoff points 25 and $30 \, \text{kg/m}^2$ used to define overweight and obesity in adults (8). National BMI-for-age charts are also available in many countries (Fig. 2). The difference between the definitions of adult and childhood obesity cannot be overlooked: in adults, obesity is defined as a risk factor for morbidity and mortality, whereas in children, obesity is defined on a population-distribution basis and/or the risk of being obese at age 18 years.

Limitations of BMI
There are a number of limitations to the use of the BMI as a measure of obesity that need to be carefully considered (11), especially since the BMI is so widely used as a phenotype in genetic studies on obesity. At individual level, the BMI does not give precise indications of body composition, i.e., it does not distinguish between weight associated with lean or fat tissue. Figure 3 illustrates the wide

TABLE 2 Classification of Weight Status in
Adults According to World Health Organization

Classification	BMI (kg/m^2)
Underweight	<18.5
Normal range	18.5–24.9
Overweight	25.0–29.9
Obese	30.0–39.9
Morbidly obese	≥40.0

Source: Adapted from Ref. 1.

variation in individual values of percent body fat for a given BMI. BMI does not capture either changes in body fat that occur with age, exercise training, or across ethnic groups (11,12). That a given BMI may not correspond to the same degree of fatness across populations is one justification for the different BMI thresholds in subjects of Asian origin mentioned above, as these individuals have a lower body fat percentage compared to Caucasians at an identical BMI (7). Thus, BMI can indeed be considered as the most useful although crude population-level indicator of obesity (1). However, it clearly does not account for the wide variation in obesity phenotypes between individuals and populations.

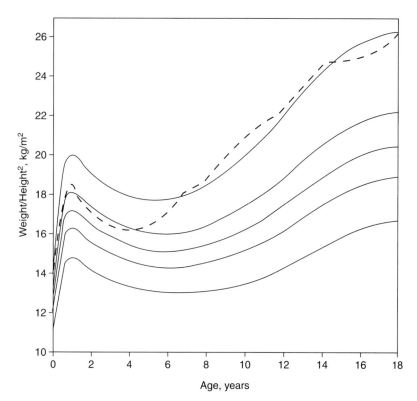

FIGURE 2 Body mass index (BMI) centile distribution in French girls according to age (from birth to 18 years) and an example of BMI development associated with an early adiposity rebound. *Source*: From Ref. 9.

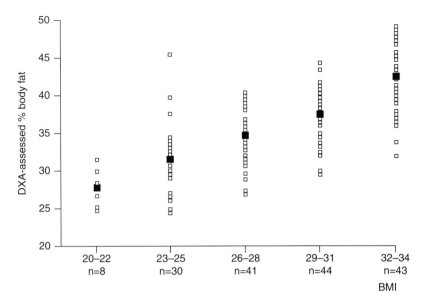

FIGURE 3 Relationship between DXA-assessed percent body fat and BMI in 166 women aged between 19 and 66 years. ■: mean percent body fat in each BMI category; □: individual percent body fat data. *Abbreviation*: DXA, dual-energy X-ray absorptiometry. *Source*: Department of Nutrition, Hôtel-Dieu Hospital, Paris, France.

Weight History

Given the natural history of obesity, some body weight values represent important phenotypes when they occur at critical time periods for body weight gain or change (10). This means that there will be special interest in body weight at birth, at puberty, at age 20 (a time when individuals are thought to remember about their weight), during pregnancy (e.g., amount of weight retained after pregnancy) and the age when the adiposity rebound took place in children; other phenotypes of interest include maximal weight during lifetime, minimal weight at adulthood, magnitude of weight change with indication of whether it corresponds to voluntary or involuntary weight loss.

Total Body Fat

As the definition of obesity specifically refers to accumulation of fat, body fat content should be a primary phenotype in genetic studies. However, to assess accurately body fat remains difficult and expensive in the clinical setting and/or in large populations (12,13). Moreover, in contrast to BMI, there are no established reference data for body fat in adults or children (11).

Importantly, health risks specifically associated with variations in body compartments (fat, lean or fat-free mass) need to be better defined (14). It is usually assumed that increased risk of morbidity and mortality associated with lower BMI is explained by decreased fat-free mass whereas increased risk associated with higher BMI is related to increased fat mass. However, research describing mortality as a function of increasing fat mass and decreasing lean mass is still at its beginning (15,16).

Table 3 lists the main methods that can be used for measuring body composition (12,13). Skinfold thicknesses measured at various locations (e.g., tricipital,

TABLE 3   Methods for Estimation of Total and Regional Body Fat

Method	Precision	Measures total fat	Measures regional fat
Anthropometry			
Height, weight, BMI	High	Yes	No
Circumferences, ratios	Moderate	No	Yes
Skinfolds	Low	Yes	Yes
Impedancemetry			
Bio-electric impedance	High	Yes	No
Absorptiometry			
Dual-energy absorptiometry	High	Yes	Yes
Densitometry			
Underwater weighing	High	Yes	No
Air-displacement plethysmography	High	Yes	No
Imaging techniques			
Computed tomography	High	No	Yes
Magnetic resonance imaging	High	Yes	Yes
Others			
Isotope dilution (e.g., deuterium)	High	Yes	No
K isotope (^{40}K)	High	Yes	No

Source: Adapted from Refs. 12, 13.

bicipital, subscapular and suprailiac skinfolds) may be used to assess total fat using various equations. The sum of such skinfolds is also considered an indicator of total subcutaneous fat. However, the interobserver variability is high when recording skinfolds and in some obese subjects skinfolds may be too large to be measured. With bioelectric impedance analysis, the impedance (or resistance) of the body to a low-intensity alternate current measured between specific locations at the extremities (arms, legs) is used to determine body water content. Assuming it has a constant hydration, fat-free mass is derived using specific equations and fat mass is calculated as body weight minus fat-free mass. The method is easy to perform, relatively cheap, repeatable, with a high precision (reproducibility) but rather moderate accuracy (validity compared to reference). Hydrostatic weighing, a method based on water displacement to assess total body density, was until recently considered the reference method against which others were validated. Once body volume is determined with the subject submerged in water, density (ratio of body mass to volume) is calculated and fat mass is derived using conversion equations. Fat-free mass is calculated as body weight minus fat mass. Precision and accuracy are high, however there are practical limitations because subjects have to climb in a water tank and then to sit still under water for several seconds. The more recent air displacement method seems a promising alternative. Dual-energy X-ray absorptiometry (DXA) is a three-compartment method that uses the differential attenuation of two low-energy X-ray beams to determine fat mass, lean body mass, and bone mineral content. DXA is increasingly considered the gold standard in body composition studies. The method gives rise to only minimal radiation, provides information about whole-body and regional body composition, has a high accuracy though decreasing with increasing body weight. Many devices do not accept subjects weighing over 150 kg. Regular cross-calibration is needed, especially in multicenter studies. Other methods using isotopes such as dilution methods or ^{40}K counting are performed only in few research centers in limited numbers of subjects.

Body Fat Distribution and Abdominal Obesity
Waist, Hip, and Waist-Hip Ratio

The concept of body fat distribution refers to the anatomical location of body fat. Since the pioneering work performed more than 60 years ago by the French physician Jean Vague (17), it is known that preferential accumulation of fat in the upper part of the body, that is at the level of trunk or abdomen, is associated with increased risk for cardiovascular and metabolic disease. Table 3 indicates from among the main body composition methods those that also allow measurement of regional fat distribution. Based on the work by Swedish investigators on cohorts of men and women from Göteborg and published during the mid-1980s, the ratio of waist-to-hip circumference, or waist-hip ratio (WHR) has been extensively used in the epidemiologic literature as indicator of body fat distribution (18). Waist circumference (WC) is measured, at the end of a gentle expiration, as the circumference midway between lower ribs and iliac crests on the midaxillary line; hip circumference is measured as the largest circumference at the trochanter level, in standing position (1). An increase in WHR is interpreted as reflecting body fat accumulation in the region of the trunk and abdomen as opposed to the extremities (limbs). Other measures of body fat distribution have been used, though less frequently, such as the ratio of iliac to thigh circumference (19) or the ratio of trunk (e.g., subscapular) to extremity (e.g., triceps) skinfolds (20).

Results of numerous prospective studies consistently indicate that an increased WHR is associated with increased risk of cardiovascular disease, especially coronary heart disease, independent of the overall level of corpulence as assessed by the BMI (21,22). Recently, results from the Interheart study, a case-control study on myocardial infarction that included 27,000 subjects in 52 countries, documented an odds-ratio of 2.52 (95% CI 2.31–2.74) when comparing the highest with the lowest WHR quintile, the latter considered as reference (23). The relation was consistent in men and women and persisted after adjustment for BMI and other risk factors. Interestingly, in that study, these relations were much stronger than that between BMI and myocardial infarction.

If the fact that the WHR is a strong risk marker for cardiovascular disease is not under debate, the biological significance of the WHR, what it means in terms of main body compartments, is not that straightforward. Indeed, as a ratio, the WHR can be elevated due to an increase in the numerator (WC) and/or a decrease in the denominator (hip circumference). For WC, it is likely that it reflects abdominal fat (without the possibility to distinguish between the subcutaneous and visceral compartments, see below). For hip circumference, bone and muscular elements at this level are likely to contribute in addition to fat. Independent of BMI and WC, enlarged hip circumferences as a marker of peripheral adiposity was shown to confer protection toward risk of cardiovascular disease and mortality (12,23,24). Recent reports using DXA to assess regional body composition indicate that in contrast to and independently of total trunk fat mass, leg fat mass displays favorable associations with several cardiovascular risk markers (12).

Although there is renewed interest in the WHR as indicator of increased cardiovascular risk in epidemiological studies (23), the WHR is not widely used in the clinical setting. One reason is that it is relatively cumbersome to measure two circumferences and compute their ratio, another is that there is no established cutoffs to denote increased values for this indicator.

Abdominal Visceral Fat

During the last 15 years or so, the development of imaging techniques [computed tomography (CT) and magnetic resonance imaging] applied to body fat assessment has led to emphasize the importance of the intra-abdominal fat compartment, or abdominal visceral fat, as opposed to abdominal subcutaneous fat (25). A large number of cross-sectional studies have documented stronger associations of abdominal visceral fat, compared to abdominal subcutaneous fat, with cardiovascular risk factors or cardiovascular events (12,21,22). Most of these risk factors are part of the "metabolic syndrome," a cluster of metabolic abnormalities closely associated with abdominal obesity, with insulin resistance as a major feature (26). However, only few prospective studies have reported positive associations of abdominal visceral fat with the incidence of coronary events, independently of other adipose compartments (27,28). In addition, an important point when documenting relationships of abdominal visceral fat with health outcomes would be to take into account the total amount of fat mass (29).

Anthropometric Indicators of Abdominal Visceral Fat

Measurement of abdominal visceral fat through imaging techniques represents the assessment of a specific adipose tissue depot, a notion which has to be differentiated from assessment of adipose tissue distribution through anthropometry. Also note that DXA allows assessment of regional body composition, e.g., fat mass in the trunk or abdominal region, but cannot differentiate between visceral and subcutaneous adiposity. For epidemiological and clinical studies, an important research question is to better define which easily obtained anthropometric indicator is best related to abdominal visceral fat content in order to identify subjects at increased cardiovascular and metabolic risk. Investigators in Quebec have shown that WC alone showed stronger correlations with CT-assessed abdominal visceral fat than WHR in adult men and women (30). It has therefore been suggested that WC may represent a better indicator for assessing intra-abdominal fat. In addition, WC is easy to assess and was shown to be independent of height (31). Cutoffs for increased WC proposed by Lean et al. (32) have been endorsed by several organizations and consensus conferences (1,26). These WC cutoffs were defined as those that would best identify subjects with increased BMI ($\geq 25 \, \text{kg/m}^2$, level 1; or $\geq 30 \, \text{kg/m}^2$, level 2) and/or increased WHR (≥ 0.95 in men and ≥ 0.85 in women) (32). Two WC levels (one for increased risk, two for substantially increased risk) were identified, separately for men and women, with reported specificity and sensitivity $\geq 96\%$: level 1 is $\geq 80 \, \text{cm}$ in women and 94 cm in men, level 2 is $\geq 88 \, \text{cm}$ in women and 102 cm in men. The same authors then showed in a sample of the general Dutch population that the odds-ratio of having at least one cardiovascular risk factor (including increased total cholesterol, increased blood pressure or decreased HDL-cholesterol level) was 4.6 in men and 2.6 in women with WC over level 2 compared to those under the cutoff value (31). Based on the relationships of WC with CT-measured abdominal visceral fat other cutoffs have been proposed (100 cm before and 90 cm after age 40, in both genders) (33).

Although WC appears better correlated to abdominal visceral fat than WHR, it has to be mentioned that WC is also correlated with abdominal subcutaneous fat (30). Therefore, WC is an important and useful anthropometric measure which is mainly an indicator of abdominal fatness. WC is of particular interest in subjects with a BMI between 25 and $35 \, \text{kg/m}^2$. When BMI is over $35 \, \text{kg/m}^2$, most subjects will have a WC over the cutoffs defined above.

Other anthropometric measures might be at least as well or better correlated with abdominal visceral fat than WC. One of these is the sagittal diameter which corresponds to abdominal height (25). For anatomical reasons, abdominal height might better reflect intra-abdominal fat content than WC. Recent data from the Paris Prospective Study showed positive associations of this indicator with death from cardiac origin (16). However, measurement of this indicator is not standardized yet and there are no published cutoffs to define values associated with increased health risks.

INTERMEDIARY PHENOTYPES: ENERGY INTAKE AND EXPENDITURE
Energy Expenditure
Components of Daily Energy Expenditure and Obesity

Daily (or total) energy expenditure in humans is usually divided in three main components: resting energy expenditure (or resting metabolic rate), thermic effect of food, and energy expenditure related to physical activity (34). Table 4 shows the relative contribution of these three components to total energy expenditure in sedentary adults, the main determinants of each component, and the effect of obesity, in absolute terms, on each component. Main determinants of energy expenditure include body dimensions (body weight), body composition (lean body mass or fat-free mass), and the habitual level of physical activity.

Resting energy expenditure accounts for the largest part of daily energy expenditure: it amounts to about two-thirds of total energy expenditure in sedentary adults (35). Resting energy expenditure is the energy expended to maintain the basal physiological functioning of the body and represents the sum of energy expenditures from tissues and organs in the postabsorptive state. The major predictor of resting energy expenditure is body weight, more specifically fat-free mass, in addition to age and sex. Taken together, age, sex, and fat-free mass account for about 80% of interindividual variations in resting energy expenditure (35). Increased resting energy expenditure in obese compared to normal-weight subjects is explained by the fact that increased body weight in the obese is associated with increased fat mass and, to a smaller but significant extent, with increased fat-free mass. There is evidence that a relatively low resting energy expenditure, after taking into account age, sex and body composition, may be a predictor of weight gain over time (36).

TABLE 4 Energy Expenditure (EE) Phenotypes: Components of Daily EE, Their Nongenetic Determinants, and Influence of Obesity

Component	% of daily EE in sedentary subjects	Main determinants	Effect of obesity (in absolute value for each component)
Resting energy expenditure	50–70	Body weight (fat-free mass) Age, sex, height Hormones (thyroid, cathecholamines)	Increased
Thermic effect of a meal	10	Total energy intake, macronutrient intakes	
Physical activity–related energy expenditure	15–20	Intensity and duration Fitness level Body weight	Increased

The thermic effect of food (or meal-induced thermogenesis) refers to the increase in metabolic rate in response to food intake (34). It accounts for only a small part of total energy expenditure. The thermic effect of food is the energy that is expended to digest, metabolize, and store ingested macronutrients. The main predictors are the total amount of energy ingested and its macronutrient composition. Whether the thermic effect of food is modified in obese subjects or whether decreased thermic effect of food could predict subsequent weight gain remain unresolved issues (37).

Energy expenditure related to physical activity is the most variable component of total energy expenditure both at the inter- and intraindividual level (34). This component can range from 15% (in sedentary subjects) to 50% (in highly trained subjects) of total energy expenditure. It represents the increase in metabolic rate that occurs during body movement of any type and corresponds primarily to energy expended for muscular contractions. The total amount of energy expended will depend on the characteristics of the activity performed (intensity and duration) and on the characteristics of the subject performing the activity (body size, level of fitness). Therefore, for given levels of corpulence and fitness, an individual will expend the same amount of energy for an activity of high intensity but short duration compared to an activity of moderate intensity and longer duration. The energy cost of weight-bearing activities is increased in obese compared to normal-weight subjects due to increased body mass to carry over (34). There is evidence that decreased physical activity–related energy expenditure is associated with weight gain over time (36).

It is well recognized that a large portion of the variability of daily energy expenditure among individuals, independent of differences in body size, is due to variability in the degree of spontaneous physical activity (35). In this field, energy expenditure of physical activities, other than volitional, sporting-like exercise, has recently been termed nonexercise activity thermogenesis (NEAT) (38). In one overfeeding study, the change in NEAT was predictive of fat gain (38).

Measurement of Energy Expenditure Phenotypes

Energy expenditure phenotypes are typically assessed by indirect calorimetry. Using this technique, energy production is measured based on respiratory gas analysis, i.e., oxygen consumption and carbon dioxide production that occur during oxidation of carbohydrates, lipids and proteins (34). Respiratory gas analysis can easily be performed over short measurement periods at rest or during exercise with a face mask or a canopy system used for gas collection. Resting metabolic rate is measured after an overnight fast, with subjects at rest lying quietly for 30 minutes. The thermic effect of a meal is typically assessed by continuous indirect calorimetry measurements for three to four hours after consumption of a test meal of known composition (note however that energy expenditure may take about six hours to go back to resting level after food ingestion). The energy expended in physical activity can also be measured under laboratory conditions by indirect calorimetry during standard activities such as treadmill walking or running. Over longer periods, measurements can be performed with the subjects living in a metabolic (or respiratory) chamber, which give more precise indication of 24-hour energy expenditure.

Another important phenotype derived from indirect calorimetry recordings is the respiratory quotient (RQ), equals to the ratio of carbon dioxide production to oxygen consumption. Interestingly, the RQ is indicative of the type of substrate being preferentially oxidized (i.e., fat vs. carbohydrate); for example, carbohydrate oxidation has an RQ of 1.0, and fat oxidation has an RQ close to 0.7. In weight-stable obese subjects, RQ has been found decreased compared to normal-weight subjects, reflecting relative increased oxidation of fat over carbohydrate. This finding is related, at least in part, to the increased fat mass inducing an increase in circulating free fatty acids which stimulates fat oxidation (39). In some studies, increased RQ was found to be a predictor of body weight gain over time (36).

The only method available to measure energy expenditure in free-living conditions is the doubly-labeled water technique (40,41). Using stable isotope methodology, carbon dioxide production rates can be measured directly and used to estimate energy expenditure over periods of 7 to 14 days. Free-living, physical activity–related energy expenditure can then be estimated by the combination of the doubly-labeled water technique to measure total energy expenditure and indirect calorimetry to measure resting energy expenditure (resting is then subtracted from total energy expenditure). Another phenotype is the physical activity level which is the ratio of total to resting energy expenditure. There are several limitations to the use of the doubly-labeled technique that prevent its applicability to large number of subjects including current difficulties in obtaining 0^{18} isotope, cost and complexity (mass spectrometry is required for isotope analysis). In addition, only carbon dioxide production is measured and an assumption on RQ is required to calculate energy expenditure. Finally, only an integrated measure of energy expenditure over the study period is obtained.

Energy Expenditure Measurements and Weight Change

An important issue to consider is whether weight is stable when energy expenditure measurements are performed. It is well recognized that weight changes (i.e., increase or decrease) are accompanied by similar changes in energy expenditure (i.e., increase or decrease) (42). Whether these changes in energy expenditure induced by weight loss are entirely explained by associated changes in body composition remains a matter of debate. Specifically, it has been hypothesized that maintenance of a reduced body weight is associated with compensatory changes in energy expenditure, which could explain the poor long-term efficacy of treatments of obesity (42). In any case, this strongly argues for performing energy expenditure measurements during periods of well-established weight stability.

Physical Activity and Eating Patterns

Eating and physical activity patterns are the most obvious mediating factors that influence energy balance. Both can be viewed as behavioral phenotypes with similar methodological problems in terms of assessment. For both phenotypes, an important feature is not only the high inter-individual but also intra-individual variability (43).

Physical Activity Levels and Obesity

Physical activity is broadly defined as "any bodily movement produced by the contraction of skeletal muscle that increases energy expenditure over resting level" (44). Main characteristics of a given physical activity are intensity (actual energy expended in kcal/min), duration, frequency and the context in which it occurs. Common categories based upon the context include leisure-time, occupational, household and transportation. Physical fitness is a different concept and is defined as a set of attributes that people have or achieve that relates to their ability to perform physical activity. Among other characteristics, health-related fitness includes cardiorespiratory fitness, muscular endurance and strength, and flexibility.

Physical activity, as defined above, and energy expenditure are not synonymous. Although physical activity–related energy expenditure is increased in obese compared to normal-weight subjects (34), the habitual level of physical activity is usually lower in obese compared to normal-weight subjects (1,3). It is generally accepted that low physical activity levels are associated with body weight gain over time (3). On the other hand, increased body weight and obesity may result in decreased physical activity (45), therefore it is a complex, and sometimes circular, relationship. Decreased levels of physical activity or fitness in obese subjects also substantially increase their risk for metabolic disease and for all-cause as well as cardiovascular mortality (46). Increasing physical activity is thus part of most weight-loss and maintenance programs (1). Sedentary behavior is another important dimension to consider. Sedentary activities include a number of occupations that have in common to expend little energy, with television/video viewing as the most widely used proxy (47). Independently of physical activity levels, television viewing has been associated with obesity (or increased BMI) in children, adolescents and adults (48).

Physical activity not only increases energy expenditure, but a major adaptation to regular exercise is the increased ability to oxidize fat relative to carbohydrate (49). The extent to which lipid or carbohydrate contribute to energy expenditure will vary according to the intensity (and duration) of physical activity performed. Fat is preferentially utilized during low- to moderate-intensity activity of prolonged duration whereas carbohydrate is the dominant fuel during high-intensity activity. Sedentary behavior is more than the inverse of physical activity and may contribute to weight gain through other means than a reduction in energy expenditure. Associations have been reported between time spent viewing television and intakes of energy-dense, high-fat foods (47).

Assessment of Physical Activity Phenotypes

Various methods are available for assessing physical activity, including questionnaires or diaries, motion counters (pedometers or accelerometers), physiologic markers such as heart-rate monitoring, or doubly-labeled water for assessment of free-living physical activity–related energy expenditure (50). Few of these instruments have been specifically designed for or studied in obese populations (51). Questionnaires represent the most widely used method to assess habitual physical activity in large numbers of subjects, as they are generally well accepted by participants and easy to administer at a low cost. Only questionnaires assess type, duration, intensity, and purpose of physical activity. To translate physical activity data from a questionnaire to energy expenditure, there are compendiums of the energy costs of various activities (leisure, sport, occupational, etc.) (52). The average metabolic costs are usually expressed using metabolic equivalent tasks (METs). An MET is the ratio of the working metabolic rate of an activity divided by the resting metabolic rate. One MET represents the metabolic rate of an individual at rest (sitting quietly) and is set at 3.5 mL of oxygen consumed per kg body mass per minute, or approximately 1 kcal/kg/hr (52). The relevance of tables reporting energy cost to obese subjects is, however, not known. Over-reporting is an important concern when assessing habitual physical activity by self-report (50).

Studies using room indirect calorimetry or the doubly-labeled water technique for measuring energy expenditure have documented that obese individuals are particularly prone to such overestimation of physical activity (53). Pedometers assess ambulatory activity as steps walked or run but give no indication about physical activity intensity. Accelerometry is based on the theoretic relationship between muscular force and body acceleration that occurs during discrete physical movements. Accelerometers assess bodily movements expressed in counts per time unit and provide data about intensity and patterns but not on physical activity types.

An important point is that each of these instruments actually measure different dimensions or aspects of physical activity (50). A major difficulty with physical activity assessment therefore remains the lack of a gold-standard method against which a given method could be validated. As mentioned, doubly-labeled water is the only method to assess energy expenditure in free-living conditions and is often taken as reference in such validation studies. However, it does not give other information than energy expended during a certain period of time. Thus, in most instances, validity is examined in an indirect fashion by comparing available techniques.

Food Intake and Obesity

When examining dietary factors associated with obesity, energy intake and macronutrient composition of the diet as well as eating patterns and eating behavior need to be taken into account. Diets that are proportionally higher in fat and proportionally lower in carbohydrate appear associated with unhealthy weight gain, although a high intake of free sugars in beverages is probably also involved (54–56). It should be noted that this knowledge comes mainly from animal experiments and physiological human studies, whereas the population-based data on dietary intake and obesity still remains a matter of much discussion (55). Results of trials in which the energy density and fat content of the diets were covertly manipulated support the notion that increased energy density, as is the case with high-fat diets, leads to a phenomenon called "passive overconsumption" (57). Moreover, when ingested in excess over energy maintenance requirements, fat intake does not promote fat oxidation, a process favoring fat storage (39). This strongly implicates dietary fat in the process of body weight and fat gain. Other dietary factors are possibly involved in unhealthy weight gain such as, for example, large portion size (58). Breastfeeding was, in contrast, found as protective in some studies (54). From a behavioral perspective, eating behaviors that have been linked to overweight and obesity include snacking/eating frequency, binge-eating patterns as well as eating out (54). In addition, certain psychological patterns such as "rigid restrain/periodic disinhibition" have been found associated with weight gain (54). Other phenotypes of interest include measures of appetite, hunger and food preferences.

Assessment of Food Intake Phenotypes

Measurement of food intake remains a challenging task, especially in human obesity (59). Various methods are available for assessing habitual food intake at individual level (60). These include techniques of direct analysis such as the use of duplicate diets, record techniques such as precise weighed record (a record is kept of all ingredients used in the preparation of meals with weight of cook items and plate waste), and interview techniques such as diet recalls, diet history or food-frequency questionnaire. A typical diet recall is the 24-hour recall for which the respondent is asked to recall all food and drinks consumed in the immediate past 24-hour period. The diet history is a more in-depth interview, usually with open-ended questions, where the respondent is asked about his/her usual eating pattern (e.g., on a 7-day period). When using food-frequency questionnaires, the respondent is presented with a list of foods and indicates how often each item is consumed over a specified length of time (i.e., times per day, week or month). To obtain long-term information about individual diets an option is to use multiple 24-hour recalls over an appropriate period of time that will allow for seasonal variation. For food-frequency questionnaire, it may be preferable to restrict their use to providing information on the long-term intake of a limited number of foods or food groups rather than use them to derive quantitative estimates of nutrient intakes at individual level.

Whatever method used, to translate food questionnaire data into energy and nutrient intake, food composition tables are needed (60). The accuracy of the calculated estimates will depend on the coding and calculation procedures used to convert the food intake data into nutrient intakes. Note that differences in food and nutrient databases across countries may represent a difficulty in international studies. Few of these instruments have been specifically designed for or studied in obese populations (59). The development of nutrient consumption biomarkers is therefore considered of importance (61). Biomarkers of energy and nutrient intake are objective measures that reflect but are independent of actual food intake. Examples are energy expenditure as measured by the doubly-labeled water method to compare with energy intake in weight-stable individuals or urinary nitrogen to assess protein intake. Under-reporting is an important concern when assessing habitual food intake and under-reporting of total energy intake has been documented in obese subjects in studies using the doubly-labeled water technique for measuring total energy expenditure (53). Using urinary nitrogen, there is also evidence for selective under-reporting of foods high in fats and/or carbohydrates in obese subjects (62). This makes the interpretation of dietary phenotypes collected in obese subjects a very complex issue. In terms of eating behaviors, a questionnaire that has been widely used to assess factors such as cognitive restraint is the Eating Inventory designed by Stunkard and Messick (63).

CONCLUSION

In this chapter we have focused on body fat phenotypes and their most proximal mediators. As shown in Table 1, there are many additional obesity phenotypes that may be dealt with in genetic studies. These phenotypes pertain to adipocyte morphology, metabolism and secretory products (adipokines), as well as to obesity comorbidities and the various consequences of obesity treatments.

Beyond increases in cell size and number, adipose-tissue modifications in obesity are numerous and may represent biological phenotypes of interest including changes in histology, vascularization and innervation, lipid and carbohydrate metabolism and endocrine functions (64,65). Second, genetic factors can influence the development of both obesity and its complications (1). It has to be realized that the presence of comorbidities may impact the clinical and biological phenotype. For example, the consequences of obesity on respiratory function and/or sleep may lead to secondary alterations in cognitive performance, mood, eating patterns, or metabolic and hormonal status (2). When studying massively obese individuals, there are also practical concerns because many body fat measurement methods we have described are not feasible (66). Finally, medical and surgical management of obesity may also lead to phenotypic modifications, weight change being the most obvious. Indeed, assessment of weight change, at least recent changes, such as in the past 3 months, whether voluntary or not, deserves great attention for interpretation of traits related to energy expenditure, metabolic status, as well as eating or physical activity habits. Going back to the temporal perspective, weight history (Fig. 1)—and more generally weight trajectories at individual and population level—emerge as major aspects of the phenotypic study of obesity.

ACKNOWLEDGMENT

The authors express their thanks to Marie-Françoise Rolland-Cachera (INSERM U 557, Paris, France) for advice on the definition of obesity in children and for providing Figure 2.

REFERENCES

1. World Health Organization. Obesity: Preventing and Managing the Global Epidemic. Report of a WHO Consultation on Obesity. Geneva: WHO Technical Report Series no. 894, 2000.
2. Basdevant A. Natural history of obesity. Bull Acad Natl Med 2003; 187:1343–52 (in French).
3. Hill JO, Wyatt HR, Reed GW et al. Obesity and the environment: where do we go from here? Science 2003; 299:853–5.
4. Willett WC. Anthropometric measures and body composition. In: Willett W, ed. Nutritional Epidemiology. 2nd ed. Oxford: Oxford University Press, 1998:244–72.
5. Troiano RP, Frongillo EA Jr, Sobal J et al. The relationship between body weight and mortality: a quantitative analysis of combined information from existing studies. Int J Obes Relat Metab Disord 1996; 20:63–75.
6. Inoue S, Zimmet P, eds. The Asia-Pacific Perspective: Redefining Obesity and Its Treatment. Hong Kong: World Health Organization/International Obesity Task Force/International Association for the Study of Obesity, 2000. Available at: http://www.idi.org.au/research/report_obesity.htm. Accessed September 29, 2006.
7. WHO Expert Consultation. Appropriate body-mass index for Asian populations and its implications for policy and intervention strategies. Lancet 2004; 363:157–63.
8. Cole TJ, Bellizzi MC, Flegal KM et al. Establishing a standard definition for child overweight and obesity worldwide: international survey. BMJ 2000; 320:1240–3.
9. Rolland-Cachera MF, Deheeger M, Bellisle F et al. Adiposity rebound in children: a simple indicator for predicting obesity. Am J Clin Nutr 1984; 39:129–35.
10. Dietz WH. Critical periods in childhood for the development of obesity. Am J Clin Nutr 1994; 59:955–9.
11. Prentice AM, Jebb SA. Beyond body mass index. Obes Rev 2001; 2:141–7.
12. Snijder MB, van Dam RM, Visser M et al. What aspects of body fat are particularly hazardous and how do we measure them? Int J Epidemiol 2006; 35:83–92.
13. Pi-Sunyer FX. Obesity: criteria and classification. Proc Nutr Soc 2000; 59:505–9.
14. Baumgartner RN, Heymsfield SB, Roche AF. Human body composition and the epidemiology of chronic disease. Obes Res 1995; 3:73–95.
15. Heitmann BL, Erikson H, Ellsinger BM et al. Mortality associated with body fat, fat-free mass and body mass index among 60-year-old Swedish men-a 22-year follow-up. The study of men born in 1913. Int J Obes 2000; 24:33–7.
16. Oppert JM, Charles AM, Thibult N et al. Anthropometric estimates of muscle and fat mass in relation to cardiac and cancer mortality in men: the Paris Prospective Study. Am J Clin Nutr 2002; 75:1107–13.

17. Vague J. The degree of masculine differentiation of obesities, a factor determining predisposition to diabetes, atherosclerosis, gout, and uric calculous disease. Am J Clin Nutr 1956; 4:20–34.

18. Larsson B, Svardsudd K, Welin L et al. Abdominal adipose tissue distribution, obesity, and risk of cardiovascular disease and death: 13 year follow up of participants in the study of men born in 1913. BMJ 1984; 288:1401–4.

19. Ducimetiere P, Richard JL. The relationship between subsets of anthropometric upper versus lower body measurements and coronary heart disease risk in middle-aged men. The Paris Prospective Study. I. Int J Obes 1989; 13:111–21.

20. Kannel WB, Cupples LA, Ramaswami R et al. Regional obesity and risk of cardiovascular disease; the Framingham Study. J Clin Epidemiol 1991; 44:183–90.

21. Bjorntorp P. Visceral obesity: a "civilization syndrome". Obes Res 1993; 1:206–22.

22. Kissebah AH, Krakower GR. Regional adiposity and morbidity. Physiol Rev 1994; 74:761–811.

23. Yusuf S, Hawken S, Ounpuu S et al. INTERHEART Study Investigators. Obesity and the risk of myocardial infarction in 27,000 participants from 52 countries: a case–control study. Lancet 2005; 366:1640–9.

24. Heitmann BL, Frederiksen P, Lissner L. Hip circumference and cardiovascular morbidity and mortality in men and women. Obes Res 2004; 12:482–7.

25. van der Kooy K, Seidell JC. Techniques for the measurement of visceral fat: a practical guide. Int J Obes Relat Metab Disord 1993; 17:187–96.

26. Expert Panel on Detection, Evaluation, and Treatment of High Blood Cholesterol in Adults. Executive Summary of the Third Report of The National Cholesterol Education Program (NCEP) Expert Panel on Detection, Evaluation, and Treatment of High Blood Cholesterol in Adults (Adult Treatment Panel III). JAMA 2001; 285:2486–97.

27. Fujimoto WY, Bergstrom RW, Boyko EJ et al. Visceral adiposity and incident coronary heart disease in Japanese-American men. The 10-year follow-up results of the Seattle Japanese-American Community Diabetes Study. Diabetes Care 1999; 22:1808–12.

28. Nicklas BJ, Penninx BW, Cesari M et al. Health, aging and body composition study. association of visceral adipose tissue with incident myocardial infarction in older men and women: the Health, Aging and Body Composition Study. Am J Epidemiol 2004; 160:741–9.

29. Seidell JC, Bouchard C. Visceral fat in relation to health: is it a major culprit or simply an innocent bystander? Int J Obes Relat Metab Disord 1997; 21:626–31.

30. Pouliot MC, Despres JP, Lemieux S et al. Waist circumference and abdominal sagittal diameter: best simple anthropometric indexes of abdominal visceral adipose tissue accumulation and related cardiovascular risk in men and women. Am J Cardiol 1994; 73:460–8.

31. Han TS, van Leer EM, Seidell JC et al. Waist circumference action levels in the identification of cardiovascular risk factors: prevalence study in a random sample. BMJ 1995; 311:1401–5.

32. Lean ME, Han TS, Morrison CE. Waist circumference as a measure for indicating need for weight management. BMJ 1995; 311:158–61.

33. Lemieux S, Prud'homme D, Bouchard C et al. A single threshold value of waist girth identifies normal-weight and overweight subjects with excess visceral adipose tissue. Am J Clin Nutr 1996; 64:685–93.

34. Jequier E, Acheson K, Schutz Y. Assessment of energy expenditure and fuel utilization in man. Annu Rev Nutr 1987; 7:187–208.

35. Ravussin E, Lillioja S, Anderson TE et al. Determinants of 24-hour energy expenditure in man. Methods and results using a respiratory chamber. J Clin Invest 1986; 78:1568–78.

36. Ravussin E, Fontvieille AM, Swinburn BA et al. Risk factors for the development of obesity. Ann N Y Acad Sci 1993; 683:141–50.

37. Laville M, Cornu C, Normand S et al. Decreased glucose-induced thermogenesis at the onset of obesity. Am J Clin Nutr 1993; 57:851–6.

38. Levine JA, Eberhardt NL, Jensen MD. Role of nonexercise activity thermogenesis in resistance to fat gain in humans. Science 2005; 307:584–6.

39. Schutz Y, Tremblay A, Weinsier RL et al. Role of fat oxidation in the long-term stabilization of body weight in obese women. Am J Clin Nutr 1992; 55:670–4.
40. Schoeller DA, Ravussin E, Schutz Y et al. Energy expenditure by doubly labeled water: validation in humans and proposed calculation. Am J Physiol 1986; 250:R823–30.
41. Ritz P, Coward WA. Doubly labelled water measurement of total energy expenditure. Diabetes Metab 1995; 21:241–51.
42. Leibel RL, Rosenbaum M, Hirsch J. Changes in energy expenditure resulting from altered body weight. N Engl J Med 1995; 332:621–8.
43. Tarasuk V, Beaton GH. The nature and individuality of within-subject variation in energy intake. Am J Clin Nutr 1991; 54:464–70.
44. US Department of Health and Human Services. Physical activity and health: a report of the Surgeon General. Atlanta, GA: USDHSS, Center for Disease Control and Prevention, National Center for Chronic Disease Prevention and Health Promotion, 1996.
45. Petersen L, Schnohr P, Sørensen TIA. Longitudinal study of the long-term relation between physical activity and obesity in adults. Int J Obes Relat Metab Disord 2004; 28:105–12.
46. Katzmarzyk PT, Church TS, Blair SN. Cardiorespiratory fitness attenuates the effects of the metabolic syndrome on all-cause and cardiovascular disease mortality in men. Arch Intern Med 2004; 164:1092–7.
47. Dietz WH. The role of lifestyle in health: the epidemiology and consequences of inactivity. Proc Nutr Soc 1996; 55:829–40.
48. Bertrais S, Beyeme-Ondoua JP, Czernichow S et al. Sedentary behaviors, physical activity, and metabolic syndrome in middle-aged French subjects. Obes Res 2005; 13:936–44.
49. Saris WH. Fit, fat and fat free: the metabolic aspects of weight control. Int J Obes Relat Metab Disord 1998; 22(Suppl. 2):S15–21.
50. Montoye HJ, Kemper HCG, Saris WHM et al. Measuring Physical Activity and Energy Expenditure. Champaign, IL: Human Kinetics, 1996.
51. Tehard B, Saris WH, Astrup A et al. Comparison of two physical activity questionnaires in obese subjects: the NUGENOB study. Med Sci Sports Exerc 2005; 37:1535–41.
52. Ainsworth BE, Haskell WL, Whitt MC et al. Compendium of physical activities: an update of activity codes and MET intensities. Med Sci Sports Exerc 2000; 32(9 Suppl.): S498–504.
53. Lichtman SW, Pisarska K, Berman ER et al. Discrepancy between self-reported and actual caloric intake and exercise in obese subjects. N Engl J Med 1992; 327:1893–8.
54. WHO. Diet, nutrition and the prevention of chronic diseases. World Health Organ Tech Rep Ser 2003; 916(i–viii):1–149.
55. Bray GA, Paeratakul S, Popkin BM. Dietary fat and obesity: a review of animal, clinical and epidemiological studies. Physiol Behav 2004; 83:549–55.
56. Ludwig DS, Peterson KE, Gortmaker SL. Relation between consumption of sugar-sweetened drinks and childhood obesity: a prospective, observational analysis. Lancet 2001; 357:505–8.
57. Blundell JE, MacDiarmid JI. Fat as a risk factor for overconsumption: satiation, satiety, and patterns of eating. J Am Diet Assoc 1997; 97(7 Suppl.):S63–9.
58. Ello-Martin JA, Ledikwe JH, Rolls BJ. The influence of food portion size and energy density on energy intake: implications for weight management. Am J Clin Nutr 2005; 82(1 Suppl.):236S–41S.
59. Lissner L. Measuring food intake in studies of obesity. Public Health Nutr 2002; 5(6A):889–92.
60. Nelson M, Bingham SA. Assessment of food consumption and nutrient intake. In: Margetts BM, Nelson M, eds. Design Concepts in Nutritional Epidemiology, Oxford University Press, 2nd ed, 1997, pp. 123–69.
61. Potischman N. Biologic and methodologic issues for nutritional biomarkers. J Nutr 2003; 133(Suppl. 3):875S–80S.
62. Heitmann BL, Lissner L. Dietary underreporting by obese individuals—is it specific or non-specific? BMJ 1995; 311:986–9.

63. Stunkard AJ, Messick S. The three-factor eating questionnaire to measure dietary restraint, disinhibition and hunger. J Psychosom Res 1985; 29(1):71–83.
64. Cancello R, Tounian A, Poitou Ch et al. Adiposity signals, genetic and body weight regulation in humans. Diabetes Metab 2004; 30:215–27.
65. Coppack SW. Adipose tissue changes in obesity. Biochem Soc Trans 2005; 33:1049–52.
66. Allison DB, Nathan JS, Albu JB et al. Measurement challenges and other practical concerns when studying massively obese individuals. Int J Eat Disord 1998; 24:275–84.

2.1 Family Studies

Finn Rasmussen
Child and Adolescent Public Health Epidemiology Group, Department of Public Health Sciences, Karolinska Institute, Stockholm, Sweden

Patrik K.E. Magnusson
Department of Medical Epidemiology and Biostatistics, Karolinska Institute, Stockholm, Sweden

Thorkild I.A. Sørensen
Institute of Preventive Medicine, Copenhagen University Hospitals, Centre for Health and Society, Copenhagen, Denmark

Obesity frequently aggregates in families. The first large family study known to the authors was published in 1923 by Davenport, who investigated more than 500 families with 3582 parent-offspring pairs (1). Familial resemblance in obesity phenotypes is caused not only by genetic factors, but also by shared environmental factors, possibly related to lifestyle and culture. Body mass index (BMI) is by far the most frequently studied measure of fatness in family studies and the present chapter focuses on this phenotype. However, other measures related to fatness such as skinfold thickness and waist circumference, are also briefly mentioned (see Chapter 1.1).

Familial resemblance is usually quantified by the intrafamilial correlation coefficient for each specific type of familial relation. Heritability is the fraction of variance in a quantitative phenotype observed in a given population that is due to interindividual differences in genetic factors. Under various assumptions, heritability of a trait, e.g., BMI, can be estimated by modeling intrafamilial correlations for different types of relatives. Since heritability is the fraction of the genetic component of variance to the total genetic and non-genetic variance, it must lie between 0 and 1. This concept, which has been used extensively in quantitative genetic studies, should be interpreted with caution. In general, greater diversity of environmental factors in a given population will lower the estimated heritability, while populations with more homogeneous environments will provide higher estimates of heritability, even though the biological mechanism underlying the trait may be identical. For this reason heritability is a population-specific concept.

Although a large number of family studies have been conducted, it is important to be aware that many of them have not been population-based. Recruitment of family members of obese-index subjects, who have received medical attention in certain health care settings, may create selection bias that is impossible to assess or control for retrospectively.

In a review paper that included a pooled analysis of 25,000 twin pairs and 50,000 biological and adoptive family members, the weighted mean BMI correlations were 0.74 for monozygotic twins, 0.32 for dizygotic twins, 0.25 for full siblings, 0.19 for parent-offspring pairs 0.06 for adoptive relatives, and 0.12 for spouses (2).

THE NUCLEAR FAMILY DESIGN

One common type of study design is based on nuclear families consisting of parents and offspring. In this setting, correlations between spouses, parent-offspring pairs, and sibling pairs are investigated. Most family studies have been based on BMI, but several studies in the literature have also analyzed family correlations in waist circumference, waist-hip ratio, skinfold thickness, or fat mass estimated by dual energy X-ray absorptiometry.

Many studies have reported *spouse correlations* in BMI and other measures of adiposity (2). Tambs et al. estimated spouse correlation in BMI to 0.12 in a large population-based Norwegian study including 23,939 pairs (3). Katzmarzyk et al. investigated spousal resemblance for adiposity and leanness in the Canadian population and the possible implications for the obesity epidemic (4). This cross-sectional study was based on parents and offspring from 1,341 families, in total 4,023 subjects comprising a subsample of the Canada Fitness Survey. Indicators of adiposity were BMI and the sum of five skinfolds. Both offspring and parents were ranked by their BMI and sums of five skinfolds percentile position in the entire study population of the Canada Fitness Survey including 15,818 subjects. Pearson correlations indicated significant spousal resemblance for both BMI ($r = 0.14$; $P < 0.0001$) and sums of five skinfolds ($r = 0.13$; $P < 0.0001$). The magnitude of the spousal correlations varied by the adiposity status of the offspring, with spousal correlations tending to be stronger in parents of lean or obese children and lower among parents of "average" children. The degree to which these similarities were due to assortative mating, loading of spouses with predisposing genes, or a shared household environment, could not be determined. An increased spousal correlation for parents ascertained by having children in the BMI tails may be expected when additive genetics influence a quantitative trait also in absence of assortative mating.

For a phenotype assumed to be highly influenced by lifestyle, like BMI, it is appropriate to consider whether the spouse correlation reflects spouse selection for the phenotype itself (phenotypic assortative mating), a consequence of social homogamy (assortment according to socioeconomic position), or convergence during marriage because of common household and living habits. Tambs et al. found no heterogeneity in BMI spousal correlation across marital duration and the results of the Norwegian study did not lend support to the suggestion of convergence during marriage (3). Instead these results seemed to reflect partner selection based on BMI. Although not analyzed or discussed in the paper, it is a possibility that assortment due to socioeconomic position may have contributed to spouse BMI correlations.

As regards *parent-offspring pairs*, Tambs et al. reported father-son, father-daughter, mother-son and mother-daughter BMI correlations in the range 0.18 to 0.20 with no obvious differences with respect to gender of the parents or the offspring (3). The pooled analysis reported by Maes et al. (2) showed a correlation of 0.19 for parent-offspring pairs. No estimates were presented for mother-daughter, mother-son, father-son and father-daughter, but in the literature review in the same paper, no clear trends were observed in the parent-offspring correlations by gender of the parents or the offspring (2). Results from the Bogalusa Heart Study including 727 11-year-old children and their parents showed that mothers' childhood-offspring BMI correlations were stronger than mothers' adulthood-offspring BMI correlations. Corresponding father-offspring correlations showed similar patterns, but the age dependence were smaller (5). These results indicate that parent-offspring associations may be age-dependent, possibly corresponding to changing degrees of shared environment between the family members.

In the Fels Longitudinal study from the United States, BMI was measured annually from birth to age 18 years among 523 pairs of full siblings and BMI correlations were calculated at the same age (6). Brother correlations varied from 0.31 to 0.49, sister correlations from 0.43 to 0.61, and brother-sister correlations varied from 0.24 to 0.44. Several other studies of pairs of full siblings have reported BMI correlations in the same range (7).

A few family studies have reported the familial resemblance of longitudinal changes in measures of fatness. One such study is the 7-year longitudinal follow-up of the Canada Fitness Survey which included 521 nuclear families with 655 women and 660 men between 7 and 69 years of age at baseline examination in 1981 (8). The results showed age-adjusted and gender-adjusted heritability at baseline, i.e., cross-sectional estimates of 0.39 (95% CI, 0.27–0.51) for BMI, 0.41 (0.29–0.53) for the sum of five skinfolds, and 0.39 (0.07–0.55) for waist circumference (8). A longitudinal familial correlation model was used and age- and gender-adjusted heritability estimates were 0.14 (0–0.30) for 7-year BMI changes, 0.12 (0–0.30) for changes of the sum of five skinfolds and 0.45 (0.19–0.71) for 7-year changes in waist circumference. The heritabilities for the 7-year changes were adjusted for baseline levels. The authors acknowledged that the estimates of heritability are influenced by common environmental factors to an unknown degree and they therefore designated these estimates as "maximal." The low heritability for change of BMI is in disagreement with the results of the Longitudinal Québec Family Study (9) which showed maximal heritability ranging from 0.33 to 0.44 for change of BMI over 12 years among 412 individuals from 105 families. The results of the follow-up of the Canada Fitness Survey are also inconsistent with the Kaiser Permanente Women Twins Study including 185 monozygotic and 130 dizygotic twin pairs followed from ages of 41 and 51 years. That study found age-adjusted heritability estimates for change in BMI ranging from 0.57 to 0.86 depending on method of estimation. However, the results of the follow-up of the Canada Fitness Survey are in accordance with a Finnish study of 5,967 adult twin pairs followed longitudinally for 6 years (10). In that study BMI changes appeared to be determined by environmental effects rather than genetic factors.

The results of the 7-year follow-up of the Canada Fitness Survey for changes in the sum of five skinfolds were of similar magnitude as found in the Longitudinal Québec Family Study (0.16) (9). The familial correlation pattern for changes in waist circumference was different than that for changes in BMI. The heritability of changes in waist circumference (0.45) was surprisingly high.

As discussed above it is impossible to disentangle the effects of shared genes from shared environment by the nuclear family design. This goal can, however, be attained by modeling correlations between various degrees of relatedness (full siblings/half siblings or monozygotic/dizygotic twins) or by comparing correlations between biological relatives with correlations between adoptees and their nonbiological parents and siblings (11).

THE EXTENDED FAMILY DESIGN

In the large population-based Norwegian study referred to above, Tambs et al. investigated BMI correlations among first- and second-degree relatives (3). This family study included 23,936 spouse pairs, 43,586 parent-offspring pairs, 19,157 sibling pairs and more than and 2,400 second-degree relatives. The mean parent-offspring correlation was 0.20 and varied little by age and sex of parents and offspring. The BMI correlation was 0.26 for same-sexed siblings, 0.20 for opposite-sexed siblings, and 0.58 for monozygotic twins, and close to zero for most second-order relatives. The authors estimated total heritability to 0.39 much of which was due to genetic dominance (3).

The authors of this section have conducted a large population-based study on resemblance of BMI for biological and non-biological family relationships in Swedish young men. A record linkage was made between the Swedish Military Service Conscription Register and the Multi-Generation Register covering individuals born 1932 or later who were registered as Swedish citizens by January 1, 1961 (8.5 million subjects year 2001). Included as index subjects in this study were males born in Sweden as singletons 1950–1982, who had participated in conscription examination at age 18 to 19 years (mean age 18.3 years), and who shared at least one parent with another conscript. More than 85% of all young men belonging to these birth cohorts had information on BMI from conscription examination. The data allowed the following three aims to be addressed. First, to estimate correlations for BMI within male full-brother pairs, maternal and paternal half-brother pairs, father-son pairs and other biological relatives as shown in Figure 1; second, to estimate BMI correlations between young adult male adoptees and their biological fathers, adopt-ive fathers, biological full brothers and biological sons of their adoptive fathers (see Chapter 2.2); and third, to estimate BMI correlations between biologically unrelated individuals such as stepsons and stepfathers, men who had sons with the same women, etc.

This large dataset includes 271,119 pairs of biological nontwin full brothers and to secure independent brother pairs, the firstborn pair in each family was selected. The dataset includes 83,646 biological father-son pairs, 31,755 biological maternal half brothers, 36,755 biological paternal half brothers, 17,136 biological paternal uncle-nephew pairs, 89,522 biological pairs of maternal cousins, and

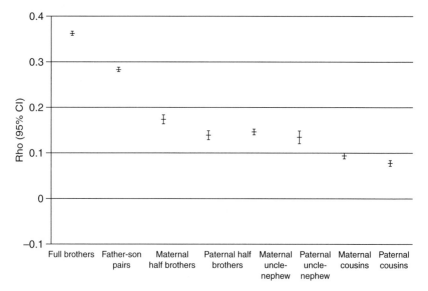

FIGURE 1 BMI correlations (95% CI) in various types of biological relatives born in Sweden 1950–1982 and participating in conscription examination at age 18 to 19 years.

56,370 biological pairs of paternal cousins. These analyses include individuals with height in the range 130 to 225 cm and weight within in the range 40 to 225 kg. The authors have previously reported results based on a smaller study population from the same information sources (12).

The Pearson correlation coefficients for the various types of family pairs were 0.36 (95% CI, 0.36–0.37) for biological full brothers, 0.28 (0.28–0.29) for biological father-son pairs, 0.17 (0.16–0.18) for biological maternal half brothers, 0.14 (0.13–0.15) for biological paternal half brothers, 0.14 (0.14–0.15) for biological maternal uncle-nephew pairs, 0.13 (0.12–0.15) for biological paternal uncle-nephew pairs, 0.09 (0.09–0.10) for biological maternal cousins, and 0.07 (0.07–0.08) for biological paternal cousins (Fig. 1). The slightly stronger BMI correlations between maternal half brothers than paternal half brothers may reflect that mothers have stronger impact on the family environment (eating habits, food choices, etc.) than fathers or in utero genetic or environmental influences. Nonpaternity is another possible explanation to consider (13). However, the authors have simulated non-paternity and the previous results showed that a highly unlikely rate (over 40%) would have to be assumed for nonpaternity to be the full explanation of the discrepancy in correlation between maternal and paternal half brothers (12).

The BMI associations between two men who have offspring with the same woman, 0.08 (95% CI, 0.02–0.15) may be due to shared environmental factors (eating habits, physical activity, etc.), assortative mating or other unrecognized environmental factors (Figs. 2 and 3). The significant BMI associations between other biologically unrelated individuals, such as son to first husband and mother–second husband to mother 0.05 (0.01–0.08), and husband to firstborn sister–husband to second born sister 0.06 (0.02–0.10) further emphasize the importance of shared environmental factors (Figs. 2 and 3).

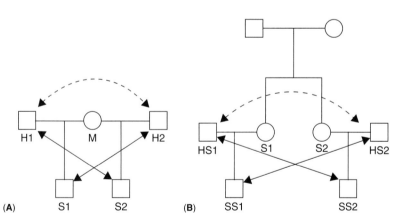

FIGURE 2 Pedigrees illustrating the nonbiological family relationships used in the analyses. (**A**) Mother (*circle*) has one son (*lower leftmost square*) with one husband (*top leftmost square*), then remarries a second husband (*top rightmost square*) and gets another son (*lower rightmost square*). Solid arrows indicate the husband1-son2 (H1-S2) and husband2-son1 (H2-S1) relations, and the dotted arrow indicates the husband1-husband2 (H1-H2) relation. (**B**) Full sisters (*middle circles*) have one son each (*bottom squares*) with unrelated men (*middle leftmost and rightmost squares*). Solid arrows indicate son to firstborn sister-husband to second born sister's husband (SS2-HS1) and vice versa (SS1-HS2). The dotted arrow indicates husband to firstborn sister-husband to second born sister (HS1-HS2).

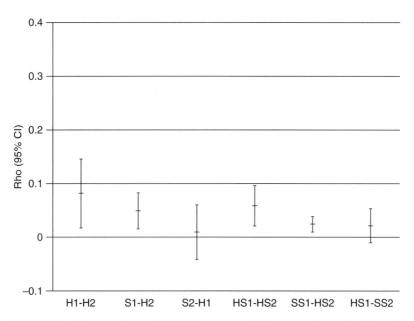

FIGURE 3 BMI correlations (95% CI) for nongenetic family relations. For illustration of H1-H2, S1-H2, and S2-H1, see Figure 2A. For illustration of HS1-HS2, SS1-HS2, and HS1-SS2, see Figure 2B.

ARE BMI CORRELATIONS STRONGER IN THE UPPER OR LOWER PARTS OF THE BMI DISTRIBUTION?

Several studies have attempted to address the intriguing question of whether there is a particular interval in the BMI spectrum where familial resemblance is increased, and therefore could be used as a suitable "phenotype" for gene-identification studies. One study with sufficient statistical power to address this question is the Canada Fitness Survey referred to above and including 15,245 participants from 6377 families (14). The authors estimated standardized risk ratios for underweight (BMI < 18.5 kg/m^2), normal weight (18.5 ≤ BMI ≤ 24.9), overweight (25.0 ≤ BMI ≤ 29.9), obesity of class I (30.0 ≤ BMI ≤ 34.9) and obesity of class II. (35 ≤ BMI < 40) among first-degree relatives of probands who belonged to one of these five BMI categories. The risk for obesity of class II was seven times increased among first-degree relatives of individuals belonging to the same BMI category compared with the risk (prevalence) in the general population. The authors concluded that genetic factors may play a more important role in more extreme levels of obesity than among normal weight subjects.

A study from the United States based on a convenience sample of 2349 parents and siblings of 840 obese probands and 5851 participants of the National Health and Nutrition Examination Survey III showed that the risk of obesity of class III (BMI ≥ 40 kg/m^2) in relatives of women with obesity of class III was six times higher than the risk among individuals in a general population sample also obtained from National Health and Nutrition Examination Survey III. The authors concluded that statistical power in gene mapping studies of obesity might be increased by focusing on family members of obese individuals (15).

The results of these two studies are comparable with a population-based study of 72,687 pairs of full brothers from Sweden (12). Probabilities were estimated for the 10 BMI decile classes among later-born brothers whose earlier-born brothers belonged to either the 1% upper tail or the 1% lower tail of the BMI distribution (Fig. 4). The probability of being among the 10% thinnest individuals was 0.42 for brothers of the 1% thinnest older brothers, while the probability of being among the 10% most obese individuals is 0.40 for brothers of the 1% most obese of the older brothers. The shape of the BMI curve based on values simulated from a bivariate normal distribution followed the empirical data fairly well (Fig. 4). These results show that the BMI of earlier born brothers influence the BMI of later born brothers in a way that would be expected if the correlation was equal over the whole spectrum. Strength of this study is that all subjects had their height and weight measured at age 18 to 19 years (mean age 18.3 years).

CONCLUSION

Families consisting of parents and offspring, so called nuclear families, are the most readily available family constellation and studies based on nuclear families can often be large enough to provide precise estimates of correlations in phenotypes related to adiposity (BMI, waist circumference, etc.) between relatives. Parent-offspring correlations and sibling correlation may arise as a consequence of shared genes and shared environment and from the nuclear family design it is impossible to separate the relative importance of the two. By investigating the correlation between spouses it is, however, possible to estimate the aggregate contribution of spouse assortment and familial environment. A number of studies of adiposity using the nuclear family design have been based on national

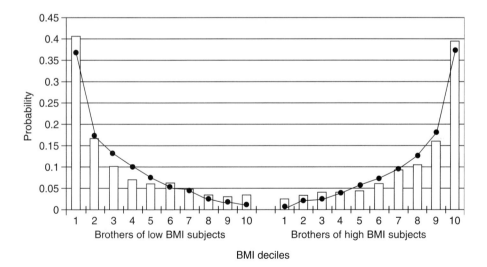

FIGURE 4 Each individual bar represents the probability that the later-born full brother belongs to BMI decile 1 to 10 (from *left* to *right*) conditional on the BMI decile of the firstborn brother (each cluster of bars, 1–10). The connected dots represent simulated probabilities according to the bivariate normal distribution, with constant correlation across the entire BMI spectrum equal to the correlation observed from the empirical data (0.36).

population registers, allowing for virtually complete ascertainment of families from particular birth cohorts. Such an approach renders unbiased estimates that are likely to be representative of the general population.

BMI correlations have consistently been found to be larger among siblings than among parent-offspring relations. Both these types of relations are of first degree with an average genetic sharing of 50%. If the BMI correlations solely reflected additive genetic influences, they would be expected to be equal. When dominance genetic factors are present, they contribute to the sibling correlation but not to the parent-offspring correlation. The observed differences between correlations in biological pairs of full brother (0.36) and father-son pairs (0.28) in the large Swedish study of conscripts (Fig. 1) may therefore indicate effects of genetic dominance. Other possible explanations for the stronger resemblance between siblings than between parents and their offspring are specific environmental influences shared by the siblings and not with the parents, maternal effects (in utero effects, genetic imprinting and mitochondrial genetic effects) or secular environmental changes making siblings, who are more equal in age, share such influences to larger degree.

Remarriages are common in most Western societies and studies on large number of families containing half siblings have been conducted. Half siblings are second-degree relatives that on average share 25% of their genes identical by descent. The BMI correlation among half siblings is typically somewhat higher for maternal than for paternal half siblings and close to half the correlation observed for full siblings. Because half siblings with mother in common share raising environment to a substantially larger degree (children tend to follow the mother upon divorce), it is possible that differences in correlations between maternal and paternal half siblings not only is due to maternal effects but also reflects influences from shared environmental components.

The nuclear family design can be extended to link relations over more than two generations. It is then possible to identify various second, third, and even higher degree, relatives. Because the correlations decrease with genetic distance between relations, large numbers of pairs are needed to establish statistically significant estimates for the more distant relations. The correlation in BMI between relatives appears to follow fairly well a pattern of a reduction by a half for each extra degree of genetic relationship, something expected if the bulk of the correlation is due to additive genetic effects.

In both the nuclear and the extended family design, it is sometimes possible to investigate similarities between nonbiological relations that arise in these families. Examples are spouses, the first and second spouse to remarried individuals, and unrelated offspring to spouses in their previous or later marriages. In the extended family design similar nonbiological relations can be found in niece/nephew–spouse to uncle/aunt. The BMI correlations between these types of relatives are typically weak, but may be explained by social homogamy, phenotypic assortative mating, or convergence due to common living habits.

A few studies have investigated whether there are parts of the adiposity spectrum in which the resemblance between relatives is particularly pronounced. The results show that the familial risk ratio increases gradually when the cut-point for fatness is moved upward and the cut-point for leanness are moved downward. To what extent this is reflecting genetic influences specific to the extreme ends of the adiposity spectrum (e.g., BMI distribution) is not known, but it is clear that there exists no threshold in the BMI distribution that can define any type of distinct genetically founded phenotype.

REFERENCES

1. Davenport CB. Body-Build and its Inheritance. Washington, DC: Carnegie Institution of Washington, 1923.
2. Maes HHM, Neale MC, Eaves LJ. Genetic end environmental factors in relative body weight and human adiposity. Behav Genet 1997; 27(4):325–51.
3. Tambs K, Moun T, Eaves L et al. Genetic and environmental contributions to variance of the body mass index in a Norwegian sample of first- and second-degree relatives. Am J Human Biol 1991; 2:257–67.
4. Katzmarzyk PT, Hebebrand J, Bouchard C. Spousal resemblance in the Canadian population: implications for the obesity epidemic. Int J Obes Relat Metab Disord 2002; 26(2):241–6.
5. Chen W, Srinivasan SR, Bao W et al. The magnitude of familial associations of cardiovascular risk factor variables between parents and offspring are influenced by age: the Bogalusa Heart Study. Ann Epidemiol 2001; 11(8):522–8.
6. Byard PJ, Siervogel RM, Roche AF. Sibling correlations for weight/stature and calf circumference: age changes and possible sex linkage. Hum Biol 1983; 55(3):677–85.
7. Rotimi C, Cooper R. Familial resemblance for anthropometric measurements and relative fat distribution among African Americans. Int J Obes Relat Metab Disord 1995; 19(12):875–80.
8. Hunt MS, Katzmarzyk PT, Perusse L et al. Familial resemblance of 7-year changes in body mass and adiposity. Obes Res 2002; 10(6):507–17.
9. Rice T, Perusse L, Bouchard C et al. Familial aggregation of body mass index and subcutaneous fat measures in the longitudinal Quebec family study. Genet Epidemiol 1999; 16(3):316–34.
10. Austin MA, Friedlander Y, Newman B et al. Genetic influences on changes in body mass index: a longitudinal analysis of women twins. Obes Res 1997; 5(4):326–31.
11. Vogler GP, Sørensen TIA, Stunkard AJ et al. Influences of genes and shared family environment on adult body mass index assessed in an adoption study by a comprehensive path model. Int J Obes Relat Metab Disord 1995; 19(1):40–5.
12. Magnusson PK, Rasmussen F. Familial resemblance of body mass index and familial risk of high and low body mass index. A study of young men in Sweden. Int J Obes Relat Metab Disord 2002; 26(9):1225–31.
13. Sykes B, Irven C. Surnames and the Y chromosome. Am J Hum Genet 2000; 66(4): 1417–9.
14. Katzmarzyk PT, Perusse L, Rao DC et al. Familial risk of overweight and obesity in the Canadian population using the WHO/NIH criteria. Obes Res 2000; 8(2):194–7.
15. Lee JH, Reed DR, Price RA. Familial risk ratios for extreme obesity: implications for mapping human obesity genes. Int J Obes Relat Metab Disord 1997; 21(10):935–40.

Adoption Studies

Thorkild I.A. Sørensen
Institute of Preventive Medicine, Copenhagen University Hospitals, Centre for Health and Society, Copenhagen, Denmark

Finn Rasmussen
Child and Adolescent Public Health Epidemiology Group, Department of Public Health Sciences, Karolinska Institute, Stockholm, Sweden

Patrik K.E. Magnusson
Department of Medical Epidemiology and Biostatistics, Karolinska Institute, Stockholm, Sweden

As described in Chapter 2.1, obesity shows a familial correlation when analyzed as a continuous trait, such as body mass index (BMI = weight/height^2, kg/m^2), and a familial aggregation when analyzed as a dichotomous trait (e.g., BMI $\geq$ 30 kg/m^2). Such resemblance of traits in nuclear families may be due to identity of genes by descent or shared family environment. The investigation of the effects of these influences can be carried out in several different ways. Studies of twin pairs and studies of extended families are addressed in other chapters in Section 2 (see Chapters 2.1 and 2.3) (1). This chapter presents adoption studies, which are studies of families in which an individual has been removed from the biological parents early in life and reared in an adoptive family. In these studies, it is a fundamental requirement that the adoptive family is genetically unrelated to the biological relatives, but how adoptive families are selected varies between countries and over time in the same country. Adoptions may take place within other branches of the family, e.g., uncles and aunts, but these types of adoptions are obviously not suitable for assessing the separated effects of genes and shared environment.

When adoptions have been to biologically unrelated families, the expectation is that the correlations (or aggregation) of the trait under investigation between the adopted-away offspring and the biological family members, parents and/or siblings, reflect the genetic influence on the trait. A correlation in the trait between the adoptive parents and the adoptee is assumed to reflect the effects of the family environment. A common question raised in interpretation of such adoption studies is whether the genetic influence is stronger or weaker than the influence of the family environment. This is answered by comparing the correlation of the adoptee to the biological parents with the correlation of the adoptee to the adoptive parents, but it should be emphasized that the primary question is whether any of the two correlations are different from 0, i.e., whether there is any genetic influence or any influence of the family environment.

A number of such studies were conducted from the 1960s through the 1990s, which have been previously reviewed (2,3). Together with family and twin studies (1), they confirmed that obesity has a genetic basis, and that the genetic influence rather than shared family environment is the major reason for the familial resemblance of obesity. The adoption studies may also be used for other purposes such as characterizing the genetic influence with regard to genetic additive versus nonadditive effects and dependence on specific aspects of the familial environmental conditions, if the relevant information is available.

COMPLETE VS. PARTIAL ADOPTION STUDIES

Two types of adoption studies have been conducted depending on whether or not the study included pertinent information about the trait under investigation among the biological relatives of the adoptee. In view of the circumstances of many adoptions and of the mere process of the adoption, it is a serious challenge to get this information on the biological relatives. The information most likely to be obtained pertains to the biological mother and sometimes the father at the time of adopting-away the child, but a few studies have had the opportunity to get trait information on earlier or later occasions also on the other offspring of the biological parents of the adoptee, including paternal and maternal half siblings. When such information is available, it is possible to estimate the genetic influences on the trait directly. This study design is called the complete adoption study.

The partial adoption study allows a direct estimation of the correlation of the trait under investigation between the adoptee and the adoptive relatives, which, by nature of the design, informs only about possible effects of shared environment. However, various attempts have been made to estimate the effects of genes indirectly from these studies (2,3). When subtracting the estimated correlation between the adoptee and the adoptive family members from the corresponding correlations in intact nuclear families, the resulting difference is assumed to be an estimate of the effect of the genetic contribution to the correlation. The estimates of the correlations in the intact nuclear families have been generated from different sets of families or from the other members of the adoptive families, which themselves, irrespective of the introduction of an adoptee, can be considered as such intact nuclear families.

ASSUMPTIONS—STRENGTH AND WEAKNESSES OF ADOPTION STUDIES

Both the strength and weaknesses of adoption studies are closely related to the fulfillment of the assumptions made for achieving sufficient internal and external validity, i.e., unbiased results that can be generalized to other populations, and especially to populations of common intact families (2,4). Most of the assumptions are implicit in the principles of the study design, and the better they are met, the higher the validity of the study results.

It is assumed that the adoptee is separated very early after birth from the biological mother and the rest of the biological family, and that he or she remains separated with no contact throughout life. Selective placement must be avoided, i.e., the adoptee should not be placed in an adoptive family that to some extent resembles the biological family with regard to the trait under study or factors determining the trait. It is assumed that there is no sustained effect on the trait of the prenatal or the preadoptive postnatal environment shared with the biological mother or with the biological father and other members of the biological family. It is assumed that the paternity is correctly assigned and that there has been no genetic assortative mating between the biological parents, i.e., they are uncorrelated with regard to the genes that may influence the trait under study.

The fulfillment of several of these assumptions can be tested in complete adoption studies, and it may be taken into account in the statistical modeling of the main effects, if they are not perfectly fulfilled.

For the partial adoption study it is implicit that the genetic and environmental influences are only additive, which may be considered a rather strict assumption. Since many adoptions take place due to difficult psychosocial circumstances for the biological parents, it is important to consider whether the results apply to the population of nonadopted subjects. The familial correlations of the trait within the biological and within the adoptive families may be compared with the familial correlations in intact nuclear families; however, similar correlations do not guarantee that there are only additive genetic and environmental influences.

RESULTS OF THE ADOPTION STUDIES
The Partial Adoption Studies
Studies from the United Kingdom, the United States, and Canada have employed the partial adoption method (2,3), where information is only available on the adoptee in childhood and adolescence and on the members of the adoptive family sharing the same household, most frequently the adoptive parents. As previously reviewed (2,3), the partial adoption studies convey a picture of rather mixed results, with some showing a great similarity in degree of fatness between the adoptee and the members of the rearing family, and other showing no such association. Conclusions about the role of genetic influences differ accordingly among these studies. Clearly, this study design is very sensitive to the selection of the families. If the study by some mechanisms tends to include families in which the adoptee and the other members of the adoptive family resemble each other, e.g., with regard to degree of obesity, it will produce an upwardly biased estimate of the influence of the shared family environment, hence, an underestimation of the genetic influence. On the other hand, most of the studies were conducted on members of the same households, where the adoptees were still in their childhood or adolescence. So, the results may suggest that the shared environment have an effect as long as it is still shared, whereas the effect fades away after the individuals have left the household (2,3).

The Complete Adoption Studies
Rather few complete adoption studies have been performed (2,3). Two studies addressed BMI in the adult adoptee, one conducted in Denmark (5–7) on the basis of the unique Danish Adoption Register (8), and one in Iowa (9). Some new, hitherto unpublished data from the Swedish Multigenerational Conscription Study (10) is presented below. The Danish study also included results on children in school age (11). Preliminary results on children from an ongoing longitudinal adoption study in Colorado have been published (12). The scarcity of studies reflects the difficulties in identifying and approaching the biological parents and their other offspring.

Studies on Adults
The Danish Adoption Study first asked about 4000 adult adoptees what their current and maximum height and weight were (5–7). To make it feasible to get data on the family members, it was necessary to select a smaller sample to work with. This selection of adoptees took place on the basis of the distributions of both

the current and the maximum BMI. Within the two genders and five age strata, the upper 8% (4% obese and 4% overweight), the 4% around the median and the 4% at the lower end of each of the two distributions were selected, allowing some adoptees belonging to both samples. The biological parents, the adoptive parents, the biological full siblings and maternal and paternal half siblings, the adoptive parents and the adoptive "siblings" were identified. Postal questionnaires were used to get data on height and weight. The parents were asked about their height and weight at the time their own children went to school, which would be at an age that corresponded to the age of the adult offspring in the study. For parents who were dead or unable to respond, the adult offspring was asked about the information, a procedure validated for the purpose of this study (13). Additional data on height and weight on the adoptees and their various types of siblings were collected from school health records (11).

In the statistical analysis, the first question was whether there were any differences in BMI between the various types of biological and adoptive relatives to the four groups of overweight, median weight and underweight adoptees. For the parents, there were clearly higher BMI of the biological parents, the higher the adoptee BMI, whereas there were no such association between adoptee BMI and BMI of the adoptive parents (5). For the adult biological siblings, there was a distinct increase in BMI of the full siblings by adoptee BMI, and, as expected, a weaker increase for the half sibling, slightly more pronounced for the maternal than for the paternal half siblings (6).

While taking into account the sampling scheme, these results could also be transformed to correlations in BMI between the adoptees and their various types of relatives (7), and to a comprehensive path analysis (14). This latter analysis showed a heritability of 0.34 ± 0.03 (SE), indicating that 34% of the total pheno-typic variance could be attributed to genetic influences. No other relationships were needed to explain the data such as shared environmental effects from parents to offspring or between siblings, specific maternal effects, assortative mating or selective placement.

The adoption study conducted in Iowa (9) was based on 357 adoptees aged 18 to 38 years, one half of whom were selected because of occurrence of psychopathology in the biological family, and the other half by gender and age-matching on adoptees from families without such records. BMI was obtained from data reported by the biological parents at the time of adoption and from data reported by the adoptees and the adoptive parents at the time of the study. The correlations in BMI on the biological side were as follows: mother-daughter, 0.40; mother-son, 0.15; father-daughter, 0.18; and father-son, 0.08, but only the first mentioned were statistically significantly different from 0. The correlations on the adoptive side were all around and not significantly different from 0 (0.06, 0.04, 0.09, and –0.09, respectively). In this study, control for age, height, and possible confounding environmental factors such as rural upbringing and disturbances in the adoptive home did not alter the results. Thus, this study essentially confirmed the results obtained in the Danish study.

Studies on Children and Adolescents

In the Danish Adoption Study, it was possible to retrieve data on a subset of 269 adoptees and their biological and adoptive siblings from the school health examinations, including measurement of height and weight, at ages 7 through 13 years (11). The parent-offspring and sibling correlations were stable across these ages.

The average correlations of BMI of the adoptees with those of the biological mothers were 0.17, of the biological fathers, 0.16, of adoptive mothers, 0.10, and of adoptive fathers, 0.03, and some of the individual age-specific correlations were significantly different from 0 for all parents except the adoptive fathers. The school data on BMI of the adoptees were also compared with those of the biological and adoptive siblings, measured at the same ages in school. The average correlations of BMI of the adoptees with those of biological full siblings were 0.59 (all individual age-specific correlations were significant), of maternal half siblings, 0.16 (some significant), of paternal half siblings, 0.08 (nonsignificant), and of adoptive siblings, 0.14 (some significant). This study thus confirmed the findings of correlations between the adult adoptees and the biological parents and siblings, but it also revealed positive correlations, some of which were statistically significant, between the adoptees and the adoptive parents and siblings, with whom they were sharing household environment, corroborating the corresponding findings in some of the partial adoption studies (2,3).

The Colorado Adoption Project included 245 adoptive and 245 nonadoptive families matched to the adoptive families by age, education, occupational status of the father, gender of the adopted child, and number of older children in the family (12). Height and weight data were available for each year from birth through 7 years and then at 9 years. Applying longitudinal modeling of the data suggested that genetic influences were strong at all ages, but the genetic factors operating were changing over time. There was only little influence of the rearing environment.

The Swedish Multigenerational Conscript Study

A large-scale, population-based Swedish study has been conducted on men whose height and weight have been measured at the military conscription examination conducted at age 18 years (see Chapter 2.1) (15). This study also includes a subset of families of male adoptees (unpublished data). The study showed correlation coefficients of 0.31 (95% CI, 0.25–0.38) for 791 biological full sibling pairs, in which one of the brothers had been adopted away to another family, and 0.30 (0.22–0.37) for 546 biological father-son pairs (sons adopted and raised apart from their biological fathers) (Fig. 1). The correlation coefficients were 0.08 (0.02–0.15) for 808 nonbiological full siblings raised in the same family (one brother adopted and the other not adopted), and 0.06 (0–0.13) for 762 nonbiological father-son pairs (adoptive fathers and adopted sons).

The correlation of 0.08 (0.02–0.15) between pairs of biologically unrelated brothers, where one was adopted and the other was biological son of adoptive parents, may reflect shared sibling environmental effects, possibly detectable because the brothers still lived in or had only recently left the same household environment. Assuming only additive effects of genes and shared environment, this correlation might be used as a correction factor for common environmental factors when estimating heritability on the basis of the various types of sibling correlations reported in Chapter 2.1. The heritability will then become $2 \cdot (0.36-0.08) = 0.56$ for full brothers raised together, and $2 \cdot (0.31-0.00) = 0.62$ for full brothers reared in different families. Applying this estimate to the half siblings, who share 25% of their genes on average, yield heritability estimates of $4 \cdot (0.17-0.08) = 0.36$ for maternal half brothers and $4 \cdot (0.14-0.08) = 0.24$ for paternal half brothers. There are several possible sources of these differences. The half siblings may not have lived as much together as full siblings, so an estimate of 0.08 for the shared environmental influence may be too high. If there are

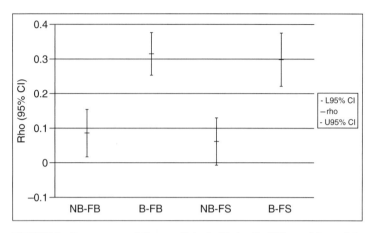

FIGURE 1 Pearson correlation coefficients (rho) with 95% confidence intervals for the association of BMI of adoptees and their biological and nonbiological relatives. Singleton men born in Sweden 1950–1982, who had participated in conscription examination at ages 18 to 19 years. *Abbreviations*: CI, confidence interval; NB-FB, nonbiological full brothers (one adopted, the other not adopted by same parents); B-FB, biological full brothers (same biological parents, one brother adopted, the other not adopted by the same parents); NB-FS, nonbiological father-son pairs (adoptive father); B-FS, biological father-son pair (son adopted).

nonadditive, so-called dominance effects (see below), which emerge among full siblings, but not among half siblings, then the estimated heritability for the full siblings will be greater than that estimated from half-sibling relationships (as from parent-offspring relationships). Both nonpaternity and specific maternal, possibly pre-adoptive, pre- or postnatal effects, may lead to greater correlations for maternal than for paternal half-sibling pairs.

When comparing the heritability of 0.34, estimated in the Danish Adoption study (14), with the results from the Swedish Multigenerational Conscription study and the heritability obtained in the large-scale family studies (see Chapter 2.1), it should be taken into account that the intra-familial correlations—and hence the heritability estimates—in the Danish study are attenuated by the measurement errors due to the use of reported rather than measured data on height and weight and by the variation due to age differences. The larger sample size of the Swedish study also produced correlations with greater precision. Generally, the results from the Swedish study confirm and refine the results of the Danish Adoption study.

ADDITIVE AND NONADDITIVE GENETIC INFLUENCES

The extended family studies strongly suggest that the heritability of BMI has additive and nonadditive genetic components, with the latter being due to dominance, which means that part of the genetic influences are only expressed if particular combinations of genes have been received from both parents (recessive transmission or intra-locus interaction, and epistasis or inter-locus interaction) (see Chapter 2.1). This may explain greater correlation in BMI between full siblings than between parents and offspring even though both types of pairs are assumed to share half of the genes. The Danish adoption study also suggested nonadditive effects (7), but they were not strong enough to be included in the general path model (14).

COMPARISON WITH TWIN STUDIES, INCLUDING STUDIES OF SEPARATED TWINS

As described in later chapters (Chapters 2.3 and 2.4), the many twin studies generally produce higher heritability estimates than the family-based studies, usually in the range of 0.65 to 0.90. There are several possible explanations of this phenomenon. The most important one is probably related to a combination of factors that may increase the intrapair correlations for monozygotic twins compared with those obtained in dizygotic twins. Thus, a contribution of dominance effects, which the family studies does suggest is present for BMI, will add relatively more to the monozygotic correlations than to the dizygotic correlations. In twin studies it is generally assumed that the possible shared environmental influences on the particular phenotype from conception until time of assessment is on average equal for monozygotic and dizygotic twin pairs. It is usually impossible to validate this assumption, and it is possible that the shared environmental influences are stronger for monozygotic than for dizygotic twin pairs. The fact that the genetic identity of the monozygotic twins makes their body appearance more similar may reinforce the parents and others, contributing to their environment in broadest sense, to treat them more equal than they would treat the more dissimilar dizygotic twins.

There are also various reasons for the dizygotic twin correlations to be higher than the full sibling correlations observed in family studies. Thus, the fact that they are assessed at exactly the same age may give rise to a greater correlation for dizygotic twins even if the age differences between full siblings are controlled for by regression methods. It seems plausible to assume that there might be a shared environmental effect that is present and perhaps is greater than it might be between full siblings, and this may also add to the correlations between dizygotic twins compared with full siblings. These effects will of course also increase the monozygotic correlations accordingly, and are therefore not expected to contribute to the greater heritability estimates obtained in twin studies.

The assessment of both the dominance effects and shared environmental effects may be possible in twin studies, where the study also includes series of monozygotic and dizygotic twin pairs where the two twins have been separated early in life and raised apart as in adoption studies. Since this separation is a rare event, especially where the separation implies placement in unrelated families as in the adoption studies, the available studies are based on fairly small series (16,17). The studies, which are further discussed in a later chapter (see Chapter 2.3), clearly support that the genetic influence is strong and includes considerable dominance effects, and none of these studies, which are all conducted in adults, suggest shared environmental effects.

ENVIRONMENTAL EFFECTS CONTROLLED FOR OR INTERACTING WITH GENETIC EFFECTS

In the prevailing paradigm for the role of genes and environment in development of obesity, there is an assumption that genes and environment interacts, meaning that the genetic effects depend on the environmental conditions and vice versa. Very few adoption studies have addressed this possibility, also because the information available about the specific environmental influences is rather sparse; moreover, the statistical power needed to provide reasonably precise estimates of such effects has been limited in the studies available.

In the Danish Adoption study, it was assessed whether the correlations between the adoptees, on one hand, and the biological parents and siblings on the other were modified by a number of environmental indicators that might influence the BMI of the adoptees, such as age at transfer to the adoptive home, region of residence, presence of adoptive siblings, and, for the adoptive parents, year of birth, age at the time of the adoption, smoking habits, BMI, and social position, assessed by the occupation of the adoptive father (18). None of these environmental indicators had any detectable effect on the correlations between the adoptee and the biological relatives. There were no such effects detectable in the Iowa study (9), where rural upbringing and disturbances in the adoptive family were investigated, both of which had their own obesity-promoting influence.

WHAT IS INHERITED?

In view of the clear support of a genetic influence on BMI throughout the range, from the very thin to the very obese, it becomes urgent to understand the mediating mechanisms behind these genetic influences. Knowledge about this would greatly facilitate the search for the specific genes and environmental factors that may lead to development of obesity. This is dealt with in other chapters of the book, and very little has been contributed to this area by adoption studies. One analysis based on the Danish Adoption Study utilized the information about occupational rating as a measure of social class among the biological and adoptive parents to see if this measure could be an indicator of the mediating mechanisms (19). Given that multiple studies shows that the occurrence of obesity is strongly inversely related to social position, it might be that some personality traits, (e.g., intelligence, which influences education and social position, and hence degree of obesity, could be the mediator. Social position, educational level (20), and a variety of personality traits (21), including intelligence (22,23), show a genetic influence. The social position of the biological father influenced the BMI of the adult adoptee, even after adjustment for his or her own and the adoptive father's social class (19). The correlation was too strong to be explained by a possible influence of the biological father's BMI on his social class. This suggests that there may be common genetic determinants of BMI and social class. Clearly, the observation needs to be confirmed and several other potential mediators, not least the biological factors regulating energy intake, energy expenditure and adipose tissue development, and fat storage, need to be further investigated.

CONCLUSION

The adoption studies have contributed by clearly demonstrating that the familial correlations of BMI or other obesity-related measures are attributable mainly to the genetic influences, even among both children and adults living in the same household. There is, however, a weak effect of the shared environment as long as the individuals live together, but no evidence supports that this effect persists after the household has been left.

REFERENCES

1. Rice T. Segregation and commingling analysis of family studies of obesity. In: Clément K, Sørensen TIA, eds. Genetics of Obesity. New York: Taylor & Francis Group, LLC, 2006: in press.
2. Sørensen TIA, Stunkard AJ. Overview of the adoption studies. In: Bouchard C, ed. The Genetics of Obesity. Boca Raton, FL: CRC Press, 1994:49–61.
3. Sørensen TIA. Adoption studies of obesity. In: Bray GA, ed. Molecular and Genetic Aspects of Obesity, Pennington Nutrition Series. Volume V. Baton Rouge, LA: Pennington Biomedical Research Foundation, 1996:462–9.
4. Sørensen TIA. Genetic epidemiology utilizing the adoption method: studies of obesity and of premature death in adults. Scand J Soc Med 1991; 19:14–9.
5. Stunkard AJ, Sørensen TIA, Hanis C1, et al. An adoption study of human obesity. N Engl J Med 1986; 314:193–8.
6. Sørensen TIA, Price RA, Stunkard AJ, et al. Genetics of obesity in adult adoptees and their biological siblings. Br Med J 1989; 298:87–90.
7. Sørensen TIA, Holst C, Stunkard AJ, et al. Correlations of body mass index of adult adoptees and their biological and adoptive relatives. Int J Obesity 1992; 16:227–36.
8. Kety SS, Rosenthal D, Wender PH, et al. The types and prevalence of mental illness in the biological and adoptive families of adopted schizophrenics. J Psychiatr Res 1967/1968; 6(Suppl. 1):345–62.
9. Price RA, Cadoret RJ, Stunkard AJ, et al. Genetic contributions to human fatness: an adoption study. Am J Psychiatry 1987; 144:1003–8.
10. Magnusson PK, Rasmussen F. Familial resemblance of body mass index and familial risk of high and low body mass index: a study of young men in Sweden. Int J Obes 2002; 26(9):1225–31.
11. Sørensen TIA, Holst C, Stunkard AJ. Childhood body mass index—genetic and familial environmental influences assessed in a longitudinal study. Int J Obesity 1992; 16:705–14.
12. Cardon LR. Genetic influences on body mass index in early childhood. In: Turner JR, Cardon LR, Hewitt JK, eds. Behavior Genetic Approaches in Behavioral Medicine. New York: Plenum Press 1995:133–43.
13. Sørensen TIA, Stunkard AJ, Teasdale TW, et al. The accuracy of reports of weight—children's recall of their parents' weight 15 years earlier. Int J Obesity 1983; 7:115–22.
14. Vogler GP, Sørensen TIA, Stunkard AJ, et al. Influences of genes and shared family environment on adult body mass index assessed in an adoption study by a comprehensive path model. Int J Obesity 1995; 19:40–5.
15. Rasmussen F, Johansson M, Hansen HA. Trends in overweight and obesity among 18-year-old males in Sweden between 1971 and 1995. Acta Paediatr 1999; 88:431–7.
16. Stunkard AJ, Harris JR, Pedersen NL, et al. The body-mass index of twins who have been reared apart. N Engl J Med 1990; 322:1483–7.
17. Allison DB, Kaprio J, Korkeila M, et al. The heritability of body mass index among an international sample of monozygotic twins reared apart. Int J Obes 1996; 20(6):501–6.
18. Sørensen TIA, Holst C, Stunkard AJ. Adoption study of environmental modifications of the genetic influences on obesity. Int J Obesity 1998; 22:73–81.
19. Teasdale TW, Sørensen TIA, Stunkard AJ. Genetic and early environmental components in socio-demographic influences on adult body fatness. Br Med J 1990; 300:1615–8.
20. Teasdale TW, Sørensen TIA. Educational attainment and social class in adoptees: genetic and environmental contributions. J Biosoc Sci 1983; 15:509–18.
21. Plomin R, Owen MJ, McGuffin P. The genetic basis of complex human behaviors. Science 1994; 264(5166):1733–9.
22. Bouchard TJ, McGue M. Familial studies of intelligence: a review. Science 1981; 212(4498):1055–9.
23. Teasdale TW, Owen DR. Heredity and familial environment in intelligence and educational level: a sibling study. Nature 1984; 309(5969):620–2.

Twin Studies

Jaakko Kaprio
Department of Public Health, University of Helsinki and Department of Mental Health and Alcohol Research, National Public Health Institute, Helsinki, Finland

Jennifer R. Harris
Department of Genes and Environment, Division of Epidemiology, Norwegian Institute of Public Health, Oslo, Norway

THE TWIN METHOD AND ASPECTS SPECIAL TO OBESITY STUDIES

Family, twin, and adoption studies have provided evidence for cultural and biological inheritance in human behavior and health (1). Because currently known genes account for only a fraction of the estimated genetic variance of obesity-related traits, more knowledge of the dynamics of gene action and of specific environmental conditions is needed. Longitudinal twin and twin-family studies with multiple measurements can permit a more detailed assessment of the developmental aspects of obesity-related factors and how the relative roles of genes and environment unfold over time.

A Brief Overview of the Analysis of Twin Data

We briefly describe the general principles of genetic data analysis for variance components, which is a first step in the exploration of the genetic architecture of a trait or disease. That is, the goal is to establish whether familial, in particular genetic factors are of relevance for the trait, and to what degree genetic variation accounts for the total variance of a trait (2).

The total variance in a behavior, trait or liability to disease can be divided into additive genetic (A), nonadditive genetic (D), common environmental (C), and unique environmental (E) variance (1,3). Additive genetic effects occur when the effects of each gene are adding up to affect the phenotype, whereas nonadditive (dominance) genetic effects denote interactions between the alleles at a genetic locus. These interactions produce deviations between the expected, additive genotypic value and actual genotypic value in the heterozygote. The additive and nonadditive effects add up over all the genes contributing to the phenotype. Interactions between genes (also known as epistatic effects) are seen as nonadditive genetic effects.

Environmental variance can be divided into shared (also called sometimes common) and unique components. Shared or common environmental effects denote all those aspects of the environment which lead family members, also co-twins to be similar. These shared effects can be derived from familial influences, such as eating habits arising from shared family meals. They can also be peer effects that both twins share as they attend the same school or from being in the same occupation. In contrast, unique environmental factors affect only one member of the family. Unique environment refers to environmental experiences and exposures that do not contribute to familial resemblance. The estimate of unique environmental variance also contains error variance, because random measurement error decreases correlations between family members. Following from this definition, the same aspect of the environment can serve as a common or unique environmental factor depending on its influence on family members. For example, parental behavior may either influence all children similarly, acting as a common environmental factor, or it may be experienced differently by each sib, thus acting as a unique environmental factor.

The twin method is based on differences between the two types of twins: monozygotic (MZ) twins, who are genetically identical, and dizygotic (DZ) twins, who share on average 50% of their segregating genes, like any other siblings. The comparison of trait similarity between the co-twins of the two types, measured using the correlations between the co-twins, provides first pass information on the genetic and environmental contribution to the phenotypic variation of that trait. A MZ twin correlation double the DZ twin correlation indicates additive genetic effects, whereas genetic dominance will reduce the DZ twin correlation to below half of the MZ twin correlation. DZ correlations more than one-half the MZ correlation provide evidence for shared environmental effects (4). While comparing MZ and DZ correlations are useful initial guides to the partitioning of variance, evaluation of different genetic models is best done by formal statistical models. Using Mx (5,6), a tailor-made program for genetically informative data, or other structural equation modeling programs, alternative models can be compared in which different components of variance are specified, and goodness-of-fit statistics assess how well the various models fit the data. Scripts for different designs and models are available at the Genomeutwin Mx-script library (http://www.psy.vu.nl/mxbib/), at the Mx home page and elsewhere.

When the data permit, the twin model can be extended to analyze more detailed questions about the variance and covariance structures in the data (1). Sex differences in the magnitude of the genetic and environmental parameters can be estimated in classical twin models, but if the data include male and female MZ and DZ pairs as well as DZ pairs where one twin is male and one twin is female, then models of sex differences permit tests of whether different sets of genes (or environments) influence phenotypic variation in males and females.

The effective genotype of MZ twins may begin to diverge over time as epigenetic and various environmental effects modifies gene expression in the twins, even though their genomic DNA remains unchanged, except for possible somatic mutations (7–9,10). This phenomenon studied in discordant MZ twin pairs provides a unique method for investigating specific genes that may influence the trait of interest and is currently being used to study genetic influences on adiposity, as described later in this chapter.

Assumptions of the Twin Method

One of the assumptions of the classic twin analysis is that there is random mating of the parents of twins with respect to the trait being studied. Under that assumption, the expected value of genetic resemblance of DZ twins is 0.5, i.e., that they share 50% of their segregating genes in common. If there is assortative mating whereby phenotypic similarities affects partner selection then the spousal correlation is greater than 0, and the parents may thus resemble each other with respect to the genes of the trait being studied. This is known as *phenotypic assortment.*

On the other hand, parents can resemble each other because they share the same social background, which causes them to resemble each other to a greater extent without being genetically more alike than expected. This is known as *social homogamy*. Assortative mating by body height and weight is well established in various populations (see Chapter 2.1), but its causal mechanisms remain poorly understood. We analyzed the effect of phenotypic assortment and social homogamy on spousal correlations for body height and body mass index (BMI, kg/m^2) (11). Our questionnaire-based data were obtained from the adult Finnish Twin Cohort; 922 MZ and 1697 DZ adult twin pairs reported in 1990 information about their body height and weight and that of their spouses. Assortative mating was evident for both body height and BMI. For body height, the effects of social homogamy and phenotypic assortment were about the same. For BMI, the effect of social homogamy was stronger (0.31 in men and 0.28 in women) than the effect of phenotypic assortment (0.13 in both men and women). When assortative mating was taken into account, shared environmental factors had no effect on phenotypic variation in body height or BMI. Thus, assortative mating needs to be considered in population genetic studies of body height and weight (11). Estimates of heritability from twin studies are nonetheless unlikely to be biased because of the relatively small role of phenotypic assortment. On the other hand, context-dependent analyses of heritability of BMI should be pursued to elucidate the nature of social homogamy.

The equal environment assumption (EEA) is a central tenet in twin studies. Briefly, the EEA posits that environmental influences that affect the trait of interest (in this case BMI) are not shared to a greater extent among MZ than DZ twins. Violation of this assumption could mean that increased similarity among MZ pairs leads to inflated estimates of genetic influences in twin studies. The tenability of the EEA is most likely phenotype-specific and should be examined for each phenotype and age group of interest. For most behavioral traits, the assumption is rarely violated (12) and the evidence regarding EEA and BMI is presented below.

Even though the growth of twins in utero differs from that of singletons, birth weight in twins weakly predicts later adiposity (13). The placentation of MZ and DZ pairs differ. MZ twins can be either monochorionic or dichorionic, while DZ pairs are always dichorionic and have their own placenta (14). In monochorionic twin pairs the risk of twin-to-twin transfusion syndrome is high resulting in large intrapair growth differences. However, the greater similarity of MZ twins in body weight compared to DZ twins is already established after the first year of life (15).

TWIN DATA ON OBESITY AND RELATED PHENOTYPES
Cross-sectional Surveys of BMI

In large population-based survey studies, adiposity is most commonly measured using BMI. Early family studies provided clear evidence that obesity tended to cluster in families, but since family members share common environmental and genetic influences, the reasons for this familial resemblance were not well understood. In 1977, the NHLBI twin study revealed the importance of genetic factors in explaining the observed familial aggregation for BMI. Since then numerous twin studies of BMI have been conducted in many countries including the United States, Canada, Europe, China and Japan (16). The findings consistently showed a significant role of genetic factors in the etiology of obesity with heritability estimates ranging from 0.50 to 0.90. As described below, these studies also highlighted a number of critical issues about the sources of individual variation in BMI which have been further investigated in twin studies using special design features or sophisticated analytic models.

It is commonly noted that twin studies yield larger heritability estimates for BMI than those derived from family studies. This raised questions regarding the applicability of the EEA. A seminal study of BMI used data from twins who were reared together and twins who were reared apart and did not find evidence that MZ twins who grew up together were more similar for adult BMI than were MZ twins who were separated shortly after birth (17). Other potential explanations for the discrepancy in heritability between twin and other family designs have emerged. Primary among these are that twin studies are more likely to reflect the effects of epistasis (gene-gene interaction) and the recognition that the effective genotype may vary across age. Twins are perfectly correlated for age and thereby for differences in gene expression that may occur as part of normal developmental trajectories. In contrast, family members, particularly parent-offspring dyads, differ widely in age and may differ in stages of body composition development that could be differentially influenced by genes (and environments) across the life course. The presence of such effects would manifest as reduced trait similarity between relatives of disparate ages. Such developmental effects are illustrated by several twin studies on growth from birth to early childhood (18) and from later childhood to adolescence (19) which show progressive changes whereby MZ twins become more similar and DZ twins become less similar in their trajectories for weight development.

Sex Differences
Characteristic male and female patterns of weight development and fat distribu-tion are well known and raise the question of sex differences in the factors influencing BMI. This issue has critical implications for health and mortality because overweight and obesity confer differential risks on health outcomes in males and females. Classical twin studies that include like-sexed MZ and DZ twins can test for differences in the magnitude of genetic and environmental influences (common sex limitation) on variation in BMI. Augmenting the data with information from unlike-sexed pairs permits tests for sex differences in the sets of genes and environments that influence variation. Studies of sex-specific effects on variation in BMI are few but the findings suggest developmental aspects. Specifically, there was no evidence for sex-specific effects based on data from a pre-adolescent sample aged 11 (20), but sex-specific genetic effects emerge in data from older samples aged 16 to 17 (21) and 18 to 25 (22). The most comprehensive effort to explore sex differences in the genetic and environmental variance architecture of BMI was conducted through the GenomEUtwin collabora-tion, which analyzed data from approximately 37,000 twin pairs from eight countries. The data were stratified into two age groups, aged 20 to 29 and aged 30 to 39, to explore potential age differences in the sex-specific effects. Findings were highly similar across the countries revealing greater variation in BMI among women than among men. In general, the variance structures were also similar across countries and across age with genetic differences explaining most of the variation in BMI. Furthermore, sex differences in the genetic and environmental variance components were consistently significant. The collective data indicate that the sets of genes influencing variation in BMI during young and middle adulthood are not fully identical for males and females (23). Although these

studies do not include measured genotype information, the results have provided insights for further genetic investigations. Results generated from molecular research are consistent with evidence of sex-specific effects for BMI and is beginning to pinpoint possible genetic loci and variants that could help explain the sex differences for BMI. For example, the twin findings prompted researchers to probe further the Xq22-24 region of the X-chromosome for genes associated with obesity. Linkage results suggested a sex-specific effect and association with the SLC6A14 gene which encodes an amino acid transporter speculated to affect appetite regulation (24). Another study examining common variants in the leptin gene and BMI revealed associations between a number of SNPs in men but not in women (25). Sex-specific findings were also reported based on a genome-wide linkage analysis of BMI and percent body fat in the HyperGen Study, with signs of linkage on 12q in women and on 15q and 3q for men. These regions harbor quantitative trait loci (QTLs) with biological relevance to body composition.

Because BMI is a ratio trait, estimates of genetic and environmental effects are a function of the separate parameters for height, weight and their covariance. An alternate strategy to studying sex-specific effects for BMI is to analyze the component elements of height and weight. This approach addresses the question of genetic pleiotropy (where the same gene or sets of genes influencing variation in more than one trait) by estimating the genetic correlation (r_g) between height and weight in males, in females, and between males and females. Results using this approach and data from the population-based registry of Norwegian twins (aged 18–32) provided further insight into the nature of these sex-specific effects. Namely, genetic covariance between weight and height is significantly larger for males ($r_g = 0.61$) than for females ($r_g = 0.46$) indicating a greater set of common genetic effects that influence height and weight development in males than in females. In contrast, height and weight development among women is more strongly influenced by genetic (A) and environmental (E) factors that are specific to each phenotype. Furthermore, cross-sex analyses reveal a greater degree of commonality between males and females for the genes influencing variation in height ($r_g = 0.86$) than for weight ($r_g = 0.66$). These results suggest that sex-specific effects found for BMI are primarily explained by general sex limitation for weight (26).

Similar analyses in a smaller and younger sample (aged 20) of Italian twins did not find sex differences in the magnitude of the genetic correlation between height and weight, but rather reported genetic correlations for the males (0.46) and females (0.42) that were quite similar to the findings for the females in the Norwegian study (27). Further studies are needed to verify whether the sex-specific effects reside in factors affecting weight development and how these may vary across development. These analyses are currently underway using data from more than 65,000 pairs in the GenomEUtwin project.

Lifestyle Factors and Moderation of Genetic Effects on BMI
Although heritability for BMI is substantial, the recent and dramatic increase in the prevalence of overweight and obesity has been attributed to lifestyle and environmental factors. Several lines of reasoning are invoked, including epidemiological findings linking health behaviors with weight development, and, that changes in the gene pool could not have occurred so quickly as to account for the rapid changes in prevalence. However, gene-environment interactions, whereby genetic differences between individuals modulate responses to obesity-promoting

behaviors and environments, are another important consideration. Gene-environment interactions are typically difficult to detect and analyze but advances in statistical modeling allow tests of the effects of moderators on heritability (28). Analyses using Norwegian twin data to test whether smoking, alcohol use, and physical activity affect the expression of genetic factors on BMI revealed that lifestyle factors differentially moderate genetic influences on BMI. Heritability increased with increasing levels of smoking, and this effect was more pronounced among the women; and heritability decreased with increasing levels of drinking and exercise. The overall findings suggest that genetic effects seem to be more susceptible to moderation by health behaviors among females than among males (29). A similar finding of moderation of the genetic effect on weight by physical activity has been reported in Finnish adult twins (30).

Longitudinal Data on Weight: Determinants of Weight Change
Longitudinal Data in Childhood and Adolescence
Data from longitudinal twin studies in Finland (13,31) have been advantageous in determining the growth trajectories from birth to early adulthood and in defining the genetic and environmental architecture responsible for height and weight development. It was shown that size at birth tracks to late adolescence and early adulthood, but the tracking of height is more substantial than the tracking of relative weight. Length at birth and parents' height were the main predictors of final height and birth weight; parents' BMI and mother's smoking during pregnancy were the most significant determinants of early adult BMI. Variation in size at birth was mostly explained by fetal environmental factors, whereas most of the variation in adolescent and adult body size was attributable to genes. Shared environmental effects for height showed considerable carry-over effects from birth to early adulthood, whereas the genetic and unique environmental effects were more age specific. In BMI, both genetic and environmental effects were changing rather than staying stable during growth. Similar results have been observed elsewhere (32–34).

The genetics of changes in weight in adults is less well known and characterized. The heritability estimate of 7-year changes in BMI among 521 Canadian families was 14% (35), while a longer term (24 years) follow-up in the Framingham family data showed a more substantial heritability (24%) for rate of weight change in adulthood (36). Twin studies have found substantial heritability (>70%) for maximum BMI and a trend to adult weight gain in 514 male twin pairs examined during military induction, at the mean age of 20 years, from the WWII veteran twin panel (37), based on four measurements during a 43-year interval. Based on two examinations of 315 female pairs, Austin et al. found a similar high heritability (from 0.57 to 0.86) of change in BMI over a decade (38).

We have used a latent growth model to estimate genetic effects on BMI level at baseline and the rate of change in BMI over a 15-year study period, based on a longitudinal cohort of Finnish twins ($N = 10,556$ individuals). They were aged 20 to 46 years at baseline and provided data on weight and height from mailed surveys in 1975, 1981, and 1990. We found a substantial genetic influence on rate of change in BMI [h^2 for men = 58% (95% CI 0.50–0.69), h^2 for women = 64% (95% CI 0.58–0.69)] (39). The genetic correlation between BMI level and rate of change was virtually zero, suggesting that the genes affecting BMI are different from those involved in weight changes in adults.

Other Study Designs

One of the few approaches by which the effects of obesity can be studied in the absence of confounding due to genetic effects is to study MZ twins discordant for obesity. The obese and the nonobese co-twins share the same genes and differ only by environmental exposures (considered in the broadest sense including epigenetic effects) and the resultant acquired obesity. Greenfield et al. examined intrapair differences in weight to associate inflammation markers with obesity (40). With this co-twin control design, we were able to identify and study 10 healthy MZ pairs with 10 to 25 kg differences in weight from the Finntwin16 studies. A control group of nine normal-weight or obesity concordant MZ pairs was also studied. These studies show that acquired obesity is associated with increased liver fat content, insulin resistance, various vascular abnormalities and several changes in adipose tissue metabolism and lipid profiles using lipidomics (41–46). This observational approach of long-term obesity discordance complements the short-term experimental studies described by Bouchard in Chapter 2.4.

PROSPECTS FOR TWIN-BASED STUDIES OF BMI

Two major challenges for future analyses to elucidate the etiology of individual differences in weight development and obesity concern: (*i*) identifying the relevant metabolic pathways and the underlying genetic influences on those pathways, and (*ii*) differential classification of obesity outcomes as they relate to genetic heterogeneity and environmental influences. Research incorporating new methodologies (i.e., transcriptomics, metabolomics and proteomics, neuroimaging) that target upstream endophenotypes of factors affecting weight development will be uniquely powerful when used in twin studies such as the discordant MZ design. In order to take into account the complexity of the phenotype it is essential to use longitudinal studies with repeated measures of biomarkers and environmental influences. This work will facilitate the identification of genes influencing BMI-related traits and diseases. Within the framework of genetically informative datasets, we need detailed phenotyping starting from gene expression studies all the way to neurobiological and social correlates of eating behavior, physical activity and other determinants of weight maintenance and weight change in relevant cultural contexts.

REFERENCES

1. Boomsma D, Busjahn A, Peltonen L. Classical twin studies and beyond. Nat Rev Genet 2002; 3(11):872–82.
2. Thomas DC. Statistical Methods in Genetic Epidemiology. Oxford: Oxford University Press, 2004.
3. Lynch M, Walsh B. Genetics and Analysis of Quantitative Traits. Sunderland, MA, U.S.A.: Sinauer Associates, Inc., 1998.
4. Posthuma D, Beem AL, De Geus EJ, et al. Theory and practice in quantitative genetics. Twin Res 2003; 6(5):361–76.
5. Neale MC, Cardon LR. Methodology for Genetic Studies of Twins and Families. Dordrecht: Kluwer Academic, 1992.
6. Mx. Statistical Modelling. Richmond, VA: Department of Psychiatry, 1994.
7. Gottesman II, Hanson DR. Human development: biological and genetic processes. Annu Rev Psychol 2005; 56:263–86.
8. Wong AH, Gottesman II, Petronis A. Phenotypic differences in genetically identical organisms: the epigenetic perspective. Hum Mol Genet 2005; 14(Suppl. 1):R11–8.

9. Martin NG, Boomsma DI, Machin G. A twin-pronged attack on complex traits. Nat Genet 1997; 17:387–92.
10. Fraga MF, Ballestar E, Paz MF, et al. Epigenetic differences arise during the lifetime of monozygotic twins. Proc Natl Acad Sci U S A 2005; 102(30):10604–9.
11. Silventoinen K, Kaprio J, Lahelma E, et al. Assortative mating by body height and BMI: Finnish twins and their spouses. Am J Hum Biol 2003; 15(5):620–7.
12. Kendler KS. Twin studies of psychiatric illness: an update. Arch Gen Psychiatry 2001; 58(11):1005–14.
13. Pietilainen KH, Kaprio J, Rasanen M, et al. Tracking of body size from birth to late adolescence: contributions of birth length, birth weight, duration of gestation, parents' body size, and twinship. Am J Epidemiol 2001; 154(1):21–9.
14. Derom R, Derom C. Placentation. In: Blickstein I, Keith LG, eds. Multiple Pregnancy: Epidemiology, Gestation and Perinatal outcome. London and New York: Taylor & Francis, 2005:157–67.
15. Silventoinen K, Pietiläinen KH, Tynolius P, Sorensen TIA, Kaprio J, Rasmussen F. Genetic and environmental factors in relative weight from birth to age 18: the Swedish young male twins study. Int J Obes 2007; 31:615–21.
16. Maes HH, Neale MC, Eaves LJ. Genetic and environmental factors in relative body weight and human adiposity. Behav Genet 1997; 27(4):325–51.
17. Stunkard AJ, Harris JR, Pedersen N, et al. The body mass index of twins who have been reared apart. N Engl J Med 1990; 322:1483–7.
18. Wilson RS. Concordance in physical growth for monozygotic and dizygotic twins. Ann Hum Biol 1976; 3(1):1–10.
19. Fischbein S. Intra-pair similarity in physical growth of monozygotic and of dizygotic twins during puberty. Ann Hum Biol 1977; 4(5):417–30.
20. Bodurtha JN, Mosteller M, Hewitt JK, et al. Genetic analysis of anthropometric measures in 11-year-old twins: the Medical College of Virginia Twin Study. Pediatr Res 1990; 28(1):1–4.
21. Pietilainen KH, Kaprio J, Rissanen A, et al. Distribution and heritability of BMI in Finnish adolescents aged 16y and 17y: a study of 4884 twins and 2509 singletons. Int J Obes Relat Metab Disord 1999; 23(2):107–15.
22. Harris JR, Tambs K, Magnus P. Sex-specific effects for body mass index in the new Norwegian twin panel. Genet Epidemiol 1995; 12:251–65.
23. Schousboe K, Willemsen G, Kyvik KO, et al. Sex differences in heritability of BMI: a comparative study of results from twin studies in eight countries. Twin Res 2003; 6(5):409–21.
24. Suviolahti E, Oksanen LJ, Ohman M, et al. The SLC6A14 gene shows evidence of association with obesity. J Clin Invest 2003; 112(11):1762–72.
25. Jiang Y, Wilk JB, Borecki I, et al. Common variants in the 5′ region of the leptin gene are associated with body mass index in men from the National Heart, Lung, and Blood Institute Family Heart Study. Am J Hum Genet 2004; 75(2):220–30.
26. Rønning T, Harris JR. Bivariate twin study of height and weight. Twin Res 2006; 7:376.
27. Fagnani C, Cirrincione R, Cotichini R, et al. A cross-sectional study of height, weight and body mass index in young adult Italian twins. Twin Res 2004; 7:346.
28. Purcell S. Variance components models for gene-environment interaction in twin analysis. Twin Res 2002; 5(6):554–71.
29. Harris JR, Rønning T. Interactions between genetic and lifestyle factors influence variation in body mass index in Norwegian twins. Behav Genet 2005; 35(6):804.
30. Heitmann BL, Kaprio J, Harris JR, et al. Are genetic determinants of weight gain modified by leisure-time physical activity? A prospective study of Finnish twins. Am J Clin Nutr 1997; 66(3):672–8.
31. Pietilainen KH, Kaprio J, Rasanen M, et al. Genetic and environmental influences on the tracking of body size from birth to early adulthood. Obes Res 2002; 10(9):875–84.
32. Johansson M, Rasmussen F. Birthweight and body mass index in young adulthood: the Swedish young male twins study. Twin Res 2001; 4(5):400–5.
33. Loos RJ, Beunen G, Fagard R, et al. Birth weight and body composition in young adult men—a prospective twin study. Int J Obes Relat Metab Disord 2001; 25(10):1537–45.

34. Whitfield JB, Treloar SA, Zhu G, et al. Genetic and non-genetic factors affecting birthweight and adult body mass index. Twin Res 2001; 4(5):365–70.
35. Hunt MS, Katzmarzyk PT, Perusse L, et al. Familial resemblance of 7-year changes in body mass and adiposity. Obes Res 2002; 10(6):507–17.
36. Fox CS, Heard-Costa NL, Vasan RS, et al. Genomewide linkage analysis of weight change in the Framingham Heart Study. J Clin Endocrinol Metab 2005; 90(6):3197–201.
37. Fabsitz RR, Sholinsky P, Carmelli D. Genetic influences on adult weight gain and maximum body mass index in male twins. Am J Epidemiol 1994; 140:711–20.
38. Austin MA, Friedlander Y, Newman B, et al. Genetic influences on changes in body mass index: a longitudinal analysis of women twins. Obes Res 1997; 5:326–31.
39. Hjelmborg JvB, Fagnani C, Silventoinen K, McGue M, Korkeila M, Christensen K, Rissanen A, Kaprio J. Genetic Influences on growth traits of body mass index. A longitudinal study of adult twins. Unpublished data.
40. Greenfield JR, Samaras K, Jenkins AB, et al. Obesity is an important determinant of baseline serum C-reactive protein concentration in monozygotic twins, independent of genetic influences. Circulation 2004; 109:3022–8.
41. Gertow K, Pietilainen KH, Yki-Jarvinen H, et al. Expression of fatty-acid-handling proteins in human adipose tissue in relation to obesity and insulin resistance. Diabetologia 2004; 47(6):1118–25.
42. Kannisto K, Pietilainen KH, Ehrenborg E, et al. Overexpression of 11beta-hydroxysteroid dehydrogenase-1 in adipose tissue is associated with acquired obesity and features of insulin resistance: studies in young adult monozygotic twins. J Clin Endocrinol Metab 2004; 89(9):4414–21.
43. Pietilainen KH, Rissanen A, Kaprio J, et al. Acquired obesity is associated with increased liver fat, intra-abdominal fat, and insulin resistance in young adult monozygotic twins. Am J Physiol Endocrinol Metab 2005; 288(4):E768–74.
44. Pietilainen KH, Rissanen A, Laamanen M, et al. Growth patterns in young adult monozygotic twin pairs discordant and concordant for obesity. Twin Res 2004; 7(5):421–9.
45. Pietiläinen KH, Kannisto K, Korsheninnikova E, et al. Acquired obesity increases CD68 and TNF-{alpha} and decreases adiponectin gene expression in adipose tissue. A study in monozygotic twins. J Clin Endocrinol Metab 2006; 91:2776–81.
46. Pietiläinen KH, Sysi-Aho M, Rissanen A, et al. Acquired obesity is associated with changes in the serum lipidomic profile independent of genetic effects—a monozygotic twin study. PLoS ONE 2007; 1:e218.

2.4 Experimental Twin Studies

Claude Bouchard and Tuomo Rankinen

Human Genomics Laboratory, Pennington Biomedical Research Center, Baton Rouge, Louisiana, U.S.A.

There are considerable individual differences in responses to various dietary manipulations, such as diets rich in cholesterol or in saturated fats. The same phenomenon has been observed in response to chronic overfeeding. For instance, in the Vermont overfeeding study, body weight gain varied among subjects and was below the expected weight gain based upon the ingested caloric surplus (1). Much has been learned from experimental overfeeding, dietary energy restriction, or exercise-induced negative energy balance studies conducted with human subjects.

However, such energy balance experiments would yield better and more powerful data if they were performed with sets of monozygotic (MZ) twins (2). A unique aspect of this research design is that it examines the issue of a genotype-environment interaction effect in response to the treatment. Environment is defined here as an overfeeding or a negative energy balance treatment. A genotype-environment interaction effect refers to a phenotype's response to an environmental challenge that is significantly influenced by the genotype (3,4).

We briefly review in this chapter the results of fully standardized and controlled experiments conducted with pairs of identical twins, and the observations made in pairs of identical twins discordant for obesity.

THE EXPERIMENTAL DESIGNS

In the experimental MZ twin design, both members of several pairs of MZ twins are subjected to the same experimental treatment (2). If there are individual differences in response to the treatment, within-pairs and between-pairs variances can be obtained. Full control over all aspects of the treatment is critical to the success of such experiments. The procedure is quite similar to that used in animal genetics when testing for a genotype-environment interaction effect by comparing various strains of a given species exposed to a given treatment. The main difference is that by using MZ twins, we have only two subjects per genotype. However, the number of genotypes (MZ pairs) can be relatively large depending on the requirements of the research.

Data gathered before and after treatment on both members of several twin pairs can be analyzed by a two-way analysis of variance for repeated measures on one factor (the treatment effect). Twins are nested in pairs. F ratios for the treatment effect and for the genotype-treatment interaction effect can be obtained. The intraclass correlation calculated with the absolute or relative response to the treatment can also be computed from the within and between pairs means of squares, without or with adjustment for the pre-treatment level (2). A larger between MZ pairs variance compared to the within-pair variance suggests that the response to the experimental treatment is more heterogeneous in subjects who are genetically different.

However, this design has important limitations. For instance, even though it is possible, at least from a theoretical point of view, to exert satisfactory experimental control and reach full standardization over energy or nutrient intake in overfeeding or underfeeding studies, it is not possible to fully standardize energy expenditure. Clamping of energy expenditure at the same level for all subjects of a given group cannot be achieved because of individual differences in resting metabolic rate, thermic response to food, fidgeting or variations in body mass that impact on the energy cost of weight maintenance. Of course, there are also limits as to the severity of the nutritional stress that can be tested as well as in the duration of the experimental treatment.

OVERFEEDING EXPERIMENTS WITH MZ TWIN PAIRS

It is generally recognized that some individuals are prone to excessive accumulation of fat, for whom losing weight represents a continuous battle, and others who seem relatively well-protected against such a menace. We have in the past investigated whether such differences could be accounted for by inherited differences. In other words, we asked whether there were differences in the sensitivity of individuals to gain fat when chronically exposed to positive energy balance or to lose fat when exposed to negative energy balance conditions and whether such differences were dependent or independent of the genotype. If the answer to these questions was affirmative, then one would have to conclude that there was a significant genotype energy-balance interaction effect.

The results from a short-term experiments (22 days) suggested that such an effect was likely to exist for body weight, body fat, fat distribution, metabolic rates and several aspects of carbohydrate and lipid metabolism (6). These results were subsequently confirmed by a long-term study which is reviewed below.

Twelve pairs of male MZ twins ate a 1000 kcal/day caloric surplus, 6 days a week, during a period of 100 days (6). Significant increases in body weight and fat mass were observed after the period of overfeeding. Data showed that there were considerable interindividual differences in the adaptation to excess calories and that the variation observed was not randomly distributed, as indicated by the significant within-pair resemblance in response. For instance, there were at least three times more variance in response between pairs than within pairs for the gains in body weight, fat mass and fat-free mass (Table 1 and Fig. 1). These data demonstrate that some individuals are more at risk than others to gain fat when energy intake surplus is clamped at the same level for everyone and when all subjects are confined to a sedentary lifestyle. The within identical twin pair response to the standardized caloric surplus suggests that the amount of fat stored is likely influenced by the genotype.

At the beginning of the overfeeding treatment, almost all the daily caloric surplus was recovered as body energy gain, but the proportion decreased to 60% at the end of the 100-day protocol (8). The weight gain pattern followed an exponential with a half-duration of about 86 days. We have estimated that the weight gain attained in the experiment reached about 55% of the anticipated maximal weight gain had the overfeeding protocol been continued indefinitely (8).

TABLE 1 Effects of the 100-Day Overfeeding Treatment and Intrapair Resemblance in the Absolute Response[a]

Variable	Before overfeeding (mean ± SD)	After overfeeding (mean ± SD)	Within-pair resemblance	
			F ratio	Intraclass
Body weight (kg)	60.3 ± 8.0	68.4 ± 8.2[c]	3.43[b]	0.55[b]
Body mass index (kg/m²)	19.7 ± 2.0	22.4 ± 2.0[c]	2.85[b]	0.48[b]
Percent fat	11.3 ± 5.0	17.8 ± 5.7[c]	2.92[b]	0.49[b]
Fat mass (kg)	6.9 ± 3.5	12.3 ± 4.5[c]	3.00[b]	0.50[b]
Fat-free mass (kg)	53.4 ± 6.6	56.1 ± 6.7[c]	2.34	0.40
Fat mass/fat-free mass	0.13 ± 0.06	0.22 ± 0.08[c]	3.30[b]	0.53[b]
Subcutaneous fat (mm)	75.9 ± 21.2	129.4 ± 32.9[c]	2.77[b]	0.47[b]
Body energy (MJ)	497 ± 142	719 ± 176[c]	3.12[b]	0.51[b]

[a]Statistical significance was established from a two-way analysis of variance for repeated measures on one factor (time). F ratio of between-pairs over within-pairs variances. Intraclass coefficient was used to assess the within-pair resemblance in response to the treatment.
[b]$p < 0.05$.
[c]$p < 0.0001$.
Source: From Ref. 7. Copyright © 2007 Massachusetts Medical Society. All rights reserved.

The mean body mass gain for the 24 subjects of the 100-day overfeeding experiment was 8.1 kg, of which 5.4 kg were fat mass and 2.7 kg were fat-free mass increases. Assuming that the energy content of body fat is about 9300 kcal/kg and that of fat-free tissue is 1020 kcal/kg, then about 63% of the excess energy intake was recovered on the average as body mass changes. This proportion is of the same order as that reported by other investigators (9,10), i.e., between 60% and 75% of total excess energy intake. There were, however, individual differences among the 24 subjects with respect to the amount of fat and fat-free tissues gained. Thus, while the mean gain of fat mass to fat-free mass ratio was 2 to 1, a ratio close to what was reported before (11), it was 1 to 2 in one subject and reached 4 to 1 in some cases. Variations in the fat mass to fat-free mass ratio changes in response to overfeeding were correlated with the changes in body weight and the coefficient reached 0.61 ($p < 0.01$) (7). In other words, about 37% of the variation in weight gain as a result of exposure to long-term overfeeding was associated with this dimension of nutrient partitioning. Those who gained more fat relative to fat-free tissues were the high gainers for body mass while those who gained relatively more lean tissues were the low gainers. Moreover, a significant genotype-overfeeding interaction effect ($p < 0.05$) was observed for the response of the fat mass (kg) to fat-free mass (kg) ratio (see Table 1).

If, on the average, 63% of the extra energy consumed was accounted for by the changes in fat mass and fat-free mass, one would be left with 29,000 kcal to be accounted for. We measured the energy content of the feces for several days before and after the overfeeding treatment in 16 of the 24 subjects. There was no significant change in the amount of energy that was not absorbed during digestion. Thus, the remaining energy must in all likelihood be associated with the costs of protein (3333 kcal) and fat (8095 kcal) tissues gained and with increases in resting metabolic rate, thermic effect of food, standard postures, moving the body around and fidgeting. In fact, we were able to account for 91% of the 84,000 kcal energy surplus ingested by the 24 young adults of the study simply through increases in body

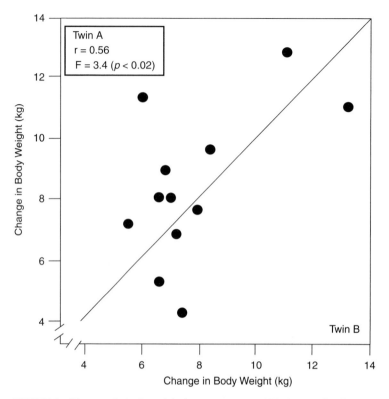

FIGURE 1 Changes in body weight in response to a 100-day overfeeding protocol in 12 pairs of young adult male identical twins. The within-pair resemblance in response is illustrated. *Source*: From Ref. 7. Copyright © 2007 Massachusetts Medical Society. All rights reserved.

energy content and costs of storage (12). One must also entertain the possibility that increases in energy expenditure for postures, bodily activities and fidgeting were present not only as a result of increases in body mass but perhaps also because of a shift in the daily pattern of activities toward a more energy-demanding profile even though subjects were kept under sedentary conditions. The remaining unexplained energy expenditure (about 9%) was likely accounted for by errors of measurement, errors in the assumptions made to estimate overall energy balance at the onset of the study, and by small differences in the daily pattern of activities over the duration of the overfeeding protocol.

The long-term overfeeding study also revealed that there was six times more variance between pairs than within pairs for the changes in upper body fat and in computerized tomography determined abdominal visceral fat when both were adjusted for the gain in total fat mass (Fig. 2) (7). These observations indicate that some individuals store fat predominantly in selected fat depots primarily as a result of undetermined genetic characteristics.

Biopsies obtained in the vastus lateralis muscle before and after the over-feeding protocol in these 24 healthy young men indicated that the weight gain was lower in those with a high proportion of type I fibers and higher levels of OGDH enzyme (alpha-ketoglutarate dehydrogenase is limiting enzyme of the tricarboxylic

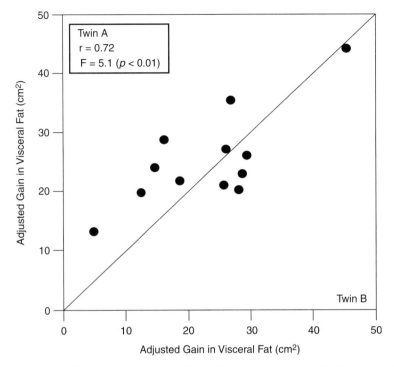

FIGURE 2 Changes in abdominal visceral fat in response to a 100-day overfeeding protocol in 12 pairs of young adult male identical twins. The within-pair resemblance in response is illustrated. *Source*: From Ref. 7. Copyright © 2007 Massachusetts Medical Society. All rights reserved.

acid cycle) activity at baseline. Overall, skeletal muscle morphological and metabolic characteristics accounted for 18% to 28% of the variance in body weight and adiposity gains with overfeeding (13). A number of candidate gene studies have been performed with the response phenotypes of these 12 pairs of MZ twins (14). In brief, markers in the adipsin (or complement factor D, *CDF*), adrenergic, beta-2-, receptor (*ADRB2*), glucocorticoid receptor (*GR*), lipoprotein lipase (*LPL*) and ATPase, Na+/K+ transporting, alpha 2 (+) polypeptide (*ATP1A2*) genes have been associated with weight gain in response to the standardized overfeeding protocol.

NEGATIVE ENERGY BALANCE EXPERIMENTS WITH MZ TWINS

Seven pairs of young adult male identical twins completed a negative energy balance protocol during which they exercised on cycle ergometers twice a day, 9 out of 10 days, over a period of 93 days while being kept on a constant daily energy and nutrient intake (15). The total energy deficit caused by exercise above the estimated energy cost of body weight maintenance reached a mean of 58,095 kcal. Baseline energy intake was estimated over a period of 17 days preceding the negative energy balance protocol. Mean body weight loss was 5.0 kg ($p < 0.001$), and it was entirely accounted for by the loss of fat mass ($p < 0.001$). Fat-free mass was unchanged. Body energy losses reached 45,476 kcal ($p < 0.001$) which represented about 78% of the estimated energy deficit. Subcutaneous fat loss was slightly more pronounced on the trunk than on the limbs as estimated from skinfolds, circumferences and computed tomography. The reduction in abdominal visceral fat was quite striking, from 81 to 52 cm^2 ($p < 0.001$). At the same submaximal power output level, subjects oxidized more lipids than carbohydrates after the program as indicated by the changes in the respiratory exchange ratio ($p < 0.05$) (15).

Figure 3 depicts the changes in body weight and in abdominal visceral fat with the negative energy balance protocol. The intrapair resemblance in response is also illustrated. The F ratio of the between-pairs to the within-pairs variances reached about 6 for the body weight changes and 11 for the changes in visceral fat. Intrapair resemblance was observed for the changes in body weight ($p < 0.05$), fat mass ($p < 0.01$), percent fat ($p < 0.01$), body energy content ($p < 0.01$), sum of 10 skinfolds ($p < 0.01$), abdominal visceral fat ($p < 0.01$), fasting plasma triglycerides ($p < 0.05$) and cholesterol ($p < 0.05$), maximal oxygen uptake ($p < 0.05$), and respiratory exchange ratio during submaximal work ($p < 0.01$) (Fig. 3) (15).

We concluded that even though there were large individual differences in response to the negative energy balance and exercise protocol, subjects with the same genotype were more alike in responses than subjects with different genotypes particularly for body fat, body energy and abdominal visceral fat changes.

These observations were supported by a weight loss experiment performed with 14 pairs of premenopausal female MZ twin pairs who were subjected to 28 days of a very low calorie diet (1.6 MJ/day) in an inpatient metabolic unit (16). Subjects lost on average 8.8 kg (SD = 1.9) with a range from 5.9 to 12.4 kg. Changes in weight were not randomly distributed among the 28 women. There was about

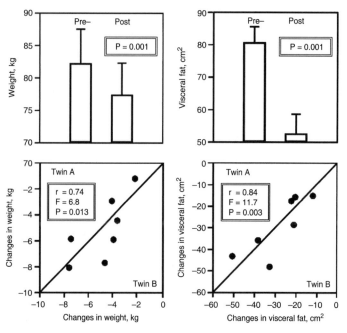

FIGURE 3 Changes in body weight (left panels) and abdominal visceral fat (right panels) in response to a 93-day negative energy balance and exercise protocol. Mean decrease and within-pair resemblance in response are illustrated. *Source*: From Ref. 15.

13 times more variability between pairs than within pairs of MZ twins for the changes in body weight (Fig. 4). The similarity among members of twin pairs of the decreases in fat mass, as assessed from underwater weighing, was even more pronounced with an F ratio of 17. The loss of fat-free mass accounted on average for 24% of the weight loss, a value comparable to other weight loss studies. High intrapair resemblance was also observed for an indicator of overall metabolic efficiency suggesting that the response to therapeutic weight loss regimen may be influenced by genetic variability (17).

OBSERVATIONS ON MZ TWINS DISCORDANT FOR BODY WEIGHT

One strategy that can be helpful in the study of the genetic and environmental conditions under which obesity may develop is based on the comparisons of MZ twin pairs whose members are discordant for weight gain or obesity in comparison to twin pairs who are concordant for the same trait. This design or a variant from it has been used with considerable success in recent years by investigators from Finland who have taken advantage of their well-curated Finnish Twin Registry. Such studies are quite powerful as MZ twins are not only identical for their genes but also for age, sex, ethnicity, and have been exposed to rather similar environmental conditions when they were raised together. However, in the Finnish Twin Registry, the numbers of pairs of MZ twins sufficiently discordant for BMI may be quite low, and therefore difficult to recruit for these studies.

In a first report, it was observed that the obese twins (mean BMI of 30 with SD=2) were not different from their normal weight MZ brothers or sisters (mean BMI of 23 with SD=1) in terms of heart rate, blood pressure or papillary responses to a number of tests (18). In a subsequent report based on 23 pairs of MZ twins discordant for obesity, with an average intrapair weight difference of 18 kg, differences in glucose metabolism and lipoproteins were investigated (19,20). The results indicated that, on a given genotype, excess adiposity and particularly excess visceral fat are associated with atherogenic and diabetogenic profiles. Plasma leptin levels were threefold higher in obese twins compared to their lean brothers or sisters (19).

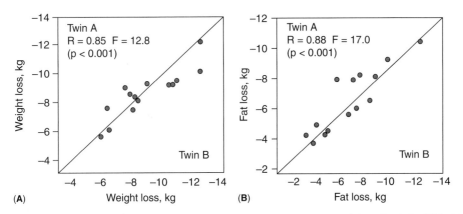

FIGURE 4 Similarity within pairs with respect to decrease in body weight (**A**) and body fat (**B**) in 14 pairs of obese female monozygotic twins in response to 28 days on a very low calorie diet (1.6 MJ/day). Each point represents one pair of twins. *Source*: From Ref. 16.

The lean cotwins were more often smokers (21) while the obese brothers and sisters consumed fatty foods three times more frequently than their lean siblings (22).

In a recent paper, the effects of acquired obesity on intra-abdominal and liver fat were examined in 19 pairs of MZ twins, aged from 24 to 27 years, 10 of which were discordant for BMI (23). The heavier twin had more intra-abdominal fat and liver fat with a higher fasting insulin and a lower insulin sensitivity compared to their lean co-twin (Fig. 5). The data suggested that intra-abdominal fat level is more influenced by acquired obesity independent of the genetic background than is liver fat.

CONCLUSIONS

Some form of biological determinism can make one more susceptible to evolve toward chronic positive or negative energy balance over prolonged periods of time. For a minority of individuals, say the high gainers in our experimental over-feeding studies or the low losers in the two negative energy balance experiments reviewed herein, the genotype seems to contribute importantly to the continuous battle they have to wage in order to maintain body mass within acceptable limits.

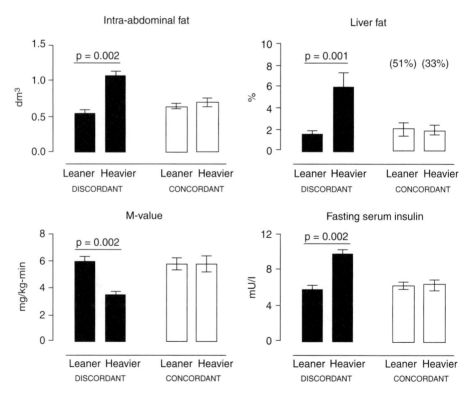

FIGURE 5 Intra-abdominal fat, liver fat, whole-body insulin sensitivity of glucose metabolism (M-value), and fasting serum insulin in leaner and heavier monozygotic twins in 10 pairs discordant for BMI and 9 pairs concordant for BMI. Twins with liver fat contents of 51% and 33% were outliers in concordant pairs. *Source*: From Ref. 23.

It is remarkable to see that such genotypes were observed in the overfeeding studies reported here despite the fact that the MZ twin pairs were not themselves at risk for obesity or obesity-related complications based on their own weight status and their family history. Also of particular importance is the general observation that about 3% of all identical twin pairs are discordant for body weight, with one brother or sister obese and the other in the normal weight range. The full significance of this observation remains to be fully understood.

The studies summarized in this paper and elsewhere demonstrate that individual differences in response to chronic alterations in energy balance are ubiquitous. They are observed for a wide variety of phenotypes including body weight, body fat content, subcutaneous fat, visceral fat, postprandial energy expenditure, resting metabolic rate, adipose tissue metabolism, and insulin, glucagon and thyroid hormone levels. The comparison of the between-pairs and within-pairs heterogeneity reveal that members of the same twin pair (twin brothers) are generally more alike in their response to variation in energy balance than people who are not related by descent. These observations support the notion that genotype–energy balance interaction effects are quite common.

The genes that are responsible for those individual differences in the sensitivity to alterations in energy balance remain to be fully identified. It would not be surprising if these genes turned out to be quite numerous considering the complexity of the biological systems that are involved in body weight homeostasis, nutrient partitioning, energy expenditure, and regulation of energy balance. A variety of genetic and molecular research strategies will be needed to identify these genes and to delineate the nature and the extent of the genetic polymorphisms involved. We believe that it would now be useful to undertake intervention studies with large number of singletons so that the full range of the heterogeneity in response to chronic alterations in energy balance can be documented. Such studies would also provide the opportunity, if the sample sizes were large enough, to investigate the molecular basis of the genotype–energy balance interaction effects.

One also needs to look beyond sequence variation to take full advantage of studies performed with identical twins. Indeed, recent data suggested that epigenetic differences arising during the lifetime of an individual are of particular interest when it comes to accounting for differences to standardized protocols or for discordance in phenotypes between brothers or sisters identical by descent. In an experiment performed on 40 pairs of MZ twins, it was observed that the patterns of epigenetic modifications diverged as they became older (24). Using a combination of whole genome and locus specific methods, it was found that about one-third of MZ pairs harbored epigenetic differences in DNA methylation and histone modification that had an impact on gene expression. These epigenetic events were more pronounced in MZ pairs who were older, had different lifestyles, and had spent less of their lives together, thus emphasizing the key role of environmental factors in fostering a different phenotype on an identical genotype (24).

REFERENCES

1. Sims EA, Goldman RF, Gluck CM et al. Experimental obesity in man. Trans Assoc Am Physicians 1968; 81:153–70.
2. Bouchard C, Pérusse L, Leblanc C. Using MZ twins in experimental research to test for the presence of a genotype-environment interaction effect. Acta Genet Med Gemellol (Roma) 1990; 39:85–9.

3. Eaves LJ. Human behavioural genetics. Proc Roy Soc Med 1976; 69:184–9.
4. Plomin R, DeFries JC, Loehlin JC. Genotype-environment interaction and correlation in the analysis of human behavior. Psychol Bull 1977; 84:309–22.
5. Berdanier CD. Nutrient-gene interactions: today and tomorrow. FASEB J 1994; 8:1.
6. Bouchard C, Tremblay A, Despres JP et al. Sensitivity to overfeeding: the Quebec experiment with identical twins. Prog Food Nutr Sci 1988; 12:45–72.
7. Bouchard C, Tremblay A, Despres JP et al. The response to long-term overfeeding in identical twins. N Engl J Med 1990; 322:1477–82.
8. Deriaz O, Tremblay A, Bouchard C. Non-linear weight gain with long-term over-feeding in man. Obes Res 1993; 1:179–85.
9. Norgan NG, Durnin JV. The effect of 6 weeks of overfeeding on the body weight, body composition, and energy metabolism of young men. Am J Clin Nutr 1980; 33:978–88.
10. Ravussin E, Schutz Y, Acheson KJ et al. Short-term, mixed-diet overfeeding in man: no evidence for "luxuskonsumption". Am J Physiol 1985; 249:E470–7.
11. Forbes GB, Brown MR, Welle SL et al. Deliberate overfeeding in women and men: energy cost and composition of the weight gain. Br J Nutr 1986; 56:1–9.
12. Tremblay A, Despres JP, Thériault G et al. Overfeeding and energy expenditure in humans. Am J Clin Nutr 1992; 56:857–62.
13. Sun G, Ukkola O, Rankinen T et al. Skeletal muscle characteristics predict body fat gain in response to overfeeding in never-obese young men. Metabolism 2002; 51:451–6.
14. Ukkola O, Bouchard C. Role of candidate genes in the responses to long-term over-feeding: review of findings. Obes Rev 2004; 5:3–12.
15. Bouchard C, Tremblay A, Despres JP et al. The response to exercise with constant energy intake in identical twins. Obes Res 1994; 2:400–10.
16. Hainer V, Stunkard AJ, Kunesova M et al. Intrapair resemblance in very low calorie diet-induced weight loss in female obese identical twins. Int J Obes Relat Metab Disord 2000; 24:1051–7.
17. Hainer V, Stunkard A, Kunesova M et al. A twin study of weight loss and metabolic efficiency. Int J Obes Relat Metab Disord 2001; 25:533–7.
18. Piha SJ, Ronnemaa T, Koskenvuo M. Autonomic nervous system function in identical twins discordant for obesity. Int J Obes Relat Metab Disord 1994; 18:547–50.
19. Ronnemaa T, Koskenvuo M, Marniemi J et al. Glucose metabolism in identical twins discordant for obesity. The critical role of visceral fat. J Clin Endocrinol Metab 1997; 82:383–7.
20. Ronnemaa T, Marniemi J, Savolainen MJ et al. Serum lipids, lipoproteins, and lipid metabolizing enzymes in identical twins discordant for obesity. J Clin Endocrinol Metab 1998; 83:2792–9.
21. Hakala P, Rissanen A, Koskenvuo M et al. Environmental factors in the development of obesity in identical twins. Int J Obes Relat Metab Disord 1999; 23:746–53.
22. Rissanen A, Hakala P, Lissner L et al. Acquired preference especially for dietary fat and obesity: a study of weight-discordant monozygotic twin pairs. Int J Obes Relat Metab Disord 2002; 26:973–7.
23. Pietilainen KH, Rissanen A, Kaprio J et al. Acquired obesity is associated with increased liver fat, intra-abdominal fat, and insulin resistance in young adult mono-zygotic twins. Am J Physiol Endocrinol Metab 2005; 288:E768–74.
24. Fraga MF, Ballestar E, Paz MF et al. Epigenetic differences arise during the lifetime of monozygotic twins. Proc Natl Acad Sci U S A 2005; 102:10604–9.

Treva Rice

Division of Biostatistics and Department of Psychiatry, Washington University in St. Louis School of Medicine, St. Louis, Missouri, U.S.A.

Commingling and segregation analyses are statistical methods that explore whether the variation in a trait is caused by a single gene. Prior to the relatively recent era of widely available DNA markers, these methods, which statistically infer the presence of major genes, were considered to be some of the most important genetic analyses and were even used by Mendel to first discover the basic laws of heredity. These methods were most useful when the trait was due primarily to a single (monogenic) segregating diallelic locus. However, when several loci and/or environmental factors impacted on the trait, they were less successful, and this led to a great deal of methodological development in expanding the "Mendelian" model so that multiple determinants (both genetic and environmental) were considered. This was extremely helpful for analyzing "complex traits" like the obesities, which are known to be determined by multiple susceptibility genes whose effects can be modified by a variety of "environmental" factors. In this chapter, we briefly describe the basic methods and models for detecting commingling and segregation and then review the available obesity literature using these models.

METHODS

There is a variety of analytical methods for exploring major gene effects for both quantitative as well as qualitative traits, although here we focus on those for continuous traits that use maximum likelihood methods. Commingling analysis (1) is a screening technique that can provide preliminary evidence of major loci by exploring the distributional properties of a trait within a population or sample. Segregation analysis (2) additionally asks whether the within family transmission is consistent with Mendelian genetic expectations. Many excellent reviews of the commingling and segregation methods are available (e.g. 3–13) so only a brief explanation is provided here. The basic model and assumptions are similar for both segregation and commingling analyses, i.e., a major gene can be parameterized in terms of the distributional properties in the sample.

Basic Model

In a simple diallelic case (alleles "A" and "a" with respective frequencies "p" and "q" in the population), we expect to see up to three distributions corresponding to genotypes AA, Aa and aa, each having a mean (μ_{AA}, μ_{Aa} and μ_{aa}) and standard deviation as shown in Figure 1. Assuming Mendelian principles including Hardy-Weinberg equilibrium, the number of individuals within each of the distributions is p^2 (in the AA distribution), $2pq$ (in Aa) and, q^2 (in aa). The number of component distributions, the proportion of individuals within each component, and the means and variances associated with each component are estimated using

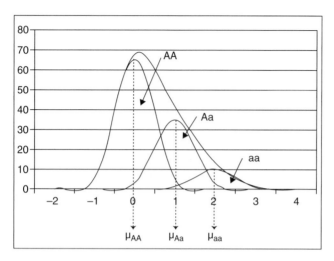

FIGURE 1 For a simple diallelic case (alleles "A" and "a" with corresponding frequencies of "p" and "q"), the frequency distribution of genotypes "AA", "Aa" and "aa" are each normally distributed with means μ_{AA}, μ_{Aa}, μ_{aa} and standard deviations of 1.0. Assuming Hardy-Weinberg equilibrium, the frequency of individuals in each distribution is p^2, 2pq and q^2. In this case, the overall distribution appears as a single skewed distribution.

maximum likelihood methods. Tests among nested models (determining the optimum number of components or the mode of inheritance) are performed using likelihood ratios. For example, a finding that two commingled distributions fits the data better than either one or three distributions is consistent with a recessive mode of inheritance, one distribution representing the combination of AA and Aa individuals and the other for aa individuals.

Commingling Analysis

In commingling analysis the primary emphasis is in determining whether one, two, or three distributions best fit the observed data. Note that the overall distribution in Figure 1 that results from combining the separate distributions can appear to be a single skewed distribution (14). Consequently, in addition to testing for the number of distributions, commingling analysis also allows for tests of whether the distributions are skewed. No assumptions or allowances are made with regard to family membership and the model may be applied to population data, case-control data or any type of family data. Moreover, simulation studies show that when commingling analyses indicate major genes (i.e., multiple distributions), segregation analysis is confirmatory 98% of the time (15).

Segregation Analysis

In segregation analysis the model requires family data structures in order to test Mendelian transmission patterns. In this case, the likelihood for a particular inheritance mode depends on three types of probability distribution functions. First are the probabilities of the genotypes among the founders (the parents), second are the probabilities of the genotypes of the nonfounders or offspring conditional on the parents' genotypes (called transmission probabilities), and finally is the distribution of the phenotype conditional on the genotype (penetrance). The founder probabilities (p and q defined above) are assumed by be drawn independently from the population. The transmission probabilities correspond to the parent-to-child transmission expectations for each genotype, where τ_{AA} is the probability that an individual with the AA genotype transmits allele A to their offspring, τ_{Aa} is the probability that an Aa individual transmits allele A, and τ_{aa} is the probability that aa transmits allele A. Under Mendelian assumptions, these three probabilities are 1, ½ and 0, respectively. The statistical support for a major gene under this model requires three basic tests to be satisfied. First, the hypothesis of no major effect must be rejected (i.e., reject the hypothesis of a single underlying distribution). Second, the hypothesis of Mendelian transmission must not be rejected (i.e., the transmission probabilities should conform to the values of 1, ½ and 0). Third, the hypothesis of no transmission of the major effect (i.e., the three transmission probabilities are equal) must be rejected. Tests on these transmission probabilities are particularly important to safeguard against falsely inferring a major gene when skewed distributions are being analyzed, when there is unaccounted excess sibling resemblance and when the null hypothesis of no major gene is true (16–18).

Model Extensions

Various extensions to the basic model were developed to better capture the variability in complex traits such as the obesities. For example, we generally expect that more than a single underlying genetic defect as well as various "environmental" factors can affect the phenotypic distribution of a given obesity phenotype. The "mixed" or "unified" model of segregation incorporates both a major segregating locus and a residual polygenic (or multifactorial) background (19–21). Other extensions allow for more than one major locus (oligogenic models), for more than two alleles at a given locus, and for the genotype to "interact" with relevant covariates (22–24). The latter effects are referred to as gene-by-environment interactions or genotype-specific effects and typically are modeled as regression coefficients on the genotype-specific means (21,22,24). For the obesities, these genotype-specific effects often depend on age and sex, although other covariates such as diet and exercise levels may be germane. Several concerns with segregation analysis should be noted. First, there is a lack of power for detecting genes with low to moderate effects. In one simulation (25), this problem was found to be more frequent for recessive models (Mendelian transmission was not resolved in 20–70% of cases) than for dominant ones (3–15% of the time). Consequently failure to detect a major gene when one exists is more frequent under recessive models.

Another widely used segregation method is the regressive models for segregation analysis, which is generally equivalent with the mixed model described above (26). The basic mixed and regressive models differ primarily in how the residual familial resemblance (after accounting for the major gene) is expressed. The mixed model of segregation uses a variance components decomposition to partition the trait variance into three primary factors due to a major gene, a residual polygenic (or multifactorial) heritability, and a residual environmental (nonfamilial) effect. Regressive models are somewhat less structured and use a successive conditioning (on ancestral genotypes) method. In practice, after inferring the major gene component, the regressive models express the residual familial resemblance simply as sib-sib, parent-offspring and spouse correlations rather than computing a residual "heritability." Class A regressive models assume that the sib-sib correlation is a function only of common parentage (ancestry), while both the mixed model and class D regressive models allow for additional sources of sib-sib resemblance. The mixed model and class D regressive methods are theoretically and numerically equivalent although different results can emerge using class A regressive models.

Twin studies may also provide evidence consistent with major gene assumptions in two ways. First, commingling analyses are valid for any type of family as well as nonfamily (case–control, population, cross-section, etc.). A finding of multiple distributions is consistent with major gene inferences. Second, provided there is a sufficient twin sample size, maximum likelihood models using structural equation methods may explore nonadditive genetic effects. While polygenic traits are expected to act strictly in an additive manner, major genes may act additively (i.e., Aa distribution mean exactly half-way between those for AA and aa) or nonadditively. Nonadditive (dominance) effects include recessive or dominant modes of transmission where the middle distribution is combined with one of the two extremes. However, nonadditive genetic effects may also be caused by other factors such as the existence of oligogenic or gene-by-gene interaction systems or by masking effects of shared environments (27). Consequently, while nonadditive effects in twin studies are consistent with major genes they are not proof and should be interpreted in light of corroborating evidence from segregation analysis of nuclear family or pedigree data. Conversely, since major genes also may act in a strictly additive fashion, additive only genetic effects in a twin design do not rule out the possibility of major genes.

EVIDENCE CONSISTENT WITH MAJOR GENES FOR OBESITY

Tables 1–3 (28–73) show the results of a Medline search by combining the obesity terms [obesity, adipose, fat, fat distribution or body mass index (BMI)] with method terms (segregation analysis, commingling analysis or major locus, twin studies), among other relevant terms. Table 1 provides results for the BMI, Table 2 for other measures of total fat or body mass components, and Table 3 for fat distribution and abdominal fat measures. In interpreting the relative importance of these studies several caveats should be kept in mind. For example, it is highly likely that the cumulative evidence from the previous literature is skewed toward positive results given the likelihood that negative results (i.e., not finding evidence for a major gene) remain unpublished. Second, from the measured gene studies we already know that there are genes for obesity so what we really want to know is whether and how the results from these inferred gene studies remain pertinent in today's climate of available DNA markers. Consequently, we will primarily review the form that the major gene takes under these inferred methods, in particular if the evidence is consistent with oligogenic and/or mixed models and if the effects of such susceptibility genes are attenuated or accentuated by "environmental" covariates such as age, sex or even dietary or activity levels. When measured gene studies report a causative gene, we can use the results from these segregation analyses to ask how much variance the measured gene accounts for, what are the likely contributory factors and is there is still remaining variance for another gene or genes?

Body Mass Index

Support for major genes for BMI, arise from twin studies where nonadditive effects account for 25% to 50% of the variance (27–28,30–31) and from a variety of designs (twin, adoptee and family) showing multiple commingled distributions (32–33,35–37). The commingling studies typically suggest that about 50% of the

(*Text continues on page 70*)

TABLE 1 Commingling and Segregation Studies for BMI

Reference	Study	Selection	Adjustments	Model	MG %Var	MG q²	MF %Var	Program
Stunkard et al. (28)	Twins reared apart and together			Substantial nonadditive + additive genetic component				
Tambs et al. (29)	Norwegian families		Age/sex	Broad h2 of 40%, mostly due to dominance effect				
Allison et al. (30)	Twins			Nonadditive genetic component				
Maes et al. (31)	Virginia 30,000 twin families 14,763 (5287)	Twins born 1915–1971	Age, sex, twin, status source	Additive (male-fem) Dominance (male-fem)	35–39% 31–26%		66–65%	Stealth and Mx (ACDE)
Jacobson et al. (27)	National Longitudinal Study of Adolescent Health (twins and families)	White M & F Black M & F	Age/sex log Tx 1408 pairs Age/sex log Tx 557 pairs	Additive only Additive only Additive only Additive + nonadditive	0 0 0 50%		80% 80% 73% 35%	Mx (ACDE)
Price and Stunkard (32)	NAS Twin 4071 pairs	Males uni & bivar	Age	Induction 2–3D; 25-yr follow up 2–3D				SKUMIX & BIVAR
Price et al. (33)	Danish adoptees 3577	Random	Age/sex	3D	51%	1%		SKUMIX Inferred %
Price et al. (34) Borecki et al. (35)	LRC QFS Fr Can 1628 (301)	Random ½ Random ½ Obese	Age/sex SES clinic Age/sex generation	2–3D BMI (parents = 3N, offspring = 1S)	14%	4%	34%	SKUMIX POINTER SKUMIX
Price et al. (36)	Pima Indians 2500	Nondiabetic	Age, on or off reservation by sex	3N or 1S distribution, inferred genetic effects	52%	1%		SKUMIX Inferred %

(Continued)

TABLE 1 Commingling and Segregation Studies for BMI (*Continued*)

Reference	Study	Selection	Adjustments	Model	MG %Var	MG q^2	MF %Var	Program
Mitchell et al. (37)	India	Random	Age/sex energy	2N	29%	12%		SKUMIX Inferred % NUCLEAR
Rao et al. (38)	Brazilian			*No MG*				
Province et al. (39)	Tecumseh, Michigan 9226 (3281)	Random	Age/sex, power Tx	Recessive MG	20%	6%	41–20% (O, P)	SKUMIX POINTER
Moll et al. (40)	Muscatine 1586 (284) Iowa families of school children		Age/sex, relative type (race not mentioned)	2D Recessive MG	35%	6%	42%	PAP
Ness et al. (41)	LRC Black 231 (60) White 3925 (961)	Random families	Age/sex, SES clinic, race, power Tx	*Black 2D non-Mendelian recessive* / White 2–3D recessive MG / Combined recessive MG	22% / 14% / 14%	4% / 4% / 4%	50% / 34% / 34%	SKUMIX POINTER
Tiret et al. (42)	Nancy Family Study	Random	Age/sex, GxE model	*Recessive vs. codominant both non-Mendelian, failure due to one family recessive and several families codominant*				PAP
Rice et al. (43)	QFS Fr Can 1628 (301)	½ random, ½ obese	Age/sex	*ME (non-Mendelian)*	<1–40%	<1–4%	42%	POINTER
Borecki et al. (44)	QFS Fr Can 1628 (301)	½ random, ½ obese	Age, polynomial by generation and sex	GxE: MG, aa negative trend w/age, AA = Aa no trend	By age & sex	6%		REGRESS
Price et al. (45)	Pima Indians	By birth cohorts						SKUMIX POINTER

Reference	Population	Sample (N)	Ascertainment	Covariates	Model				Method
Price et al. (46)	LRC	Black 95 (29), White 1206 (403)	Random, within birth cohort	Age/sex, temporal trends; Interactions between early-vs.-late born cohorts and Tx for MG inference	Black recessive MG	35%	7%	53%	SKUMIX POINTER
					White recessive MG	10%	4%	66%	
Hasstedt et al. (47)	Utah	White 446 (42)	T2DM families	Age/sex	Combined recessive MG	12%	4%	66%	PAP
					Recessive MG (extreme)		8%	33% 1L	
					2nd recessive MG (moderate)		18%	0 2L	
					Combined	(68%)			
Borecki et al. (48)	NHLBI FHS	White 2461 (541)	Random	Age, polynomial by sex	Multiple maxima: recessive (d = 0.09); MG vs. ambiguous	44%	9%	24%	POINTER
Ginsburg et al. (49)	5 ethnically distinct populations	Kirghizian 397 (74) age/sex		Age/sex	MG+MF additive 3D	17%	3%	0	MAN regressive model
		Turkmenian 558 (19) age/sex			MG+MF additive 3D	40%	10%	0	
		Chuvashian 516 (135) age/sex			MG-MF additive 3D	40%	56%	0	
		Israeli 672 (165) age/sex			MG-MF recessive 2D	29%	30%	0	
		Mexican 1742 (280) age/sex			MG-MF additive 3D +r(sib)	15%	8%	18%	
Rice et al. (50)	SOS (Swedish) families	Obese probands		Age/sex	GxE (age) co-dominance MG	8–34%	1%	17–24%	SKUMIX PAP
Colilla et al. (51)	Htn in African Americans Black 315(95)	Hyperten proband		Age/sex, SBP, diabetes, smoke, education	Black (codominance) MG	52%	6%		S.A.G.E. REGC
	Nigerian 1159(400)				*Nigerian non-Mendelian ME*	42%	30%		
Feitosa et al. (52)	India 1691 (432)	Random		Age/sex Age/sex/EE/EI	Codominant MG	37%	6%	32%	POINTER
					Non-Mendelian recessive, ME	0.5–21%	<1%	15–81%	

(Continued)

TABLE 1 Commingling and Segregation Studies for BMI (*Continued*)

Reference	Study	Selection	Adjustments	Model	MG %Var	MG q^2	MF %Var	Program
Nath et al. (53)	GenNet FBPP White (261)	Hyperten proband	Age, relative type asct correction on BP of proband	2D recessive MG	43%	40%		S.A.G.E. Class D
Skaric-Juric et al. (54)	Croatia (Island)		Age/sex	MG	39–50%			
Liu et al. (55)	Han Chinese 1190 (392)	Osteoporosis	Age/sex	Codominant ME *(reject Mendelian)*	16%	25%		S.A.G.E. Class D

Abbreviations: 1D–3D, 1 through 3 distributions; 1N–3N, 1 through 3 normal distributions; 1S–3S, 1 through 3 skewed distributions; asct, ascertainment; Bivar, bivariate; BP, blood pressure; Can, Canadian; EE, energy expenditure; EI, energy intake; FBPP, Family Blood Pressure Program; FHS, Family Heart Study; Fr, French; GxE, gene by environment interaction; h2, heritability; Htn, hypertension; Hypertens, hypertensive; LRC, Lipid Research Clinic; ME, major effect; MF, multifactorial effect; NHLBI, National Heart, Lung, and Blood Institute; NAS, National Academy of Sciences; O and P, offspring and parent; q2, genotype frequency in upper distribution; QFS, Quebec Family Study; SAFHS, San Antonio Family Heart Study; Tx, transformation; M & F, male & female; SBP, systolic blood pressure; SES, socioeconomic status. MG, major gene; SOS, Swedish Obese Subjects; T2DM, type 2 diabetes mellitus; Uni, univariate; %Var, percentage of variance due to MG effect;

TABLE 2 Commingling and Segregation Studies for Measures of Overall Adiposity (Primary Weight Partitions)—Percent BF (body fat), FM (fat mass) and FFM (fat-free mass)

Reference	Study	Selection	Adjustments	Model	MG %Var	MG q^2	MF %Var	Program
Borecki et al. (35)	QFS Fr Can 1628 (301)	½ random, ½ obese	Age/sex generation	FM (P=1S, O=1S) FM/FFM (P=2N, O=1S) FM/height (P=1S, O=1S)				SKUMIX
Rice et al. (56)	QFS Fr Can 1628 (301)	½ random, ½ obese	Age/sex generation	FM, recessive MG	45%	9%	22%	POINTER
Comuzzie et al. (57)	SAFHS Hispanics	Random	Age/sex	FM GxE (male–female) MG	37–43%	6%	18–35%	PAP
Lecomte et al. (58)	Stanislas White		Age/sex height GxE (age, sex)	FM GxE, codominant non-Mendelian				REGRESS
Rice et al. (59)	HERITAGE	Sedentary	Age/sex generation	FM codominant MG	64%	6%	0%	POINTER
Rice et al. (60)	HERITAGE (response to exercise training)	Exercise training response	Age/sex	ΔFM dominant MG	31%	49%		POINTER
Borecki et al. (35)	QFS Fr Can 1628 (301)	½ random, ½ obese	Age/sex generation	% BF (parent = 2N, offspring = 1S)				SKUMIX
Rice et al. (56)	QFS Fr Can 1628 (301)	½ random, ½ obese	Age/sex generation	% BF recessive MG	45%	12%	26%	POINTER
Borecki et al. (60)	QFS Fr Can 1628 (301)	½ random, ½ obese	Age/sex generation	FFM (All = 1N)				SKUMIX
Rice et al. (56)	QFS Fr Can 1628 (301)	½ random, ½ obese	Age/sex generation	FFM non-Mendelian (ME)	59%	29%	0	POINTER
Lecomte et al. (58)	Stanislas White		Age/sex height	FFM GxE, recessive non-Mendelian				REGRESS

Note: See Table 1 for abbreviations. Δ denotes change from pre- to postexercise training conditions.

TABLE 3 Commingling and Segregation Studies for Fat Distribution and Abdominal Adipose Measures

Reference	Study	Selection	Adjustments	Model	MG %Var	MG q^2	MF %Var	Program
Bouchard et al. (61)	QFS	½ random ½ obese	Age/sex	AVF recessive MG	51%	10%	21%	POINTER
			Age/sex FM	*AVF-f non-Mendelian*				
Rice et al. (59)	HERITAGE	Sedentary	Age/sex	AVF recessive MG	54%	8%	17%	POINTER
			Age/sex FM	*AVF-f non-Mendelian*	28%	5%	42%	
Rice et al. (60)	HERITAGE (response to exercise training)	Exercise training response	Age/sex	Δ AVF recessive MG	18%	1%		POINTER
			Age/sex FM	Δ AVF-f recessive MG	26%	3%		
Sharma et al. (62)	India	Random	Age/sex	Hip circumference (2N)	19%	2%		SKUMIX
				Waist circumference (1N)	0	0		Inferred %
An et al. (63)	HERITAGE	Sedentary	Age/sex	WHR codominant MG	48%	15%	0	POINTER
			Age/sex SF8	*WHR-f—no major effect*	0%	–	50%	
Feitosa et al. (64)	NHLBI FHS	Random	Age/sex	WHR additive MG	35%	30%	0	POINTER
			Age/sex BMI	*WHR-f additive (or MF)*	34%	36%	0	
Olson et al. (65)	Minnesota Breast Cancer Family Study	Family history of breast cancer	Age BMI education contraception & others (e.g., menopause smoke, etc.)	WHR additive MG among postmenopausal women and families BUT *non-Mendelian among premenopausal families*	42%	7%		S.A.G.E. RegC
Jee et al. (66)	Korean nationwide family study	Random	Age/sex BMI alcohol smoke exercise	Waist dominant MG *hip non-Mendelian WHR non-Mendelian*	22%	58%		S.A.G.E. RegD
Rice et al. (67)	QFS Fr Can	½ random ½ obese	Age/sex FM	TER-f	39%	15%		SKUMIX Inferred %
Mitchell et al. (37)	India	Random	Age/sex EE EI	TER-e (2N)	39%	14%		SKUMIX Inferred %
Borecki et al. (68)	QFS Fr Can	½ random ½ obese	Age/sex FM	TER-f recessive MG	37%	12%	29%	POINTER Inferred %
Feitosa et al. (69)	India	Random	Age/sex	TER recessive MG	34%	13%	25%	POINTER
			Age/sex EE EI	TER-e recessive MG	38%	13%	21%	skew
			Age/sex SF6	TER-f recessive non-Mendelian	35–51%	2%	61–17%	Tx remove ME

Reference	Cohort	Design	Adjustment	Model	%	%	%	Method
An et al. (63)	HERITAGE	Sedentary	Age/sex	TER codominant MG	54%	10%	17%	POINTER
				TER-f codominant MG	56%	10%	18%	Inferred %
Rice et al. (67)	QFS Fr Can	½ random, ½ obese	Age/sex SF8	SF6-f 2D	27%	5%		SKUMIX; Inferred %
Mitchell et al. (37)	India	Random	Age/sex EE EI	SF6 (2S)	42%	81%		POINTER; Inferred %
Borecki et al. (68)	QFS Fr Can	½ random, ½ obese	Age/sex FM	SF6 recessive MG or equal taus	34%	6%	36%	POINTER
An et al. (63)	HERITAGE	Sedentary	Age/sex	SF8 recessive (equal taus)	47%	16%	30%	POINTER; Inferred %
Sharma et al. (62)	India	Random	Age/sex	Biceps (3S)	67%	6%		SKUMIX; Inferred %
				triceps (1N)	0	0		
Rice et al. (67)	QFS Fr Can	½ random, ½ obese	Age/sex FM	TSF3-f 3D	53%	1%		SKUMIX; Inferred %
Mitchell et al. (37)	India	Random	Age/sex EE EI	TSF3-e (3S)	59%	74%		SKUMIX; Inferred %
Borecki et al. (68)	QFS Fr Can	½ random, ½ obese	Age/sex FM	TSF3-f recessive MG or equal taus	28%	2%	44%	POINTER
Hasstedt et al. (70)	Utah pedigrees	Htn and CHD pedigrees	Age/sex	RFPI recessive MG	42%	22%	10%	PAP
Rice et al. (67)	QFS Fr Can	½ random, ½ obese	Age/sex FM	RFPI-f male	60%	73%		SKUMIX; Inferred %
				RFPI-f female	30%	88%		
Mitchell et al. (37)	India	Random	Age/sex energy	RFPI (2N)	9%	2%		SKUMIX; Inferred %
Allison et al. (71)	NHANES II	Multiracial	Age/sex Box-Cox Tx to remove skewness	BMI, subcutaneous/triceps skinfold				KMM (commingling)
Borecki et al. (72)	QFS Fr Can	½ random, ½ obese	Age/sex	BMI and fat mass	64%			PAP
				2 recessive pleiotropic loci	47%			
				Covariance 2 recessive loci	73%		8%	
Cheng et al. (73)	Israeli	Random	Age/sex and gene age	SBP and BMI, pleiotropic codominant locus	8%	6%		PAP

Abbreviations: (See also *Tables 1 and 2*): AVF, abdominal visceral fat; AVF-f, AVF with additional adjustment for total fat; ΔAVF change in pre- to postexercise training; BMI, body mass index; CHD, coronary heart disease. RFPI, relative fat pattern index from skinfolds = subscapular/(subscapular + suprailiac); RFPI-f, RFPI additionally adjusted for total fat; SF6, sum of 6 skinfolds; SF6-f, SF6 with additional adjustment for total fat; SF8, sum of eight skinfolds; TER, trunk-to-extremity skinfold ratio; TER-e, TER with additional adjustment for energy measures; TER-f, TER with additional adjustment for total fat; TSF3, sum of three trunk skinfolds; TSF3-e, TSF3 with additional adjustment for energy measures; TSF3-f, TSF3 with additional adjustment for total fat; WHR, waist-to-hip ratio; WHR-f, WHR with additional adjustment for total fat.

BMI variance in the sample can be accounted for by two to three admixed distributions. While these studies provide evidence that is consistent with that expected if BMI is influenced by one or more major genes, the results could also be due to other factors such as oligogenic effects, gene–gene interactions and major environmental factors. Segregation analysis provides more direct evidence that is consistent with major gene hypotheses since the transmission patterns between parents and offspring are also tested for Mendelian patterns.

The primary results for BMI using segregation analysis fit one of two patterns, either a recessive or codominant major gene. The recessive hypothesis was found in a variety of studies and the percentage of variance that was due to this putative recessive locus was variable. For example, a recessive locus accounted for nearly 45% of the variance in a random sample of Caucasian families from the Family Heart study (48) and families of hypertensive probands in GenNet (53). However, the percentage of individuals in the upper distribution (presumably overweight to obese having the recessive "aa" genotype) was lower in the randomly selected families (9%) than in the hypertensive (40%) families. Since there is a positive and significant correlation between obesity and blood pressure (BP), the higher allele frequency in the hypertensive families may indicate that this putative BMI locus is pleiotropic with or closely linked to a gene for hypertension. At least one study has explicitly tested this pleiotropic BMI-BP hypothesis (73) in a random sample of Israeli families. Systolic blood pressure was the primary analysis target and BMI was a significant covariate. Subsequent bivariate segregation analysis suggested that a single pleiotropic locus accounted for the covariance between the traits, with no residual genetic correlation due to other factors such as polygenic or familial environmental. About 6% of the sample was in the upper distribution, and the variance attributed to the pleiotropic locus increased with age for BP and decreased with age for BMI. Several other randomly ascertained family samples (African Americans and Caucasians) provided evidence consistent with a major effect gene having similar characteristics that accounted for somewhat less variance (12–35%) but with 4% to 7% of the individuals in the upper distribution (39–41,46). Most of these studies that used the mixed model also reported that another 30% to 50% of the variance was due to a multifactorial (polygenic and/or familial environmental) factors.

A second genetic pattern commonly reported in the literature involves a codominant or additive major gene effect for BMI (49–52,55). These studies varied greatly in terms of sample selection (random, obese, hypertensive) and ethnicity (Kirghizian, Turkmenian, Chuvashian, Mexican, Swedish, Nigerian, Eastern Indian and Han Chinese). The characteristics of this codominant or additive locus were also quite variable, accounting for between 15% to over 50% of the variance and with the frequency of individuals in the upper distribution being quite variable as well (from <1% to over 56%). So, the combined evidence across all of these BMI studies is consistent with the hypothesis of at least two major genes for BMI and a few studies have explicitly investigated this issue. For example, in both a random sample of French families (42) and in a random sample of U.S. Caucasians (72) numerical convergence led to two different solutions in each study, one for a recessive and another for a codominant major effect. In two other studies using bivariate segregation methods, two loci also were reported; one for extreme and another for moderate levels of obesity (47,48). In each study the pair of genes acted in a recessive manner with the combined two-locus model accounting for about 70% of the variance in BMI levels. Interestingly, when only a single locus was considered there were both major and multifactorial effects (the mixed model), but when the second locus was sequentially introduced the multifactorial effect disappeared (47).

Additional findings from these studies relate to the interacting effects of specific covariates. For example, in the Quebec Family Study there was a major effect having an ambiguous transmission pattern that accounted for more variance in offspring than parents (43). Mendelian transmission was not clearly supported until genotype-specific effects of age were included in the model (44), and consistent with the earlier study the variance due to the major gene decreased as a function of age. Other studies suggesting age-specific genotype and/or birth cohort trends include findings from the Swedish Obese Subjects study (50) and in obese Pima Indians (45). In summary, these findings for the BMI suggest that there are multiple genes (i.e., oligogenic) some acting in a recessive manner and others in a codominant or additive manner, some influencing extreme obesity while others influence moderate levels of overweight, and that age is an important player in determining not only the magnitude of effect but also whether there is an effect at all.

TOTAL FAT

While the BMI is a widely used measure of total adiposity or obesity, more specific measures of total body composition are available such as fat mass, percent body fat and fat-free mass using various methods such as underwater weighing or bioimpedence. While these measures are considered more valid than the BMI in terms of indexing total body composition, studies of these specific measures are under-represented in the literature, presumably because they are harder and/or more expensive to measure reported (all details regarding phenotype issues are provided in Chapter 1.1). For fat mass, both recessive and codominant modes of transmission have been reported. A recessive Mendelian hypothesis was supported in the Quebec Family Study (56) and in the San Antonio Family Heart Study (57), and the effect of this gene depended on age in the latter sample. In both cases the major effect accounted for over 40% of the variance with 6% to 9% of the sample in the upper (obese) distribution. These characteristics are remarkably similar to those for the recessive BMI gene reported earlier. However, in a specific test of whether the two genes are the same, a bivariate study suggested two recessive pleiotropic loci, each having effects on both BMI and fat mass (48). In two other studies (58,59), a codominant major gene was reported that accounted for somewhat more variance (nearly 65%) with about 6% of the sample in the upper distribution. For percent body fat, a recessive locus was reported in the Quebec Family Study that accounted for 45% of the variance (35,56). Finally, for fat-free mass, the evidence is consistent across studies for a single component that accounts for about 60% of the variance (35,56,58). However, whether the component is a major non-Mendelian factor or is multifactorial is not clear. In summary, the limited results for fat mass and percent body fat are consistent in suggesting the presence of at least two major genes with effects that are remarkably similar to those reported for the BMI. However, explicit tests suggest that different genes may be involved in determining the different phenotypes.

Fat Distribution

Fat distribution measures are important phenotypes since the abdominal obesity is implicated as an important risk factor for cardiovascular disease and diabetes.

Whether the pertinent abdominal component is in the visceral or subcutaneous compartments is also under discussion although the visceral component is more often linked to some diseases, in particular diabetes (see Chapter 1.1). Only two studies were found that reported segregation analyses for specific measures of abdominal visceral fat measured with computed tomography scan (59,61). Both found a major recessive gene that accounted for about 50% of the variance in abdominal visceral fat, with 8% to 10% of the sample in the upper distribution. An additional ~20% of the variance was due to multifactorial effects. Again, this major gene characteristic is reminiscent of the recessive locus commonly reported for BMI and/or fat mass. This possibility has not been ruled out since analyses of the residual abdominal visceral component after adjusting for the amount of total fat led to dissipation of the major gene evidence. However, an explicit test of this hypothesis using bivariate segregation methods was not found in the literature. Together, these results suggest that there is at least one putative recessive gene that may be pleiotropic with respect to total fat and fat deposition to the abdominal visceral component.

More common measures of abdominal fat include the waist circumference and waist-to-hip ratio, although these measures do not separate the specific visceral (deep) from subcutaneous (surface) fat components (details regarding fat repartition phenotypes are provided in Chapter 1.1). In contrast to the finding of a recessive gene for abdominal visceral fat reported above, the circumference measures typically exhibit an additive or codominant mode of transmission (63–66). Adjusting for the amount of total adiposity obliterated the major effect in one study of sedentary U.S. Caucasians (63) had little effect in the random subsample of the Family Heart Study (64), and in randomly selected Korean families the major gene was apparent only after preadjusting for total adiposity (66). In another study of U.S. women and their families (65), the additive major gene was found only among post-menopausal (but not premenopausal) women and their families. These findings are again consistent with more than one major gene for abdominal fat, one being recessive in nature and perhaps pleiotropic with respect to both total body fat and the abdominal visceral component, and the other gene being codominant in nature. It is not clear whether the second gene is specific to subcutaneous abdominal fat or to overall visceral plus subcutaneous abdominal fat. More work remains to be explored in this area, for example in assessing how age, hormone and overall adiposity levels interact with fat deposition patterns specifically for each of the visceral from subcutaneous compartments.

Other reported segregation studies use skinfold measures which specifically capture the subcutaneous compartment. Some index abdominal subcutaneous fat, for example trunk-to-extremity skinfold ratio (TER) and relative fat pattern index (RFPI). Others index absolute amounts of total overall (SF) and total truncal (TSF) subcutaneous fat. The trunk-to-extremity skinfold ratio has been analyzed both before and after adjusting for specific covariates including total fat (TER-f) and energy intake and expenditure measures (TER-e). The adjustment scheme has remarkably little effect on the characteristics of the major gene for trunk-to-extremity skinfold ratio. A recessive locus was reported in two studies (25,69) and a codominant locus in another (63). The recessive locus accounted for 35% to 38% of the variance with over 10% of the sample in the upper distribution, while the codominant locus accounted for over 50% of the locus with about 10% of the sample in the upper distribution. For the RFPI [subscapular/(subscapular + suprailiac)] one study reported a recessively segregating locus accounting for 42%

of the variance with 22% of the sample in the upper distribution (70). However, a commingling analysis in another sample was consistent with a major effect accounting for 30% to 60% of the variance (males–females) with well over 70% of the sample in the upper distribution (67). This latter finding suggests that the rarer allele is for low (rather than high) values. For the sum of several skinfolds (total and truncal) the results were somewhat ambiguous. In two studies (63,68) there was a major effect that accounted for about 40% of the variance but it was unclear whether the effect was Mendelian or not. In general, the skinfold studies are inconclusive primarily because there is little overlap across studies in terms of the exact skinfold sites that are measured. Consequently, there is little ability to make cross-study comparisons for generalizing the results.

CONCLUSION

These combined results are consistent with our expectation that the obesities are influenced by oligogenic and polygenic systems whose effects are mediated by various other factors. Some genes appear to act in a recessive manner while others are codominant or additive. Moreover, some genes are specific to given obesity traits while others appear to be pleiotropic across traits particularly with regard to measures of total fat versus fat distribution and total fat versus BP. An integrated approach (e.g., 74) will be required to take into account the constellation of factors that impact on the gene expression such as age, hormone levels, habitual activity levels and nutrition (to name a few). These factors are likely to be quite important in determining the direction and level of effect for given susceptibility genes and should be used in interpreting the results from analyses of measured genes and in designing future studies. For example, do the linkage studies account for the complete variance as suggested by segregation analysis? If not, the linkage analysis may need to continue to look for additional (oligogenic) loci in order to fully explain the genetic variance. Is the linkage signal more likely to be detected if certain genotype-specific effects are allowed in the model? And, are some genes more likely to be detected using bivariate methods, particularly pleiotropic genes in samples with low power (i.e., smaller samples). Commingling and segregation studies continue to provide insights both in terms of their past and potential future contributions in discovering the genes for the obesities.

REFERENCES

1. MacLean CJ, Morton NE, Elston RC et al. Skewness in commingled distributions. Biometrics 1976; 32:695–9.
2. Elston RC, Stewart J. A general model for the genetic analysis of pedigree data. Hum Hered 1971; 21:523–42.
3. Morton NE, Yee S, Lew R. Complex segregation analysis. Am J Hum Genet 1971; 23(6):602–11.
4. Elandt-Johnson RC. Complex segregation analysis. II. Multiple classification. Am J Hum Genet 1971; 23(1):17–32.
5. Rao DC, Elandt-Johnson RC. Complex segregation analysis. Am J Hum Genet 1971; 23(3):325–6.
6. Boyle CR, Elston RC. Multifactorial genetic models for quantitative traits in humans. Biometrics 1979; 35:55–68.
7. Zhao LP. Segregation analysis of human pedigrees using estimating equations. Biometrika 1994; 81:197–209.

8. Elston RC. Segregation ratios. In: Armitage P, Colton T, eds. Encyclopedia of Biostatistics. Vol. 5. New York: Wiley & Sons, 1998:4044–5.

9. Blangero J. Complex segregation analysis. In: Armitage P, Colton T, eds. Encyclopedia of Biostatistics. Vol. 5. New York: Wiley & Sons, 1998:4032–44.

10. Jarvik GP. Complex segregation analyses: uses and limitations. Am J Hum Genet 1998; 63:942–6.

11. Majumder PP. Classical segregation analysis. In: Armitage P, Colton T, eds. Encyclopedia of Biostatistics. Vol. 5. New York: Wiley & Sons, 1998:4029–32.

12. Mendell NR, Finch SJ. Commingling analysis. In: Armitage P, Colton T, eds. Encyclopedia of Biostatistics. Vol. 5. New York: Wiley & Sons, 1998:789–91.

13. Elston RC. Introduction and overview: statistical methods in genetic epidemiology. Stat Methods Med Res 2000; 9:527–41.

14. Chakraborty R, Hanis CL. Nonrandom sampling in human genetics: skewness and kurtosis. Genet Epidemiol 1987; 4(2):87–101.

15. Kwon JM, Boehnke M, Burns TL et al. Commingling and segregation analyses: comparison of results from a simulation study of a quantitative trait. Genet Epidemiol 1990; 7(1):57–68.

16. Demenais FM, Lathrop M, Lalouel JM. Robustness and power of the unified model in the analysis of quantitative measurements. Am J Hum Genet 1986; 38:228–34.

17. Demenais FM, Murigande C, Bonney GE. Search for faster methods of fitting the regressive models to quantitative traits. Genet Epidemiol 1990; 7:319–34.

18. Demenais F, Martinez M, Andrieu N. The transmission probability model is useful to prevent false inference. Am J Hum Genet 1993; 52:441–2.

19. Morton NE, MacLean CJ. Analysis of family resemblance. III. Complex segregation of quantitative traits. Am J Hum Genet 1974; 26:489–503.

20. Lalouel JM, Rao DC, Morton NE et al. A unified model for complex segregation analysis. Am J Hum Genet 1983; 35:816–26.

21. Bonney GE, Lathrop GM, Lalouel J-M. Combined linkage and segregation analysis using regressive models. Am J Hum Genet 1988; 43:29–37.

22. Konigsberg LW, Blangero J, Kammerer CM et al. Mixed model segregation analysis of LDL-c concentration with genotype-covariate interaction. Genet Epidemiol 1991; 8:69–80.

23. Blangero J, Konigsberg LW. Multivariate segregation analysis using the mixed model. Genet Epidemiol 1991; 8:299–316.

24. Blangero J. Statistical genetic approaches to human adaptability. Hum Biol 1993; 65:941–66.

25. Borecki IB, Province MA, Rao DC. Inferring a major gene for quantitative traits by using segregation analysis with tests on transmission probabilities: how often do we miss? Am J Hum Genet 1995; 56:319–26.

26. Demenais FM, Bonney GE. Equivalence of the mixed and regressive models for genetic analysis. I. Continuous traits. Genet Epidemiol 1989; 6:597–617.

27. Jacobson KC, Rowe DC. Genetic and shared environmental influences on adolescent BMI: interactions with race and sex. Behav Genet 1998; 28:265–78.

28. Stunkard AJ, Harris JR, Pedersen NL et al. The body-mass index of twins who have been reared apart. N Engl J Med 1990; 322:1483–7.

29. Tambs K, Mourn T, Eaves L et al. Genetic and environmental contributions to the variance of the body mass index in a Norwegian sample of first- and second-degree relatives. Am J Human Biol 1991; 3:257–67.

30. Allison DB, Heshka S, Neale MC et al. Race effects in the genetics of adolescents' body mass index. Int J Obes 1994; 18:363–8.

31. Maes HHM, Neale MC, Eaves LJ. Genetic and environmental factors in relative body weight and human adiposity. Behav Genet 1997; 27(4):325–51.

32. Price RA, Stunkard AJ. Commingling analysis of obesity in twins. Hum Hered 1989; 39(3):121–35.

33. Price RA, Stunkard AJ, Sørensen TIA et al. Component distributions of body mass index defining moderate and extreme overweight in Danish women and men. Am J Epidemiol 1989; 130:193–201.

34. Price RA, Ness R, Laskarzewski P. Common major gene inheritance of extreme overweight. Hum Biol 1990; 62(6):747–65.
35. Borecki IB, Rice T, Bouchard C et al. Commingling analysis of generalized body mass and composition measures: the Quebec Family Study. Int J Obes 1991; 15(11):763–73.
36. Price RA, Lunetta K, Ness R et al. Obesity in Pima Indians. Distribution characteristics and possible thresholds for genetic studies. Int J Obes 1992; 16(11):851–7.
37. Mitchell LE, Nirmala A, Rice T et al. Commingling analysis of adiposity in an Indian population. Int J Obes 1994; 18(1):1–8.
38. Rao DC, MacLean CJ, Morton NE et al. Analysis of family resemblance. V. Height and weight in northeastern Brazil. Am J Hum Genet 1975; 27:509–20.
39. Province MA, Arnqvist P, Keller J et al. Strong evidence for a major gene for obesity in the large, unselected, total Community Health Study of Tecumseh. Am J Hum Genet 1990; 47(Suppl.):A143.
40. Moll PP, Burns TL, Lauer RM. The genetic and environmental sources of body mass index variability: the Muscatine Ponderosity Family Study. Am J Hum Genet 1991; 49(6):1243–55.
41. Ness R, Laskarzewski P, Price RA. Inheritance of extreme overweight in black families. Hum Biol 1991; 63(1):39–52.
42. Tiret L, Andre JL, Ducimetiere P et al. Segregation analysis of height-adjusted weight with generation- and age-dependent effects: the Nancy Family Study. Genet Epidemiol 1992; 9(6):389–403.
43. Rice T, Borecki IB, Bouchard C et al. Segregation analysis of body mass index in an unselected French-Canadian samples: the Quebec Family Study. Obes Res 1993; 1(4):288–94.
44. Borecki IB, Bonney GE, Rice T et al. Influence of genotype-dependent effects of covariates on the outcome of segregation analysis of the body mass index. Am J Hum Genet 1993; 53(3):676–87.
45. Price RA, Charles MA, Pettitt DJ et al. Obesity in Pima Indians: genetic segregation analysis of body mass index complicated by temporal increases in obesity. Hum Biol 1994; 66(2):251–74.
46. Price RA. Within birth cohort segregation analyses support recessive inheritance of body mass index in white and African-American families. Int J Obes 1996; 20(11):1044–7.
47. Hasstedt SJ, Hoffman M, Leppert MF et al. Recessive inheritance of obesity in familial non-insulin-dependent diabetes mellitus, and lack of linkage to nine candidate genes. Am J Hum Genet 1997; 61(3):668–77.
48. Borecki IB, Higgins M, Schreiner PJ et al. Evidence for multiple determinants of the body mass index: the National Heart, Lung, and Blood Institute Family Heart Study. Obes Res 1998; 6(2):107–14.
49. Ginsburg E, Livshits G, Yakovenko K et al. Major gene control of human body height, weight and BMI in five ethnically different populations. Ann Hum Genet 1998; 62(Pt 4):307–22.
50. Rice T, Sjostrom CD, Perusse L et al. Segregation analysis of body mass index in a large sample selected for obesity: the Swedish Obese Subjects study. Obes Res 1999; 7(3):246–55.
51. Colilla S, Rotimi C, Cooper R et al. Genetic inheritance of body mass index in African-American and African families. Genet Epidemiol 2000; 18(4):360–76.
52. Feitosa MF, Rice T, Nirmala A et al. Major gene effect on body mass index: the role of energy intake and energy expenditure. Hum Biol 2000; 72(5):781–99.
53. Nath SK, Chakravarti A, Chen CH et al. Segregation analysis of blood pressure and body mass index in a rural US community. Hum Biol 2002; 74(1):11–23.
54. Skaric-Juric T, Ginsburg E, Kobyliansky E et al. Complex segregation analysis of body height, weight and BMI in pedigree data from Middle Dalmatia, Croatia. Colleg Antro 2003; 27(1):135–49.
55. Liu PY, Li YM, Li MX et al. Lack of evidence for a major gene in the Mendelian transmission of BMI in Chinese. Obes Res 2004; 12(12):1967–73.

56. Rice T, Borecki IB, Bouchard C et al. Segregation analysis of fat mass and other body composition measures derived from underwater weighing. Am J Hum Genet 1993; 52(5):967–73.

57. Comuzzie AG, Blangero J, Mahaney MC et al. Major gene with sex-specific effects influences fat mass in Mexican Americans. Genet Epidemiol 1995; 12(5):475–88.

58. Lecomte E, Herbeth B, Nicaud V et al. Segregation analysis of fat mass and fat-free mass with age- and sex-dependent effects: the Stanislas Family Study. Genet Epidemiol 1997; 14(1):51–62.

59. Rice T, Despres JP, Perusse L et al. Segregation analysis of abdominal visceral fat: the HERITAGE Family Study. Obes Res 1997; 5(5):417–24.

60. Rice T, Hong Y, Perusse L et al. Total body fat and abdominal visceral fat response to exercise training in the HERITAGE Family Study: evidence for major locus but no multifactorial effects. Metabolism 1999; 48(10):1278–86.

61. Bouchard C, Rice T, Lemieux S et al. Major gene for abdominal visceral fat area in the Quebec Family Study. Int J Obes 1996; 20(5):420–7.

62. Sharma K, Byard PJ, Rao DC. Commingling in the distributions of fat-related measures in Punjabi families. Hum Hered 1984; 34(5):278–84.

63. An P, Rice T, Borecki IB et al. Major gene effect on subcutaneous at distribution in a sedentary population and its response to exercise training: the HERITAGE Family Study. Am J Hum Biol 2000; 12:600–9.

64. Feitosa MF, Borecki I, Hunt SC et al. Inheritance of the waist-to-hip ratio in the National Heart, Lung, and Blood Institute Family Heart Study. Obes Res 2000; 8(4):294–301.

65. Olson JE, Atwood LD, Grabrick DM et al. Evidence for a major gene influence on abdominal fat distribution: the Minnesota Breast Cancer Family Study. Genet Epidemiol 2001; 20(4):458–78.

66. Jee SH, Kim MT, Lee SY et al. Segregation analysis of waist circumference, hip circumference and waist-to-hip ratio in the Korean Nationwide Family Study. Int J Obes 2002; 26(2):228–33.

67. Rice T, Borecki IB, Bouchard C et al. Commingling analysis of regional fat distribution measures: the Quebec Family Study. Int J Obes 1992; 16(10):831–44.

68. Borecki IB, Rice T, Perusse L et al. Major gene influence on the propensity to store fat in trunk versus extremity depots: evidence from the Quebec Family Study. Obes Res 1995; 3(1):1–8.

69. Feitosa MF, Rice T, Nirmala-Reddy A et al. Segregation analysis of regional fat distribution in families from Andhra Pradesh, India. Int J Obes 1999; 23(8):874–80.

70. Hasstedt SJ, Ramirez ME, Kuida H et al. Recessive inheritance of a relative fat pattern. Am J Hum Genet 1989; 45:917–25.

71. Allison DB, Heshka S, Heymsfield SB. Evidence of a major gene with pleiotropic action for a cardiovascular disease risk syndrome in children younger than 14 years. Am J Diseases Child 1993; 147(12):1298–302.

72. Borecki IB, Blangero J, Rice T et al. Evidence for at least two major loci influencing human fatness. Am J Hum Genet 1998; 63(3):831–8.

73. Cheng LS, Livshits G, Carmelli D et al. Segregation analysis reveals a major gene effect controlling systolic blood pressure and BMI in an Israeli population. Hum Biol 1998; 70(1):59–75.

74. Clement K. Genetics of human obesity. Proc Nutr Soc 2005; 64:133–42.

3.1 Natural Monogenic Models

Allison W. Xu
Diabetes Center and Department of Anatomy, University of California, San Francisco, San Francisco, California, U.S.A.

Andrew A. Butler
Pennington Biomedical Research Center, Louisiana State University System, Baton Rouge, Louisiana, U.S.A.

Gregory S. Barsh
Department of Genetics, Stanford University School of Medicine, Stanford, California, U.S.A.

Over the past decade, significant breakthroughs have been made in identifying genes critical in regulating energy balance and obesity, and most of these advances have relied upon the utilization of both forward and reverse genetics in mice. Forward genetics goes from phenotype to genotype by means of positional cloning and candidate gene analyses, and this approach has led to the cloning of leptin and leptin receptor genes. Conversely, reverse genetics goes from genotype to phenotype by means of gene targeting, transgenic manipulation of gene expression, or expression knockdown by RNA interference. Reverse genetics in rodents has revealed the critical role the central melanocortin system plays in energy homeostasis and its function in obesity development. To date, mutations in the central melanocortin pathways constitute the most prevalent forms of monogenic obesity seen in rodents and humans.

The central melanocortin pathway consists of neurons that express proopiomelanocortin (POMC), Agouti-related peptide (AgRP), melanocortin 3 receptor (MC3R) and melanocortin 4 receptor (MC4R) (Fig. 1). POMC neurons secrete the neuropeptide alpha-melanocyte stimulating hormone (α-MSH), which serves as the ligand for MC3R and MC4R. On the other hand, a counter regulatory system exists which is based on the AgRP and neuropeptide Y (NPY) neurons. AgRP is released by neurons, and acts as an antagonist and inverse agonist for MC3R and MC4R.

POMP and AgRP neurons are located in the arcuate nucleus of the hypothalamus, which is in close approximation to the median eminence, a circumventricular organ that is considered "outside" the blood-brain barrier. Consequently, the POMC and AgRP neurons are uniquely positioned to sample blood-borne hormones such as leptin. Leptin receptors are expressed in both the POMC and AgRP neurons and they are considered key target neurons of leptin regulation. Loss of function of leptin, leptin receptor, POMC or MC4R gene results in the most profound obesity caused by mutation of a single gene. Thus, the leptin (LEP) $\rightarrow$ leptin receptor (LEPR) $\rightarrow$ POMC, AgRP neurons $\rightarrow$ MC3R, MC4R pathway represents one of the most important neuronal circuits in body weight regulation. There are five classical murine model of obesity that result from spontaneous mutations, and whose effects on body weight appear to involve abnormal CNS control of energy balance.

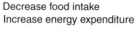

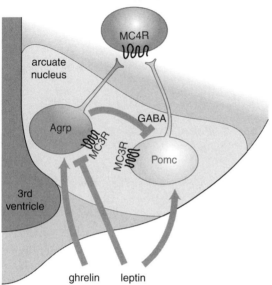

FIGURE 1 Central melanocortin system and its integration with peripheral hormones. Central melanocortin system consists in POMC and AgRP expressing neurons and neurons expressing their receptors MC3R and MC4R in the hypothalamus. POMC neurons also express CART, another anorectic peptide that is not represented here. α-MSH secreted from the POMC/CART neurons activates MC4R to promote negative energy balance, while AgRP inhibits MC4R to promote positive energy balance. These two pathways act reciprocally to increase and decrease food intake, respectively, and to transduce outflow signals regulating body fat stores. POMC neurons also receive inhibitory GABAergic input from AgRP neurons. POMC and AgRP neurons are regulated by adiposity signals such as leptin and insulin in an opposite manner, while AgRP neurons are stimulated by the gut-derived hormone ghrelin. Thus, the central melanocortin system senses and integrates peripheral hormonal signals to control energy homeostasis.

OB/OB MICE AND LEPTIN

In 1950, mice carrying the *obese* (ob/ob) mutation were first reported by Ingalls at the Jackson Laboratory (1). It was a spontaneous mutation that arose from the C57BL/6J strain. ob/ob mice develop obesity from 4 weeks of age, and their body weight eventually reaches approximately three times the normal weight of wild-type controls. ob/ob mice exhibit hyperphagia, reduced energy expenditure, hyperinsulinemia and impaired glucose tolerance.

In 1953, Kennedy hypothesized that circulating signals produced by, or in proportion to, adipose tissue mass act within the brain to reduce food intake (2).

In 1973, Coleman from the Jackson Laboratory reported the classical para-biosis experiment, in which the vascular systems of ob/ob mice and normal mice were surgically joined together and the ob/ob mice lost weight as a result (3). Coleman predicted that the *obese* gene product was a circulating factor. Not until two decades later, in 1994, was the *obese* gene positionally cloned by Zhang et al., confirming it was indeed a circulating hormone (4). Lep^{ob}/Lep^{ob} mice carry a C→T mutation at position 105, converting an arginine residue to a premature stop codon in the leptin gene, and resulting in a truncated and nonfunctional protein (4).

The 16 kDa hormone, termed leptin, is undetectable in the ob/ob mice. Leptin administration completely normalizes the obesity phenotype of ob/ob mice and also leads to anorexia and body weight loss in normal mice (5–8).

Leptin is secreted mainly from adipocytes. Circulating leptin levels generally correlate with the amount of white adipose tissue. Leptin levels fall during fasting and are normalized upon refeeding (9). In most forms of obesity including diet-induced obesity, leptin levels are high, a condition called hyperleptinemia; and leptin is less effective in causing anorexia and body weight loss. This condition is termed "leptin resistance." The gut may also be an important source of leptin (10), where leptin secreted by cells in the gastric mucosa possibly behaves as a "satiety" signal acting on vagal afferents after ingestion of a meal (10,11).

Leptin crosses the blood brain barrier by a saturable mechanism (12) and acts on neurons in the hypothalamus that express their receptors. Central melano-cortinergic POMC and AgRP neurons are two of the most important "first-order" neurons that are regulated by leptin.

Leptin fulfills the following criteria as being an adiposity signal: it circulates in proportion to body fat mass, it induces negative energy balance, and its mutation leads to obesity. Another hormone that fulfills these criteria is insulin, although the obesity phenotype caused by brain insulin receptor knockout is relatively mild (13). In addition to leptin's role in regulating energy homeostasis, recent studies suggest additional biological functions. Leptin acts as a neuro-trophic factor to control development of the hypothalamus (14), it modulates neuronal plasticity of the feeding circuits (15), it acts in the hypothalamus to regulate glucose homeostasis (16–18), and it affects bone density (19) and repro-duction (20,21).

db/db Mice and Leptin Receptor

The spontaneous *diabetes* mutation, db/db, was first reported by Hummel et al. in 1966 (22). db/db mice are obese, hyperinsulinemic and hyperglycemic, and the severity of these phenotypes is markedly influenced by genetic background. In C57BLKS background, from which the db mutation originally arose, db/db mice exhibit uncontrolled diabetes, depletion of pancreatic β cells and die by 10 months of age. In contrast, db/db mice on C57BL6 background exhibit compensatory hyperplasia in β-cell growth and consequently are able to survive up to 20 months. The marked influence of genetic background on obesity and diabetes phenotypes indicates the complex interactions between various quantitative trait loci in differ-ent backgrounds.

In Coleman's parabiosis experiment reported in 1973, surgical connection of db/db with ob/ob or normal mice caused the ob/ob mice or normal mice to die of starvation while db/db mice showed no changes. Coleman wrote: "It is postulated that the ob/ob mouse is unable to produce sufficient satiety factor to regulate its food consumption, whereas the db/db mouse produces satiety factor, but cannot respond to it because of a defective satiety center" (3). Coleman's prediction once again was fulfilled two decades later with the positional cloning of the db gene, using cDNA from the mouse plexus choroids, discovering it encoded the leptin receptor (23–26). Leptin receptor, a single transmembrane protein is a member of the gp130 cytokine receptor family, and binds leptin with nanomolar affinity (26).

Several spontaneous *Lepr* mutant models have been described. *Lepr^db/Lepr^db* mice are deficient for functional leptin receptors. The *Lepr^db* mutation is due to a G→T point mutation, leading to the insertion of a 106 nucleotide insert and expression of a premature stop codon (24,25). This mutation occurs in the Ob-Rb isoform of the leptin receptor; the longest and functionally most important of five leptin receptor isoforms (24) (see details below). Other *Lepr* gene mutations have been identified. The *db^3J* mutation is due to a 17 base pair deletion beginning at G^1874 (Ser^625), resulting in a frameshift and premature stop codon 11 amino acids after the deletion site (27). The *db^PAS* mutation is a duplication of exons 4 and 5, leading to the introduction of a premature stop codon and production of a truncated 281 amino acid receptor (28). Comparable mutations of the leptin receptor gene have also been described in rats. The Zucker rat *fatty* mutation (*Lepr^fa*) is an A→C point mutation resulting in a Gln^269Pro substitution (29). The *Lepr^fa* mutation leads to reduced leptin signaling, probably by affecting protein folding or receptor transport to the cell surface. The Koletsky rat has a separate mutation in the leptin receptor gene (*Lepr^fak*) resulting in a Tyr^763Stop nonsense mutation and complete absence of functional receptor (30,31).

Leptin-deficient and leptin receptor-deficient rodent models are extreme examples of obesity, exhibiting hyperphagia, earlyonset obesity, insulin resistance, hyperlipidemia and diabetes (4,26). Much of the obese phenotype can be ascribed to hypercorticosteronemia, with adrenalectomy and glucocorticoid antagonists able to block the development of obesity and diabetes (32).

Leptin receptor gene is alternatively spliced to produce multiple isoforms (33,34). Only the isoform b, known as the long form, has an intact intracellular domain and is capable of mediating leptin signaling. Leptin binding to leptin receptor activates the Jak-Stat3 signaling pathway (35). Mice carrying a mutated leptin receptor unable to activate Stat3 signaling are obese (36). Leptin activation also leads to increased expression of suppressor of cytokine signaling 3 (Socs3), which is a downstream transcriptional product of Jak-Stat3 signaling and a negative feedback regulator. Heterozygous deletion of Socs3 or neuronal deletion of Socs3 results in increased leptin sensitivity and resistance to diet-induced obesity, indicating the Socs3 might be an important mediator of leptin resistance. In addition to the Jak-Stat3 signaling pathway, pharmacological study has shown that phosphatidylinositol 3-kinase (PI3K) activity in the hypothalamus is required for leptin's anorexic effect (37) and that leptin stimulates PI3K activity in key leptin target neurons (38).

The long form of the leptin receptor is primarily expressed in the hypothalamus. It is densely concentrated in the arcuate nucleus (ARC), and is expressed at lower levels in other hypothalamic sites including the dorsomedial hypothalamus (DMH), ventromedial hypothalamus (VMH), and lateral hypothalamic area (LHA) (39). The enrichment of leptin receptor long form in the hypothalamus suggests that leptin mainly exerts its effects centrally. Indeed, the obesity, diabetes and infertility phenotypes seen in db/db mice can be completely rescued by neuron-specific expression of the leptin receptor gene (40). By using a genetic approach, researchers have created transgenic mice that specifically delete leptin receptor function in only a subset of neurons, with the goal to assess the relative importance of each neuronal subtype in mediating leptin function (41,42). If mutant mice that lack leptin receptor in specific neuronal subtypes develop obesity, one can conclude that those neuronal subtypes play key roles in normal regulation of energy balance. Negative results are more difficult to interpret, however, since alternative circuits or other signaling pathways can underlie compensatory mechanisms.

PROOPIOMELANOCORTIN

Through post-translational modification, the POMC gene produces multiple peptides which include alpha-, beta-, gamma-melanocyte stimulating hormone (α-, β-, γ-MSH), adrenocorticotropin (ACTH) and beta-endorphin. POMC derived peptides have diverse biological activities. ACTH is mainly released from the anterior pituitary and it acts on the adrenal gland to regulate glucocorticoid secretion in response to stress. In the brain, POMC expressing neurons are found mainly in the arcuate nucleus of the hypothalamus, and a small number of the POMC neurons are also found in the nucleus of the solitary tract (NTS) in the brain stem. α-MSH, the neuropeptide secreted by POMC neurons, is essential for body weight regulation. Injection of alpha-MSH or its analog MTII into the brain inhibits food intake and decreases energy expenditure.

POMC expression is positively regulated by leptin in the hypothalamus. *POMC* mRNA expression is decreased in ob/ob or db/db mice, and is normalized by leptin injection (43–45). Leptin also increases the firing rate of the POMC neurons (46). The leptin receptor is expressed in the majority of POMC neurons (47,48), and leptin administration activates Stat3 and PI3K in POMC neurons (38,49). These observations have led to the conclusion that POMC neurons are direct targets of leptin regulation.

The absolute requirement for POMC in energy homeostasis was established when a null mutation of the *POMC* gene was created by gene targeting in embryonic stem cells (50). These mice were hyperphagic and develop morbid obesity (see detailed phenotypic description in Chapter 3.2). Recently, a cell ablation model has been developed in which the POMC neurons have been genetically ablated by either deleting an essential gene (51) or by introducing a toxic gene (52) into the POMC neurons. Mice with the ablation of POMC neurons are again hyperphagic, obese, and exhibit defects in compensatory refeeding following fasting (51). However, the above manipulations via gene targeting or transgenic ablation also abolish pituitary *POMC* expression in addition to brain *POMC* expression and lack of pituitary *POMC* expression leads to corticosterone deficiency in these mice. Recently, transgenic mice have been produced in which a *POMC* transgene is expressed in the pituitary in an otherwise POMC null background. Compared with the POMC null mice, the pituitary-rescued POMC knockout mice have restored peripheral melanorcortin and corticosterone secretion, but exhibit increased food intake, enhanced feeding efficiency, reduced energy expenditure and higher degree of obesity (53). These results confirm that POMC exerts its function in energy homeostasis by acting in the hypothalamus.

LETHAL YELLOW (A^Y) MICE AND AGOUTI-RELATED PEPTIDE

One of the first mouse models of obesity described was the naturally occurring *lethal yellow* agouti (A^y/a) mouse (54,55). *Lethal yellow* (A^y) is an unusual dominant mutation in which a large deletion fuses the promoter of a ubiquitously expressed gene (*Raly*) to protein-coding sequences for the *Agouti* coat color gene, simultaneously creating a gain-of-function allele for *Agouti* and a loss-of-function allele for *Raly* (56,57). Homozygous mutation for A^y is lethal due to the loss of *Raly* function, but heterozygous A^y mice are yellow due to the expression of Agouti protein throughout the entire hair cycle and inhibition of melanocortin-1 receptor (MC1R) in the skin. In addition, A^y mice are obese, hyperinsulinemic and insulin resistant, exhibit impaired glucose tolerance and mild hyperglycemia, and demonstrate increased longitudinal growth (58) A^y/a mice were also shown to be hyperleptinemic and leptin resistant (59), correlating with increased expression of Socs3 in the mediobasal hypothalamus. As described above, this component of intracellular signal transduction is known to inhibit leptin receptor signaling (60).

The obesity phenotype associated with hyperphagia is now known to be due to ectopic expression of *Agouti* in the hypothalamus, leading to inhibition of the MC3R and MC4R receptors. Subsequent studies demonstrated that the suppression of food intake associated with the icv injection of a synthetic α-MSH analogue, melanotan-II (MTII), a non-selective melanocortin receptor agonist, was inhibited by the co-administration of SHU9119, a synthetic non-selective antagonist of the MC3R and MC4R (45). Moreover, icv injection of SHU9119 was shown to potently increase food intake, suggesting a central melanocortinergic tone that can be modulated to affect ingestive behavior. These works led furthermore to the identification of AgRP, a homolog of Agouti protein that is normally expressed in the hypothalamus and functions as the natural antagonist for MC3R and MC4R (described in Chapter 3.2).

Fat and Tubby

Fat

The recessive *fat* mutation, characterized by lateonset obesity and hyperinsulinemia, arose at The Jackson Laboratory in 1974 (61). The *fat* locus encodes carboxypeptidase E (*Cpe*), a prohormone processing exopeptidase found in secretory granules of endocrine and neuroendocrine cells. The Cpe^{fat} mutation is a missense mutation leading to a Ser^{202}Pro substitution, resulting in an unstable and enzymatically inactive CPE molecule (62). Cpe^{fat}/Cpe^{fat} mice have undetectable levels of CPE-mediated peptide processing in all tissues (63). Cpe^{fat}/Cpe^{fat} mice have very high levels of proinsulin, indicating a role for CPE in functional insulin processing. Mice deficient for *Cpe* have been created, and exhibit many endocrine and neural abnormalities including obesity and insulin resistance (64). CPE is necessary for the correct processing of several prohormones apart from insulin, including POMC (65,66), progonadotropin releasing hormone (67), progastrin (68), and proneurotensin (69). The molecular mechanism responsible for the development of obesity in Cpe^{fat}/Cpe^{fat} mice is unknown due to the functional diversity of carboxypeptidase E, although loss of POMC has also been observed to cause severe obesity (50,70).

Tubby

Tubby mice exhibit lateonset obesity and hyperinsulinemia, as well as sensory neural defects, due to an autosomal recessive loss-of-function mutation in the *tub* gene (61,71). The *tub* mutation is located on chromosome 7 (72,73), and since the identification of the gene three other tubby-like proteins (TULPs) have been identified (*Tulp1-3*) (74,75). *Tub* knockout mice exhibit a similar phenotype of lateonset obesity and hyperinsulinemia, confirming the *tub* mutation as responsible for the obesity of tubby mice (76). *Tulp1* knockout mice, however, do not exhibit obesity but are instead models of retinal degredation (77), and *Tulp3*-deficient mice die in utero due to neural tube develoment defects (78). The specific function of *tub*, and of the TULPs, is not yet completely understood. However, *tub* may play a role in insulin signaling as it is a target of the insulin receptor tyrosine kinase (79). Tub may therefore function as an adaptor protein that is able to mediate some of insulin's effects on energy balance in the brain.

INTEGRATION OF CENTRAL MELANOCORTIN SYSTEM WITH HORMONAL SIGNALS

Leptin and insulin are adiposity signals that act directly on melanocortin neurons. In both rodents and humans, loss of function of either *LEP, LEPR, POMC* or *MC4R* results in morbid obesity, which are the most profound monogenic obesities identified to date.

Thus, the neuronal circuit of leptin→leptin receptor→POMC→MC4R is one of the most important neuronal circuits in energy balance regulation. In addition to mediating the function of adiposity signals, central melanocortin neurons also integrate signals originated from the gastrointestinal tract. One of these hormones is ghrelin, which is secreted from the gut and is thought to be a meal-initiating signal. However, it is still unclear how the activated MC4R transmits the received signals to the downstream endophentoypes related to obesity. Mice doubly null for both *AgRP* and *NPY* are not responsive to the orexigenic effect of ghrelin (80), suggesting that AgRP/NPY neurons are the neuronal substrate that mediates ghrelin action in the hypothalamus. Within the arcuate nucleus, POMC neurons receive inhibitory GABAergic inputs from the neighboring AgrRP/NPY neurons (46,81). Thus, POMC neurons receive direct and indirect inputs from peripheral hormones such as leptin and ghrelin, whereas AgRP inhibits MC4R directly and indirectly through regulation of POMC (Fig. 1). Proper communication between the periphery and the brain and an intricate balance between multiple neuropeptides is required to maintain energy homeostasis. Additional understanding of genes and pathways involved in the central regulation of energy expenditure was brought by the detailed studies of transgenic rodents as described in the next chapter (Chapter 3.2).

REFERENCES

1. Ingalls AM, Dickie MM, Snell GD. Obese, a new mutation in the house mouse. J Hered 1950; 41:317–8.
2. Kennedy GC. The role of depot fat in the hypothalamic control of food intake in the rat. Proc R Soc Lond B Biol Sci 1953; 140:578–96.
3. Coleman DL. Effects of parabiosis of obese with diabetes and normal mice. Diabetologia 1973; 9:294–8.
4. Zhang Y, Proenca R, Maffei M, Barone M, Leopold L, Friedman JM. Positional cloning of the mouse obese gene and its human homologue. Nature 1994; 372:425–32.
5. Pelleymounter MA, Cullen MJ, Baker MB, et al. Effects of the obese gene product on body weight regulation in ob/ob mice. Science 1995; 269:540–3.
6. Halaas JL, Gajiwala KS, Maffei M, et al. Weight-reducing effects of the plasma protein encoded by the obese gene. Science 1995; 269:543–6.
7. Rentsch J, Levens N, Chiesi M. Recombinant ob-gene product reduces food intake in fasted mice. Biochem Biophys Res Commun 1995; 214:131–6.
8. Weigle DS, Bukowski TR, Foster DC, et al. Recombinant ob protein reduces feeding and body weight in the ob/ob mouse. J Clin Invest 1995; 96:2065–70.

9. Trayhurn P, Thomas ME, Duncan JS, Rayner DV. Effects of fasting and refeeding on ob gene expression in white adipose tissue of lean and obese (oblob) mice. FEBS Lett 1995; 368:488–90.

10. Bado A, Levasseur S, Attoub S, et al. The stomach is a source of leptin. Nature 1998; 394:790–3.

11. Peters JH, McKay BM, Simasko SM, Ritter RC. Leptin-induced satiation mediated by abdominal vagal afferents. Am J Physiol Regul Integr Comp Physiol 2005; 288: R879–84.

12. Banks WA, Kastin AJ, Huang W, Jaspan JB, Maness LM. Leptin enters the brain by a saturable system independent of insulin. Peptides 1996; 17:305–11.

13. Bruning JC, Gautam D, Burks DJ, et al. Role of brain insulin receptor in control of body weight and reproduction. Science 2000; 289:2122–5.

14. Bouret SG, Draper SJ, Simerly RB. Trophic action of leptin on hypothalamic neurons that regulate feeding. Science 2004; 304:108–10.

15. Pinto S, Roseberry AG, Liu H, et al. Rapid rewiring of arcuate nucleus feeding circuits by leptin. Science 2004; 304:110–5.

16. Coppari R, Ichinose M, Lee CE, et al. The hypothalamic arcuate nucleus: a key site for mediating leptin's effects on glucose homeostasis and locomotor activity. Cell Metab 2005; 1:63–72.

17. Morton GJ, Gelling RW, Niswender KD, Morrison CD, Rhodes CJ, Schwartz MW. Leptin regulates insulin sensitivity via phosphatidylinositol-3-OH kinase signaling in mediobasal hypothalamic neurons. Cell Metab 2005; 2:411–20.

18. Bates SH, Kulkarni RN, Seifert M, Myers MG, Jr. Roles for leptin receptor/STAT3-dependent and -independent signals in the regulation of glucose homeostasis. Cell Metab 2005; 1:169–78.

19. Ducy P, Amling M, Takeda S, et al. Leptin inhibits bone formation through a hypothalamic relay: a central control of bone mass. Cell 2000; 100:197–207.

20. Ahima RS, Prabakaran D, Mantzoros C, et al. Role of leptin in the neuroendocrine response to fasting. Nature 1996; 382:250–2.

21. Ahima RS, Dushay J, Flier SN, Prabakaran D, Flier JS. Leptin accelerates the onset of puberty in normal female mice. J Clin Invest 1997; 99:391–5.

22. Hummel KP, Dickie MM, Coleman DL. Diabetes, a new mutation in the mouse. Science 1966; 153:1127–8.

23. Chua SC, Jr., Chung WK, Wu-Peng XS, et al. Phenotypes of mouse diabetes and rat fatty due to mutations in the OB (leptin) receptor. Science 1996; 271:994–6.

24. Lee GH, Proenca R, Montez JM, et al. Abnormal splicing of the leptin receptor in diabetic mice. Nature 1996; 379:632–5.

25. Chen H, Charlat O, Tartaglia LA, et al. Evidence that the diabetes gene encodes the leptin receptor: identification of a mutation in the leptin receptor gene in db/db mice. Cell 1996; 84:491–5.

26. Tartaglia LA, Dembski M, Weng X, et al. Identification and expression cloning of a leptin receptor, OB-R. Cell 1995; 83:1263–71.

27. Lee G, Li C, Montez J, Halaas J, Darvishzadeh J, Friedman JM. Leptin receptor mutations in 129 db3J/db3J mice and NIH facp/facp rats. Mamm Genome 1997; 8:445–7.

28. Li C, Ioffe E, Fidahusein N, Connolly E, Friedman JM. Absence of soluble leptin receptor in plasma from dbPas/dbPas and other db/db mice. J Biol Chem 1998; 273:10078–82.

29. Phillips MS, Liu Q, Hammond HA, et al. Leptin receptor missense mutation in the fatty Zucker rat. Nat Genet 1996; 13:18–9.

30. Takaya K, Ogawa Y, Hiraoka J, et al. Nonsense mutation of leptin receptor in the obese spontaneously hypertensive Koletsky rat. Nat Genet 1996; 14:130–1.

31. Wu-Peng XS, Chua SC Jr., Okada N, Liu SM, Nicolson M, Leibel RL. Phenotype of the obese Koletsky (f) rat due to Tyr763Stop mutation in the extracellular domain of the leptin receptor (Lepr): evidence for deficient plasma-to-CSF transport of leptin in both the Zucker and Koletsky obese rat. Diabetes 1997; 46:513–8.

32. Freedman MR, Horwitz BA, Stern JS. Effect of adrenalectomy and glucocorticoid replacement on development of obesity. Am J Physiol 1986; 250(4 Pt 2):R595–607.

33. Guan XM, Hess JF, Yu H, Hey PJ, van der Ploeg LH. Differential expression of mRNA for leptin receptor isoforms in the rat brain. Mol Cell Endocrinol 1997; 133:1–7.

34. Lollmann B, Gruninger S, Stricker-Krongrad A, Chiesi M. Detection and quantification of the leptin receptor splice variants Ob-Ra, b, and, e in different mouse tissues. Biochem Biophys Res Commun 1997; 238:648–52.

35. Vaisse C, Halaas JL, Horvath CM, Darnell JE, Jr., Stoffel M, Friedman JM. Leptin activation of Stat3 in the hypothalamus of wild-type and ob/ob mice but not db/db mice. Nat Genet 1996; 14:95–7.

36. Bates SH, Stearns WH, Dundon TA, et al. STAT3 signalling is required for leptin regulation of energy balance but not reproduction. Nature 2003; 421:856–9.

37. Niswender KD, Morton GJ, Stearns WH, Rhodes CJ, Myers MG, Jr., Schwartz MW. Intracellular signalling. Key enzyme in leptin-induced anorexia. Nature 2001; 413:794–5.

38. Xu AW, Kaelin CB, Takeda K, Akira S, Schwartz MW, Barsh GS. PI3K integrates the action of insulin and leptin on hypothalamic neurons. J Clin Invest 2005; 115:951–8.

39. Schwartz MW, Seeley RJ, Campfield LA, Burn P, Baskin DG. Identification of targets of leptin action in rat hypothalamus. J Clin Invest 1996; 98:1101–6.

40. de Luca C, Kowalski TJ, Zhang Y, et al. Complete rescue of obesity, diabetes, and infertility in db/db mice by neuron-specific LEPR-B transgenes. J Clin Invest 2005; 115:3484–93.

41. Balthasar N, Coppari R, McMinn J, et al. Leptin receptor signaling in POMC neurons is required for normal body weight homeostasis. Neuron 2004; 42:983–91.

42. Dhillon H, Zigman JM, Ye C, et al. Leptin directly activates SF1 neurons in the VMH, and this action by leptin is required for normal body-weight homeostasis. Neuron 2006; 49:191–203.

43. Mizuno TM, Kleopoulos SP, Bergen HT, Roberts JL, Priest CA, Mobbs CV. Hypothalamic proopiomelanocortin mRNA is reduced by fasting and [corrected] in ob/ob and db/db mice, but is stimulated by leptin. Diabetes 1998; 47:294–7.

44. Schwartz MW, Seeley RJ, Woods SC, et al. Leptin increases hypothalamic proopiomelanocortin mRNA expression in the rostral arcuate nucleus. Diabetes 1997; 46:2119–23.

45. Fan W, Boston BA, Kesterson RA, Hruby VJ, Cone RD. Role of melanocortinergic neurons in feeding and the agouti obesity syndrome. Nature 1997; 385:165–8.

46. Cowley MA, Smart JL, Rubinstein M, et al. Leptin activates anorexigenic POMC neurons through a neural network in the arcuate nucleus. Nature 2001; 411:480–4.

47. Baskin DG, Breininger JF, Schwartz MW. Leptin receptor mRNA identifies a subpopulation of neuropeptide Y neurons activated by fasting in rat hypothalamus. Diabetes 1999; 48:828–33.

48. Cheung CC, Clifton DK, Steiner RA. Proopiomelanocortin neurons are direct targets for leptin in the hypothalamus. Endocrinology 1997; 138:4489–92.

49. Munzberg H, Huo L, Nillni EA, Hollenberg AN, Bjorbaek C. Role of signal transducer and activator of transcription 3 in regulation of hypothalamic proopiomelanocortin gene expression by leptin. Endocrinology 2003; 144:2121–31.

50. Yaswen L, Diehl N, Brennan MB, Hochgeschwender U. Obesity in the mouse model of proopiomelanocortin deficiency responds to peripheral melanocortin. Nat Med 1999; 5:1066–70.

51. Xu AW, Kaelin CB, Morton GJ, et al. Effects of hypothalamic neurodegeneration on energy balance. PLoS Biol 2005; 3:e415.

52. Gropp E, Shanabrough M, Borok E, et al. Agouti-related peptide-expressing neurons are mandatory for feeding. Nat Neurosci 2005; 8:1289–91.

53. Smart JL, Tolle V, Low MJ. Glucocorticoids exacerbate obesity and insulin resistance in neuron-specific proopiomelanocortin-deficient mice. J Clin Invest 2006; 116:495–505.

54. Bultman SJ, Michaud EJ, Woychik RP. Molecular characterization of the mouse agouti locus. Cell 1992; 71:1195–204.

55. Miller MW, Duhl DM, Vrieling H, et al. Cloning of the mouse agouti gene predicts a secreted protein ubiquitously expressed in mice carrying the lethal yellow mutation. Genes Dev 1993; 7:454–67.

56. Michaud EJ, Bultman SJ, Stubbs LJ, Woychik RP. The embryonic lethality of homozygous lethal yellow mice (Ay/Ay) is associated with the disruption of a novel RNA-binding protein. Genes Dev 1993; 7:1203–13.

57. Michaud EJ, Bultman SJ, Klebig ML, et al. A molecular model for the genetic and phenotypic characteristics of the mouse lethal yellow (Ay) mutation. Proc Natl Acad Sci USA 1994; 91:2562–6.

58. Wolff GL, Roberts DW, Mountjoy KG. Physiological consequences of ectopic agouti gene expression: the yellow obese mouse syndrome. Physiol Genomics 1999;151–63.

59. Halaas JL, Boozer C, Blair-West J, Fidahusein N, Denton DA, Friedman JM. Physiological response to long-term peripheral and central leptin infusion in lean and obese mice. Proc Natl Acad Sci USA 1997; 94:8878–83.

60. Bjorbaek C, Elmquist JK, Frantz JD, Shoelson SE, Flier JS. Identification of SOCS-3 as a potential mediator of central leptin resistance. Mol Cell 1998; 1:619–25.

61. Coleman DL, Eicher EM. Fat (fat) and tubby (tub): two autosomal recessive mutations causing obesity syndromes in the mouse. J Hered 1990; 81:424–7.

62. Naggert JK, Fricker LD, Varlamov O, et al. Hyperproinsulinaemia in obese fat/fat mice associated with a carboxypeptidase E mutation which reduces enzyme activity. Nat Genet 1995; 10:135–42.

63. Fricker LD, Berman YL, Leiter EH, Devi LA. Carboxypeptidase E activity is deficient in mice with the fat mutation. Effect on peptide processing. J Biol Chem 1996; 271:30619–24.

64. Cawley NX, Zhou J, Hill JM, et al. The carboxypeptidase E knockout mouse exhibits endocrinological and behavioral deficits. Endocrinology 2004; 145:5807–19.

65. Cool DR, Normant E, Shen F, et al. Carboxypeptidase E is a regulated secretory pathway sorting receptor: genetic obliteration leads to endocrine disorders in Cpe(fat) mice. Cell 1997; 88:73–83.

66. Shen FS, Loh YP. Intracellular misrouting and abnormal secretion of adrenocorticotropin and growth hormone in cpefat mice associated with a carboxypeptidase E mutation. Proc Natl Acad Sci USA 1997; 94:5314–9.

67. Srinivasan S, Bunch DO, Feng Y, et al. Deficits in reproduction and pro-gonadotropin-releasing hormone processing in male Cpefat mice. Endocrinology 2004; 145:2023–34.

68. Udupi V, Gomez P, Song L, et al. Effect of carboxypeptidase E deficiency on progastrin processing and gastrin messenger ribonucleic acid expression in mice with the fat mutation. Endocrinology 1997; 138:1959–63.

69. Rovere C, Viale A, Nahon J, Kitabgi P. Impaired processing of brain proneurotensin and promelanin-concentrating hormone in obese fat/fat mice. Endocrinology 1996; 137:2954–8.

70. Challis BG, Coll AP, Yeo GS, et al. Mice lacking proopiomelanocortin are sensitive to high-fat feeding but respond normally to the acute anorectic effects of peptide-YY (3-36). Proc Natl Acad Sci USA 2004; 101:4695–700.

71. Ohlemiller KK, Hughes RM, Mosinger-Ogilvie J, Speck JD, Grosof DH, Silverman MS. Cochlear and retinal degeneration in the tubby mouse. Neuroreport 1995; 6:845–9.

72. Kleyn PW, Fan W, Kovats SG, et al. Identification and characterization of the mouse obesity gene tubby: a member of a novel gene family. Cell 1996; 85:281–90.

73. Noben-Trauth K, Naggert JK, North MA, Nishina PM. A candidate gene for the mouse mutation tubby. Nature 1996; 380:534–8.

74. Nishina PM, North MA, Ikeda A, Yan Y, Naggert JK. Molecular characterization of a novel tubby gene family member, TULP3, in mouse and humans. Genomics 1998; 54:215–20.

75. North MA, Naggert JK, Yan Y, Noben-Trauth K, Nishina PM. Molecular characterization of TUB, TULP1, and TULP2, members of the novel tubby gene family and their possible relation to ocular diseases. Proc Natl Acad Sci USA 1997; 94:3128–33.

76. Stubdal H, Lynch CA, Moriarty A, et al. Targeted deletion of the tub mouse obesity gene reveals that tubby is a loss-of-function mutation. Mol Cell Biol 2000; 20:878–82.

77. Ikeda S, Shiva N, Ikeda A, et al. Retinal degeneration but not obesity is observed in null mutants of the tubby-like protein 1 gene. Hum Mol Genet 2000; 9:155–63.

78. Ikeda A, Ikeda S, Gridley T, Nishina PM, Naggert JK. Neural tube defects and neuroepithelial cell death in Tulp3 knockout mice. Hum Mol Genet 2001; 10:1325–34.

79. Kapeller R, Moriarty A, Strauss A, et al. Tyrosine phosphorylation of tub and its association with Src homology 2 domain-containing proteins implicate tub in intracellular signaling by insulin. J Biol Chem 1999; 274:24980–6.

80. Chen HY, Trumbauer ME, Chen AS, et al. Orexigenic action of peripheral ghrelin is mediated by neuropeptide Y and agouti-related protein. Endocrinology 2004; 145:2607–12.
81. Roseberry AG, Liu H, Jackson AC, Cai X, Friedman JM. Neuropeptide Y-mediated inhibition of proopiomelanocortin neurons in the arcuate nucleus shows enhanced desensitization in ob/ob mice. Neuron 2004; 41:711–22.

Transgenic Models Targeting the Central Nervous System

James L. Trevaskis and Gregory M. Sutton
Pennington Biomedical Research Center, Louisiana State University System, Baton Rouge, Louisiana, U.S.A.

Allison W. Xu
Diabetes Center and Department of Anatomy, University of California, San Francisco, San Francisco, California, U.S.A.

Andrew A. Butler
Pennington Biomedical Research Center, Louisiana State University System, Baton Rouge, Louisiana, U.S.A.

Significant advances in our understanding of the regulation of energy balance have been achieved through combining molecular biology and physiology. The initial stimulus driving much of these advances involved the characterization of a small number of spontaneous mouse mutants with altered metabolic phenotypes leading to obesity described in Chapter 3.1. Our understanding of the mechanisms by which genetics maintains body weight is partly due to increased use of transgenic mouse models. The development of technology enabling the manipulation of gene expression, either by over expression or through targeted gene inactivation, has resulted in the creation of many new mutant strains that either develop obesity, or are protected from diet-induced obesity. Transgenic techniques are now widely used for the study of physiological processes and disease states (1).

Mice are the most commonly used vector for transgenic experiments, owing to nearly a century of knowledge gained from the study of mouse physiology and genetics, the availability of oocytes and embryonic stem cells for manipulation and creation of transgenic animals, and low cost of maintenance (1). A growing repertoire of tissue-specific promoters are used to control expression of transgenes in a cell-specific, tissue-specific, or ubiquitous manner thus leading to restricted or widespread alteration of expression of the gene of interest. Homologous recombination in embryonic stem (ES) cells to introduce foreign DNA into target genes to create models with a null allele has now been largely superseded by methods incorporating the Cre-*lox*P system from bacteriophage P1 (2), and the Flp-*FRT* system from the yeast organism *S. cerevisiae* (3,4). A detailed technical explanation regarding can be found on the Jackson laboratory web site (http://jaxmice.jax.org/models/cre_intro.html). Briefly, these tools can be adapted to conditionally either activate or inactivate gene expression. To create a knockout mouse using the Cre-*lox*P system, transgenic mice which have *lox*P sites flanking the target gene (a so-called "floxed" gene) are crossed with transgenic mice expressing the Cre recombinase gene (5). Another variation is the use of intracerebroventricular (i.c.v.) administration of an adenovirus expressing Cre to regulate the expression of a floxed gene in target brain areas of adult mice, thus reducing any possible compensatory effects of gene deletion at the embryonic stage. These and other variations have been used to generate spatial-, temporal- and tissue-specific gene knockout models (5).

CENTRAL CONTROL OF ENERGY BALANCE

Sites within the central nervous system (CNS), and in the hypothalamus in particular, are important for regulating ingestive behaviors and metabolic efficiency. Molecular biology has led to insights into mechanisms, and a more accurate appreciation of the neuroanatomal distribution, of the sites involved in the central control of energy balance. In this chapter, we will introduce some of the transgenic mouse models currently in use that exhibit a phenotype of disturbed energy balance after insertion of a transgene into the CNS. In order to accomplish this a basic understanding of the role of the CNS in the regulation of energy balance is required.

Energy homeostasis, the maintenance of energy stored primarily as triglyceride in adipocytes over the lifespan of an organism, is a complex process. This process involves the integration of neural pathways affecting ingestive behaviors and peripheral metabolism through autonomic and neuroendocrine outputs, with inputs derived from peripheral signaling systems sensing and relaying information about energy stores (6). Within the CNS, areas distributed throughout the forebrain and caudal brainstem are important for regulating feeding behavior (7,8). Hypothalamic neurons transform sensory and endocrine signals into outputs that influence both behavioral and physiological responses. Early lesioning studies suggested that normal function of the hypothalamus is critical for energy homeostasis (9). However, interpretation of knife and chemical lesion experiments investigating specific hypothalamic nuclei is confounded by destruction of axonal fibers passing through the affected area.

It is now possible to target specific neurons, either at the level of gene expression, or through targeted ablation of specific neurons using "suicide" genes. While elegant, the interpretation of some of these recent experiments has again been questioned, with the possibility that the disruption of some genes might affect the development of axonal projections between critical areas of the central nervous system (10–12). Nevertheless, based on the information provided by these tools, it is now thought that hypothalamic neurons may respond to a milieu of metabolites as well as hormones secreted from the gut and adipose tissue that affect energy balance [e.g., leptin, peptide YY_{3-36} (PYY_{3-36}), insulin, ghrelin, cholecystokinin].

TRANSGENIC NEUROPEPTIDE MODELS OF OBESITY—THE MELANOCORTIN SYSTEM

Two populations of melanocortin neurons have been the most intensively analyzed, and are critically important for integrating inputs and output in response to peripheral and central signals affecting energy homeostasis. One population of neurons found in the arcuate nucleus (ARC) of the hypothalamus coexpress neuropeptide Y (NPY) and agouti-related peptide (AGRP), neuropeptides that stimulate food intake and therefore promote weight gain. Another population of neurons expressing proopiomelanocortin (POMC) is located in the ARC of the hypothalamus. A small number of POMC neurons are detected in the nucleus tractus solitarius of the brainstem (NTS). Melanocortin neurons in the brain stem respond to cholecystokinin (CCK), a satiety factor secreted from the gut that reduces food intake through activation of MC4R (13).

As described in Chapter 3.1 POMC is a precursor for several peptides involved in regulating energy homeostasis and analgesia, including the melano-cyte-stimulating hormones (α-,β-, and γ-MSH) that are agonists of the melanocortin receptors (MC1-5R) (7,14). Central administration of α- and β-MSH suppresses food intake, likely through the activation of MC4R. γ-MSH is distinguished from α- and β-MSH in being a selective MC3R agonist (15,16), while i.c.v. administration of γ-MSH peptide has no or only minimal effects on feeding behavior (17,18). In addition, several other experiments using melanocortin receptor knockout mice have demonstrated the dependency of melanocortin agonists, and factors such as serotonin that regulate appetite through melanocortin neurons, on functional MC4R (19–23).

Melanocortin neurons in the hypothalamus are direct targets of leptin. POMC and AgRP neurons express *Lepr-b* mRNA (24,25). Moreover, inhibition of central melanocortin receptors can attenuate the anorectic response to leptin (26). Hypothalamic melanocortin neurons are now also thought to be targets of several peripheral hormones that regulate energy balance, including insulin, ghrelin, and PYY. Several detailed reviews of this topic have recently been published (6,7,27–30). In the following sections, we will briefly discuss animal models that have manipulated components of this system that present phenotypes of disturbed energy balance. A summary of transgenic and knockout mice where manipulation of genes expressed in the CNS affects energy balance and metabolism is provided in Table 1.

POMC and AGRP Transgenics
POMC
Two groups independently created POMC knockout (*Pomc*–/–) mice, which exhibit obesity and hyperphagia (31,32). *Pomc*–/– mice are hyperinsulinemic, have undetectable levels of corticosterone owing to loss of ACTH, and have disturbed pigmentation. The obese phenotype observed in mice with homozygous or heterozygous null *Pomc* genes is comparable to the obesity syndrome observed in humans with spontaneous loss of function mutations in the *POMC* gene (see Chapter 5.5) (14). Rescuing *Pomc* gene expression specifically in the pituitary of POMC knockout mice rescues adrenal function, but is associated with hypercorticosteronemia, which exacerbates the obese phenotype (33).

To investigate whether chronic activation of melanocortin receptors can protect against obesity and insulin resistance, transgenic strains over expressing *Pomc* have also been created.

In one line, over expression utilized a cytomegalovirus (CMV) promoter to express an N-terminal fragment of *Pomc*, including the sequence encoding γ-MSH and α-MSH (34). The levels of γ-MSH and α-MSH were increased two-fold in the hypothalamus of CMV-POMC transgenic mice, resulting in a lean phenotype, and attenuating obesity and improving glucose tolerance of genetic models of obesity (A^y/a, $Lepr^{db3J}$). Overexpression of a full length *Pomc* specifically in neurons using the enolase promoter had similar effects, attenuating obesity and significantly improving glucose metabolism in leptin deficient mice (35).

AgRP
AgRP neurons are also found in the ARC of the hypothalamus, with POMC and AgRP neurons sending projections to hypothalamic and extrahypothalamic

TABLE 1 Phenotypes of Mouse Models with Transgenic Modulation of Central Nervous System Targets

Gene	Modulation	Phenotype	Ref.
AgRP	Ubiquitous overexpression	Obesity, hyperphagia, increased longitudinal growth	(38,41)
	Knockout	No phenotype	(42)
		Age-related lean phenotype	(47)
	Cre-*lox*P-mediated ablation of AgRP/NPY neurons after diptheria toxin administration	Loss of body weight, hypophagia, hypoglycemia	(45)
	Transgenic expression of the neurotoxin ataxin-3 in AgRP neurons, reducing AgRP neurons by 47%	Reduced body weight, hypophagia, hypoinsulinemia	(46)
Mc4r	Knockout	Obesity, hyperphagia, increased feed efficiency, hyperinsulinemia, hyperleptinemia; increased lipogenic gene expression, reduced energy expenditure, enlarged liver and hepatic steatosis; increased longitudinal growth	(52,53, 135)
Mc3r	Knockout	Increased adiposity, diet-dependent obesity, increased feed efficiency.	(21,60, 62)
Pomc	Knockout	Obesity, hyperphagia, hyperinsulinemia, severe adrenal dysfunction. Increased longitudinal growth	(31,32, 136)
	Cre-*lox*P-mediated ablation of POMC neurons after diptheria toxin administration	Delayed onset hyperphagia, moderate weight gain	(45)
Npy	Knockout	No phenotype or very mild obesity	(68,69)
	Cre-*lox*P-mediated ablation of AgRP/NPY neurons after diptheria toxin administration	Loss of body weight, hypophagia, hypoglycemia	(45)
Mch	Transgenic overexpression	Moderate hyperphagia and obesity, insulin resistant, hyperleptinemia	(77)
	Knockout	Hypophagia, lower body weight, increased energy expenditure	(78)
Mchr1	Knockout	Hypophagic and lean phenotype	(79,80)
Bdnf	Heterozygous	Obesity, hyperphagia, aggressive behavior	(82)
	Conditional knockout	Late-onset obesity, increased longitudinal growth	(83)
5-ht2Cr	Knockout	Late-onset obesity, hyperphagia; seizures	(88)
Socs3	Haploinsufficient	Resistant to high fat diet-induced obesity, hyperinsulinemia, hyperleptinemia; hypersensitive to exogenous leptin treatment	(105)
	Neural-specific conditional knockout using Cre-*lox*P	Resistant to high fat diet-induced obesity and hyperleptinemia; also hypersensitive to exogenous leptin treatment	(106)

(Continued)

TABLE 1 Phenotypes of Mouse Models with Transgenic Modulation of Central Nervous System Targets (*Continued*)

Gene	Modulation	Phenotype	Ref.
Irs2	Global knockout	Insulin resistant, pancreatic failure	(113)
	Neuron-specific knockout (NIRKO)	Moderate late-onset obesity sensitive to diet, insulin resistant, elevated serum insulin and leptin levels	(111)
	Hypothalamic-specific deletion	Obesity; leptin and insulin resistant	(114)
	Deleted from pancreatic β-cells and a population of hypothalamic neurons (*RipCreIrs2KO*); neuron-specific deletion (*NesCreIrs2KO*)	Obesity, hyperphagia, increased longitudinal growth; not leptin resistant	(117)

regions of the central nervous system (7). While a small amount of *Agrp* expression is also found in some peripheral tissues, such as the adrenal gland, the role of AGRP in the periphery is currently unknown.

In the brain, most of the AgRP neurons in the ARC also express another neuropeptide NPY. AgRP is negatively regulated by leptin. The firing rates of AgRP neurons are indeed inhibited by leptin administration (36). Intracerebroventricular injection of AgRP potently stimulates feeding and antagonizes the anorexic effects of i.c.v. α-MSH (37). AgRP acts as a natural antagonist of melanocortin receptors, specifically the MC3R, MC4R and probably MC5R (38,39). *Agrp* mRNA expression is increased with fasting, and in the ARC of leptin-deficent (e.g., Lep^{ob}/Lep^{ob}) mice, and might be a factor causing hyperphagia and obesity in the leptin-deficient state (38,40). Transgenic mice ubiquitously over expressing *Agrp* are obese compared to nontransgenic littermates (38,41).

While overexpression of *Agrp* gene has been shown to stimulate feeding and increase body weight gain by both pharmacological and genetic approaches, *Agrp* loss of function mutation in mice has yielded surprising results. AgRP knockout mice were initially reported to have no phenotype, being normoinsulinemic and responding normally to leptin, diet-induced obesity and exhibiting a normal refeeding response after fasting (42). Since *Agrp* and *Npy* co-express in the same neurons within the ARC, it is thus possible that NPY and AGRP exhibit redundant function but mice doubly null for both *Agrp* and *Npy* were generated and surprisingly these mice also exhibited normal body weight (42).

In sharp contrast, the genetic ablation of the AgRP neurons postnatally leads to hypophagia and reduced adiposity, suggesting that the AgRP neurons themselves are essential in regulating feeding behaviors (43–46). The lean phenotype is more evident in older mice, associated with increased metabolic rate (47). Indeed Gropp et al. recently used the Cre-*lox*P system to activate the expression of the diptheria toxin receptor in neurons expressing AgRP, and then administered diptheria toxin to inducibly ablate AgRP neuronal populations. Loss of AgRP neurons in adult mice was associated with a significant reduction in body weight and inhibition of food intake with concomitant reductions in insulin, leptin and blood glucose concentrations (45).

Similar results have been reported by a separate group using another neurotoxin, a mutant of the Ataxin-3 gene that is mildly neurotoxic causing a gradual decline in the number of neurons expressing the protein, to ablate AgRP neurons (46). Conditional loss of AgRP neurons in adult mice is therefore able to alter energy balance, whereas mice completely deficient for AgRP from birth were able to compensate for loss of AgRP and exhibited a normal phenotype. Further studies are needed to investigate the developmental compensatory mechanisms and determine whether additional molecules in the AgRP neurons are required for energy homeostasis.

MELANOCORTIN-RECEPTOR KNOCKOUT MICE

There are five melanocortin receptors identified to date. They are G-protein coupled receptors, whose activation leads to stimulation of intracellular cyclic amp. Three of the melanocortin receptor genes (MC3R, MC4R, and MC5R) have been knocked out in mice, with two of the melanocortin receptor family (MC3R, MC4R) appearing to have a significant role in energy homeostasis (48). The melanocortin-3 receptor and melanocortin-4 receptors are the endogenous receptors for α-MSH and AGRP in the brain. α-MSH is the ligand and AGRP serves as an inverse ligand and antagonist for the same receptors. MC4R is expressed in multiple regions in the central nervous system, including the cortex, thalamus, hypothalamus, brainstem and spinal cord (49). Within the hypothalamus, MC4R is expressed in the paraventricular nucleus (PVN), a site that is densely innervated by the POMC and AgRP neuronal projections (50).

MC3R expresses primarily in the ARC and at lower levels in the ventromedial hypothalamus (VMH) (21,51). In the ARC, MC3R is expressed by approximately 31% of POMC neurons and 44% of AgRP neurons. In contrast, neither POMC nor AgRP neurons express *Mc4r* mRNA (51). It is therefore possible that MC3R mediates cross-talks between the POMC and AgRP neurons or serves as an auto-receptor for POMC and AgRP neurons themselves. The role of MC4R in energy balance has been established by genetic studies decribed below.

Melanocortin-4 Receptor Gene

Confirmation of the key role of MC4R in the regulation of energy homeostasis by melanocortins occurred with the creation of MC4R knockout mice (*Mc4r–/–* mice) (52). *Mc4r–/–* mice exhibited a syndrome of hyperphagia, obesity and accelerated longitudinal growth very similar to that observed for A^y/a mice, with the exception that coat color was normal (52). The phenotype of *Mc4r–/–* mice implied that obesity of A^y/a mice was likely due to loss of central melanocortin signaling associated with inhibition of the MC4R. Subsequent experiments demonstrated that the obese phenotype of *Mc4r–/–* mice is due to a combination of hyperphagia and enhanced metabolic efficiency, perhaps coupled with reduced energy expenditure (53,54). *Mc4r–/–* mice were used to demonstrate that the inhibition of food intake and stimulation of energy expenditure observed after i.c.v. injection of nonselective melanocortin receptor agonists required the MC4R (22,23). A critical role for the MC4R in the suppression of food intake by cholecystokin (CCK), mediated by melanocortin neurons in the brain stem, was also demonstrated using *Mc4r–/–* mice (13).

Early results indicated that inhibition of central melanocortin receptors could block the anorectic actions of leptin (26). However, the development of obesity-related leptin resistance complicates the analysis of the response of *Mc4r–/–* mice to leptin. Young "pre-obese" *Mc4r–/–* mice, and *Mc4r–/–* mice crossed onto the Lep^{ob}/Lep^{ob} background exhibit a modest resistance to the inhibition of food intake and weight loss associated with leptin replacement therapy (22,55). However, another study using young lean *Mc4r–/–* mice on a different genetic background did not observe a reduced efficacy of leptin to reduce food intake (56). Several studies by independent groups, using *Mc4r–/–* mice developed independently on different genetic backgrounds and using a variety of readouts, have demonstrated a crucial role for the MC4R in stimulating nervous activity in response to melanocortin agonists or leptin (54,56–58). In addition, due to the wide-spread expression of MC4R, recent studies have employed a gene reactivation strategy to restore MC4R function in specific regions of the brain in an otherwise MC4R null animal. Such studies have led to the discovery that MC4R neurons within the PVN and a subpopulation of amygdala neurons regulate food intake while MC4R neurons elsewhere control energy expenditure (59).

Melanocortin-3 Receptor Gene

MC3R-deficient (*Mc3r–/–*) mice exhibit a very different syndrome of metabolic disturbance compared to POMC and MC4R knockout mice. *Mc3r–/–* mice were originally reported to be not significantly heavier than wild type littermates on standard chow diet, but did exhibit greater fat mass (21,60). On high fat diets, *Mc3r–/–* mice were significantly heavier than wild type controls beginning at about two months of age (60,61). On either diet, *Mc3r–/–* mice demonstrated increased adiposity. Coupled with the observations that food intake was not altered, it was suggested that *Mc3r–/–* mice are models of enhanced metabolic efficiency (gain in body mass energy per kilo Joules consumed) (21,60). These mice also exhibit a reduction in motor activity, which could also be a contributing factor for the increase in adiposity (21,60). While loss of MC3R is associated with increased metabolic efficiency, the specific functions of MC3R in the regulation of energy balance remain unclear.

More recently, A. Butler's group compared the obese insulin resistant phenotype of *Mc3r–/–*. *Mc4r–/–* mice fed purified low or high fat diets (LFD, HFD) using mice backcrossed onto the C57BL/6J background (61,62). The results of these studies have confirmed previous results indicating that increased weight gain of *Mc3r–/–* is dependent on high fat diets. Indeed, when obesity is defined as body fat content, there is little difference between *Mc3r–/–* mice and *Mc4r–/–* mice. In males, the increased metabolic efficiency of *Mc3r–/–* mice on LFD is intermediate compared to that observed for *Mc4r–/–* mice; however on HFD the metabolic efficiency of *Mc3r–/–* and *Mc4r–/–* mice is similarly increased (20%, compared to 9% for wild type controls). Moreover, while *Mc3r–/–* and *Mc4r–/–* mice fed HFD exhibited a comparable obesity, insulin resistance and the development of hepatic steatosis was far more severe with loss of MC4R. Overall, the results of these experiments suggest that, while loss of MC3R and MC4R can both result in marked obesity in certain conditions, loss of MC4R is associated with a more severe deterioration of glucose homeostasis.

TRANSGENIC NEUROPEPTIDE MODELS OF OBESITY—OTHER NEUROPEPTIDES

Neuropeptide Y

A role for NPY, a 36-residue polypeptide widely expressed in the CNS, in the regulation of energy homeostasis was suggested after the observations that fasting induced its expression in the hypothalamus (63). Administration of NPY into the cerebral ventricles, or directly into the PVN, is associated with hyperphagia and increased adiposity (64–67). Surprisingly, *Npy* knockout mice exhibit normal body weight (68), or were only slightly obese on the obesity-prone C57BL/6J genetic background (69). NPY deficiency, however, attenuates the obese phenotype of leptin-deficient Lep^{ob}/Lep^{ob} mice (70), indicating that NPY plays some role in energy balance regulation, possibly downstream of leptin signaling. Moreover, transgenic mice that overexpress NPY in the brain exhibit mild hyperphagia and obesity when fed a high-sucrose diet (71). As discussed earlier, specific ablation of AgRP neurons, which co-express NPY, is associated with hypophagia and loss of body weight, indicating that NPY/AgRP neurons are critical for normal energy homeostasis. As with any gene knockout model, the possibility exists that other genes may compensate for the loss of a single molecule from an early age, and that this may therefore attenuate the phenotype that may result from deletion of the gene from an adult system.

Six NPY receptors have been identified, with the Y1, Y2 and Y5 isoforms deleted by homologous recombination in mice (72–74). In each of these knockout mice, and surprisingly for loss of an orexigenic signal, a mild form of lateonset obesity was observed. The effects of each knockout were subtle and varied. For example, hyperphagia was evident in Y5 knockout mice but not in Y1-deficient mice. Y1 and Y2 knockout mice also exhibited a normal hyperphagic response to NPY administration whereas Y5 knockout mice did not. Moreover, while NPY deficiency attenuates obesity of Lep^{ob}/Lep^{ob} mice, loss of the NPY Y5 receptor has no effect on obesity of Lep^{ob}/Lep^{ob} mice (73). The different NPY knockout models also exhibited varying degrees of reduced energy expenditure, sexual dimorphism, and susceptibility to diet-induced obesity. The body of work to date suggests a complex role for NPY and its receptors in energy balance regulation.

Melanin-Concentrating Hormone

Melanin-concentrating hormone (MCH) is a lateral hypothalamic cyclic neuropeptide that was first proposed to have a role in energy balance after the discovery that its expression was increased in the brain of Lep^{ob}/Lep^{ob} mice compared to wild type littermates (75). Furthermore, acute i.c.v. administration of MCH resulted in rapid hyperphagia (75), and chronic i.c.v. infusion resulted in profound hyperphagia associated with increased body weight in mice (76).

A transgenic mouse model that over expresses *Mch* was created by insertion of a large 70 kb section of DNA containing the *Mch* gene into ES cells and subsequent injection of positive clones into the pronucleus of fertilized oocytes from FVB mice. The transgene was later backcrossed onto the C57Bl6/J background. In both strains *Mch* overexpression resulted in increased food intake and moderate obesity compared to nontransgenic mice (77). These mice also exhibited insulin resistance, hyperglycemia and hyperleptinemia (77). Conversely, mice with targeted deletion of the *Mch* gene were lean, and exhibited hypophagia and elevated resting energy expenditure (78). Inactivation of the *Mch* gene in Lep^{ob}/Lep^{ob} mice also attenuated the obese phenotype without resolving the hyperphagia (69).

MCH functions via two G-protein coupled receptors, MCH1R and MCH2R. To further investigate the role of MCH in energy balance Marsh et al. ablated *Mch1* in mice (*Mch1r–/–* mice) and observed that while body weight was unaffected, *Mchr1–/–* mice had reduced adiposity, but were hyperphagic (79). These results were recapitulated by Chen et al. who also observed that *Mchr1–/–* mice were resistant to obesity induced by high fat diet (80). Furthermore *Mchr1–/–* mice demonstrated increased locomotor activity which might contribute to their elevated energy expenditure and lean phenotype (79–81).

Brain-Derived Neurotrophic Factor

Brain-derived neurotrophic factor (BDNF) and its receptor neurotrophic tyrosine kinase, receptor, type 2 (TRKB) are widely expressed in the CNS. Homozygous knockout mice are embryonic lethal, however mice that are haploinsufficient for *Bdnf* are obese and hyperphagic, coupled with aggressive behavior, presumably associated with dysfunctional serotonin receptors (82). A conditional knockout model of *Bdnf* using Cre-*lox*P produced a very similar model of late onset obesity; however, these mice exhibited hyperactivity and anxiety-like behavior instead of being aggressive (83). Conditional *Bdnf* knockouts also exhibited high levels of insulin, glucose, leptin, and cholesterol, and reminiscent of mouse models of melanocortin system blockade, they also exhibited increased longitudinal growth (83).

Recently, the link between BDNF/TRKB signaling and the melanocortin system has been further explored using mice with a hypomorphic allele of *TrkB*. *TrkB* hypomorphs express *TrkB* at 25% of normal levels in a normal distribution throughout the brain (84). *TrkB* hypomorphs developed a mature-onset obesity associated with hyperphagia, and also demonstrated increased longitudinal growth (85). MC4R signaling was shown to regulate *Bdnf* expression in the VMH, and i.c.v. administration of BDNF peptide to A^y/a mice, a model of melanocortin receptor antagonism, blocked the hyperphagia of this model (85). Chronic subcutaneous administration of BDNF is also able to reverse the hyperphagia and obesity of A^y/a and diet-induced obese mice (86). Together these data imply that BDNF/TRKB signaling is a component of the MC4R-mediated pathway that regulates energy balance.

Serotonin Receptor 2C (HTR2C)

The effect of the central neurotransmitter serotonin (5-hydroxytryptamine, 5HT) on the regulation of feeding behavior is strongly indicated by the anorectic effect of compounds that stimulate 5HT receptors (87). 5-hydroxytryptamine (serotonin) receptor 2C (HTR2C)-specific agonists such as dexfenfluramine (d-FEN) reduce food intake, with a marked attenuation of this action observed after administration of HTR2C-specific antagonists. Mice deficient for 5-hydroxytryptamine (serotonin) receptor 2C developed lateonset obesity driven by hyperphagia (88). Mutant mice, however, responded normally to the anorectic effect of exogenous leptin administration, but this response deteriorated over time as the mice became more insulin resistant and glucose intolerant (89). This result suggested that HTR2C are not required for leptin action, and that the obese phenotype of *Htr2c*-deficient mice was probably not mediated by perturbed leptin signaling.

Muscarinic 3 Receptor (M3R)

The muscarinic acetylcholine receptors (M1-5R) are involved in the regulation of many physiological functions. Deletion of *M3r* in mice (*M3R–/–* mice) reduced food intake and body weight, and reduced insulin, leptin and triglyceride levels (90). *Mch* gene expression in the hypothalamus was lower in *M3R–/–* mice, and

M3R–/– mice were also unresponsive to exogenous administration of an AgRP analogue. It appeared that low *Mch* expression coupled with reduced efficacy of AgRP at central melanocortin receptors were the strongest contributing factors to the hypophagic and lean phenotype of *M3R–/–* mice (90). Recent analysis of *M3R–/–* mice revealed reduced plasma glucagon levels and attenuated insulin response to an oral glucose load suggesting that loss of M3R in peripheral tissues, particularly the pancreas, may also be contributing to their phenotype (91).

TRANSGENIC NEUROPEPTIDE MODELS OF OBESITY—LEPTIN AND INSULIN SIGNALING

Two of the most well characterized endocrine signals that target arcuate NPY/ AgRP and POMC neurons are leptin and insulin. In this section, we will discuss the central molecular pathways of leptin and insulin signaling and how modulation of these mechanisms can affect body weight.

Leptin Receptor (LEPR)

As described earlier, $Lepr^{db}/Lepr^{db}$ mice are monogenic models of obesity as a result of a mutation that leads to production of nonfunctional leptin receptor. However, *Lepr* is expressed in a wide variety of tissues indicating possible peripheral effects of reduced leptin signaling in the development of obesity. To address this Cohen et al. used the Cre-*lox*P system to specifically delete *Lepr* from neurons using the synapsin-1 promoter, as well as from hepatocytes using the albumin promoter. Although the degree of Cre-mediated recombination in neurons was variable, the investigators were able to conclude that in those mice in which *Lepr* mRNA was reduced by 85% or more, obesity was also observed. These mice were hyperleptinemic, hyperinsulinemic, hyperglycemic and had markedly enlarged livers with severe steatosis (92). Selective deletion of *Lepr* from the liver, however, did not affect body weight, adiposity or liver phenotype (92). Another model of neuron-specific *Lepr* deletion was able to recapitulate the obese, hyperleptinemic, hyper-insulinemic and glucose intolerant phenotype (93). Conversely, homozygous expression of a neural-specific *Lepr* transgene, using the neural-specific enolase (NSE) promoter, almost fully corrects the excessive body weight and adiposity of $Lepr^{db}/Lepr^{db}$ mice (94). Furthermore, restoration of leptin signaling in the ARC of another model of Flp-mediated neuronal-specific *Lepr* deletion, reduced the hyper-insulinemia and normalized glucose levels of these mice, and was coupled with mild reductions in body weight and food intake (95).

The Cre/*lox*P system was also used to generate mice with leptin receptors deleted specifically from POMC-expressing neurons (96). These mice exhibited a mild form of obesity and hyperleptinemia, confirming that whilst leptin signaling via hypothalamic POMC neurons is necessary for some of leptin's effects on body weight, other leptin-independent signals are required.

Taken together, results from studies investigating condition *Lepr* mutants and infusion of leptin directly into ventricles strongly indicate an important role for the hypothalamus in mediating the functions of leptin in energy homeostasis.

Leptin Receptor Signaling Pathways

Specific hypothalamic targets of leptin have now been identified. Leptin is known to directly activate POMC neurons (97,98), and inhibit NPY/AgRP neurons (99) in the ARC of the hypothalamus. Therefore reduced central leptin signaling is proposed to lead to increased levels of NPY and reduced melanocortin tone which manifests as positive energy balance, increased feeding behavior and ultimately profound Metabolic Syndrome.

The neural response to leptin receptor activation primarily involves activation of the Janus kinase (JAK) and signal transducer and activator of transcription pathway (STAT) pathway, and also the molecule suppressor of cytokine signaling-3 (SOCS3), which inhibits leptin-mediated JAK/STAT activation (100,101). SOCS3, activated by leptin-receptor induced activation of STAT3 (102), is purported to act as a feedback inhibitor of leptin signaling (103,104). In agreement with this prescribed function, mice with heterozygous *Socs3* deficiency (*Socs3*$^{+/-}$ mice) displayed greater sensitivity to chronic leptin administration (105). In addition, *Socs3*$^{+/-}$ mice were resistant to high fat diet-induced obesity, hyperphagia, hyper-leptinemia and hyperinsulinemia (105). Similar phenotypes were also reported in mice with targeted deletion of *Socs3* specifically in neurons using the Cre-*loxP* system (106). Socs3 is therefore an important molecular mediator of neuronal leptin sensitivity.

The activation of STAT3 by leptin is similarly critical for appropriate leptin signaling. Neuronal deletion of *Stat3* (*Stat3*$^{N-/-}$ mice) recapitulated the leptin-deficient phenotype of *Lep*^{ob}/*Lep*^{ob} and *Lepr*^{db}/*Lepr*^{db} mice including hyperphagia, obesity, diabetes, hepatic steatosis and hepatomegaly, and hyperlipidemia (107). *Stat3*$^{N-/-}$ mice also exhibited reduced energy expenditure and were shorter than wild type littermates. Bates et al. created a mouse model with a Tyr^{1138}Ser substitution in the leptin receptor protein, so-called *s/s* mice (102). The tyrosine residue at 1138 is specifically required for leptin receptor mediated activation of STAT3. These mice displayed a phenotype similar to *Lepr*^{db}/*Lepr*^{db} mice including hyperphagia, obesity, hyperinsulinemia and hyperleptinemia. Later studies revealed that *s/s* mice were not as insulin resistant or as hyperglycemic as *Lep*^{ob}/*Lep*^{ob} or *Lepr*^{db}/*Lepr*^{db} mice (108). Although STAT3 is clearly important in the regulation of central leptin sensitivity via its activity on SOCS3 and therefore feeding and adiposity, leptin/STAT3-independent signals may be involved in the regulation of glucose metabolism.

Insulin Receptor Signaling

Insulin was one of the earliest afferent signals proposed to be an adiposity feedback mechanism to the brain when it was observed that central injections of insulin inhibited food intake in primates (109). Insulin, like leptin, circulates in proportion to body fat stores, is transported into the brain, and its receptor is located in discrete brain regions associated with feeding behavior (110). To show that the CNS is a key regulator of insulin-mediated effects on body weight homeostasis mice with downregulation of insulin receptors in the ARC by transgenic neuronal-specific deletion—mice known as NIRKO mice—were created. NIRKO mice exhibited moderate late onset obesity and dysregulated glucose homeostasis, as well as impaired reproductive capacity (111). Insulin signaling in the brain is clearly able to regulate energy homeostasis.

The primary pathway of insulin signal transduction is thought to be mediated by activation of the insulin receptor substrate-phosphatidylinositol 3-OH kinase (IRS-PI3K) pathway (112). Indeed, global deletion of IRS2 leads to diabetes and insulin resistance due to pancreatic -cell dysfunction (113), and targeted deletion of IRS2 specifically from hypothalamic neurons results in obesity, and insulin and leptin resistance (114). Recent evidence suggests that leptin is also able to activate the IRS-PI3K pathway, which may be necessary for its ability to inhibit NPY/AgRP neurons (115,116). A recent elegant study using the Cre-*lox*P system showed that specific deletion of IRS2 from a poorly characterized population of hypothalamic neurons and pancreatic β cells (*RipCreIrs2KO* mice), as well as deletion of IRS2 from all neurons (*NesCreIrs2KO* mice) resulted in obesity, hyperphagia and increased body length, but that deletion of IRS2 from POMC-expressing arcuate neurons did not (117). Furthermore, *RipCreIrs2KO* and *NesCreIrs2KO* mice were not leptin resistant, suggesting that the IRS-PI3K pathway may not be a requirement for leptin-mediated effects on energy balance.

It is clear that leptin and insulin overlap at multiple levels in neuronal pathways important for the regulation of energy balance. Specific animal models that have one or more of these components deleted from specific neuronal populations are, and will continue to be, useful in determining the precise mechanisms of central leptin and insulin signaling.

TRANSGENIC NEUROPEPTIDE MODELS OF OBESITY—EMERGING TARGETS

SH2B Adaptor Protein 1 (SH2B)

In a yeast two-hybrid screen for proteins that interact with JAK2, a member of the Jak family of tyrosine kinases, Rui et al. isolated a novel protein termed SH2B (118). Targeted deletion of *Sh2B* by homologous recombination resulted in a mouse that displayed insulin resistance and diabetes (119), as well as marked obesity due to severe hyperphagia, hyperleptinemia, hyperlipidemia and hepatic steatosis (120). SH2B was proposed to act as a mediator of leptin signaling via its interaction with JAK2, and the ability of high levels of SH2B to restore blocked leptin signaling in cell culture supports this hypothesis. If SH2B is to be an important central component of the leptin signaling pathway that regulates body weight transgenic overexpression of *Sh2B* in mice should enhance, or mimic, leptin's effects and result in a lean phenotype.

SHP2 or Protein Tyrosine Phosphatase, Non-receptor Type 11 (PTPN11)

Neuronal SHP2 is a Src-homology 2-containing tyrosine phosphatase (also called protein tyrosine phosphatase, nonreceptor type 11) that has been implicated in a variety of growth factor and cytokine signaling pathways, although its specific physiological function remains largely unknown. SHP2 is recruited to the leptin receptor upon phosphorylation of the tyrosine residue at position 985 where it subsequently activates the ERK/*c-fos* signaling pathway (121). Recently, the Cre-*lox*P system was utilized to generate conditional neuronal specific *Shp2* knockout mice, (CaMKIIα-Cre:Shp2$^{flox/flox}$, or CaSKO mice) (122). These mice were characterized by earlyonset obesity without hyperphagia, increased levels of insulin, glucose, leptin and triglycerides, and exhibited hepatomegaly and hepatic steatosis (12). CaSKO mice also exhibited increased expression of the lipogenic genes *Fasn* and *Scd1*. The ability of leptin to induce ERK activity in the ARC was severely abrogated in CaSKO mice, whereas hypothalamic JAK2 and STAT3 tyrosine phosphorylation levels were modestly enhanced (122). These data suggest a key role for SHP2 in mediating hypothalamic leptin signaling by suppressing JAK-STAT activation by leptin while at the same time promoting ERK activity.

Protein Tyrosine Phosphatase 1B (PTP1B)

PTP1B is a tyrosine phosphatase implicated in the negative feedback of signaling from receptor tyrosine kinases such as the insulin receptor (123), and also the leptin receptor. Mice deficient for *Ptp1b* (*Ptp1b–/–* mice) have enhanced insulin sensitivity, and are also resistant to diet-induced obesity (124). Insulin receptor phosphorylation in liver and muscle of *Ptp1b–/–* mice was significantly increased, further indicating a role for PTP1B as a negative regulator of insulin signaling. Recent studies however, have also shown that PTP1B regulates leptin signaling, primarily by dephosphorylating Janus kinase 2 (a protein tyrosine kinase) (JAK2) (125,126), and signal transducer and activator of transcription 3 (STAT3) (127). Inhibitors of PTP1B signaling may therefore be useful as therapeutic tools for the treatment of obesity and diabetes.

Syndecan 1 (SDC1) and 3 (SDC3)

The syndecans are a family of heparin sulfate proteoglycans that are implicated in melanocortin signaling, particularly the neural member, syndecan-3, which is proposed to facilitate and potentiate AgRP signaling (128). A transgenic mouse overexpressing syndecan-1 in the hypothalamus was created and resulted in lateonset obesity and hyperphagia (129). *Sdc3* null mice fail to respond to fasting-induced hyperphagia, and are resistant to diet-induced obesity (130). Investigating the function of the syndecans, and SDC3 in particular, will add to our understanding of melanocortin signaling and regulation of energy balance.

Neuromedin U

Neuromedin U (NMU) is one of a family of new peptides that is linked to the central regulation of body weight. Administration of NMU centrally to rats resulted in reduced body weight. *Nmu* null mice are obese, exhibit reduced energy expenditure, and have elevated insulin, leptin, triglyceride and free fatty acid levels (131). Conversely, transgenic overexpression of *Nmu* in the brain caused leanness and hypophagia (132). NMU functions via two differentially expressed receptors (133), although its specific signaling pathways remain unknown. NMU, or even other members of the neuromedin family (134), may be critically involved in the regulation of feeding behavior.

CONCLUSION

We have provided a broad outline of the current knowledge and transgenic tools used for investigation of the molecular machinery of the hypothalamic neuronal circuitry underlying energy balance regulation. The creation of transgenic animals, using models involving the over expression or targeted deletion of genes, has greatly enhanced our knowledge base. A great deal of work remains, however, in order to generate a complete and integrated understanding of how these central molecules interact with peripheral signaling factors. Our ability to manipulate genes will no doubt accelerate this process.

REFERENCES

1. van der Weyden L, Adams DJ, Bradley A. Tools for targeted manipulation of the mouse genome. Physiol Genomics 2002; 11:133–64.

2. Sauer B, Henderson N. Cre-stimulated recombination at loxP-containing DNA sequences placed into the mammalian genome. Nucleic Acids Res 1989; 17:147–61.
3. Dymecki SM. Flp recombinase promotes site-specific DNA recombination in embryonic stem cells and transgenic mice. Proc Natl Acad Sci USA 1996; 93:6191–6.
4. Rodriguez CI, Buchholz F, Galloway J, et al. High-efficiency deleter mice show that FLPe is an alternative to Cre-loxP. Nat Genet 2000; 25:139–40.
5. Le Y, Sauer B. Conditional gene knockout using cre recombinase. Methods Mol Biol 2000; 136:477–85.
6. Saper C, Chou T, Elmquist J. The need to feed. Homeostatic and hedonic control of eating. Neuron 2002; 36:199.
7. Cone RD. Anatomy and regulation of the central melanocortin system. Nat Neurosci 2005; 8:571–8.
8. Grill HJ, Kaplan JM. The neuroanatomical axis for control of energy balance. Front Neuroendocrinol 2002; 23:2–40.
9. Cone RD, Low MJ, Elmquist JK, et al. Neuroendocrinology. In: Larsen PR, Kronenberg HM, Melmed S, Polonsky KS, eds. Williams Textbook of Endocrinology. 10th ed. Philadelphia: Saunders, 2003:81–176.
10. Bouret SG, Draper SJ, Simerly RB. Trophic action of leptin on hypothalamic neurons that regulate feeding. Science 2004; 304:108–10.
11. Bouret SG, Draper SJ, Simerly RB. Formation of projection pathways from the arcuate nucleus of the hypothalamus to hypothalamic regions implicated in the neural control of feeding behavior in mice. J Neurosci 2004; 24:2797–805.
12. Bouret SG, Simerly RB. Minireview: Leptin and development of hypothalamic feeding circuits. Endocrinology 2004; 145:1–6.
13. Fan W, Ellacott KL, Halatchev IG, et al. Cholecystokinin-mediated suppression of feeding involves the brainstem melanocortin system. Nat Neurosci 2004; 7:335–6.
14. Coll AP, Farooqi IS, Challis BG, et al. Proopiomelanocortin and energy balance: insights from human and murine genetics. J Clin Endocrinol Metab 2004; 89:2557–62.
15. Cone RD, Mountjoy KG, Robbins LS, et al. Cloning and functional characterization of a family of receptors for the melanotropic peptides. Ann N Y Acad Sci 1993; 680: 342–63.
16. Roselli-Rehfuss L, Mountjoy KG, Robbins LS, et al. Identification of a receptor for gamma melanotropin and other proopiomelanocortin peptides in the hypothalamus and limbic system. Proc Natl Acad Sci U S A 1993; 90:8856–60.
17. Abbott CR, Rossi M, Kim M, et al. Investigation of the melanocyte stimulating hormones on food intake. Lack Of evidence to support a role for the melanocortin-3-receptor. Brain Res 2000; 869:203–10.
18. Tung YC, Piper SJ, Yeung D, et al. A comparative study of the central effects of specific POMC-derived melanocortin peptides on food intake and body weight in Pomc null mice. Endocrinology 2006; 147(12):5940–7.
19. Heisler LK, Cowley MA, Tecott LH, et al. Activation of central melanocortin pathways by fenfluramine. Science 2002; 297:609–11.
20. Heisler LK, Jobst EE, Sutton GM, et al. Serotonin reciprocally regulates melanocortin neurons to modulate food intake. Neuron 2006; 51:239–49.
21. Chen AS, Marsh DJ, Trumbauer ME, et al. Inactivation of the mouse melanocortin-3 receptor results in increased fat mass and reduced lean body mass. Nat Genet 2000; 26:97–102.
22. Marsh DJ, Hollopeter G, Huszar D, et al. Response of melanocortin-4 receptor-deficient mice to anorectic and orexigenic peptides. Nat Genet 1999; 21:119–22.
23. Chen AS, Metzger JM, Trumbauer ME, et al. Role of the melanocortin-4 receptor in metabolic rate and food intake in mice. Transgenic Res 2000; 9:145–54.
24. Cheung CC, Clifton DK, Steiner RA. Proopiomelanocortin neurons are direct targets for leptin in the hypothalamus. Endocrinology 1997; 138:4489–92.
25. Wilson BD, Bagnol D, Kaelin CB, et al. Physiological and anatomical circuitry between Agouti-related protein and leptin signaling. Endocrinology 1999; 140:2387–97.
26. Seeley RJ, Yagaloff KA, Fisher SL, et al. Melanocortin receptors in leptin effects. Nature 1997; 390:349.

27. Barsh GS, Schwartz MW. Genetic approaches to studying energy balance: perception and integration. Nat Rev Genet 2002; 3:589–600.

28. Jobst EE, Enriori PJ, Cowley MA. The electrophysiology of feeding circuits. Trends Endocrinol Metab 2004; 15:488–99.

29. Schwartz MW, Porte D. Diabetes, obesity, and the brain. Science 2005; 307:375–9.

30. Zigman JM, Elmquist JK. Minireview: From anorexia to obesity—the yin and yang of body weight control. Endocrinology 2003; 144:3749–56.

31. Challis BG, Coll AP, Yeo GS, et al. Mice lacking proopiomelanocortin are sensitive to high-fat feeding but respond normally to the acute anorectic effects of peptide-YY (3-36). Proc Natl Acad Sci USA 2004; 101:4695–700.

32. Yaswen L, Diehl N, Brennan MB, et al. Obesity in the mouse model of pro-opiomelanocortin deficiency responds to peripheral melanocortin. Nat Med 1999; 5:1066–70.

33. Smart JL, Tolle V, Low MJ. Glucocorticoids exacerbate obesity and insulin resistance in neuron-specific proopiomelanocortin-deficient mice. J Clin Invest 2006; 116: 495–505.

34. Savontaus E, Breen TL, Kim A, et al. Metabolic effects of transgenic melanocyte-stimulating hormone overexpression in lean and obese mice. Endocrinology 2004; 145:3881–91.

35. Mizuno TM, Kelley KA, Pasinetti GM, et al. Transgenic neuronal expression of proopiomelanocortin attenuates hyperphagic response to fasting and reverses meta-bolic impairments in leptin-deficient obese mice. Diabetes 2003; 52:2675–683.

36. van den Top M, Lee K, Whyment AD, et al. Orexigen-sensitive NPY/AgRP pace-maker neurons in the hypothalamic arcuate nucleus. Nat Neurosci 2004; 7:493–4.

37. Rossi M, Kim MS, Morgan DG, et al. A C-terminal fragment of Agouti-related protein increases feeding and antagonizes the effect of alpha-melanocyte stimulating hormone in vivo. Endocrinology 1998; 139:4428–31.

38. Ollmann MM, Wilson BD, Yang YK, et al. Antagonism of central melanocortin receptors in vitro and in vivo by agouti-related protein. Science 1997; 278:135–8.

39. Yang YK, Thompson DA, Dickinson CJ, et al. Characterization of Agouti-related protein binding to melanocortin receptors. Mol Endocrinol 1999; 13:148–55.

40. Shutter JR, Graham M, Kinsey AC, et al. Hypothalamic expression of ART, a novel gene related to agouti, is up-regulated in obese and diabetic mutant mice. Genes Dev 1997; 11:593–602.

41. Graham M, Shutter JR, Sarmiento U, et al. Overexpression of Agrt leads to obesity in transgenic mice. Nat Genet 1997; 17:273–4.

42. Qian S, Chen H, Weingarth D, et al. Neither agouti-related protein nor neuropeptide Y is critically required for the regulation of energy homeostasis in mice. Mol Cell Biol 2002; 22:5027–35.

43. Xu AW, Kaelin CB, Morton GJ, et al. Effects of hypothalamic neurodegeneration on energy balance. PLoS Biol 2005; 3(12):2168–76.

44. Luquet S, Perez FA, Hnasko TS, et al. NPY/AgRP neurons are essential for feeding in adult mice but can be ablated in neonates. Science 2005; 310:683–5.

45. Gropp E, Shanabrough M, Borok E, et al. Agouti-related peptide-expressing neurons are mandatory for feeding. Nat Neurosci 2005; 8:1289–91.

46. Bewick GA, Gardiner JV, Dhillo WS, et al. Post-embryonic ablation of AgRP neurons in mice leads to a lean, hypophagic phenotype. FASEB J 2005; 19(12):1680–2.

47. Wortley KE, Anderson KD, Yasenchak J, et al. Agouti-related protein-deficient mice display an age-related lean phenotype. Cell Metab 2005; 2:421–7.

48. Butler AA, Cone R. The melanocortin receptors: lessons from knockout models. Neuropeptides 2002; 36:77–84.

49. Mountjoy KG, Mortrud MT, Low MJ, et al. Localization of the melanocortin-4 receptor (MC4-R) in neuroendocrine and autonomic control circuits in the brain. Mol Endocrinol 1994; 8:1298–308.

50. Cowley MA, Pronchuk N, Fan W, et al. Integration of NPY, AGRP, and melanocortin signals in the hypothalamic paraventricular nucleus: evidence of a cellular basis for the adipostat. Neuron 1999; 24:155–63.

51. Bagnol D, Lu XY, Kaelin CB, et al. Anatomy of an endogenous antagonist: relationship between Agouti-related protein and proopiomelanocortin in brain. J Neurosci 1999; 19:RC26.

52. Huszar D, Lynch CA, Fairchild-Huntress V, et al. Targeted disruption of the melanocortin-4 receptor results in obesity in mice. Cell 1997; 88:131–41.

53. Butler AA, Marks DL, Fan W, et al. Melanocortin-4 receptor is required for acute homeostatic responses to increased dietary fat. Nat Neurosci 2001; 4:605–11.

54. Ste Marie L, Miura GI, Marsh DJ, et al. A metabolic defect promotes obesity in mice lacking melanocortin-4 receptors. Proc Natl Acad Sci USA 2000; 97:12339–44.

55. Trevaskis JL, Butler AA. Double leptin and melanocortin-4 receptor gene mutations have an additive effect on fat mass and are associated with reduced effects of leptin on weight loss and food intake. Endocrinology 2005; 146:4257–65.

56. Zhang Y, Kilroy GE, Henagan TM, et al. Targeted deletion of melanocortin receptor subtypes 3 and 4, but not CART, alters nutrient partitioning and compromises behavioral and metabolic responses to leptin. FASEB J 2005; 19:1482–91.

57. Rahmouni K, Haynes WG, Morgan DA, et al. Role of melanocortin-4 receptors in mediating renal sympathoactivation to leptin and insulin. J Neurosci 2003; 23:5998–6004.

58. Ni XP, Butler AA, Cone RD, et al. Central receptors mediating the cardiovascular actions of melanocyte stimulating hormones. J Hypertens 2006; 24:2239–46.

59. Balthasar N, Dalgaard LT, Lee CE, et al. Divergence of melanocortin pathways in the control of food intake and energy expenditure. Cell 2005; 123:493–505.

60. Butler AA, Kesterson RA, Khong K, et al. A unique metabolic syndrome causes obesity in the melanocortin-3 receptor-deficient mouse. Endocrinology 2000; 141(9):3518–21.

61. Butler AA. The melanocortin system and energy balance. Peptides 2006; 27(2):281–90.

62. Sutton GM, Trevaskis JL, Hulver MW, et al. Diet-genotype interactions in the development of the obese, insulin-resistant phenotype of C57BL/6J mice lacking melanocortin-3 or -4 receptors. Endocrinology 2006; 147:2183–96.

63. Brady LS, Smith MA, Gold PW, et al. Altered expression of hypothalamic neuropeptide mRNAs in food-restricted and food-deprived rats. Neuroendocrinology 1990; 52:441–7.

64. Raposinho PD, Pierroz DD, Broqua P, et al. Chronic administration of neuropeptide Y into the lateral ventricle of C57BL/6J male mice produces an obesity syndrome including hyperphagia, hyperleptinemia, insulin resistance, and hypogonadism. Mol Cell Endocrinol 2001; 185:195–204.

65. Stanley BG, Kyrkouli SE, Lampert S, et al. Neuropeptide Y chronically injected into the hypothalamus: a powerful neurochemical inducer of hyperphagia and obesity. Peptides 1986; 7:1189–92.

66. Vettor R, Zarjevski N, Cusin I, et al. Induction and reversibility of an obesity syndrome by intracerebroventricular neuropeptide Y administration to normal rats. Diabetologia 1994; 37:1202–8.

67. Zarjevski N, Cusin I, Vettor R, et al. Chronic intracerebroventricular neuropeptide-Y administration to normal rats mimics hormonal and metabolic changes of obesity. Endocrinology 1993; 133:1753–8.

68. Erickson JC, Clegg KE, Palmiter RD. Sensitivity to leptin and susceptibility to seizures of mice lacking neuropeptide Y. Nature 1996; 381:415–21.

69. Segal-Lieberman G, Trombly DJ, Juthani V, et al. NPY ablation in C57BL/6 mice leads to mild obesity and to an impaired refeeding response to fasting. Am J Physiol Endocrinol Metab 2003; 284:E1131–9.

70. Erickson JC, Hollopeter G, Palmiter RD. Attenuation of the obesity syndrome of ob/ob mice by the loss of neuropeptide Y. Science 1996; 274:1704–7.

71. Kaga T, Inui A, Okita M, et al. Modest overexpression of neuropeptide Y in the brain leads to obesity after high-sucrose feeding. Diabetes 2001; 50:1206–10.

72. Kushi A, Sasai H, Koizumi H, et al. Obesity and mild hyperinsulinemia found in neuropeptide Y-Y1 receptor-deficient mice. Proc Natl Acad Sci USA 1998; 95:15659–64.

73. Marsh DJ, Hollopeter G, Kafer KE, et al. Role of the Y5 neuropeptide Y receptor in feeding and obesity. Nat Med 1998; 4:718–21.

74. Naveilhan P, Hassani H, Canals JM, et al. Normal feeding behavior, body weight and leptin response require the neuropeptide Y Y2 receptor. Nat Med 1999; 5: 1188–93.

75. Qu D, Ludwig DS, Gammeltoft S, et al. A role for melanin-concentrating hormone in the central regulation of feeding behavior. Nature 1996; 380:243–7.

76. Gomori A, Ishihara A, Ito M, et al. Chronic intracerebroventricular infusion of MCH causes obesity in mice. Melanin-concentrating hormone. Am J Physiol Endocrinol Metab 2003; 284:E583–8.

77. Ludwig DS, Tritos NA, Mastaitis JW, et al. Melanin-concentrating hormone over-expression in transgenic mice leads to obesity and insulin resistance. J Clin Invest 2001; 107:379–86.

78. Shimada M, Tritos NA, Lowell BB, et al. Mice lacking melanin-concentrating hormone are hypophagic and lean. Nature 1998; 396:670–4.

79. Marsh DJ, Weingarth DT, Novi DE, et al. Melanin-concentrating hormone 1 receptor-deficient mice are lean, hyperactive, and hyperphagic and have altered metabolism. Proc Natl Acad Sci USA 2002; 99:3240–5.

80. Chen Y, Hu C, Hsu CK, et al. Targeted disruption of the melanin-concentrating hormone receptor-1 results in hyperphagia and resistance to diet-induced obesity. Endocrinology 2002; 143:2469–77.

81. Kokkotou E, Jeon JY, Wang X, et al. Mice with MCH ablation resist diet-induced obesity through strain-specific mechanisms. Am J Physiol Regul Integr Comp Physiol 2005; 289:R117–24.

82. Lyons WE, Mamounas LA, Ricaurte GA, et al. Brain-derived neurotrophic factor-deficient mice develop aggressiveness and hyperphagia in conjunction with brain serotonergic abnormalities. Proc Natl Acad Sci USA 1999; 96:15239–44.

83. Rios M, Fan G, Fekete C, et al. Conditional deletion of brain-derived neurotrophic factor in the postnatal brain leads to obesity and hyperactivity. Mol Endocrinol 2001; 15:1748–57.

84. Xu B, Zang K, Ruff NL, et al. Cortical degeneration in the absence of neurotrophin signaling: dendritic retraction and neuronal loss after removal of the receptor TrkB. Neuron 2000; 26:233–45.

85. Xu B, Goulding EH, Zang K, et al. Brain-derived neurotrophic factor regulates energy balance downstream of melanocortin-4 receptor. Nat Neurosci 2003; 6:736–42.

86. Nakagawa T, Ogawa Y, Ebihara K, et al. Anti-obesity and anti-diabetic effects of brain-derived neurotrophic factor in rodent models of leptin resistance. Int J Obes Relat Metab Disord 2003; 27:557–65.

87. Blundell JE, Lawton CL, Halford JC. Serotonin, eating behavior, and fat intake. Obes Res 1995; 3(Suppl. 4):471S–6S.

88. Tecott LH, Sun LM, Akana SF, et al. Eating disorder and epilepsy in mice lacking 5-HT2c serotonin receptors. Nature 1995; 374:542–6.

89. Nonogaki K, Strack AM, Dallman MF, et al. Leptin-independent hyperphagia and type 2 diabetes in mice with a mutated serotonin 5-HT2C receptor gene. Nat Med 1998; 4:1152–6.

90. Yamada M, Miyakawa T, Duttaroy A, et al. Mice lacking the M3 muscarinic acetylcholine receptor are hypophagic and lean. Nature 2001; 410:207–12.

91. Duttaroy A, Zimliki CL, Gautam D, et al. Muscarinic stimulation of pancreatic insulin and glucagon release is abolished in m3 muscarinic acetylcholine receptor-deficient mice. Diabetes 2004; 53:1714–20.

92. Cohen P, Zhao C, Cai X, et al. Selective deletion of leptin receptor in neurons leads to obesity. J Clin Invest 2001; 108:1113–21.

93. McMinn JE, Liu SM, Liu H, et al. Neuronal deletion of Lepr elicits diabesity in mice without affecting cold tolerance or fertility. Am J Physiol Endocrinol Metab 2005; 289: E403–11.

94. Chua SC, Liu SM, Li Q, et al. Transgenic complementation of leptin receptor deficiency. II. Increased leptin receptor transgene dose effects on obesity/diabetes and fertility/lactation in lepr-db/db mice. Am J Physiol Endocrinol Metab 2004; 286:E384–92.

95. Coppari R, Ichinose M, Lee CE, et al. The hypothalamic arcuate nucleus: a key site for mediating leptin's effects on glucose homeostasis and locomotor activity. Cell Metab 2005; 1:63–72.

96. Balthasar N, Coppari R, McMinn J, et al. Leptin receptor signaling in POMC neurons is required for normal body weight homeostasis. Neuron 2004; 42:983–91.

97. Cowley MA, Smart JL, Rubinstein M, et al. Leptin activates anorexigenic POMC neurons through a neural network in the arcuate nucleus. Nature 2001; 411:480–4.

98. Schwartz MW, Seeley RJ, Woods SC, et al. Leptin increases hypothalamic proopiomelanocortin mRNA expression in the rostral arcuate nucleus. Diabetes 1997; 46:2119–23.

99. Schwartz MW, Seeley RJ, Campfield LA, et al. Identification of targets of leptin action in rat hypothalamus. J Clin Invest 1996; 98:1101–06.

100. Bates SH, Myers MG. The role of leptin—STAT3 signaling in neuroendocrine function: an integrative perspective. J Mol Med 2004; 82:12–20.

101. Bjorbaek C, Elmquist JK, Frantz JD, et al. Identification of SOCS-3 as a potential mediator of central leptin resistance. Mol Cell 1998; 1:619–25.

102. Bates SH, Dundon TA, Seifert M, et al. LRb-STAT3 signaling is required for the neuroendocrine regulation of energy expenditure by leptin. Diabetes 2004; 53:3067–73.

103. Dunn SL, Bjornholm M, Bates SH, et al. Feedback inhibition of leptin receptor/Jak2 signaling via Tyr1138 of the leptin receptor and suppressor of cytokine signaling 3. Mol Endocrinol 2005; 19:92538.

104. Munzberg H, Flier JS, Bjorbaek C. Region-specific leptin resistance within the hypothalamus of diet-induced obese mice. Endocrinology 2004; 145:4880–9.

105. Howard JK, Cave BJ, Oksanen LJ, et al. Enhanced leptin sensitivity and attenuation of diet-induced obesity in mice with haploinsufficiency of Socs3. Nat Med 2004; 10: 734–8.

106. Mori H, Hanada R, Hanada T, et al. Socs3 deficiency in the brain elevates leptin sensitivity and confers resistance to diet-induced obesity. Nat Med 2004; 10:739–43.

107. Gao Q, Wolfgang MJ, Neschen S, et al. Disruption of neural signal transducer and activator of transcription 3 causes obesity, diabetes, infertility, and thermal dysregulation. Proc Natl Acad Sci USA 2004; 101:4661–6.

108. Bates SH, Kulkarni RN, Seifert M, et al. Roles for leptin receptor/STAT3-dependent and -independent signals in the regulation of glucose homeostasis. Cell Metab 2005; 1:169–78.

109. Woods SC, Lotter EC, McKay LD, et al. Chronic intracerebroventricular infusion of insulin reduces food intake and body weight of baboons. Nature 1979; 282:503–5.

110. Schwartz MW, Figlewicz DP, Baskin DG, et al. Insulin in the brain: a hormonal regulator of energy balance. Endocr Rev 1992; 13:387–414.

111. Bruning JC, Gautam D, Burks DJ, et al. Role of brain insulin receptor in control of body weight and reproduction. Science 2000; 289:2122–5.

112. Niswender KD, Morrison CD, Clegg DJ, et al. Insulin activation of phosphatidylinositol 3-kinase in the hypothalamic arcuate nucleus: a key mediator of insulin-induced anorexia. Diabetes 2003; 52:227–31.

113. Withers DJ, Gutierrez JS, Towery H, et al. Disruption of IRS-2 causes type 2 diabetes in mice. Nature 1998; 391:900–4.

114. Kubota N, Terauchi Y, Tobe K, et al. Insulin receptor substrate 2 plays a crucial role in beta cells and the hypothalamus. J Clin Invest 2004; 114:917–27.

115. Morrison CD, Morton GJ, Niswender KD, et al. Leptin inhibits hypothalamic Npy and Agrp gene expression via a mechanism that requires phosphatidylinositol 3-OH-kinase signaling. Am J Physiol Endocrinol Metab 2005.

116. Niswender KD, Morton GJ, Stearns WH, et al. Intracellular signalling. Key enzyme in leptin-induced anorexia. Nature 2001; 413:794–5.

117. Choudhury AI, Heffron H, Smith MA, et al. The role of insulin receptor substrate 2 in hypothalamic and beta cell function. J Clin Invest 2005; 115:940–50.

118. Rui L, Mathews LS, Hotta K, et al. Identification of SH2-Bbeta as a substrate of the tyrosine kinase JAK2 involved in growth hormone signaling. Mol Cell Biol 1997; 17:6633–44.

119. Duan C, Yang H, White MF, et al. Disruption of the SH2-B gene causes age-dependent insulin resistance and glucose intolerance. Mol Cell Biol 2004; 24:7435–43.

120. Ren D, Li M, Duan C, et al. Identification of SH2-B as a key regulator of leptin sensitivity, energy balance, and body weight in mice. Cell Metab 2005; 2:95–104.

121. Banks AS, Davis SM, Bates SH, et al. Activation of downstream signals by the long form of the leptin receptor. J Biol Chem 2000; 275:14563–72.

122. Zhang EE, Chapeau E, Hagihara K, et al. Neuronal Shp2 tyrosine phosphatase controls energy balance and metabolism. Proc Natl Acad Sci USA 2004; 101:16064–9.

123. Salmeen A, Andersen JN, Myers MP, et al. Molecular basis for the dephosphorylation of the activation segment of the insulin receptor by protein tyrosine phosphatase 1B. Mol Cell 2000; 6:1401–2.

124. Elchebly M, Payette P, Michaliszyn E, et al. Increased insulin sensitivity and obesity resistance in mice lacking the protein tyrosine phosphatase-1B gene. Science 1999; 283:1544–8.

125. Cheng A, Uetani N, Simoncic PD, et al. Attenuation of leptin action and regulation of obesity by protein tyrosine phosphatase 1B. Dev Cell 2002; 2:497–503.

126. Zabolotny JM, Bence-Hanulec KK, Stricker-Krongrad A, et al. PTP1B regulates leptin signal transduction in vivo. Dev Cell 2002; 2:489–95.

127. Lund IK, Hansen JA, Andersen HS, et al. Mechanism of protein tyrosine phosphatase 1B-mediated inhibition of leptin signalling. J Mol Endocrinol 2005; 34:339–51.

128. Reizes O, Benoit SC, Strader AD, et al. Syndecan-3 modulates food intake by interacting with the melanocortin/AgRP pathway. Ann N Y Acad Sci 2003; 994:66–73.

129. Reizes O, Lincecum J, Wang Z, et al. Transgenic expression of syndecan-1 uncovers a physiological control of feeding behavior by syndecan-3. Cell 2001; 106:105–16.

130. Strader AD, Reizes O, Woods SC, et al. Mice lacking the syndecan-3 gene are resistant to diet-induced obesity. J Clin Invest 2004; 114:1354–60.

131. Hanada R, Teranishi H, Pearson JT, et al. Neuromedin U has a novel anorexigenic effect independent of the leptin signaling pathway. Nat Med 2004; 10:1067–73.

132. Kowalski TJ, Spar BD, Markowitz L, et al. Transgenic overexpression of neuromedin U promotes leanness and hypophagia in mice. J Endocrinol 2005; 185:151–64.

133. Raddatz R, Wilson AE, Artymyshyn R, et al. Identification and characterization of two neuromedin U receptors differentially expressed in peripheral tissues and the central nervous system. J Biol Chem 2000; 275:32452–9.

134. Ida T, Mori K, Miyazato M, et al. Neuromedin s is a novel anorexigenic hormone. Endocrinology 2005; 146:4217–23.

135. Albarado DC, McClaine J, Stephens JM, et al. Impaired coordination of nutrient intake and substrate oxidation in melanocortin-4 receptor knockout mice. Endocrinology 2004; 145:243–52.

136. Smart JL, Low MJ. Lack of proopiomelanocortin peptides results in obesity and defective adrenal function but normal melanocyte pigmentation in the murine C57BL/6 genetic background. Ann N Y Acad Sci 2003; 994:202–10.

3.3   Transgenic Models in the Periphery

Isabelle Castan-Laurell, Jérémie Boucher, Cédric Dray, and Philippe Valet
INSERM, U858, Institut de Médecine Moléculaire de Rangueil and Institut Louis Bugnard, Université Paul Sabatier, Toulouse, France

Transgenesis has contributed to a better understanding of adipose tissue homeostasis and development mechanisms (1). A very large number of transgenic animal models have been created to study the involvement of adipose tissue proteins in obesity. The aim of the present chapter is to give an overview of the transgenic studies performed in this field. The application of transgenic mouse technology to the study of insulin resistance has been extensively reviewed (2,3) and will not be considered herein. We focus on genes expressed in adipose tissue that cover the main functions of white adipose tissue (WAT), from the classical metabolic functions (lipolysis, lipogenesis, etc.) to the new established endocrine function (adipokine production). Animal models created to understand adipose tissue development will be also discussed.

METABOLIC FUNCTIONS
Lipolysis

Hormone-sensitive lipase (HSL) is classically considered as the key enzyme catalyzing the rate-limiting step of the hydrolysis of triglycerides (lipolysis) resulting in the release of free fatty acids and glycerol (4). This view is supported by numerous biochemical, physiological, and clinical studies. However, recent data from HSL deficient mice led to a reassessment of the role of HSL in WAT and brown adipose tissue (BAT) fat mobilization (5,6). Although no major change in the weight of fat pads was observed, lipid metabolism was altered in the knockout mice. WAT from HSL-deficient mice accumulated diglycerides, demonstrating that the enzyme catalyzed the rate-limiting step in diglyceride catabolism (7). Catecholamine-induced lipolysis is markedly blunted as expected, but basal (or unstimulated) lipolysis is unaltered in isolated adipocytes suggesting the existence of a lipase different from HSL. A novel lipase, termed adipose triglyceride lipase, has been identified. ATGL belongs to a family of closely related hydrolases that contain patatin-like domain. Several members of this family are expressed in WAT (8). Thus, the knockout of HSL led to the discovery that HSL is no more the only enzyme involved in the lipolysis of adipose tissue triglycerides. The generation and characterization of mouse overexpressing or lacking *Atgl* (or patatin-like phospholipase domain containing 2 *Pnpla2*) will provide new insights in the concept of fat mobilization (Fig. 1).

ALBP

Proper activation of lipolysis also relies upon proteins that are not directly involved in the catalytic process. Adipocyte lipid binding protein (ALBP/aP2) is an intracellular fatty acid-binding protein highly expressed in adipocytes. Its

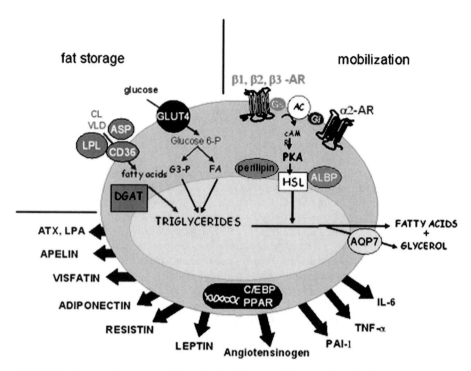

FIGURE 1 Schematic representation of adipokines and elements involved in white adipocyte metabolism and adipogenesis. *Lipolysis:* The β1-3- and the α2-adrenergic receptors are, respectively, positively and negatively coupled to adenylyl cyclase (AC) and to cAMP; production by heterotrimeric G proteins (Gs and Gi); cAMP in turns activates protein kinase A (PKA), which stimulates hormone-sensitive lipase (HSL) and catalyzes the hydrolysis of triglycerides. Aquaporin 7 (AQP7) transports the glycerol. Perilipins and adipocyte lipid binding protein (ALBP) are members of the lipase complex influencing lipolytic capacity. *Glucose transport:* The glucose transporter 4 (GLUT4) is translocated to the membrane in response to insulin. Glucose will be transformed into glycerol 3-P (G3-P) and fatty acids (FA) to generate triglycerides. *Uptake of lipids:* triglycerides contained in chylomicrons (CL) and VLDL are hydrolized by the lipoprotein lipase (LPL). The released fatty acids are re-esterified for storage as triglycerides by the diacylglyceroltransferase (DGAT). CD36/FAT and acylation-stimulating protein (ASP) are proteins involved in fatty acid uptake. *Note:* C/EBP and PPAR symbolized the main transcription factors involved in adipogenesis (common gene symbols are used in this figure). *Abbreviation:* cAMP, cyclic adenosine monophosphate.

interaction with HSL N-terminal region may avoid local accumulation of fatty acid during lipolysis and prevent their deleterious effects. It would also allow the fatty acids to be shuttled out of adipose tissue. Consistent with such a role for ALBP is the observation that ALBP-null mice exhibit a decreased lipolytic capacity (9,10). The ALBP-deficient mice show minor alterations of lipid metabolism under a standard chow diet as a consequence of functional compensation by the keratino-cyte fatty acid binding protein (11,12). However, the lack of ALBP protects against hyperinsulinemia and insulin resistance in high fat diet -induced or genetically obese mice (11,13).

Perilipin (PLIN)
Access to the lipid droplet constitutes another potential mechanism for the control of lipolysis. Perilipins are proteins covering the large lipid droplets in adipocytes.

They shield stored triglycerides from cytosolic lipases. It has been hypothesized that, upon phosphorylation, perilipins allow access to the lipid droplet and thereby allow lipases to interact with their substrates. In two independent studies, ablation of *Plin* results in mice with decreased fat mass and increased lean body mass (14,15). The mice are resistant to diet-induced obesity. Moreover, breeding *Plin*–/– alleles into *lepr* deficient mice reverses the obesity phenotype. No hepatic steatosis or alteration of the lipid profile was observed which might be due to the increased metabolic rate of the mutant animals. Basal lipolysis is increased in perilipin-deficient adipocytes, which is in line with a role of perilipin as a suppressor of lipolysis in quiescent cells. However, the results of β-adrenergic stimulated lipolysis differ between the two studies. Martinez-Botas et al. observed that the basal lipolysis in *Plin*–/– mice was similar to the maximal lipolytic capacity of wild type fat cells and that there was no further stimulation by a β-adrenergic agonist (15). The data suggest that, without perilipin, adipocytes have a permanent lipolytic drive. In contrast, Tansey et al. report that the increase of glycerol and free fatty acid release induced by a β-adrenergic agonist was markedly blunted in perilipin–/– adipocytes, which would indicate that perilipin is a necessary cofactor for full lipolytic stimulation (14). The reasons for the discrepancy are unclear. However, the issue needs to be solved as it implies different functions for perilipin.

Protein Kinase A

Surprisingly, adipocyte adenylyl cyclase, one of the major components of trans-membrane signalling associated to the control of lipolysis has not been investigated using transgenic techniques. Stimulation of the lipolytic cascade involves the phosphorylation of HSL by the cAMP-activated protein kinase which is composed of two regulatory and two catalytic subunits. Among the four regulatory subunit genes, the RIIβ isoform is abundant in BAT, WAT and brain. Targeted disruption of the RIIβ subunit produces lean mice resistant to obesity when fed a high fat diet (16–18). In both brown and white adipocytes, a compensatory rise in the RIα subunit has been described. This isoform switch is associated to an increased UCP1 expression in BAT and basal lipolysis in WAT due to the higher binding capacity of RIα to cAMP. The disruption of both RIβ and RIIβ genes leads to the same preservation of cAMP-dependent regulation by the compensatory rise in RIα protein half-life without a change in gene transcription. However, the ability of β-AR agonists to stimulate lipolysis is strongly compromised in WAT. Finally, RIα null mice show early embryonic lethality with severe developmental abnormalities confirming RIα modulation as an essential mechanism in the safeguard of pleiotropic cAMP cellular responses (19).

Adrenergic Receptors

Among the nine pharmacologically and genetically distinct adrenergic receptors (ADR), four are expressed in adipocytes. The adrenergic, alpha-2 and beta receptors (common gene symbol α_2- and β-ADRs) have opposite signal transduction pathways and are known to participate in the regulation of BAT and WAT development and metabolism (20). In addition to variations in receptor number, lipolytic rates in adipose tissue are thought to be affected by the expression of particular adrenergic beta receptors subtypes and by the ratio of alpha/beta adrenergic receptors. Transgenic mice overexpressing the human adrenergic, beta-1-, receptor (ADRB1) specifically in adipose tissue have been generated (21).

Transgenic mice gained weight more slowly and had reduced adipose stores compared to transgenic littermates, especially in response to a high fat diet. Moreover, brown adipocytes appeared in the subcutaneous white fat pads. The in vivo phenotypic effects are in agreement with the in vitro responses to adrenergic, beta-1-, receptor stimulation in isolated fat cells i.e., increased lipolytic activity of the adipocytes and greater energy expenditure through heat production by the additional population of brown adipocytes.

In rodents, the adrenergic, beta-3-, receptor (ADRB3) is expressed in fat at a much higher level than beta 2 and beta 1 receptors (22) and has therefore been proposed to be the major regulator of adrenergic responses in spite of its lower affinity for endogenous catecholamines. Although beta 3 adrenergic receptor agonists have been described as potent anti-obesity drugs in rodents, their importance remains questionable in humans. To study the physiological relevance of ADRB3, mice lacking the receptor were generated (23,24). Surprisingly, *Adrb3*–/– mice show only a modest tendency to become overweight even when fed a HIGH FAT DIET. However, a rise in total body fat was observed. Decreased action of the beta 3 adrenergic receptor was once thought to be responsible for the development of obesity. It is clear now that the absence of the receptor is not sufficient. Specific expression of *Adrb3* in BAT) or BAT and WAT confirmed that the expression of ADRB3 was indispensable in white and brown adipocytes to rescue the effects of beta 3 adrenergic receptor agonists on oxygen consumption, insulin secretion and food intake and that ADRB3 in other tissues were not required (25). The generation of mice lacking the three beta adrenergic receptors (26) confirms that beta adrenergic signalling is required for thermogenic function of brown adipocytes. When fed a high fat diet, these mice developed massive obesity (25 g weight gain in 8 weeks) due to a defect in diet-induced thermogenesis.

In human white adipocytes, the beta-adrenergic response to catecholamines can be totally counteracted by the α_2-adrenergic pathway. A large body of evidence indicates that the ratio of α_2/β-adrenergic receptor in different fat pad depots affects the lipolytic rate and is closely associated to the enlargement of adipose tissue in obese subjects (20). Because of the high levels of ADRB3 and the very low expression of α_2-ADRs, rodents do not mimic human adrenergic receptivity. To assess the importance of the α_2/beta-ADR balance in vivo, gene targeting and transgenic approaches were combined to create mice with increased α_2/β-ADR balance in adipose tissue (27,28). Expression of human adrenergic, alpha-2A-, receptor (ADRA2A) was targeted in the *Adrb3* null mouse adipose tissue. Such "human-like" mice developed high fat diet-induced obesity associated to adipocyte hyperplasia rather than hypertrophy. No apparent phenotype was observed in mice maintained in normal diet whereas when fed a HIGH FAT DIET, transgenic mice increased significantly body weight and fat mass. Thus, this obese phenotype required the interactions between two genes and diet, i.e., the presence of alpha2-adrenergic receptor, the absence of ADRB3 and a HIGH FAT DIET.

Aquaporin 7 (AQP7) is a member of aquaglyceroproteins that transport water and glycerol. The molecular mechanism involved in the transport of glycerol from adipocytes remains unclear. To verify that AQP7 might function as a glycerol channel molecule in adipose tissue, mice lacking AQP7 were generated (29). *Aqp7*–/– mice have low plasma glycerol concentration and decreased release of glycerol after β3-adrenergic agonist-induced lipolysis. In addition, knockout mice showed impaired adaptation to fasting and exhibited profound hypoglycemia.

Another group reported in older *Aqp7–/–* mice a marked adipocyte hypertrophy and increased body fat (30). AQP 7 deficiency was associated with development of obesity through activation of adipose glycerol kinase and accelerated triglycerides synthesis in adipocytes (31).

FATTY ACID TRANSPORT AND METABOLISM

The lipoprotein lipase (LPL), located on the capillary endothelium of extrahepatic tissues, catalyses the rate-limiting step in the hydrolysis of triglycerides from circulating chylomicrons and VLDL. Most LPL is found in adipose tissue and skeletal muscle, where the released free fatty acids are stored or oxidized, respectively. LPL-deficient mice are normal at birth, but develop lethal hypertriglyceridemia within the first day of life (32). To directly assess the role of LPL in adipose tissue, *Lpl* heterozygous knockout mice have been crossed with transgenic mice expressing human *LPL* in skeletal muscle and heart (33). Through backcross, mice expressing *Lpl* exclusively in muscle were obtained. Growth and body composition were not altered by the lack of LPL in adipose tissue on a standard genetic background. However, when adipose tissue LPL deficiency was obtained on the leptin deficient *ob/ob* mice, the rate of weight gain was decreased due to an impaired accumulation of lipid in adipose tissue. Triglyceride content was increased in skeletal muscle suggesting partial reallocation of dietary fat storage from adipose tissue to skeletal muscle. The chemical nature of the lipid stored in adipose tissue was markedly modified in adipose tissue from adipose tissue *Lpl* deficient mice and suggested that the development of fat stores in adipose tissue *Lpl* deficient mice relies on endogenous fat synthesis.

Acylation-stimulating protein (ASP) is a cleavage product of complement component 3 C3 produced by the adipocyte that promotes fatty acid reesterification and inhibits lipolysis. Knockout of the *C3* gene has provided a model of ASP deficiency (34,35). The knockout mice show a delay in postprandial triglyceride clearance and an increase in plasma nonesterified fatty acid levels. A moderate decrease in fat depot weights is observed on both high and low fat diets. The data suggest that ASP may play a role in fat partitioning.

CD36 molecule (thrombospondin receptor). Another potential gatekeeper of fatty acid entry into adipose cells is the transporter CD36/FAT. CD36 is expressed in tissues with a high metabolic capacity for fatty acid such as adipose tissue, skeletal muscle and heart. The adipocytes of *Cd36* null mice lack the high affinity component of long chain fatty acid transport observed in wild type fat cells (36). Furthermore, there is a defective in vivo uptake of fatty acid in adipose tissue and skeletal muscle, which results in impaired triglyceride synthesis in the two tissues (37). The defective fatty acid esterification is most likely due to a limiting supply of acylCoA which impairs conversion of diglyceride to triglyceride at the level of diacylglycerolacyltransferase (DGAT), suggesting a regulatory role for this enzyme in vivo.

Diacylglycerol O-acyltransferase homolog 1 and acetyl-Coenzyme A carboxylase beta (ACC2). Mice lacking DGAT are viable and fertile (38). The animals are capable of synthesizing triglycerides and have normal body weight on a standard chow diet. The fat pad weights are slightly lower than in wild-type control mice. However, *Dgat*-deficient mice are resistant to diet-induced obesity, which appears to be due to, increased energy expenditure. Puzzlingly, the study also shows that triglyceride synthesis can occur without DGAT. This suggests the existence of another enzyme with DGAT activity. Indeed, such an enzyme has recently been characterized and may partially compensate for the lack of DGAT (39). Increased fatty acid oxidation may also lead to reduced fat storage. This is best exemplified by the phenotype of *Acc2* deficient mice (40). The lack of ACC2 leads to a reduction of malonyl-CoA levels in heart and skeletal muscle and increased fatty acid oxidation in these tissues. The *Acc2* null mice consume more food than wild type mice, yet have a reduction in fat pad sizes.

AMP-activated protein kinase (AMPK) is viewed as a fuel sensor for glucose and lipid metabolism. The role of AMPK in adipose tissue was studied in knock-out mouse where the α2 catalytic subunit was deleted (41). The *Prkaa2* (protein kinase, AMP-activated, alpha 2 catalytic subunit) knockout mice fed with a high fat diet fed exhibited increased body weight and fat mass. The increase in adipose tissue mass was due to the enlargement of the preexisting adipocytes with increased accumulation. In addtion, *Prkaa2* KO did not show differences in glucose tolerance and insulin sensitivity. These results suggest that lack of the alpha2 subunit of AMPK could contribute to the development of obesity.

GLUCOSE METABOLISM

The glucose transporter GLUT4 [Official name and symbol: solute carrier family 2 (facilitated glucose transporter), member 4 or SLC2A4] is the major transporter in tissues in which glucose uptake is stimulated by insulin such as skeletal muscle and white adipose tissue. A decrease in GLUT4 level might therefore be responsible for the insulin resistance observed in type 2 diabetes. Skeletal muscle accounts for most of the mass of insulin-responsive tissues. Hence, it has been postulated that in vivo alterations in glucose disposal is due to skeletal muscle. Indeed, *Slc2a4* heterozygous knockout mice develop muscle insulin resistance and diabetes, which is prevented by transgenic complementation of GLUT4 in skeletal muscle (42,43). However, the amount of GLUT4 is decreased in fat cells of diabetic patients but not in muscle cells. Transgenic techniques have therefore been used to modify the level of *Slc2a4* expression in white adipose tissue. The increased *Slc2a4* expression in white adipose tissue resulted in increased basal and insulin-stimulated glucose transport. In vivo glucose tolerance is enhanced in transgenic mice. Interestingly, young transgenic mice showed increased fat mass resulting from an increase in fat cell number without a change in fat cell size. However, in old female mice, adipocyte size increases (44). To gain further insight into the role of adipose GLUT4, inactivation of the *Slc2a4* was performed selectively in WAT and BAT. *Slc2a4* levels were reduced by more than 70% in BAT and WAT without change in solute carrier family 2 (facilitated glucose transporter), member 1 expression. *Slc2a4* expression was preserved in skeletal muscle and heart. No apparent growth retardation or cardiac abnormalities were observed in contrast to mice totally deficient in SLC2A4 (45). Unlike overexpression, *Slc2a4* targeting in adipose tissue does not affect body weight or fat mass of mice eating a standard chow diet. Reduced basal and markedly blunted insulin-stimulated glucose uptake was observed in isolated adipocytes but not in skeletal muscle ex vivo. In vivo, the animals were intolerant to glucose and resistant to insulin. Insulin-stimulated whole-body glucose uptake was decreased. As expected, in vivo insulin-stimulated glucose transport was reduced in WAT and BAT but, surprisingly, the impairment was also observed in skeletal muscle despite normal *Slc2a4* expression. The data clearly suggest that impaired expression of *Slc2a4* in adipose tissue may lead to insulin resistance in WAT but also in skeletal muscle and liver leading to glucose intolerance and hyperinsulinemia. This provocative discovery renews the interest in the role of WAT GLUT4 in the development of type II diabetes but also questions the transmission of impaired insulin action from adipose tissue to skeletal muscle and liver. Recently, retinol binding protein-4 (RBP4) was identified as a secreted protein that is regulated in adipose tissue of mice overexpressing *Slc2a4* or those lacking *Slc2a4*. The authors proposed RBP4 as a potential link between *Slc2a4* suppression in adipose tissue and insulin resistance (46).

ADIPOCYTE SECRETIONS: ADIPOKINES

Adipose tissue is now recognised as a major endocrine and secretory organ, releasing a wide range of protein factors called adipokines. The number of adipokines is continuously expanding (47). We selected here a restricted number of adipokines linked to insulin sensitivity, inflammation or adipose tissue development for which the knockout or the overexpression was realized.

Leptin was the first established hormone secreted by adipose tissue. Several studies have been performed to modify plasma leptin levels since it is considered as a major regulator of the body weight set point. Mice lacking leptin such as $lep^{ob}llep^{ob}$ mice are obese. Transgenic *ob/ob* mice expressing leptin in adipose tissue under the control of aP2/ALBP promoter show a moderately obese phenotype. The infertility and several endocrine abnormalities associated to leptin deficiency were normalized (48). Hyperleptinemia has also been obtained in normal mice using the same approach (49). The mice exhibit low body weight at a young age and an increase in body weight, accumulation of adipose mass and lipid-filled adipocytes at older age (33–37 weeks). In transgenic skinny mice overexpressing leptin in the liver, a complete disappearance of white and brown adipose tissue was observed. Such a phenotype might not occur if the transgene expression is targeted to the adipose tissue (50). In addition, they exhibited increased glucose metabolism independently of body weight change, so leptin can thus be viewed as an adipocyte-derived antidiabetic hormone in vivo.

Inflammatory Cytokines

Tumor necrosis factor (TNF superfamily, member 2, TNFA or common gene symbol TNFα) is overexpressed in a variety of experimental obesity models and is a potential candidate for obesity-induced insulin resistance since knockout mice for either the gene encoding TNFA or the two TNFA receptors (p55 and p75) are protected from obesity-induced insulin resistance (51,52) and exhibit lower plasma leptin levels (53). However, this hypothesis is still open to debate since results obtained in p55 and/or p75 TNFA receptor null mice do not support the concept (54). The lack of TNF receptors did not improve insulin sensitivity or glucose tolerance of mice fed a high fat diet. The lack of receptors has been studied in genetically $lep^{ob}llep^{ob}$ obese mice (55). The absence of p55 improved insulin sensitivity while p75 deficiency did not modify insulin resistance.

Interleukin 6 (IL6) is secreted from adipose tissue during non-inflammatory conditions in humans and raised levels of IL6 are seen in obese subjects (56). Surprisingly, *Il6* deficient mice developed mature-onset obesity with mainly an increase in subcutaneous fat depot mass. The obesity was partly reversed by IL6 replacement (57). In addition, metabolic perturbations (increased circulating triglycerides levels and decreased glucose tolerance) and leptin insensitivity were observed in obese mice. These data suggest an anti-obesity effect of IL6 but mainly exerted at the level of the central nervous system.

Increased levels of plasminogen activator inhibitor-1 (PAI) [gene name: serpin peptidase inhibitor, clade E (nexin, plasminogen activator inhibitor type 1), member 1] have been linked not only to thrombosis but also to insulin resistance. PAI1 is overexpressed in adipose tissue of obese mice and humans (47) and adipocyte PAI1 may contribute to the elevated PAI1 levels. *Pai* deficient mice submitted to high-fat diet gained weight faster (between 3 and 8 weeks of the diet) than *Pai+/+* mice. After 17 weeks of high-fat diet, there were no more differences. Obese *Pai–/–* displayed higher triglyceride and lower glucose levels than *Pai+/+* mice (58). Another study showed that obesity and insulin resistance was completely prevented in *Pai–/–* mice on a high-fat diet. PAI1 deficiency also enhanced glucose uptake in adipocytes in vitro (59).

Resistin (RETN1) was initially identified as a hormone potentially linking obesity with insulin resistance (60). Subsequent studies have reported a severe down-regulation of resistin mRNA expression in rodent obesity (61–63). Recently, mice deficient in *Retn1* were generated in order to know the normal physiological function of resistin and to have a clear view of its role in glucose metabolism (64). *Retn1–/–* mice had similar gain weight than control mice fed normal chow or high-fat diet. However, a decrease of blood glucose levels after fasting specially in obese mice was obseved suggesting that absence of resistin protects against fasting hyperglycemia associated with obesity.

Adiponectin (ADIPOQ) produced exclusively by adipocytes, is considered as an insulin sensitizer and low plasma levels of adiponectin are found in diabetic patients. Three reports described mouse models with a disruption of the adiponectin locus (65–67). KO mice showed high levels of TNF alpha, increased insulin resistance and susceptibility to atherosclerosis. Additionally, transgenic mice overexpressing a truncated form of adiponectin (68) or with a deletion in the collagenous domain of adiponectin (69) exhibit amelioration of insulin sensitivity.

Angiotensinogen

The renin-angiotensin system with its active metabolite angiotensin II has been related to hypertension but also to obesity and insulin resistance. Angiotensinogen (AGT) is the precursor of angiotensin II and its production by adipose tissue is increased in the obese state. *Agt* null mice fed standard chow diet or a high fat diet gain less weight than wild-type mice (70). Adipose tissue mass was specifically altered in *Agt–/–* mice due to hypotrophy and a decrease of the fatty acid synthase activity. AGT appears to be involved in the regulation of fat mass through a combination of decreased lipogenesis and increased locomotor activity. Transgenic mice overexpressing adipose *Agt* or in which *Agt* is restricted to adipose tissue were also generated (71). In both models, increased fat mass was observed. The partial rescue of *Agt* deficiency through specific expression of *Agt* in adipose tissue led to a return to normal plasma AGT level. However, the associated increase in body weight did not reach wild-type values. Mice overexpressing adipose of *Agt* have increased levels of circulating AGT and are hypertensive.

Angiotensin II acts through two major subtypes of membrane receptors angiotensin II receptor, type 1 (AGTR1) and angiotensin II receptor, type 2 (AGTR2). *Atgr1–/–* mice exhibit attenuation of diet-induced weight gain and adiposity through increased energy expenditure (72). No difference in the ability to differentiate into adipocytes was observed between *Agtr1–/–* and wild type mice. *Agtr2–/–* mice develop normal adipose mass in spite of adipocyte hypotrophy because of an increased number of adipocytes (73). In addition, *Agtr2–/–* mice exhibit an increased lipid oxidation capacity and are protected from high-fat diet-induced obesity and insulin resistance.

Newly emergent adipokines: Autotaxin (ATX) catalyses a lysophospholipase D-activity leading to the production of lysophosphatidic acid (LPA), a bioactive phospholipid. ATX and LPA are produced by adipocytes. The expression of ATX is increased in the adipocytes of *Lepr* deficient mice but not in other obese mouse models (74). LPA by acting through LPA1 receptor is involved in preadipocyte proliferation. However LPA impairs adipogenesis. Conversely, the anti-adipogenic activity of LPA1 was not observed in primary preadipocytes from LPA1 receptor KO mice, which, in parallel exhibited a higher adiposity than wild type mice (75).

Visfatin was identified as an adipokine more expressed in visceral fat of both humans and mice with increased circulating levels during the development of obesity (76). Visfatin exerted insulin-mimetic effects. Visfatin–/– mice died during early embryogenesis, so heterozygous mice were analyzed. Visfatin+/– mice had similar total body and fat weight than control mice. They exhibed modestly higher plasma glucose levels and similar insulin levels indicating that, like insulin, visfatin lowered plasma glucose levels.

Apelin production and secretion by the mature adipocyte in both mouse and man was recently demonstrated by Boucher et al. (77). Apelin was first identified as the endogenous ligand of the orphan G protein-coupled receptor APJ. Apelin and *Apj* mRNA are widely expressed in several rat and human tissues and have functional effects in both the central nervous system and periphery. Apelin expression and circulating levels are increased in different mouse models of obesity associated with hyperinsulinemia including in humans. *Apj* -deficient mice were generated in order to study the role of apelin in the cardiovascular system. *Apj* -deficient mice do not have apparent phenotype and do not show any difference in the base-line systolic blood pressure but had increased vasopressor response to angiotensin II (78).

TRANSCRIPTION FACTORS AND REGULATION OF ADIPOGENESIS

A tremendous amount of information has been collected on the molecular regulation of adipocyte differentiation on preadipocyte cell lines. Despite the wealth of information obtained on these models, it is important to keep in mind the inherent differences with in vivo adipose tissue development. The immortalized preadipocyte cells are aneuploid. This property may induce differences in gene expression compared to adipocytes. Moreover, the cells are cultured out of the normal environment for AT, e.g. normal extracellular matrix in the presence of several cell types which can interact with each other. In that respect, the recent production of animal models with altered expression of key transcription factors for fat cell development has provided essential support for the current model of adipocyte differentiation. Several classes of transcription factors and nuclear factors have been implicated in the control of adipocyte differentiation (79). We focused on two groups of factors that appear to be essential: CCAAT-enhancer binding proteins (C/EBPs) and peroxisome-proliferator activated receptors (PPARs).

The CCAAT/enhancer binding proteins (C/EBPs) belong to the basic-leucine zipper class of transcription factors. Six isoforms that play a role in the differentiation of several cell types have been characterized. In culture systems of adipocyte differentiation, CCAAT/enhancer binding protein (C/EBP), alpha (CEBPA) and the CCAAT/enhancer binding protein (C/EBP), beta CEBPB (common symbol *C/EBP* α and C/EBPβ, respectively) are expressed early but transiently. The factors have been shown to transactivate the *CEBPA* and *PPARG* genes. *CEBPA* is induced later than CEBPB and CCAAT/enhancer binding protein (C/EBP), delta (CEBPD) (common symbol C/EBPδ). Its expression precedes the induction of many genes characteristic of the adipocytes. A severe phenotype is observed in mice lacking CEBPD and CEBPD (80). 85% of the pups die within 24 hours after birth. The survivors show markedly decreased accumulation of lipid and low expression of UCP1 in BAT. Epididymal WAT is reduced in adults but, unexpectedly, there is no alteration of CEBPA and *PPARG* gene expression or fat cell size. The decreased fat pad weight may therefore result from a lower number of adipocytes in knockout animals. However, embryonic fibroblasts derived from CEBPB and CEBPD-null mice cannot differentiate into adipocytes and do not express *Cebpa* and *Pparg*. These findings suggest that, in vivo, some alternative pathways compensate for the lack of CEBPB and CEBPD. The phenotype of *Cebpa* null mice is also severe (81). The pups die within 8 hours postpartum. Decreased expression of glucose 6-phosphatase and phosphoenolpyruvate carboxykinase 2 (mitochondrial) (PCK2) in liver may explain the hypoglycemia observed at birth. Unlike wild type mice, the *Cebpa* null pups do not accumulate lipid in BAT and WAT. Fibroblasts from *Cebpa*−/− mice have been used to investigate in vitro the role of the transcription factor in adipose tissue differentiation (82). Through induced expression and activation of PPARG, the cells undergo differentiation but they accumulate fewer lipids than wild type cells due to a defective induction of lipogenic genes. No induction of endogenous *Pparg* gene expression in CEPA−/− adipose tissue is observed indicating the occurrence of cross-regulation between CEBPA and PPARG. Another clear defect is the absence of insulin-stimulated glucose transport, which is partly explained by a decreased expression of the insulin receptor and insulin receptor substrate 1. To improve the survival of the animals, transgenic mice that express C/EBPA in liver under the control of the albumin enhancer/promoter were crossed with *Cebpa*−/− mice (83). *Cebpa* expression in liver restored the mRNA levels of known hepatic gene targets of CEBPA. The presence of the transgene improved the survival of *Cebpa*−/− mice which were investigated at 7 days of age. The knockout animals showed a complete lack of subcutaneous and visceral WAT. Interscapular BAT was present and contained more lipid than wild-type BAT. Surprisingly, mammary gland WAT developed normally. The data demonstrate that CEBPA is required for the differentiation of preadipocytes to white fat cells in most WAT depots. However, the transcription factor is dispensable for the development of BAT and mammary gland WAT. The nature of the compensatory mechanisms is presently unknown.

PPARs are members of the nuclear receptor superfamily. PPARs heterodimerize with retinoid X receptor (RXR) to bind DNA and activate transcription. Peroxisome proliferator-activated receptor gamma (PPARG) has been shown to play a critical role in adipocyte differentiation. Two protein isoforms that differ in their amino terminus region have been characterized. Peroxisome proliferator-activated receptor gamma (PPARG1) is expressed in several cell types including adipocyte cells. Peroxisome proliferator-activated receptor gamma (PPARG2) is almost exclusively expressed in adipose tissue. Targeted disruption of the *Pparg* gene provokes cardiac malformation around embryonic day 10 due to a placental defect and in utero lethality (84–86). To bypass this developmental stage that precedes the appearance of adipose tissue, three different approaches have been used which showed that PPARG was essential for adipose tissue development. First, to rescue the placental defect, chimeric embryos were produced with diploid *Pparg*–/– cells and wild type tetraploid cells that develop into extraembryonic lineages, such as placenta, but cannot contribute to the embryo formation (84). One homozygous animal developed to term. Although it had several defects and died shortly, the pup lacked BAT. Second, a study of *Pparg*–/– chimeric mice showed that adipocytes in WAT came exclusively from wild type cells whereas other organs contained a mix of wild type and –/– cells (86). Third, ES cells (embryonic stem cells) or embryonic fibroblasts from *Pparg* null mice did not differentiate into adipocytes (86). Cells from heterozygous animals had impaired lipid accumulation with decreased expression of CEBPA, indicating that the cross talk between the two factors works in both directions (85). Furthermore, cell lines null for PPARG were generated from mouse embryonic fibroblasts containing a floxed allele and a null allele (87). After immortalization, cells were infected with adenovirus expressing Cre recombinase to inactivate the floxed allele. In these cells, PPARG but not CEBPA restored adipogenesis. The data strongly suggest that PPARG is the direct modulator of adipogenesis CEBPA primary role is maintenance of PPARG level. The phenotype of heterozygous mice proved to be very informative (85,88). Fed a standard diet, the animals had similar weight gain and fat mass as wild type mice. However, they were resistant to high fat diet-induced obesity. Besides a direct role of PPARG on the development of adipocyte maturity, the phenotype may result from an increased expression of leptin accompanied by a decrease of food intake and an increase in energy expenditure. This is somewhat paradoxical because leptin production is usually proportional to adipocyte size. However, it has been shown that PPARG agonists repress the leptin promoter activity.

The ubiquitously expressed peroxisome proliferator-activated receptor delta (PPARD) has also been proposed to play a role in adipocyte differentiation. *Ppard* null mice develop normally except that they are smaller than wild type littermates (89,90). Gonadal fat stores are reduced because of a decrease in cell number rather than cell size. To determine whether the reduction in fat pad mass was due to a loss of PPARD function in adipocytes, mice with a selective depletion of PPARD in adipose tissue were produced (91). No difference was observed between wild type and transgenic animals indicating that the decrease of fat mass in *Ppard*–/– mice was a consequence of its expression in other tissues than adipose tissue.

As stated above, RXRs are the indispensable partners of PPARs. WAT expresses high levels of retinoid X receptor, alpha (RXRA, Common name RXRα). However, its role cannot be investigated in RXRA–/– mice because the fetuses die in utero (92,93). To alleviate this problem, specific ablation of RXRA was performed in adipose tissue using the/lox system (94). Mice with adipocyte ablation of RXRA did not develop obesity under HIGH FAT DIET or administration of monosodium glutamate, which provokes lesions in the hypothalamus. Adipocyte RXRA null mice had an impaired increase in plasma free fatty acid levels during fasting. The phenotype of high fat diet fed mice is reminiscent of that of PPARD +/– mice suggesting that PPARG/RXRA heterodimers are indeed essential for the formation of mature adipocytes. Data in fasted mice reveal that RXRA is not only important for fat accretion but also for fat mobilization.

REFERENCES

1. Valet P, Tavernier G, Castan-Laurell I, et al. Understanding adipose tissue development from transgenic animal models. J Lipid Res 2002; 43:835–60.
2. Nandi A, Kitamura Y, Kahn CR, et al. Mouse models of insulin resistance. Physiol Rev 2003; 84:623–47.
3. Kadowaki T. Insights into insulin resistance and type 2 diabetes from knockout mouse models. J Clin Invest 2000; 106:459–65.
4. Holm C, Osterlund T, Laurell H, et al. Molecular mechanisms regulating hormone-sensitive lipase and lipolysis. Annu Rev Nutr 2000; 20:365–93.
5. Osuga J, Ishibashi S, Oka T, et al. Targeted disruption of hormone-sensitive lipase results in male sterility and adipocyte hypertrophy, but not in obesity. Proc Natl Acad Sci U S A 2000; 97:787–92.
6. Wang SP, Laurin N, Himms-Hagen J, et al. The adipose tissue phenotype of hormone-sensitive lipase deficiency in mice. Obesity Res 2001; 9:119–28.
7. Haemmerle G, Zimmermann R, Hayn M, et al. Hormone-sensitive lipase deficiency in mice causes diglyceride accumulation in adipose tissue, muscle and testis. J Biol Chem 2002; 277:4806–15.
8. Zechner R, Strauss JG, Haemmerle G, et al. Lipolysis: pathway under construction. Curr Opin Lipidol 2005; 16:333–40.
9. Coe NR, Simpson MA, Bernlohr DA. Targeted disruption of the adipocyte lipid-binding protein (a P2 protein) gene impairs fat cell lipolysis and increases cellular fatty acid levels. J Lipid Res 1999; 40:967–72.
10. Scheja L, Makowski L, Uysal KT, et al. Altered insulin secretion associated with reduced lipolytic efficiency in aP2–/– mice. Diabetes 1999; 48:1987–94.
11. Hotamisligil GS, Johnson RS, Distel RJ, et al. Uncoupling of obesity from insulin resistance through a targeted mutation in aP2, the adipocyte fatty acid binding protein. Science 1996; 274:1377–9.
12. Shaughnessy S, Smith ER, Kodukula S, et al. Adipocyte metabolism in adipocyte fatty acid binding protein knockout (aP2–/–) mice after short-term high-fat feeding. Functional compensation by keritinocyte fatty acid binding protein. Diabetes 2000; 49:904–11.
13. Uysal KT, Scheja L, Wiesbrock SM, et al. Improved glucose and lipid metabolism in genetically obese mice lacking aP2. Endocrinology 2000; 141:3388–96.
14. Martinez-Botas J, Anderson JB, Tessier D, et al. Absence of perilipin results in leanness and reverses obesity in Lepr$^{db/db}$ mice. Nat Genet 2000; 26:474–9.
15. Tansey JT, Sztalryd C, Gruia-Gray J, et al. Perilipin ablation results in a lean mouse with aberrant adipocyte lipolysis, enhanced leptin production, and resistance to diet-induced obesity. Proc Natl Acad Sci U S A 2001; 98:6494–9.
16. Brandon EP, Zhuo M, Huang YY, et al. Hippocampal long-term depression and depotentiation are defective in mice carrying a targeted disruption of the gene encoding the RIβ subunit of cAMP-dependent protein kinase. Proc Natl Acad Sci U S A 1995; 92:8851–5.
17. Cummings DE, Brandon EP, Planas JV, et al. Genetically lean mice result from targeted disruption of the RIIβ subunit of protein kinase A. Nature 1996; 382:622–6.
18. Planas JV, Cummings DE, Idzerda RL, et al. Mutation of the RIIβsubunit of protein kinase A differentially affects lipolysis but not gene induction in white adipose tissue. J Biol Chem 1999; 274:36281–7.
19. Amieux PS, Cummings DE, Motamed K, et al. Compensatory regulation of RIalpha protein levels in protein kinase A mutant mice. J Biol Chem 1997; 272:3993–8.
20. Lafontan M, Berlan M. Fat cell adrenergic receptors and the control of white and brown fat cell function. J Lipid Res 1993; 34:1057–91.
21. Soloveva V, Graves RA, Rasenick MM, et al. Transgenic mice overexpressing the β1-adrenergic receptor in adipose tissue are resistant to obesity. Mol Endocrinol 1997; 11:27–38.
22. Collins S, Daniel KW, Rohlfs EM, et al. Impaired expression and functional activity of the β3- and β1-adrenergic receptors in adipose tissue of congenitally obese (C57BL/6J *ob/ob*) mice. Mol Endocrinol 1994; 8:518–27.

23. Susulic VS, Frederich RC, Lawitts J, et al. Targeted disruption of the β3-adrenergic receptor gene. J Biol Chem 1995; 270:29483–92.
24. Revelli JP, Preitner F, Samec S, et al. Targeted gene disruption reveals a leptin-independent role for the mouse β3-adrenoceptor in the regulation of body composition. J Clin Invest 1997; 100:1098–106.
25. Grujic D, Susulic VS, Harper ME, et al. Beta3-adrenergic receptors on white and brown adipocytes mediate beta3-selective agonist-induced effects on energy expenditure, insulin secretion, and food intake. A study using transgenic and gene knockout mice. J Biol Chem 1997; 272:17686–93.
26. Bachman ES, Dhillon H, Zhang CY, et al. BetaAR signaling required for diet-induced thermogenesis and obesity resistance. Science 2002; 297:843–5.
27. Valet P, Grujic D, Wade J, et al. Expression of human alpha 2-adrenergic receptors in adipose tissue of beta 3-adrenergic receptor-deficient mice promotes diet-induced obesity. J Biol Chem 2000; 275:34797–802.
28. Boucher J, Castan-Laurell I, Le Lay S, et al. Human alpha 2A-adrenergic receptor gene expressed in transgenic mouse adipose tissue under the control of its regulatory elements. J Mol Endocrinol 2002; 29:251–64.
29. Maeda N, Funahashi T, Hibuse T, et al. Adaptation to fasting by glycerol transport through aquaporin 7 in adipose tissue. Proc Natl Acad Sci USA 2005; 101:17801–6.
30. Hara-Chikuma M, Sohara E, Rai T, et al. Progressive adipocyte hypertrophy in aquaporin-7-deficient mice: adipocyte glycerol permeability as a novel regulator of fat accumulation. J Biol Chem 2005; 280:15493–6.
31. Hibuse T, Maeda N, Funahashi T, et al. Aquaporin 7 deficiency is associated with development of obesity through activation of adipose glycerol kinase. Proc Natl Acad Sci U S A 2005; 102:10993–8.
32. Weinstock PH, Bisgaier CL, Aalto-Setälä K, et al. Severe hypertriglyceridemia, reduced high density lipoprotein, and neonatal death in lipoprotein lipase knockout mice. Mild hypertriglyceridemia with impaired very low density lipoprotein clearance in heterozygotes. J Clin Invest 1995; 96:2555–68.
33. Weinstock PH, Levak-Frank S, Hudgins LC, et al. Lipoprotein lipase controls fatty acid entry into adipose tissue, but fat mass is preserved by endogenous synthesis in mice deficient in adipose tissue lipoprotein lipase. Proc Natl Acad Sci U S A 1997; 94:10261–6.
34. Murray I, Sniderman AD, Cianflone K. Mice lacking acylation stimulating protein (ASP) have delayed postprandial triglyceride clearance. J Lipid Res 1999; 40: 1671–6.
35. Murray I, Sniderman AD, Havel PJ, et al. Acylation stimulating protein (ASP) deficiency alters postprandial and adipose tissue metabolism in male mice. J Biol Chem 1999; 274:36219–25.
36. Febbraio M, Abumrad NA, Hajjar DP, et al. A null mutation in murine CD36 reveals an important role in fatty acid and lipoprotein metabolism. J Biol Chem 1999; 274: 19055–62.
37. Coburn CT, Knapp FF, Febbraio M, et al. Defective uptake and utilization of long chain fatty acids in muscle and adipose tissues of CD36 knockout mice. J Biol Chem 2000; 275:32523–9.
38. Smith SJ, Cases S, Jensen DR, et al. Obesity resistance and multiple mechanisms of triglyceride synthesis in mice lacking DGAT. Nat Genet 2000; 25:87–90.
39. Cases S, Stone S, Zhou P, et al. Cloning of DGAT2, a second mammalian diacylglycerol acyltransferase, and related family members. J Biol Chem 2001; 276:38870–6.
40. Abu-Elheiga L, Matzuk MM, Abo-Hashema KAH, et al. Continuous fatty acid oxidation and reduced fat storage in mice lacking acetyl-CoA carboxylase 2. Science 2001; 291:2613–6.
41. Villena JA, Viollet B, Andreelli F, et al. Induced adiposity and adipocyte hypertrophy in mice lacking the AMP-activated protein kinase-alpha2 subunit. Diabetes 2004; 53:2242–9.
42. Stenbit AE, Tsao TS, Li J, et al. GLUT4 heterozygous knockout mice develop muscle insulin resistance and diabetes. Nat Med 1997; 3:1096–101.

43. Tsao TS, Stenbit AE, Factor SM, et al. Prevention of insulin resistance and diabetes in mice heterozygous for GLUT4 ablation by transgenic complementation of GLUT4 in skeletal muscle. Diabetes 1999; 48:775–82.

44. Shepherd PR, Gnudi L, Tozzo E, et al. Adipose cell hyperplasia and enhanced glucose disposal in transgenic mice overexpressing GLUT4 selectively in adipose tissue. J Biol Chem 1993; 268:22243–6.

45. Katz EB, Stenbit AE, Hatton K, et al. Cardiac and adipose tissue abnormalities but not diabetes in mice deficient in GLUT4. Nature 1995; 377:151–5.

46. Yang Q, Graham TE, Mody N, et al. Serum retinol binding protein 4 contributes to insulin resistance in obesity and type 2 diabetes. Nature 2005; 436:356–62.

47. Kershaw EE, Flier JS. Adipose tissue as an endocrine organ. J Clin Endocrinol Metab 2004; 89:2548–56.

48. Ioffe E, Moon B, Connolly E, et al. Abnormal regulation of the leptin gene in the pathogenesis of obesity. Proc Natl Acad Sci U S A 1998; 95:11852–7.

49. Qiu J, Ogus S, Lu R, et al. Transgenic mice overexpressing leptin accumulate adipose mass at an older, but not younger age. Endocrinology 2001; 142:348–58.

50. Ogawa Y, Masuzaki H, Hosoda K, et al. Increased glucose metabolism and insulin sensitivity in transgenic skinny mice overexpressing leptin. Diabetes 1999; 48:1822–9.

51. Marino MW, Dunn A, Grail D, et al. Characterization of tumor necrosis factor-deficient mice. Proc Natl Acad Sci U S A 1997; 94:8093–8.

52. Uysal KT, Wiesbrock SM, Marino MW, et al. Protection from obesity-induced insulin resistance in mice lacking TNF-α function. Nature 1997; 389:610–4.

53. Kirchgessner TG, Uysal KT, Wiesbrock SM, et al. Tumor necrosis factor-α contributes to obesity-related hyperleptinemia by regulating leptin release from adipocytes. J Clin Invest 1997; 100:2777–82.

54. Schreyer SA, Chua SC, LeBoeuf R. Obesity and diabetes in TNF-α receptor-deficient mice. J Clin Invest 1998; 102:402–11.

55. Uysal KT, Wiesbrock SM, Hotamisligil GS. Functional analysis of tumor necrosis factor (TNF) receptors in TNF-α-mediated insulin resistance in genetic obesity. Endocrinology 1998; 139:4832–8.

56. Fried SK, Bunkin DA, Greenberg AS. Omental and subcutaneous adipose tissues of obese subjects release interleukin-6: depot difference and regulation by glucocorticoid. J Clin Endocrinol Metab 1998; 83:847–50.

57. Wallenius V, Wallenius K, Ahren B, et al. Interleukin-6-deficient mice develop mature-onset obesity. Nat Med 2002; 8:75–9.

58. Morange PE, Lijnen HR, Alessi MC, et al. Influence of PAI-1 on adipose tissue growth and metabolic parameters in a murine model of diet-induced obesity. Arterioscler Thromb Vasc Biol 2000; 20:1150–4.

59. Ma LJ, Mao SL, Taylor KL, et al. Prevention of obesity and insulin resistance in mice lacking plasminogen activator inhibitor 1. Diabetes 2004; 53:336–46.

60. Steppan CM, Bailey ST, Bhat S, et al. The hormone resistin links obesity to diabetes. Nature 2001; 409:307–12.

61. Way JM, Gorgun CZ, Tong Q, et al. Adipose tissue resistin expression is severely suppressed in obesity and stimulated by peroxisome proliferator-activated receptor gamma agonists. J Biol Chem 2001; 276:25651–3.

62. Le Lay S, Boucher J, Rey A, et al. Decreased resistin expression in mice with different sensitivities to a high-fat diet. Biochem Biophys Res Commun 2001; 289:564–7.

63. Rajala MW, Qi Y, Patel HR, et al. Regulation of resistin expression and circulating levels in obesity, diabetes and fasting. Diabetes 2004; 53:1671–9.

64. Banerjee RR, Rangwala SM, Shapiro JS, et al. Regulation of fasted blood glucose by resistin. Science 2004; 303:1195–8.

65. Maeda N, Shimomura I, Kishida K, et al. Diet-induced insulin resistance in mice lacking adiponectin/ACRP30. Nat Med 2002; 8:731–7.

66. Kubota N, Terauchi Y, Yamauchi T, et al. Disruption of adiponectin causes insulin resistance and neointimal formation. J Biol Chem 2002; 277:25863–6.

67. Ma K, Cabrero A, Saha PK, et al. Increased beta -oxidation but no insulin resistance or glucose intolerance in mice lacking adiponectin. J Biol Chem 2002; 277:34658–61.

68. Yamauchi T, Kamon J, Waki H, et al. The fat-derived hormone adiponectin reverses insulin resistance associated with both lipoatrophy and obesity. Nat Med 2001; 7: 941–6.

69. Combs TP, Pajvani UB, Berg AH, et al. A transgenic mouse with a deletion in the collagenous domain of adiponectin displays elevated circulating adiponectin and improved insulin sensitivity. Endocrinology 2004; 145:367–83.

70. Massiera F, Seydoux J, Geloen A, et al. Angiotensinogen-deficient mice exhibit impairment of diet-induced weight gain with alteration in adipose tissue development and increased locomotor activity. Endocrinology 2001; 142:5220–5.

71. Massiera F, Bloch-Faure M, Ceiler D, et al. Adipose angiotensinogen is involved in adipose tissue growth and blood pressure regulation. FASEB J 2001; 15:2727–9.

72. Kouyama R, Suganami T, Nishida J, et al. Attenuation of diet-induced weight gain and adiposity through increased energy expenditure in mice lacking angiotensin II type 1a receptor. Endocrinology 2005; 146:3481–9.

73. Yvan-Charvet L, Even P, Bloch-Faure M, et al. Deletion of the angiotensin type 2 receptor (AT2R) reduces adipose cell size and protects from diet-induced obesity and insulin resistance. Diabetes 2005; 54:991–9.

74. Boucher J, Quilliot D, Praderes JP, et al. Potential involvement of adipocyte insulin resistance in obesity-associated up-regulation of adipocyte lysophospholipase D/autotaxin expression. Diabetologia 2005; 48:569–77.

75. Simon MF, Daviaud D, Pradere JP, et al. Lysophosphatidic acid inhibits adipocyte differentiation via lysophosphatidic acid 1 receptor-dependent down-regulation of peroxisome proliferator-activated receptor gamma2. J Biol Chem 2005; 280:14656–62.

76. Boucher J, Masri B, Daviaud D, et al. Apelin, a newly identified adipokine up-regulated by insulin and obesity. Endocrinology 2005; 146:1764–71.

77. Fukuhara A, Matsuda M, Nishizawa M, et al. Visfatin: a protein secreted by visceral fat that mimics the effects of insulin. Science 2005; 307:426–30.

78. Ishida J, Hashimoto T, Hashimoto Y, et al. Regulatory roles for APJ, a seven-transmembrane receptor related to AT1, in blood pressure in vivo. J Biol Chem 2004; 279:26274–9.

79. Rosen ED, Walkey CJ, Puigserver P, et al. Transcriptional regulation of adipogenesis. Genes Dev 2000; 14:1293–307.

80. Tanaka T, Yoshida N, Kishimoto T, et al. Defective adipocyte differentiation in mice lacking the C/EBPβ and/or C/EBPδ gene. EMBO J 1997; 16:7432–43.

81. Wang ND, Finegold MJ, Bradley A, et al. Impaired energy homeostasis in C/EBPα knockout mice. Science 1995; 269:1108–12.

82. Wu Z, Rosen ED, Brun R, et al. Cross-regulation of C/EBPα and PPARγ controls the transcriptional pathway of adipogenesis and insulin sensitivity. Mol Cell 1999; 3:151–8.

83. Linhart HG, Ishimura-Oka K, DeMayo F, et al. C/EBPalpha is required for differentiation of white, but not brown, adipose tissue. Proc Natl Acad Sci U S A 2001; 98: 12532–7.

84. Barak Y, Nelson MC, Ong ES, et al. PPARγ is required for placental, cardiac, and adipose tissue development. Mol Cell 1999; 4:585–95.

85. Kubota N, Terauchi Y, Miki H, et al. PPARγ mediates high-fat diet-induced adipocyte hypertrophy and insulin resistance. Mol Cell 1999; 4:597–609.

86. Rosen ED, Sarraf P, Troy AE, et al. PPARγ is required for the differentiation of adipose tissue in vivo and in vitro. Mol Cell 1999; 4:611–7.

87. Rosen ED, Hsu CH, Wang X, et al. C/EBPalpha induces adipogenesis through PPARgamma: a unified pathway. Genes Dev 2002; 16:22–6.

88. Miles PDG, Barak Y, He W, et al. Improved insulin-sensitivity in mice heterozygous for PPAR-γ deficiency. J Clin Invest 2000; 105:287–92.

89. Peters JM, Lee SST, Li W, et al. Growth, adipose, brain, and skin alterations resulting from targeted disruption of the mouse peroxisome proliferator-activated receptor β(δ). Mol Cell Biol 2000; 20:5119–28.

90. Barak Y, Liao D, He W, et al. Effects of peroxisome proliferator-activated receptor delta on placentation, adiposity, and colorectal cancer. Proc Natl Acad Sci U S A 2002; 99:303–8.

91. Kastner P, Grondona JM, Mark M, et al. Genetic analysis of RXR alpha developmental function: convergence of RXR and RAR signaling pathways in heart and eye morphogenesis. Cell 1994; 78:987–1003.
92. Sucov HM, Dyson E, Gumeringer CL, et al. RXR alpha mutant mice establish a genetic basis for vitamin A signaling in heart morphogenesis. Genes Dev 1994; 8:1007–18.
93. Mynatt RL, Stephens JM. Agouti regulates adipocyte transcription factors. Am J Physiol 2001; 280:C954–61.
94. Imai T, Jiang M, Chambon P, et al. Impaired adipogenesis and lipolysis in the mouse upon selective ablation of the retinoid X receptor α mediated by a tamoxifen-inducible chimeric Cre recombinase (Cre-ER^{T2}) in adipocytes. Proc Natl Acad Sci USA 2001; 98:224–8.

3.4 Natural Polygenic Models

Daniel Pomp

Departments of Nutrition and Cell and Molecular Physiology, The University of North Carolina at Chapel Hill, Chapel Hill, North Carolina, U.S.A.

In addition to the many mouse models of obesity caused by spontaneous mutations, gene knockouts and gene insertions, the commonly used inbred laboratory strains of mice constitute the primary mammalian model system and are an integral component of obesity research. Within these lines, and their derivatives such as recombinant inbred lines, genome-wide congenic strains, chromosome substitution lines, advanced intercross lines, long-term selection lines, and heterogeneous stocks (HS) there exists a vast array of obesity-relevant genetic and phenotypic variation. The study of such variation, in the form of complex trait analysis including candidate gene analysis, quantitative trait loci (QTL)/eQTL mapping, and systems biology, has shed significant light on the genetic and genomic architecture of nearly all aspects of energy balance regulation and how body weight and body fat are controlled.

We initially reviewed general strategies for use of natural polygenic mouse models in obesity genetics research ten years ago (1), and more advanced strategies, incorporating many advances in both available resources and methods of analysis, were recently summarized (2). In this chapter, we focus on describing the wide variety of polygenic models that currently exist (or will exist in the near future) for the ongoing challenge of dissecting the complex nature of obesity in mice. Although a thorough review of findings (e.g., QTL detection for obesity) using these models is beyond the purview of this review, summaries of the models used in such studies (Table 1) and a consensus schematic of results (Fig. 1) are provided.

TYPES OF MODELS
Inbred Lines
Nearly 500 strains of mice have been documented in the Mouse Genome Informatics database (http://www.informatics.jax.org/) (3), although many of these are closely related and some are extinct. Phenotypic surveys of inbred lines have been instrumental is shedding early light on the extent of genetic variation in obesity related traits. For example, West et al. (4) showed that some inbred mouse strains are sensitive to dietary obesity, while others are resistant. This relatively straightforward phenotypic survey of genetic variation across standard inbred lines has spurred major activity in analysis of the consequences of high fat intake in mice, leading to many significant findings on the metabolic and genetic basis of dietary-induced obesity.

Recently, phenotypic survey of inbred lines has been formally championed by The Mouse Phenome Project (5), an international collaborative effort, promoting the comprehensive characterization of a set of 40 commonly used and genetically diverse inbred strains and their derivatives. The phenomic approach will capture complexities of entire pathways that are simply not accessible through

(Text continues on page 131)

TABLE 1 Various Polygenic Mouse Models Developed to Detect QTL for Traits Related to Obesity (Through Early 2006)

Year	Authors	PubMed accession	Lines used	Model[a]	No.	Sex	Diet[b]	Age[c]	Phenotypes measured[d]
1993	Collins et al.	8374208	QS/C57BL/6J	BC	?	?	?	?	BW
1994	West et al.	7929816	AKR/J/SWR/J	F2	931	M	H	17–18 wks	BW, FPW, adip
1994	West et al.	7929816		BC	375				
1997	York et al.	9321464		F2	931				
1995	Warden et al.	7706460	C57BL/6J/SPRET	BC(2)	402	M/F	V	17+ wks	BW, BL, BMI, FPW, adip, TG, chol, HDL, glycerol, F-FA, hepatic lipase activity, glu, ins, corticosteroids
1995	Dragani et al.	8597632	(A/J x SPRET)/C57BL/6J	?	?	?	?	?	BW
1996	Keightley et al.	8770600	DBA/2J	F2	?	M/F	U	?	(1) ? (2) ? (3) BW, tail length, adip
1998	Keightley et al.	9885188			?			?	
1999	Morris et al.	10051315			927			10 wks	
1996	Taylor and Phillips	8786140	129/Sv/EL/Suz	F2	93	M/F	H	16 wks	BW, BL, BMI, FPW, adip, glu
1996	York et al.	8703121	CAST/Ei		?	?	?	?	(1) ?, (2) BW, BL, FPW, adip, lip, ins, HDL, glu, lep, HLA (3) BW, FPW, glu, FI, diet preference
1998	Mehrabian et al.	9616220	C57BL/6J		200	M/F	H	6 mos	
2002	S R et al.	12388789		F2	502	M	V	9–13 wks	
1996	Cheverud et al.	8846907	LG/J/SM/J	F2	535	M/F	L	10 wks	(1) BW (2) BW, growth rate (3) BW, tail length, FPW, adip (4), growth 7–14 days, maternal effect (5), BW, FPW, adip, growth rate, TG, F-FA, chol, ins, IPGTT, LW, HW, KW,SW
1999	Vaughn et al.	10689807		F2	1045		U	10 wks	
2001	Cheverud et al.	11178736		F2	510		L	10 wks	
2002	Wolf et al.	12242647		F2	510		U	10 wks	
2005	Ehrich et al.	15919810		AIL	1011		L	20 wks	

1997	Chung et al.	9169130	AKR/J/C57L/J	F2	339	M/F	H	16 wks	BW, BL, BMI, FPW, adip, glu
1997	Taylor and Phillips	9268627		F2	84	F	H	8 mos	BW, BMI, FPW, fat, adip, ins
1997	Lembertas et al.	9276742	NZB/BINJ/SM/J	F2	334	M/F	U	10 wks	BW, FPW, adip
1997	Rance et al.	9449188 / 9449189	H/L	F2 / BC	794	M/F	L	10 wks	BW, FPW, adip
1998	Suto et al.	9657845	C57BL/6J/KK-Ay	F2	192	M/F	L	6 mos	(1) BW, fat, adip (2) BW, lip, TG, chol, HDL, F-FA, phos (3) glu, ins, IPGTT
1999		10101257			190	M/F		6 mos	
2002		12439655			91	F		20 wks	
1998	Brockmann et al.	9725853	DU6/DUKs	F2	341	M/F	L	6 wks	BW, FPW, LW, KW, SW
1999	Ueda et al.	10331425	NSY/C3H/He	F2	93	M/F	L	48 wks	BW, BL, BMI, FPW, ins, IPGTT, TCF2 expression
1999	Hirayama et al.	10331427	TSOD/BALB/cA	F2	144	M	L	9 wks	BW, glu, ins, IPGTT
1999	Moody et al.	10353911	BL/MH	F2	560	M/F	U	12–14 wks	BW, FPW, LW, HW, FM, HL, FI
1999	Moody et al.	10353911	MH/ML	F2	560	M/F	L	12–14 wks	BW, FPW, LW, HW, FM, HL, FI
1999	Mu et al.	10393218	C57BL/6J-db/db/ BKS (F2-db/db)	F2	99	F	H	6–8 mos	TG, chol, HDL, non-HDL, glu, lesion size
1999	Taylor et al.	10501964	C57BL/6J/KK	F2	320	M/F	H	16 wks	BW, BL, FPW, adip, glu, lep
2000	Horvat et al.	10602985	F/L	F2	436	M/F	L	14 wks	BW, DM, adip
2000	Ishikawa et al.	11003694	Wild/C57BL/6J	BC	387	M/F	U	10 wks	BW
2000	Leamy et al.	11006632	Cast/Ei/M16i	BC	400	M/F	U	12 wks	(1) mandible characters, DA, FA (2) BW, HW, LW, SW, KW, limb lengths
2002		12118102							
2000	Reifsnyder et al.	11042154	NZO/HiLt/NON/Lt	BC	203	M	L	24 wks	BW, BMI, FPW, adip, glu, ins, lep
2000	Stoehr et al.	11078464	BTBR/C57BL/6J-ob/+(F2-ob/ob)	F2	350	M/F	L	14 wks	glu, ins, pancreatic morphology

(Continued)

TABLE 1 Various Polygenic Mouse Models Developed to Detect QTL for Traits Related to Obesity (Through Early 2006) (Continued)

Year	Authors	PubMed accession	Lines used	Model[a]	No.	Sex	Diet[b]	Age[c]	Phenotypes measured[d]
2000 2001	Anunciado et al. Kobayashi et al.	11109545 12502510	SM/J/A/J(SMXA)	RIL(21) RIL(19)	20-56/s 7-16/s	M/F	U	20 wks 10 wks	(1) BW, TG, chol, phospholipids, ins (2) BW, BL, BMI, glu, IPGTT
2000	Brockmann et al.	11116089	DU6i/DBA/2	F2	411	M/F	L	6 wks	BW, FPW, adip, MW, LW, KW, SW, ins, lep, IGF-1
2001	Taylor et al.	11210195	NZO/SM	F2	328	M/F	H	16 wks	BW, BL, BMI, FPW, adip, glu
2001	Corva et al.	11309659	C57BL/6J-hg/hg/ CAST/Ei	F2	1132	M/F	L	9 wks	BW, ash mass, carcass protein, femur length, adip
2001	Kim et al.	11414755	TH/C57BL/6J	BC	206	M	L	26 wks	BW, BL, BMI, FPW, adip, glu, ins, TG, chol, HDL, F-FA
2001	Kim et al.	11414755	TH/CAST/Ei	BC	95	M	L	28 wks	BW, BL, BMI, FPW, adip, glu, ins, TG, chol, HDL, NEFA
2001 2003	Anunciado et al.	11515095 12638235	SM/J/A/J	F2	321	M/F	U	10 wks	(1) BW (2) TG, chol, phos, ins
2002	Reifsnyder et al.	11872687	NZO/HILt/NON/Lt (NONcNZO)	RIL(10)	216	M	L	24 wks	BW, BMI, FPW, adip, glu, ins, lep
2002	Masinde et al.	12185457 12185459	MRL/MpJ/SJL/J	F2	633	M/F	U	7 wks	(1) BL, LBM (2) BL, muscle size
2003	Geisen et al.	12727230	SJL/NBom/ NZO/HIBom	BC	523	M/F	V	22 wks	BW, BL, BMI, TG, chol, glu, ins, FI
2003	Almind et al.	12765967	C57BL/6J-IR/ IRS-1 DH/129S6/Sv	F2	60	M/F	H	6 mos	glu, ins, lep
2003	Wang et al.	12805272	C57BL/6J x NZB/ BINJ	BC	104	F	V	23 wks	Chol, HDL, non-HDL, aortic lesion size

Year	Author	PMID	Cross	Design	N	Sex		Age	Traits
2003	Wang et al.	12805272	C57BL/6J x NZB/BlNJ	AIL	345	F	V	10 wks	Chol, HDL, non-HDL
2003	Zhang and Gershenfeld	12855751	A/J/C57BL/6J	F2BC	514223	M/F	L	10 wks	BW, 2 wk weight gain, exploratory behavior
2003	Reed et al.	12856282	129P3/J/C57BL/6ByJ	F2	457	M/F	L	~9 mos	BW, BL, FPW, Adip
2003	Lionikas et al.	14679300	C57BL/6J/DBA/2J	F2	380	M/F	U	26–31 wks	BW, BL, MW
2003	Lionikas et al.	14679300	C57BL/6J/DBA/2J(BXD)	RIL(23)	500	M/F	U	26–31 wks	BW, BL, MW
2004	Lyons et al.	14701919	129S1/SvlmJ and CAST/Ei	F2	277	M	H	16–18 wks	chol, HDL, non-HDL
2002	Pitman et al.	12006675		BC	89	F	V	24–26 wks	(1) Chol, HDL, non-HDL, SR-B1 (2) Chol, HDL (3) BW, FPW, fat, LBM
2004	Korstanje et al.	14993241		F2	513	M/F	H	24 wks	
2006	Stylianou et al.	16416088	SM/J x NZB/BlNJ	F2	513	M/F	H	24 wks	
2004	Rocha et al.	15058380 15058381 15672592	M16i/L6	F2	990 552 439	M/F MF	U	10 wks	(1) BW, tail length, early and late growth rate (2) BW, FPW, adip, Fat, HW, KW, LW, SW (3) OR, LF, DF, PRES, POSTS, TOTS
2004	Ishimori et al.	15210844	C57BL/6J/129S1/SvlmJ	F2	294	F	H	20 wks	BW, BL, BMI, adip, TG, Chol, HDL, non-HDL
2004	Brockmann et al.	15457339	NMRI8/DBA/2	F2	275	M/F	L	6 wks	BW, FPW, adip, MW, KW, LW, SW
2004	Jerez-Timaure et al.	15483205	MB2/M16i (F2/C57BL/6J) (F2/M16i)	F2 F3 F3	1200 424 241	M	U	12 wks	BW, fat, LBM, BMD, FPW, LW, glu
2004	Cheverud et al.	15561968	LG/J/SM/J (LGXSM)	RIL(8)	256	M/F	V	20 wks	BW, growth rate, FPW, LW, SW, HW, KW, TG, chol, F-FA, lep, ins, glu, IPGTT

(Continued)

TABLE 1 Various Polygenic Mouse Models Developed to Detect QTL for Traits Related to Obesity (Through Early 2006) (*Continued*)

Year	Authors	PubMed accession	Lines used	Model[a]	No.	Sex	Diet[b]	Age[c]	Phenotypes measured[d]
2005	Yaguchi et al.	15820311	BKS.Cg-Lepr(db)+/+m/DBA/2	F2	113	F	U	9 wks	BW, FPW, LW, MW, glu, IGPTT
2005	Collin et al.	15870393	BKS.HRS-fat/fat and HRS-+/+	F2	282	M	L	24–30 wks	BW, BL, girth, FPW, BAW, FPW, TG, chol, HDL, glu, ins
2005	Allan et al.	15944354	M16/ICR	F2	1181	M/F	L	8 wks	BW, FPW, weight gain, fat, adip, LW, FI, glu, ins, lep, TNFα, IL6,
2005	Rance et al.	16180138	MH/ML	F2	515	M/F	U	18 wks	BW

[a]Models: BC, backcross; F2, F2 cross; AIL, advanced intercross line; RIL, recombinant inbred lines; RPT, recombinant progeny testing (/s per strain).
[b]Diets: L, less than or equal to 6.5% fat; H, greater than or equal to 9% fat; U, unspecified; V, diet was a variable.
[c]Phenotypes: adip, adiposity index or % fat; ALT, alanine aminotransferase; BAW, brown adipose weight; BMD, bone mineral density; BMI, body mass index; BW, body weight; chol, cholesterol; DA, directional asymmetry; DM, dry mass; FA, fluctuating asymmetry; Fat, fat mass; F-FA, nonesterified fatty acids or free fatty acids; FI, food intake; FPW, fat pad weight; HDL, HDL cholesterol; Heat, heat loss; HL, hepatic lipase activity; HW, heart weight; IGPTT, intraperitoneal glucose tolerance test; KW, kidney weight; LBM, lean body mass; Lep, leptin; Lip, total plasma lipid concentration; LW, liver weight; MW, muscle weight; NAL, nasoanal length; Non-HDL, non-HDL cholesterol; OR, number of *corpora lutea*; Phos, phospholipids; SW, spleen weight; Temp, rectal temperature; TG, triglycerides.
[d]Age for phenotypic measurements is only for final measurements (obesity data).

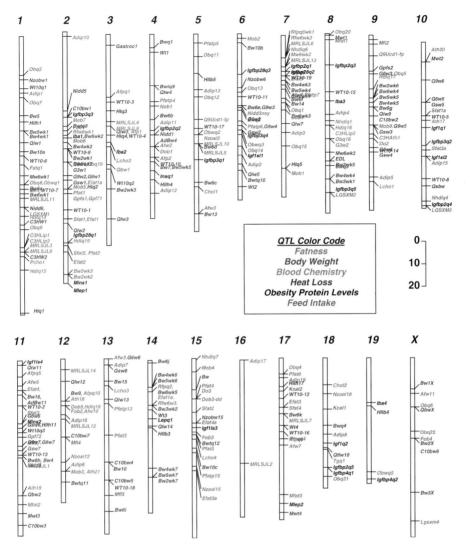

FIGURE 1 (*See color insert.*) Consensus predisposition (QTL) map for obesity-related traits in the mouse (through June 2006), representing most of the loci from the experiments detailed. *Abbreviation*: QTL, quantitative trait loci.

conventional approaches. The mouse phenome database [(MPD), www.jax.org/phenome] (6) is being populated with data relevant to many complex human diseases, including most aspects of the metabolic syndrome. Data are available for metabolism, activity, food intake, body composition, effects of atherogenic diet, leptin and insulin levels, and other biological parameters that are being used to identify and characterize new mouse models for obesity research (Fig. 2). The MPD website has a set of analysis tools for data mining, and data sets can be downloaded for custom analysis. Data are publicly available in standardized formats on a set of genetically defined and genomically stable strains. Research

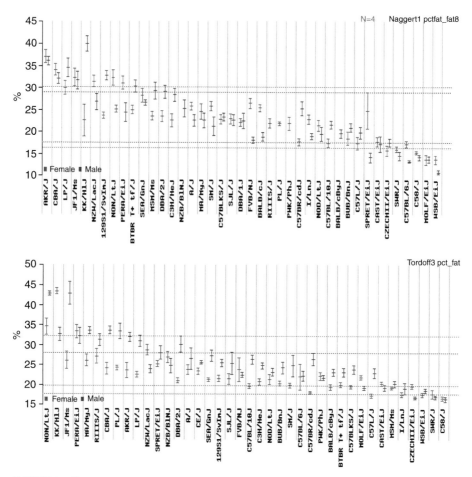

FIGURE 2 (*See color insert.*) Percent body fat after high fat (*top*) (6) and normal fat (*bottom*) (3) diets from the 40 inbred lines of the Mouse Phenome Project.

groups are moving well beyond the proof-of-principal stage by demonstrating in silico methods of identifying genes contributing to complex traits. Recent examples include identifying tumor necrosis factor (ligand) superfamily, member 4 (tax-transcriptionally activated glycoprotein 1, 34 kDa) (*Tnsf4*) as influencing athero-sclerosis susceptibility (7) and insulin induced gene 2 (*Insig2*) as a susceptibility gene for plasma cholesterol levels (8).

DERIVATIVES OF INBRED LINES—RECOMBINANT INBRED LINES

The power of the genotypic/phenotypic diversity found across inbred lines can be amplified synergistically by using them to create new polygenic models based on various strategies of crossbreeding (Fig. 3). Recombinant inbred lines were derived primarily to ease constraints of generation time and population size in genetic mapping experiments (9). There have been a large number of recombinant inbred lines created, most originating from the crossing of two inbred lines. The power of recombinant inbred lines lies primarily in that they are immortalized, and thus represent fixed polygenic models that can be

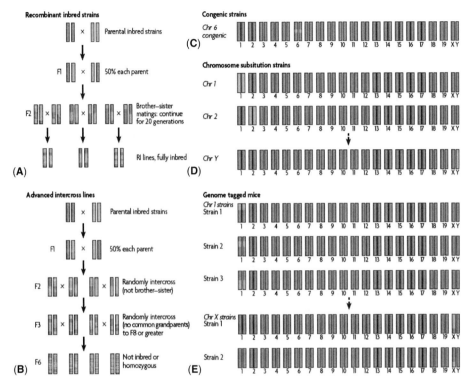

FIGURE 3 (*See color insert.*) Derivatives of inbred strains. (**A**) Recombinant inbred strains are developed by crossing two different inbred parental strains to produce F1 offspring (obligate heterozygotes at all loci). From there, a series of brother-sister matings are established, and their offspring are repeatedly intercrossed for at least 20 generations. This produces fully inbred strains, each of which is homozygous at all loci for a unique combination of the original parental genomes. (**B**) In advanced intercross lines (AILs), the goal is to increase recombination frequency, so matings between siblings and cousins are avoided. By providing large numbers of animals that carry many additional genetic breakpoints, AILs were particularly useful in narrowing quantitative trait loci (QTL) confidence intervals. (**C**) Congenic strains are produced with the goal of transferring a single locus, such as a mutant gene, from one genetic background to another. In this example, a chromosome 6 (chr 6) locus is illustrated. The mouse carrying the locus to be transferred is mated, or "outcrossed," to the strain of choice to produce obligate heterozygotes. The heterozygotes are then intercrossed, and the process of outcrossing and intercrossing, with selection for the locus of interest at all outcross generations, is repeated. (**D**) In chromosome-substitution strains (CSS, formerly called consomic strains), one chromosome in its entirety is transferred from one strain background to another. (**E**) Genome tagged mice (GTM) are similar in concept to a congenic strain, but the idea is to not only transfer a single locus to another genetic background, but to transfer large, overlapping regions of each chromosome from one strain to another, and to build up a collection of such strains that covers the whole genome. *Source*: From Ref. 2.

phenotyped deeply and in many different environments by multiple investigators. Recombinant inbred linescan also be centrally genotyped and analyzed,
and their power can be significantly extended by the use of recombinant inbred
intercross mapping (10).

Although the use of recombinant inbred lines in mapping of genes and
QTL specifically for obesity (Table 1) (11) has been relatively limited, that is
likely to change dramatically in the next several years. A new paradigm for
complex trait analysis, the "Collaborative Cross" (12), is a large panel of
recombinant inbred lines derived from a genetically diverse set of eight founder
strains (Fig. 4). By providing a large, common set of genetically defined mice,
the "Collaborative Cross" may become a focal point for cumulative and
integrated data collection for traits related to obesity in mice, giving rise to
networks of functionally important relationships within and among diverse sets
of biological and physiological phenotypes that can be altered by external
factors such as diet and exercise. Furthermore, the "Collaborative Cross" has
the potential to support studies by the larger scientific community incorporating multiple genetic, environmental, and developmental variables into comprehensive statistical models describing obesity susceptibility and progression.
Equally important, the "Collaborative Cross" will be ideal as a test bed for
predictive, or more accurately, probabilistic medicine, which will be essential
for the deployment of personalized medicine.

Although the ~1000 recombinant inbred lines that will make up the "Collaborative Cross" will not be completed until ~2009, data on most of the eight
parental inbred lines (A/J, C57BL/6J, 129S1/SvImJ, NOD/LtJ, NZO/HiLtJ,
CAST/Ei, PWK/PhJ, and WSB/EiJ, capturing over 90% of the known variation
present in laboratory mouse strains) are available within the Mouse Phenome
Project, and show a wide distribution of obesity related phenotypes. Furthermore,
data on adiposity in the many F1 hybrid combinations resulting from crossing of
the eight parental strains demonstrate broad variability (Fig. 5), indicating that the
"Collaborative Cross" will represent an excellent resource for identifying genes
controlling predisposition to obesity, and understanding the pathways, networks
and systems that control obesity.

DERIVATIVES OF INBRED LINES—GENOME-TAGGED AND CONSOMIC (CHROMOSOME SUBSTITUTION) STRAINS

Traditional congenic strains are constructed by repeated backcrossing to the background strain with selection at each generation for the presence of a donor
chromosomal region. This is a time consuming process, and is also generally used
on a case by case basis to isolate specific loci influencing obesity (13). A more
global and powerful approach is to construct a library of congenic strains encompassing the entire genome of one strain on the background of the other. Iakoubova
et al. (14) employed marker-assisted breeding to construct two sets of overlapping
congenic strains, called genome-tagged mice (GTMs), which span the entire mouse
genome. Both congenic genome-tagged mice sets contain more than 60 mouse
strains, each with an average of 23 cm introgressed segment (range 8–58 cm).
C57BL/6J was utilized as a background strain for both genome-tagged mice sets
with either DBA/2J or CAST/Ei as the donor strain.

Chromosome substitution strains (CSS, also called consomic strains) are
strains in which a single, full length chromosome from one inbred strain has been

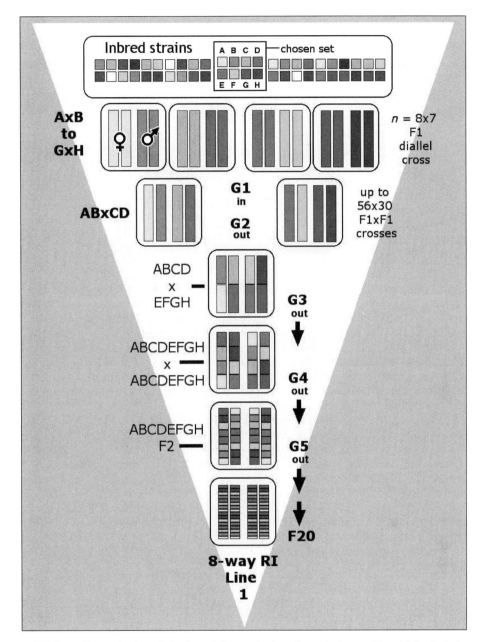

FIGURE 4 *(See color insert.)* Outline of the production of a set of recombinant inbred strains originating from a cross of eight inbred lines (The Collaborative Cross). Production of approximately 1000 such recombinant inbred strains will enable very high-resolution mapping of QTL, effective dissection of epistatic interactions, powerful analysis of gene × environment interactions, and application of systems biology to the dissection of complex traits. *Abbreviation*: QTL, quantitative trait loci.

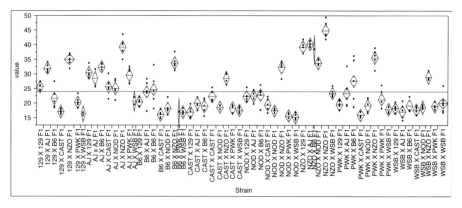

FIGURE 5 Percent body fat among male F1 hybrids of the Collaborative Cross C parental strains. Mice were 16 weeks of age and had been fed a standard chow diet. The horizontal line represents the overall mean. *Source*: Courtesy of Gary Churchill and Randy Smith.

transferred onto the genetic background of a second strain by repeated backcrossing. Phenotypic analysis of a chromosome substitution strains panel allows rapid association of a phenotypic trait with a particular chromosome (15). CSS exhibiting the trait of interest can then be used to generate a series of congenic strains that subdivide the chromosome into segments and thus refine the position of the causative locus. If two or more genes on the same chromosome interact to influence a phenotype, these additive or epistatic allele combinations will be detected in the consomic strain bearing the donor chromosome of interest and will be separated in the congenic strains thus generated.

Since construction of CSS resources requires significant time and effort, their use in obesity research is just beginning to be realized. In a CSS panel where each strain carries a single chromosome substituted from A/J mice onto C57BL/6J, a survey of 53 traits revealed evidence for many QTLs affecting diet-induced obesity (16). Another interesting example is a set of Chromosome substitution strains developed by transfer of chromosomes from DU6i, a line with extreme body weight phenotypes developed by long-term selection, to a DBA/2 genetic background (17). All analyzed chromosomes affected body weight and weight gain either directly or in interaction with sex or parent of origin. The effects were age specific, with some chromosomes showing opposite effects at different stages of development.

DERIVATIVES OF INBRED LINES—ADVANCED INTERCROSS LINES AND HETEROGENEOUS STOCKS

One of the most significant drawbacks of QTL mapping approaches is that loci are mapped broadly within relatively wide confidence intervals. This has seriously hampered translation of QTL into specific genes and mechanisms. Although QTL mapping resolution using the "Collaborative Cross" will be immensely finer, that resource is not yet available and may not readily capture some of the QTL that have already been mapped and that are awaiting identification. Two types of models have been implemented to address this problem. An Advanced intercross line (AIL) is an intercross between two lines that has been extended well beyond the normal F2 generation traditionally used for initial QTL mapping. By allowing the accumulation of recombination through intentional outbreeding over the course of many generations, the genome is "stretched," and dense genotyping can enhance QTL mapping resolution several fold (18). Several AIL have been developed from a variety of combinations of pairs of inbred lines. Two AIL with direct relevance to obesity research have been produced, including one originating from crossing of the large and small lines LG/J and SM/J (19) and another from a cross between lines selected for high and low heat loss as a proxy for basal metabolic rate (20).

A broadly powerful extension of the AIL concept is creation of HS (Fig. 6). In this case, QTL can be very finely mapped by exploiting historical recombinants that have accumulated in a genetically HS of mice descended from eight inbred progenitor strains [e.g., A/J, AKR/J, BALBc/J, CBA/J, C3H/HeJ, C57BL/6J, DBA/2J and LP/J; (21)]. This HSs resource has now been outbred for over 50 generations. Although both AIL and HSs were initially intended for fine-mapping of specific QTL regions, the current availability of very dense SNPs, and affordable high throughput genotyping, facilitates use of these models for whole-genome discovery approaches. Using the HSs, Valdar et al. (22) robustly mapped 843 QTLs with an average 95% confidence interval of 2.8 Mb. Many of these QTL contribute to variation in obesity-relevant traits, including body weight gain, activity, type-2 diabetes, and blood chemistry (e.g., high density lipoprotein, low density lipoprotein, total cholesterol, triglycerides).

LONG-TERM SELECTION LINES

Although the vast majority of mouse research employs inbred lines and their derivatives, a special class of polygenic mouse models has been instrumental in shedding light on the quantitative genetics and genetic architecture of obesity. These are the specialized lines that have been developed through long-term selective breeding for a wide variety of phenotypes related to regulation of components of energy balance, body weight and obesity. The origins of selection for obesity-related traits dates back to John MacArthur in the late 1930s and

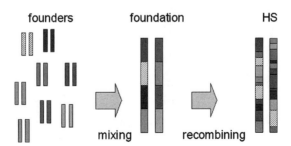

FIGURE 6 (*See color insert.*) Construction of the heterogeneous stock (HS) mice, showing one chromosome pair from each of the eight founder inbred strains and how they eventually recombine into one chromosome pair from an HS mouse that is a mosaic of the progenitors. *Source*: Courtesy of William Valdar and Richard Mott.

selective breeding for 60 day weight, while Falconer (23) pioneered the modern analysis of selection using quantitative genetic methods.

Starting from either outbred strains (e.g., ICR) or crosses of inbred lines that have been allowed to recombine, dozens of selection lines have been developed with extreme phenotypes for traits such as body weight (24), body fat (25), metabolic rate (26), appetite (27), voluntary exercise (28) and Type-2 diabetes (29), among others. Several of these lines were brought together and inbred to characterize them jointly and develop models for gene mapping (30). The range of body weights in the high growth lines is from 40 to 83 grams, with an average of 60 g (Fig. 7), a ∼3-fold increase over many widely used common inbred lines. In addition, most lines selected for high growth also have significant increase in fatness, making them useful obesity models (24).

While many of these selection lines were initially developed as models for growth and development of agriculturally relevant species such as pigs and cows, they have more recently become powerful tools for QTL detection (Table 1) (31,32) and understanding the physiological pathways controlling obesity (33). In addition, selection lines have been instrumental in testing quantitative genetic theory (34) and for estimating genetic parameters such as heritabilities for and correlations among obesity traits. At a time when such estimates in human populations were inherently very broad, heritability for fatness in mice was estimated with high precision to be in the moderate range of 50%, and genetic correlations between fat and weight, fat and feed intake, and fat and lean were accurately estimated [see review in Ref. (35)]. Selection lines were also instrumental in expanding such estimates to many other components of energy balance (20).

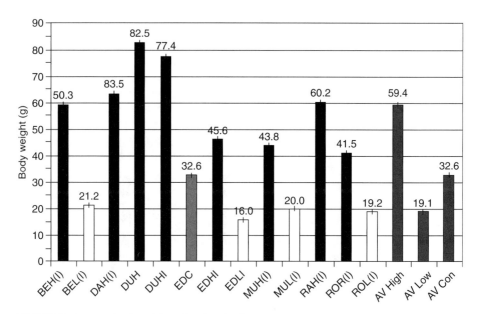

FIGURE 7 Average body weights of male mice from an assortment of lines that have undergone long-term selective breeding for high/low body weight phenotypes.

CONCLUSION

The mouse is the premier model for study of most biomedically relevant complex traits, including obesity (36). An excellent summary of resources available to use mouse models to investigate complex traits was recently provided by Peters et al. (2). The vast arsenal of polygenic models available for dissecting the genetic architecture of obesity has been instrumental is developing gene/QTL maps (Table 1, Fig. 1), which are updated annually in the journal *Obesity* (37) as part of an overall summary of the human obesity genome. The critical step of moving from QTLs to underlying genes to pathways and systems regulating obesity as a complex trait is likely to become much more feasible in the next several years with new models such as the Collaborative Cross being developed. In addition, the genomic tools available to drill down into polygenic models are developing rapidly, and with full genome sequence available for many strains and dense SNP genotyping for others, the ability to perform in-silico (haplotype association mapping) analysis of complex traits gains power (38), using the array of inbred lines already available and being phenotyped. There is reason to have significant optimism that, in regard to the genetics of obesity, we are on the cusp of progressing from the QTL era to a period of finding causal genes, understanding how they interact with each other and with the environment, and applying this knowledge to understanding predisposition to, and treatment of, body weight disregulation.

ACKNOWLEDGMENTS

The author thanks Molly Bogue, who contributed information regarding the Mouse Phenome Project; Kunjie Hua, who assisted with formatting; and John Hartmann, who was instrumental in compiling Table 1 and Figure 1.

REFERENCES

1. Pomp D. Genetic dissection of obesity in polygenic animal models. Behav Genet 1997; 27:285–306.
2. Peters LL, Robledo RF, Bult CJ et al. The mouse as a model for human biology: a resource guide for complex trait analysis. Nat Rev Genet 2007; 8:58–69.
3. Tordoff MG, Bachmanoy AA. Survey of calcium & sodium intake and metabolism with bone and body composition data. MPD:103. Mouse Phenome Database Web Site, The Jackson Laboratory, Bar Harbor, Maine, U.S.A. World Wide Web (URL: http://www.jax.org/phenome, January 2007).
4. West DB, Boozer CN, Moody DL et al. Dietary obesity in nine inbred mouse strains. Am J Physiol 1992; 262:R1025–32.
5. Bogue MA, Grubb SC. The Mouse Phenome Project. Genetica 2004; 122:71–4.
6. Naggert JK, Svenson LK, Smith RV et al. Diet effects on bone mineral density and content, body composition, and plasma glucose, leptin, and insulin levels. MPD:143. Mouse Phenome Database Web Site, The Jackson Laboratory, Bar Harbor, Maine USA. World Wide Web (URL: http://www.jax.org/phenome, January 2007).
7. Wang X, Ria M, Kelmenson PM et al. Positional identification of TNFSF4, encoding OX40 ligand, as a gene that influences atherosclerosis susceptibility. Nat Genet 2005; 37:365–72 (Epub 2005 Mar 6).
8. Cervino AC, Li G, Edwards S et al. Integrating QTL and high-density SNP analyses in mice to identify Insig2 as a susceptibility gene for plasma cholesterol levels. Genomics 2005; 86:505–17 (Epub 2005 Aug 29).

9.   Paigen K. One hundred years of mouse genetics: an intellectual history. I. The classical period (1902–1980). Genetics 2003; 163:1–7.

10. Zou F, Gelfond JA, Airey DC. Quantitative trait locus analysis using recombinant inbred intercrosses: theoretical and empirical considerations. Genetics 2005; 170:1299–311 (Epub 2005 May 6).

11. Hrbek T, de Brito RA, Wang B et al. Genetic characterization of a new set of recombinant inbred lines (LGXSM) formed from the inter-cross of SM/J and LG/J inbred mouse strains. Mamm Genome 2006; 17:417–29.

12. Churchill GA, Airey DC, Allayee H et al. The Collaborative Cross, a community resource for the genetic analysis of complex traits. Nat Genet 2004; 36:1133–7.

13. Jerez-Timaure NC, Kearney F, Simpson EB et al. Characterization of QTL with major effects on fatness and growth on mouse chromosome 2. Obes Res 2004; 12:1408–20.

14. Iakoubova OA, Olsson CL, Dains KM et al. Genome-tagged mice (GTM): two sets of genome-wide congenic strains. Genomics 2001; 74:89–104.

15. Hill AE, Lander ES, Nadeau JH. Chromosome substitution strains: a new way to study genetically complex traits. Methods Mol Med 2006; 128:153–72.

16. Singer JB, Hill AE, Burrage LC et al. Genetic dissection of complex traits with chromosome substitution strains of mice. Science 2004; 304:445–8 (Epub 2004 Mar 18).

17. Bevova MR, Aulchenko YS, Aksu S et al. Chromosome-wise dissection of the genome of the extremely big mouse line DU6i. Genetics 2006; 172:401–10 (Epub 2005 Sep 12).

18. Darvasi A, Soller M. Advanced intercross lines, an experimental population for fine genetic mapping. Genetics 1995; 141:1199–207.

19. Ehrich TH, Hrbek T, Kenney-Hunt JP et al. Fine-mapping gene-by-diet interactions on chromosome 13 in a LG/J x SM/J murine model of obesity. Diabetes 2005; 54:1863–72.

20. Leamy LJ, Elo K, Nielsen MK et al. Genetic variance and covariance patterns for body weight and energy balance characters in an advanced intercross population of mice. Genet Sel Evol 2005; 37:151–73.

21. Demarest K, Koyner J, McCaughran J Jr et al. Further characterization and high-resolution mapping of quantitative trait loci for ethanol-induced locomotor activity. Behav Genet 2001; 31:79–91.

22. Valdar W, Solberg LC, Gauguier D et al. Genome-wide genetic association of complex traits in heterogeneous stock mice. Nat Genet 2006; 38:879–87 (Epub 2006 Jul 9).

23. Falconer DS. Patterns of response in selection experiments with mice. Cold Spring Harb Symp Quant Biol 1955; 20:178–96.

24. Allan MF, Eisen EJ, Pomp D. The M16 mouse: an outbred animal model of early onset polygenic obesity and diabesity. Obes Res 2004; 12:1397–407.

25. Bünger L, Hill WG. Inbred lines of mice derived from long-term divergent selection on fat content and body weight. Mamm Genome 1999; 10:645–8.

26. Nielsen MK, Jones LD, Freking BA et al. Divergent selection for heat loss in mice: I. Selection applied and direct response through fifteen generations. J Anim Sci 1997; 75:1461–8.

27. Sharp GL, Hill WG, Robertson A. Effects of selection on growth, body composition and food intake in mice. I. Responses in selected traits. Genet Res 1984; 43:75–92.

28. Swallow JG, Carter PA, Garland T Jr. Artificial selection for increased wheel-running behavior in house mice. Behav Genet 1998; 28:227–37.

29. Ueda H, Ikegami H, Yamato E et al. The NSY mouse: a new animal model of spontaneous NIDDM with moderate obesity. Diabetologia 1995; 38:503–8.

30. Bünger L, Laidlaw A, Bulfield G et al. Inbred lines of mice derived from long-term growth selected lines: unique resources for mapping growth genes. Mamm Genome 2001; 12:678–86.

31. Rocha JL, Eisen EJ, Van Vleck LD et al. A large-sample QTL study in mice: I. Growth. Mamm Genome 2004; 15:83–99.

32. Rocha JL, Eisen EJ, Van Vleck LD et al. A large-sample QTL study in mice: II. Bodycomposition. Mamm Genome 2004; 15:100–13.

33. Bünger L, Forsting J, McDonald KL et al. Long-term divergent selection on fatness in mice indicates a regulation system independent of leptin production and reception. FASEB J 2003; 17:85–7 (Epub 2002 Nov 1).

34. Eisen EJ. Testing quantitative genetic selection theory. In: Eisen EJ, ed. The Mouse in Animal Genetics and Breeding Research. London: Imperial College Press, 2005:9–27.
35. Eisen EJ. Selection experiments for body composition in mice and rats. Livest Prod Sci 1989; 23:17–32.
36. Kozak LP, Rossmeisl M. Adiposity and the development of diabetes in mouse genetic models. Ann N Y Acad Sci 2002; 967:80–7.
37. Rankinen T, Zuberi A, Chagnon YC et al. The human obesity gene map: the 2005 update. Obesity 2006; 14:529–644.
38. Cervino AC, Gosink M, Fallahi M et al. A comprehensive mouse IBD database for the efficient localization of quantitative trait loci. Mamm Genome 2006; 17:565–74 (Epub 2006 Jun 12).

4.1 Will Fatty Worms or Flies Help Discover the Mechanism of Human Obesity?

Sona Kang, Vernon Dolinsky, and Ormond A. MacDougald

Department of Molecular and Integrative Physiology, University of Michigan Medical Center, Ann Arbor, Michigan, U.S.A.

Recent advances have made screening of model organisms a practical alternative for understanding genes and pathways involved in energy storage and utilization, as well as life span. For example, *Caenorhabditis elegans*, *Drosophila*, and zebrafish are highly amenable to genetic screening, and mutant animals can be further analyzed with high throughput transcriptomics, proteomics and metabolomics. Thus, these species promise to guide work in higher organisms on complex interactions between nutritional environment and the genome, epigenome, and proteome. Whole-body energy balance is influenced by appetite, digestion and absorption of nutrients, as well as metabolism, and these ancient processes tend to be highly conserved across species. Research on model organisms, especially in conjunction with research on rodents, provides important information on basic mechanisms of energy balance, and holds the promise of speeding development of new treatments for obesity and diabetes in humans. However, probably the greatest potential insight from model systems will come from processes that we would not necessarily be able to predict. For example, the discovery of micro-RNAs, which appear to be important regulators of gene expression in mammals, came about from unexplained genetic observations in plants. In addition, model systems have helped guide research in higher animals in the area of aging, where complex genetics and long life span limit work in mammals. Of the model organisms, we will review the potential for *C. elegans*, *Drosophila* and zebrafish to provide insights into basic metabolic processes as well as insight into obesity.

CAENORHABDITIS ELEGANS

C. elegans are free-living soil nematodes. Morphology and eating behavior suggest they largely feed on bacteria, and food intake occurs via pumping, peristaltic contractions of muscles in the corpus, the anterior isthmus, and the terminal bulb of the pharynx. *C. elegans* take up a suspension, and retain the particles while spitting out the liquid. Particles are ground and debris is passed into the intestine, which is composed of a one-cell-thick epithelial tube that runs most of the body length. Intestinal cells probably secrete nutrients through the basal surface into the pseudocoelomic fluid, which contacts all tissues. Defecation is effected by periodic muscle contractions. Food is detected via olfactory and chemosensory perception, which occurs via chemosensory organs in the head region. The ciliated endings of sensory neurons allow these nematodes to respond to changes in the environment. As detailed below some regulators of food intake and metabolism are shared between *C. elegans* and mammals.

Advantages and Disadvantages

One of the biggest benefits of *C. elegans* is the low cost of housing and maintenance compared to mammalian models. In addition, *C. elegans* reproduce rapidly and live only a few weeks. This short life span greatly decreases the time required for developmental and aging research. Furthermore, genetic information has been superior to other organisms as *C. elegans* was the first organism to have its entire genome sequenced (1). From an experimental perspective, gain- and loss-of-function studies are more easily carried out than in the gold standard for mammalian models—the mouse. In addition, systematic knocking down of several genes can be achieved in *C. elegans* by feeding *Escherichia coli* that express double-stranded siRNAs. Examination of polygenic regulators of energy balance can also be approached by screening for loci that functionally interact with known regulators to influence storage of fat (2). Also, reproducible protocols for dietary restriction make *C. elegans* useful for exploration of genetic responses to dietary manipulations. For instance, fat storage can be easily evaluated by staining whole animals with the fluorescent lipid soluble dye, Nile Red. Therefore, this organism has been broadly used to study disorders related to metabolism and aging. However, its relevance as a model organism for human obesity is less than ideal as nematodes lack adipocytes *per se*. For example, a "worm" leptin molecule has not been identified and fat storage does not occur in adipose tissues, but is instead mediated by intestines. Finally, *C. elegans* express more than 35 insulin-like peptides, suggesting that roles for the insulin and insulin-like growth factor 1 (IGF-1) signaling pathways are probably different, and potentially are more complicated than in mammalian systems.

Studies on Energy Balance, Storage of Fat, and Aging

Food Intake and Neuroendocrine Signaling

In mice and humans, it is well established that leptin, insulin, and several neuropeptides in the central nervous system are involved in control of food consumption (3,4). For instance, decreased central insulin signaling by deletion of insulin receptor in brain increases food intake of female mice, suggesting that insulin receptor-mediated signaling in the central nervous system regulates feeding behavior (5). Many other pathways including signaling by serotonin are also known to regulate satiety and food intake in mice. Furthermore, mutations in these pathways (e.g., serotonin receptor; HTR2C) can cause obesity in mice (6–8). Many but not all of these pathways appear to be conserved in *C. elegans*.

Despite the fact that *C. elegans* do not contain an identifiable leptin, there appears to be linkage between total fat content and neuroendocrine system. Probably other signaling pathways, including that of insulin, tubby, and serotonin, are the major regulators of food intake and energy balance. For example, deletion mutants of tryptophan hydroxylase 1 gene, the key serotonin biosynthetic enzyme, have increased lipid accumulation (9). Abnormalities in sensation and ingestion of food may partly be due to downregulation of transforming growth factor beta and insulin-like neuroendocrine signals (9). To explore these relationships further, Ashrafi et al. (10) screened genes that may play roles in food sensation and fat metabolism by systemically knocking down 16,757 genes using RNAi and evaluating fat storage by Nile Red staining of whole animals. They found that 7% (305) of genes caused a reduction of fat or distorted fat deposition, and 1.8% (112) of genes caused accumulation of lipid. Among these, knocking down the potential glutamine receptor and a homolog of rat somatostatin receptor increased fat content.

Conversely, knocking down the homolog of glutaminyl cyclase, an enzyme for pyroglutamyl peptide biosynthesis, and dopamine receptor, D2-like receptor, reduced lipid content. These suggest that glutaminergic and dopaminergic signaling pathways are implicated in regulation of fat storage, and likely affect feeding behavior of worms centrally in the brain.

In mice, a protein called Tubby (TUB) (see Chapter 3.1) is expressed in the brain including hypothalamus and hippocampus, suggesting that it controls food intake. Consistent with this idea, mutation of tubby causes an obesity phenotype in mice (11). However, mechanisms by which tubby regulates feeding behavior in the neuronal system are not well understood. A recent study using *C. elegans* suggests that TUB might be involved in neuronal trafficking processes, including the ciliated neurons involved in sensing external and internal nutrient levels (2). As in mice, mutation of TUB1 in worms also causes an increase in fat content. Mukhopadhyay et al. identified a RabGAP protein called RabGTPase-activating protein (RBG3) that interacts with TUB1 (12). The expression of these two proteins occurs in the same neuronal population. Moreover, knockdown of RBG3 reverses the accumulation of lipid observed in TUB1 mutants, suggesting that RBG3 might be a downstream target of TUB1. This basic mechanistic work may have relevance to humans since alterations of small GTPases, including Rabs are implicated in human diseases such as Bardet-Biedl syndrome (Chapter 5.3), where affected individuals are obese and have retinal degeneration (13).

Digestion and Absorption of Nutrients

Although model organisms should be ideal for providing insights into such ancient processes as digestion and absorption of nutrients, there has been a paucity of studies in this area. A functional link between digestion of nutrients in *C. elegans* and fat stores was made by Nehrke (14), who found that disruption of proton-mediated absorption of dipeptides leads to a functional caloric restriction followed by loss of lipid stores and an increase in longevity.

Metabolism

Insulin is a key player in metabolism of glucose and lipid in diverse organisms. It not only regulates activities of a number of metabolic enzymes, but also regulates their transcription and translation, and thereby controls glucose and fat metabolism in liver, muscle, and adipose tissue. Moreover, molecular components of the signaling pathway for insulin/IGF are highly conserved between organisms. Insulin promotes biosynthesis of fat and inhibits degradation. Mice without insulin receptors in white adipose tissue have reduced fat mass, and are protected from age- and genetic-induced obesity (15) and decreased metabolism in these mice is associated with increased longevity (15). Despite the fact that the insulin/IGF signaling pathway is highly conserved between organisms, the role of insulin signaling for energy homeostasis is very different in mammals compared to worms. Metabolism in mammals involves interplay between many tissues and organs, and many of these processes are regulated by insulin. For example, muscle-specific insulin receptor knockout mice have increased lipid accumulation in adipose tissue, but exhibit normal glucose tolerance (16), suggesting that while muscle is a significant site of glucose disposal, other tissues are critical for glucose tolerance after fasting. Consistent with this idea, mice with liver-specific insulin receptor knockout are glucose intolerant due to severe insulin resistance (17), suggesting that insulin signaling in liver plays an important role for maintenance of blood glucose.

Analysis of *C. elegans* indicates that there is not a simple correlation between loss of insulin/IGF signaling and lipid accumulation. This is because in response to food limitation or crowding, *C. elegans* enters an arrested developmental state referred to as dauer (18). In this alternative developmental stage, metabolism is shifted toward production and storage of fat. For example, inactivation of the insulin receptor homolog, Daf2, causes *C. elegans* to enter dauer and accumulate lipid (19), as do appropriate gain- or loss-of-function mutations in downstream signaling molecules, including the forkhead box O (FOXO) homolog, Daf16 (20–23). However, analysis of genes downstream of insulin/IGF signaling in *C. elegans* revealed genes involved in amino acid metabolism (*asp* genes), lipid transport (*vit2, vit5* genes) and fatty acid (*fat1, fat3* genes) metabolism, many of which are also known to be regulated in higher organisms (20,24,25).

Basic work in *C. elegans* (and yeast) has often led to insights in mammalian physiology. For example, functional and physical interactions between Daf16 and the NAD-dependent histone deacetylase, sirtuin (silent mating type information regulation 2 homolog) 2 (Sirt2), served as precedent for the mammalian homologs of these proteins regulating many aspects of cell biology including differentiation, metabolism and response to oxidative stress (26,27).

It is now well established that mammalian nuclear receptors such as peroxisome-proliferator activated receptors (PPARs) and nuclear receptor subfamily 1, group H, member 1 and 2 (LXRs) are key regulators of fat metabolism. *C. elegans* contains 248 nuclear receptors in the genome and 15 of these are conserved in mammals (28). Comparison of complete nuclear receptor sets from the human, *C. elegans* and *Drosophila* genomes suggests that the nuclear receptor superfamily has undergone extensive proliferation and diversification in nematodes (29). Van Gilst et al. examined genes that are involved in glucose and fat metabolism in response to fasting in *C. elegans*. As expected, genes that are involved in fat mobilization including β-oxidation genes and stearoyl-CoA desaturase upon food deprivation were identified (30). In addition, they found that a nuclear hormone receptor Nhr49 is responsible for induction of the fasting response genes (30,31). Further investigation revealed that an Nhr49 deletion mutant increases fat content, suggesting it plays a key role in fat metabolism (31). Decreased expression of acs-2 (acyl Co-A synthetase) and ech-1 (β-oxidation) suggests that Nhr49 controls oxidation, synthesis and saturation of fatty acids (30,31). Although Nhr49 is related to hepatocyte nuclear receptor 4 by sequence identity, the function of it appears closer to PPAR*A* and PPAR*D*. This is a nice example of how the role of nuclear receptors in energy homeostasis was elucidated using a model organism; however, given the potential for these receptors to influence human health, there is already tremendous pharmacological, structural, and genetic tools available to study functional aspects of mammalian receptors. Thus, the potential insight from future work on *C. elegans* in this area may be limited.

Development of "Adipocytes"

Although *C. elegans* lack adipocytes, they do contain lipid storing cells which share many properties of mammalian adipocytes. Thus, McKay et al. evaluated the potential of *C. elegans* as a model for fat development (32). To validate *C. elegans* as a model system, they generated worms lacking sterol regulatory element binding transcription factor (lpd1) or CCAAT/enhancer binding protein (lpd2), which are well known for their importance for adipocyte development and lipid metabolism in mammalian systems (see Section 9). The resulting mutant worms were pale, skinny and had reduced lipid stores, due in part to reduced expression of several lipogenic enzymes (acetyl-coenzyme A carboxylase, ATP citrate lyase, fatty acid synthase, glyceraldehyde 3-phosphate dehydrogenase and malic enzyme). They then performed large-scale RNAi screens and scored for lipid-depleted phenotypes to identify other genes that regulate fat storage. One of these, lpd3, was found to have a human homolog expressed in fat, brain, and testis, and the mouse lpd3 was highly expressed in embryonic fat, with lower levels in differentiated fat cells. Knocking down lpd3 in preadipocytes suppressed their ability to undergo differentiation. Therefore, lpd3 is expressed in fat storing tissues from worms to humans, and its expression is highest in developing adipose tissue (32).

Inflammation

The link between obesity and insulin resistance has been extensively studied in mammalian systems. One promising model suggests that increased production of reactive oxygen species in mitochondria both in adipocytes and adjacent endothelial cells stimulates inflammatory signaling and contributes to insulin resistance (33). *Caenorhabditis elegans* may provide an additional model to study aspects of these fundamental processes since their immune response seems to be highly regulated by insulin/IGF signaling pathways. For instance, loss of function in the homologs of insulin receptor (Daf2) and phosphatidylinositol-3-kinase (Age1) increases survival after challenge with bacterial pathogens (34). Murphy et al. identified genes that act downstream of Daf16 in *C. elegans* using microarrays and observed regulation of a group of genes coding for antimicrobial proteins (20). In addition, loss of function of Daf16 caused reduction of several stress-response genes such as ctl1, ctl2, and sod3, and the production of catalase and superoxide dismutase (20). These studies suggest that *C. elegans* can be used to identify genes regulating the immune response and to gain insight into the relationship between the innate immune system and nutrition.

Aging

The driving force for much of our insight into factors that regulate longevity comes from work in model organisms, and in particular *C. elegans* (35). Mechanisms that control aging are immensely complex, and are extremely difficult to unravel at the molecular level. Thus, simple organisms provide tremendous benefit for probing these fundamental questions. It now appears that three genetic networks regulate the aging process, with signaling contributions from the insulin/IGF pathway, the mitochondrial electron transport chain, and in response to dietary restriction. Considerable evidence now points to insulin/IGF signaling as an important contributor to the aging process. The initial observations were that mutation of Daf2 decreased insulin/IGF signaling and extended life in *C. elegans*. Subsequent work demonstrated that mutation of Age1, equivalent to phosphatidylinositol-3 kinase, doubles life span and causes dauer formation in worms, suggesting Age1 mediates insulin signaling to control life span and diapause (state of arrested development which synchronizes insect activity cycles) (36). Further, PTEN homolog Daf18 was identified to suppress Daf2 dependent signaling through a genetic screen (22). The FOXO homolog Daf16 also plays an essential role as a downstream effector of insulin/IGF signaling in *C. elegans*, and signaling through this molecule regulates life span (20,21). Likewise, the relationship between insulin/IGF signaling and aging appears to be conserved between organisms and fatty tissue seems to play an important and common role. For instance, mice without insulin receptors in white adipose tissue live 18% longer than wild type animals, have reduced fat mass, and are protected from age-related and genetic-induced obesity (15). In worms, over-expression of the FOXO homolog (Daf16) in intestine, primary site for fat storage is sufficient to increase life span (37). However, further investigations are necessary to determine conclusively whether or not insulin/IGF signaling regulates aging in invertebrates and vertebrates by shared mechanisms.

Although it has been known for many decades that reduced food intake extends mammalian life span, the mechanisms have been difficult to discern and remain unknown. There may be contributions from reduced insulin/IGF signaling as well as improved electron transport efficiency, with commensurate decreases in production of reactive oxygen species. However, recent work in C. *elegans* also suggests a key role for signaling through target of rapamycin (TOR), which senses the energy state of the cells, and regulates cell growth by controlling transcription, translation, and protein degradation. These mechanisms will be a focal point for research performed over the next decade.

DROSOPHILA

Drosophila melanogaster, commonly known as the fruit fly, is one of the most extensively researched insects in the world. Like C. *elegans*, *Drosophila* has a short life cycle and reproduces rapidly, with all the inherent advantages for developmental, aging and other types of research. About 1 day after fertilization, *Drosophila* embryos develop and hatch into worm-like larva. Larvae eat and grow continuously, molting 1 day, 2 days, and 4 days after hatching (i.e., first, second and third instars). After 2 days as a third instar larva, they molt one more time to form an immobile pupa. Over the next 4 days, the body is completely remodeled to give the winged form of the adult. After hatching from the pupal case, flies can live for 2 or 3 weeks and females will lay eggs for most of this period. They are attracted to fermenting fruit and other substances and lay their eggs in splits in the skin of overripe fruit. Fruit flies in the laboratory normally eat a nutritious mix of sugar and yeast meant to mimic their natural diet of rotting fruit and the yeast fermenting it.

Advantages and Disadvantages

Drosophila has been used as a model research organism for almost a century; thus, there is a tremendous amount known about their handling and care. In addition, the sophisticated genetics associated with a species with small genome size, high fecundity, low cost, and short generation time provides considerable research advantage. The *Drosophila* genome was completed in 2000 (38), and more than half of the *Drosophila* genes have been knocked out with transposition insertions and chemical mutagenesis (39,40). Although systematic global knockdown of genes by RNAi as used in C. *elegans* is not feasible in *Drosophila* because of the labor involved, large-scale knockdown of ~91% of the fly genome has been performed in cultured *Drosophila* cell lines (41).

As a model organism for obesity, *Drosophila* is especially appealing because they contain "fat bodies," which have some adipocyte characteristics, including a lipid transport system analogous to humans. Metabolic and signaling pathways involved in fat metabolism and the mechanism of fat storage are conserved. Therefore, *Drosophila* is a reasonable model to explore factors that influence energy balance, as well as connections between longevity and metabolism. One drawback to this model is that *Drosophila* are invertebrates and thus have some fundamental differences in physiology compared to humans. However, unlike yeast or *C. elegans*, but similar to humans, *Drosophila* are obligate aerobes, which may have a bearing on metabolism and aging-related mechanisms. Finally, flies have separate males and females (i.e., dioecious), and can therefore be used to investigate sex differences in processes associated with energy balance and aging.

Studies on Energy Balance, Adipogenesis, and Aging
Regulation of Food Intake
Several neuropeptide signaling pathways are conserved between flies and mammals. Since anatomy and signaling of the neuronal system is relatively simple in flies, *Drosophila* is a useful model organism to delineate these pathways and assess their functions. For instance in mice, neuropeptide Y (NPY) is known to have orexigenic effects such that intracerebroventricular injection induces food intake (42,43). NPY mediates its signaling through at least five different receptors with different affinities and these receptors are shared with other ligands (44), which make it challenging to delineate effects of NPY on energy balance. However, *Drosophila* has one NPY-like protein (neuropeptide F) and a single receptor. Wu et al. showed that *Drosophila* neuropeptide F receptor regulates feeding behavior in a manner analogous to that observed in mammals (45,46). Overexpression of neuropeptide F in brain of larvae increases attraction to food while downregulation causes food aversion (46). Similarly, neuropeptide F receptor regulates the response to noxious food (45). While ectopic expression of neuropeptide F receptor causes larvae to more readily take in noxious food, loss of receptor signaling increases aversion (45). Upregulation of insulin-like receptor signaling in cells overexpressing neuropeptide F receptor suppresses the feeding response to noxious food, suggesting that coordinated activities of these conserved systems are essential for regulation of food intake (45).

In addition to NPY, neurotransmitters such as serotonin, dopamine, and norepinephrine are well-known to regulate feeding behavior in the central nervous system of mammals (3,4). In *Drosophila*, dopamine and serotonin are found in distinctive cell populations in the nervous system (47) and both affect feeding behavior. In flies, the olfactory system plays an important regulatory role in appetite (48). For instance, Schwaerzel et al. (49) suggested that octopamine, the presumed homolog of norepinephrine, is necessary for the acquisition of sugar memory. They report that mutant flies without octopamine synthesis have reduced attraction to sugar, and that the "sugar reward" is dependent on cAMP signaling.

Metabolism and its Regulation
Our understanding of lipid metabolism in mammalian systems has been greatly advanced by embryonic fibroblasts that undergo differentiation into adipocytes, where metabolism can subsequently be studied. In mammalian systems, it has been found that proteins that coat lipid droplets in adipocytes contain a PAT domain, and the prototypical protein in this class is perilipin. The function of these proteins appears to be conserved across species. The *Drosophila* homologs of

perilipin, Lsd1, Lsd2 (lysine specific demethylase 1) were identified by genomic analysis. Lsd2 is localized on the surface of lipid droplets, and Lsd2 mutants have lower triglyceride content in embryos (50). Loss-of-function Lsd2 mutants are lean and overexpression causes obesity (51). Recently, a protein called Brummer was identified by Gronke et al. Brummer is a triacylglycerol lipase and homolog of human adipocyte triglyceride lipase. This protein antagonizes the function of Lsd2 (52). Overexpression of Brummer depletes fat storage, and a loss-of-function mutation causes obesity in flies (52). In mammals, one of the PAT domain proteins surrounding lipid storage droplets is perilipin, and mice devoid of perilipin have less fat and are resistant to induced obesity due to increased lipolysis (53).

A WD40/tetratricopeptide-repeat-domain protein *adipose* was first found to regulate fat metabolism in *Drosophila* in 1960. Loss of *adipose* activity almost doubles fat storage and extends life span under starvation condition. Triglyceride levels were reduced by ectopic expression of *adipose* in the fat depot, but not by neuronal-specific expression (54). Two mammalian cDNAs for *adipose* have been identified and they are expressed in a ubiquitous manner (54). Although further work is required to establish the role of these proteins in the regulation of energy balance in mammals, this line of research underscores the power of model systems for understanding lipid accumulation in higher organisms.

Whole-Body Metabolism

In mice, TOR-dependent signaling plays an important role in whole-body metabolism. For example, mice lacking S6 kinase are protected against diet- and age-induced obesity (55,56). The other effector of mTOR, eukaryotic translation initiation factor 4E binding protein 3 (4E-BP1), seems to have unique roles for regulation of fat metabolism as well. *4e-bp3*-deficient mice manifest decreased adiposity and knockout males show increased metabolic rate with increased expression of uncoupling protein in white adipose tissue (57). In *Drosophila*, signaling through dTOR-dependent pathways also appears to regulate fat metabolism. Loss of dTOR phenocopies caloric restriction such that lipid mobilization is increased from the larval fat (58). Although the fat body of 4E-BP1 null flies has unaltered levels of triglyceride under normal nutritional conditions, mutant flies have an accelerated loss of fat compared to controls. Increasing activity of 4E-BP3 by rapamycin or expression of a constitutively-active mutant elevates total fat content, further suggesting that 4E-BP1 is a key regulator of fat metabolism (59). It is clear that the TOR pathway helps coordinate the cellular response to changing energy status in both mice and *Drosophila*. Additional work in *Drosophila* may provide further insight into this pathway and lipid metabolism in mammals. Several proteins in *Drosophila* were recently shown to regulate fat accumulation by regulating the dTOR-dependent pathway. For example, *slimfast* is an amino acid transporter expressed in the fat depot of *Drosophila*, and this protein acts as a nutrient sensor through a dTOR-dependent mechanism (60). Colombani et al. showed that inhibiting expression of *slimfast* in the fat body causes a systemic larval growth defect and decreases the size of fat body, similar to effects of amino acid deprivation or mutation of dTOR (58). In addition, a protein called Melted interacts with tuberous sclerosis 1 (TSC1) and FOXO, and recruits them to the cellular membrane (61). Mutation of Melted causes a reduction in TOR and an increase in FOXO activity, which mimics nutrient deprivation. These altered activities of TOR and FOXO seem to contribute to a decrease in fat content. A microarray study supports this idea by identifying downregulation of several genes related to triglyceride accumulation including phosphoenolpyruvate carboxykinase. In mice, loss of phosphoenolpyruvate carboxykinase causes lipodystrophy, while gain of function causes obesity. Of note, Melted is conserved in mammals and its human ortholog rescues mutant phenotype in flies (61). Finally, LK6 kinase has also been shown to regulate fat metabolism through dTOR-dependent signaling. LK6 kinase, homologous to mammalian MAP-kinase signal-integrating kinase, Mnk, has been shown to phosphorylate and stimulate eukaryotic translation initiation factor 4E activity. LK6 mutant flies are smaller and contain elevated lipid content (62). Thus, the similarities in regulation of lipid metabolism in *Drosophila* and mammals suggest that work in *Drosophila* may provide important insights into the signaling pathways that regulate mammalian metabolism and physiology.

Fat Development

There are considerable similarities in development of lipid storing cells in *Drosophila* and mammals. In both cases, fat tissue is of mesenchymal origin and adipogenesis is regulated by common signaling pathways, including those initiated by wingless-type MMTV integration site family (WNTs) and Hedgehogs. In addition, control of adipogenesis at the molecular level shares some similarities. For example, serpent is a GATA-like transcription factor necessary for embryonic fat cell differentiation in *Drosophila* (63). Forced expression of serpent in mesoderm causes the production of ectopic fat cells that were not derived from proliferation of preexisting fat cells. Thus serpent seems to induce fat cells from non-adipose precursor cells, and also controls cell fate choices between fat cells and somatic gonadal precursors (64). Based upon work in *Drosophila*, the role of GATA transcription factors was further explored in mammalian systems of adipogenesis. Overexpression of *Gata2* and *3* inhibits fat cell conversion in a murine preadipocyte cell line (65). In addition, embryonic stem cells from *Gata3*-deficient mice possess a higher potential to differentiate into adipocytes, suggesting that GATAs are negative regulators of adipocyte development (65). Recently, Suh et al. screened for regulators of fat body formation and reported that loss- and gain-of-function mutations in Hedgehog signaling influence fat formation and that this regulation is mediated through GATA factors (66). Moreover, they demonstrated that Hedgehog signaling is conserved in mouse model and regulates an early stage of fat cell conversion. It will be intriguing to explore roles for Hedgehog signaling in whole-body metabolism given that there is decreased expression of Hedgehog signaling molecules in *ob/ob* and diet-induced obese mice (66).

Inflammation

Obesity is positively associated with an increased level of inflammation and this leads to several adverse effects including atherosclerosis, insulin resistance, and type 2 diabetes. Increased lipid levels, including nonesterified fatty acids, triglycerides and cholesterol, contribute to development of atherosclerosis and production of inflammatory cytokines such as tumor necrosis factor alpha and interleukin 6 from adipose tissue. Further, preadipocytes and macrophages may under some circumstances have the ability to transdifferentiate between phenotypes, suggesting that these two cell types may share roles within the immune response. Thus, reduction of inflammation is considered an alternative approach to treat obesity-related diseases (33).

This tight link between inflammation and metabolic conditions appears to be at the cellular and perhaps molecular levels. For example, the fat body in *Drosophila* functions, not only in energy storage, but also in the innate immune response. As described above, *serpent* plays a role in specification of the fat body, and Petersen et al. showed that *serpent* regulates immune function of *Drosophila* in part through transcriptional regulation of Cecropin A1, an antimicrobial peptide (67). Another link may be through TOR. Signaling through TOR regulates cellular response to changing energy status (68), but is also upregulated upon bacterial infection, participating in host immune response (69).

Aging

Although critical studies on aging have largely come from yeast and *C. elegans*, *Drosophila* provide yet another model for probing the relationship between insulin signaling and longevity. Mutations of the insulin receptor homolog (dINR) and insulin receptor substrate homolog (*Chico*) extended life span of flies (70,71). Furthermore, decreased insulin signaling by overexpressing dFOXO increased life span (72). Finally, suppression of dTOR activity by overexpressing TSC1/2 or dominant-negative forms of dTOR or dS6 kinase all cause life span extension (73), indicating that decreased insulin signaling is associated with increased longevity in *Drosophila*.

ZEBRAFISH

Danio rerio are freshwater fish originally found in slow streams, rice paddies and in the Ganges River in East India and Burma. They have been used as a model for studying vertebrate development and genetics since the early 1970s.

Advantages and Disadvantages

As with the other model organisms, zebrafish are relatively easy to maintain, inexpensive to house and care for, and they reproduce rapidly. Moreover, their transparent bodies enable phenotypic changes to be easily visualized. The biggest advantage of zebrafish as a model organism is that they are vertebrates, and thus are far closer to human physiology than either *C. elegans* or *Drosophila*. The zebrafish genome is being sequenced and extensive mapping has already been performed. In addition, genes can be silenced with antisense morpholino oligonucleotides. Although zebrafish have been used extensively for in vivo drug screening, there have been relatively few experiments on energy balance and aging in this species. While well-established assays and approaches are still under development for zebrafish, it should be possible to develop high-throughput drug screening for drugs that regulate important physiological processes.

Studies on Energy Balance, Adipogenesis, and Aging

Food Intake and Neuroendocrine Signaling

Although regulation of energy balance has not been extensively studied in zebrafish, the relationship between food intake and physical activity seems to be similar to that observed in mammalian systems (74). A genetic screen for regulators of food intake was performed and although not yet published, some interesting lines of insatiable fish were identified. One of them was dubbed *jumbo*, and fish with this mutation grow considerably larger than normal zebrafish. Another mutant was called *fressack* (which is hearty eater in German) and despite considerable gluttony, these fish do not grow larger than normal. Further work will be required to establish the potential relevance of these mutants for mammalian energy balance (75).

Lipid Metabolism

The transparent bodies of zebrafish provide a considerable advantage for screening of drugs that influence fat metabolism. For example, Farber et al. developed fluorescent substrates for phospholipase A_2, an important enzyme for lipid signaling, which emit distinct fluorescent profiles before and after cleavage (76). The fluorescent lipid labeling enables activity to phospholipase A_2 to be visualized within organs and cells. This lipid reporter system was not only successfully used for biochemical drug screening but also useful for identifying genetic mutations in ENU mutants (e.g., *canola, fat free*) with perturbed lipid metabolism (ENU is an alkylating agent now currently used in different systems that is a powerful mutagen, producing single locus mutations).

CONCLUSION

The use of invertebrate model organisms to dissect the molecular details of energy balance holds great potential, and has already been invaluable for our understanding of the aging process and its regulation. Over the next 10 years, we will see a dramatic improvement in our understanding of interactions between environment and loci to influence energy storage. From control of energy balance to regulation of aging, we are quickly learning that these pathways are conserved from model organisms to mice, and are perhaps universal in the animal kingdom. This holds great promise then that orthologs of G-protein-coupled receptors, nuclear hormone receptors and other targets identified in *C. elegans*, or the *adipose* gene identified in *Drosophila* may play important roles in higher organisms. Only time will tell whether these lines of research will influence our understanding and treatment of obesity in humans. It will be very interesting to learn whether synergy observed among pathways in invertebrates to create exceptionally long-lived animals will be recapitulated in mouse models, perhaps leading to a pushing back or even doubling of the age boundary.

REFERENCES

1. Consortium TCeS. Genome sequence of the nematode *C. elegans*: a platform for investigating biology. Science 1998; 282(5396):2012–8.
2. Mak HY, Nelson LS, Basson M et al. Polygenic control of *Caenorhabditis elegans* fat storage. Nat Genet 2006; 38(3):363–8.
3. Porte D Jr, Baskin DG, Schwartz MW. Insulin signaling in the central nervous system: a critical role in metabolic homeostasis and disease from *C. elegans* to humans. Diabetes 2005; 54(5):1264–76.
4. Schwartz MW. Brain pathways controlling food intake and body weight. Exp Biol Med (Maywood) 2001; 226(11):978–81.
5. Bruning JC, Gautam D, Burks JD et al. Role of brain insulin receptor in control of body weight and reproduction. Science 2000; 289(5487):2122–5.
6. Heisler LK, Chu HM, Tecott LH. Epilepsy and obesity in serotonin 5-HT2C receptor mutant mice. Ann N Y Acad Sci 1998; 861:74–8.
7. Tecott LH, Sun LM, Akana SF et al. Eating disorder and epilepsy in mice lacking 5-HT2c serotonin receptors. Nature 1995; 374(6522):542–6.
8. Vickers SP, Dourish CT. Serotonin receptor ligands and the treatment of obesity. Curr Opin Invest Drugs 2004; 5(4):377–88.
9. Sze JY, Victor M, Loer C et al. Food and metabolic signalling defects in a *Caenorhabditis elegans* serotonin-synthesis mutant. Nature 2000; 403(6769):560–4.
10. Ashrafi K, Chang FY, Watts JL et al. Genome-wide RNAi analysis of *Caenorhabditis elegans* fat regulatory genes. Nature 2003; 421(6920):268–72.

11. Noben-Trauth K, Naggert JK, North MA et al. A candidate gene for the mouse mutation tubby. Nature 1996; 380(6574):534–8.

12. Mukhopadhyay A, Walhout AJ, Tissenbaum HA. *C. elegans* tubby regulates life span and fat storage by two independent mechanisms. Cell Metab 2005; 2(1):35–42.

13. Fan Y, Esmail MA, Ansley SJ et al. Mutations in a member of the Ras superfamily of small GTP-binding proteins causes Bardet-Biedl syndrome. Nat Genet 2004; 36(9): 989–93.

14. Nehrke K. A reduction in intestinal cell pHi due to loss of the *Caenorhabditis elegans* Na+/H+ exchanger NHX-2 increases life span. J Biol Chem 2003; 278(45):44657–66.

15. Bluher M, Michael MD, Peroni OD et al. Adipose tissue selective insulin receptor knockout protects against obesity and obesity-related glucose intolerance. Dev Cell 2002; 3(1):25–38.

16. Bruning JC, Michael MD, Winnay JN et al. A muscle-specific insulin receptor knockout exhibits features of the metabolic syndrome of NIDDM without altering glucose tolerance. Mol Cell 1998; 2(5):559–69.

17. Michael MD, Kulkarni RN, Postic C et al. Loss of insulin signaling in hepatocytes leads to severe insulin resistance and progressive hepatic dysfunction. Mol Cell 2000; 6(1):87–97.

18. Kenyon C, Chang J, Gensch E et al. A *C. elegans* mutant that lives twice as long as wild type. Nature 1993; 366(6454):461–4.

19. Kimura KD, Tissenbaum HA, Liu Y et al. Daf-2, an insulin receptor-like gene that regulates longevity and diapause in *Caenorhabditis elegans*. Science 1997; 277(5328):942–6.

20. Murphy CT, McCarroll SA, Bargmann CI et al. Genes that act downstream of DAF-16 to influence the lifespan of *Caenorhabditis elegans*. Nature 2003; 424(6946):277–83.

21. Ogg S, Paradis S, Gootlieb D et al. The Fork head transcription factor DAF-16 transduces insulin-like metabolic and longevity signals in *C. elegans*. Nature 1997; 389(6654):994–9.

22. Ogg S, Ruvkun G. The *C. elegans* PTEN homolog, DAF-18, acts in the insulin receptor-like metabolic signaling pathway. Mol Cell 1998; 2(6):887–93.

23. Paradis S, Ailion M, Toker A et al. A PDK1 homolog is necessary and sufficient to transduce AGE-1 PI3 kinase signals that regulate diapause in *Caenorhabditis elegans*. Genes Dev 1999; 13(11):1438–52.

24. Halaschek-Wiener J, McKay S, Pouzyrev A et al. Analysis of long-lived *C. elegans* daf-2 mutants using serial analysis of gene expression. Genome Res 2005; 15(5):603–15.

25. McElwee J, Thomas JH. Transcriptional outputs of the *Caenorhabditis elegans* forkhead protein DAF-16. Aging Cell 2003; 2(2):111–21.

26. Brunet A, Swenney LB, Sturgill JF et al. Stress-dependent regulation of FOXO transcription factors by the SIRT1 deacetylase. Science 2004; 303(5666):2011–5.

27. Guarante LP. Regulation of Aging by SIR2. Ann N Y Acad Sci 2005; 1055:222.

28. Maglich JM, Sluder A, Guan X et al. Comparison of complete nuclear receptor sets from the human, *Caenorhabditis elegans* and *Drosophila* genomes. Genome Biol 2001; 2(8):RESEARCH0029.

29. Sluder AE, Mathews SW, Hough D et al. The nuclear receptor superfamily has undergone extensive proliferation and diversification in nematodes. Genome Res 1999; 9(2):103–20.

30. Van Gilst MR, Hadjivassiliou H, Yamamoto KR. A *Caenorhabditis elegans* nutrient response system partially dependent on nuclear receptor NHR-49. Proc Natl Acad Sci U S A 2005; 102(38):13496–501.

31. Van Gilst MR, Hadjivassiliou H, Jolly A et al. Nuclear hormone receptor NHR-49 controls fat consumption and fatty acid composition in *C. elegans*. PLoS Biol 2005; 3(2):e53.

32. McKay RM, McKay JP, Avery L et al. *C. elegans*: a model for exploring the genetics of fat storage. Dev Cell 2003; 4(1):131–42.

33. Wellen KE, Hotamisligil GS. Inflammation, stress, and diabetes. J Clin Invest 2005; 115(5):1111–9.

34. Garsin DA, Villanueva JM, Begun J et al. Long-lived *C. elegans* daf-2 mutants are resistant to bacterial pathogens. Science 2003; 300(5627):1921.

35. Kenyon C. A conserved regulatory system for aging. Cell 2001; 105(2):165–8.

36. Morris JZ, Tissenbaum HA, Ruvkun G. A phosphatidylinositol-3-OH kinase family member regulating longevity and diapause in *Caenorhabditis elegans*. Nature 1996; 382(6591):536–9.
37. Libina N, Berman JR, Kenyon C. Tissue-specific activities of *C. elegans* DAF-16 in the regulation of lifespan. Cell 2003; 115(4):489–502.
38. Adams MD, Celniker SE, Holt RA et al. The genome sequence of *Drosophila melanogaster*. Science 2000; 287(5461):2185–95.
39. Parks AL, Cook KR, Belvin M et al. Systematic generation of high-resolution deletion coverage of the *Drosophila melanogaster* genome. Nat Genet 2004; 36(3):288–92.
40. Rubin GM, Lewis EB. A brief history of *Drosophila*`s contributions to genome research. Science 2000; 287(5461):2216–8.
41. Armknecht S, Boutros M, Kiger A et al. High-throughput RNA interference screens in *Drosophila* tissue culture cells. Methods Enzymol 2005; 392:55–73.
42. Kalra SP, Clark JT, Sahu A et al. Control of feeding and sexual behaviors by neuropeptide Y: physiological implications. Synapse 1988; 2(3):254–7.
43. Clark JT, Kalra PS, Crowley WR et al. Neuropeptide Y and human pancreatic polypeptide stimulate feeding behavior in rats. Endocrinology 1984; 115(1):427–9.
44. Herzog H. Neuropeptide Y and energy homeostasis: insights from Y receptor knockout models. Eur J Pharmacol 2003; 480(1–3):21–9.
45. Wu Q, Zhao Z, Shen P. Regulation of aversion to noxious food by *Drosophila* neuropeptide Y- and insulin-like systems. Nat Neurosci 2005; 8(10):1350–5.
46. Wu Q, Wen T, Lee G et al. Developmental control of foraging and social behavior by the *Drosophila* neuropeptide Y-like system. Neuron 2003; 39(1):147–61.
47. Monastirioti M. Biogenic amine systems in the fruit fly *Drosophila melanogaster*. Microsc Res Tech 1999; 45(2):106–21.
48. Heisenberg M, Borst A, Wagner S et al. *Drosophila* mushroom body mutants are deficient in olfactory learning. J Neurogenet 1985; 2(1):1–30.
49. Schwaerzel M, Monastirioti M, Scholz H et al. Dopamine and octopamine differentiate between aversive and appetitive olfactory memories in *Drosophila*. J Neurosci 2003; 23(33):10495–502.
50. Teixeira L, Rabouille C, Rorth P et al. *Drosophila* Perilipin/ADRP homologue Lsd2 regulates lipid metabolism. Mech Dev 2003; 120(9):1071–81.
51. Gronke S, Beller M, Fellert S et al. Control of fat storage by a *Drosophila* PAT domain protein. Curr Biol 2003; 13(7):603–6.
52. Gronke S, Mildner A, Fellert S et al. Brummer lipase is an evolutionary conserved fat storage regulator in *Drosophila*. Cell Metab 2005; 1(5):323–30.
53. Martinez-Botas J, Anderson JB, Tessier D et al. Absence of perilipin results in leanness and reverses obesity in Lepr(db/db) mice. Nat Genet 2000; 26(4):474–9.
54. Hader T, Muller S, Aquilera M et al. Control of triglyceride storage by a WD40/TPR-domain protein. EMBO Rep 2003; 4(5):511–6.
55. Pende M, Kozma SC, Jaquet M et al. Hypoinsulinaemia, glucose intolerance and diminished beta-cell size in S6K1-deficient mice. Nature 2000; 408(6815):994–7.
56. Um SH, Frigerio F, Watanabe M et al. Absence of S6K1 protects against age- and diet-induced obesity while enhancing insulin sensitivity. Nature 2004; 431(7005):200–5.
57. Tsukiyama-Kohara K, Poulin F, Kohara M et al. Adipose tissue reduction in mice lacking the translational inhibitor 4E-BP1. Nat Med 2001; 7(10):1128–32.
58. Zhang H, Stallock JP, Ng JC et al. Regulation of cellular growth by the *Drosophila* target of rapamycin dTOR. Genes Dev 2000; 14(21):2712–24.
59. Teleman AA, Chen YW, Cohen SM. 4E-BP functions as a metabolic brake used under stress conditions but not during normal growth. Genes Dev 2005; 19(16):1844–8.
60. Colombani J, Raisin S, Pantalacci S et al. A nutrient sensor mechanism controls *Drosophila* growth. Cell 2003; 114(6):739–49.
61. Teleman AA, Chen YW, Cohen SM. *Drosophila* Melted modulates FOXO and TOR activity. Dev Cell 2005; 9(2):271–81.
62. Arquier N, Bourouis M, Colombani J et al. *Drosophila* Lk6 kinase controls phosphorylation of eukaryotic translation initiation factor 4E and promotes normal growth and development. Curr Biol 2005; 15(1):19–23.

63. Sam S, Leise W, Hoshizaki DK. The serpent gene is necessary for progression through the early stages of fat-body development. Mech Dev 1996; 60(2):197–205.

64. Moore LA, Broihier HT, Van Doren M et al. Gonadal mesoderm and fat body initially follow a common developmental path in *Drosophila*. Development 1998; 125(5):837–44.

65. Tong Q, Dalgin G, Xu H et al. Function of GATA transcription factors in preadipocyte-adipocyte transition. Science 2000; 290(5489):134–8.

66. Suh JM, Gao X, McKay J et al. Hedgehog signaling plays a conserved role in inhibiting fat formation. Cell Metab 2006; 3(1):25–34.

67. Petersen UM, Kadalayil L, Rehorn KP et al. Serpent regulates *Drosophila* immunity genes in the larval fat body through an essential GATA motif. EMBO J 1999; 18(14):4013–22.

68. Zinke I, Schutz CS, Katzenberger JD et al. Nutrient control of gene expression in *Drosophila*: microarray analysis of starvation and sugar-dependent response. EMBO J 2002; 21(22):6162–73.

69. Bernal A, Kimbrell DA. *Drosophila* Thor participates in host immune defense and connects a translational regulator with innate immunity. Proc Natl Acad Sci U S A 2000; 97(11):6019–24.

70. Clancy DJ, Gems D, Harshman LG et al. Extension of life-span by loss of CHICO, a *Drosophila* insulin receptor substrate protein. Science 2001; 292(5514):104–6.

71. Tatar M, Kopelman A, Epstein D et al. A mutant *Drosophila* insulin receptor homolog that extends life-span and impairs neuroendocrine function. Science 2001; 292(5514):107–10.

72. Hwangbo DS, Gershman B, Tu MP et al. *Drosophila* dFOXO controls lifespan and regulates insulin signalling in brain and fat body. Nature 2004; 429(6991):562–6.

73. Kapahi P, Zid BM, Harper T et al. Regulation of lifespan in *Drosophila* by modulation of genes in the TOR signaling pathway. Curr Biol 2004; 14(10):885–90.

74. Novak CM, Jiang X, Wang C et al. Caloric restriction and physical activity in zebrafish (*Danio rerio*). Neurosci Lett 2005; 383(1–2):99–104.

75. Vogel G. Zebrafish earns its stripes in genetic screens. Science 2000; 288(5469):1160–1.

76. Farber SA et al. Genetic analysis of digestive physiology using fluorescent phospholipid reporters. Science 2001; 292(5520):1385–8.

5.1 Overview of Human Monogenic, Nonsyndromic, and Syndromic Obesity

Wendy K. Chung and Rudolph L. Leibel
Division of Molecular Genetics and The Naomi Berrie Diabetes Center, Columbia University Medical College, New York, New York, U.S.A.

Body weight and fat stores are determined by the net excess or deficit of food intake over energy expenditure. The hypothalamus acts centrally to integrate redundant signaling pathways involving the neuroendocrine and autonomic nervous systems to determine food intake, energy expenditure, and nutrient partitioning. Leptin and insulin are secreted in proportion to peripheral fat mass, and signal the hypothalamus regarding the state of long-term energy stores (Fig. 1) (1). Leptin appears to act primarily to signal critical minimal energy (triglyceride) reserves for functions such as reproduction (2). Low concentrations of leptin and insulin generate an anabolic signal to increase food intake and reduce energy expenditure (3). Leptin and insulin bind to receptors on neurons in the arcuate nucleus, which is partially outside of the blood brain barrier. As detailed in Chapters 3.1 and 3.2. The arcuate nucleus contains two discrete neuronal populations producing either Agouti-related protein (AgRP) and Neuropeptide Y (NPY), or proopiomelanocortin (POMC) and cocaine and amphetamine regulated transcript (CART) that act reciprocally to increase and decrease food intake, respectively, and to transduce outflow signals regulating body fat stores (1). Leptin and insulin inhibit the NPY/AgRP neurons and reciprocally stimulate the POMC/CART neurons. Agouti-related protein is the naturally occurring inverse agonist of MC3R and MC4R (melanocortin 3 and 4 receptors) and is expressed in cell bodies in the arcuate that coexpress NPY and that project to "second order" nuclei expressing MC3R and MC4R to stimulate food intake. The "default" action of this neural system is to generate a net anabolic signal unless leptin and insulin signal sufficient energy stores. Both sets of neurons respond vigorously to starvation, but only the POMC/CART neurons respond to excess energy intake in part explaining why it is easier for individuals to gain rather than lose weight. Energy expenditure is then coordinated through the autonomic nervous system and hypothalamic control of thyroid function.

Human adiposity resolves complex interactions among genetic, developmental, behavioral, and environmental influences. Evidence for potent genetic contributions to human obesity is provided by familial clustering of increased adiposity, including a 3- to 7-fold increased relative risk among siblings (4) as well as estimates of heritability (the fraction of the total phenotypic variance of a quantitative trait caused by genes in a specified environment) for fat mass between 40% and 70% in twin studies (5,6). Clearly, genetic change cannot account for the recent trends toward increased adiposity. However, what is likely genetically determined is the relative rank of adiposity of an individual within a population living in a specific environment. As the environment becomes more, or less, conducive to the development of obesity (ease of access to food, need for physical

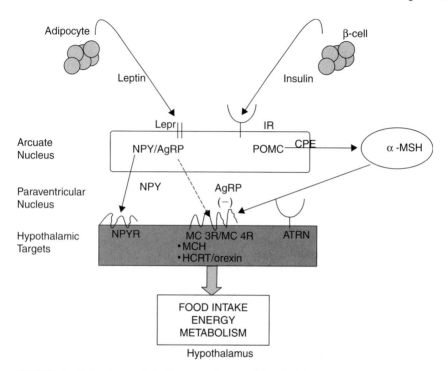

FIGURE 1 Molecular control of energy homeostasis. Peripheral signals, including leptin and insulin, bind to receptors on cell bodies in the arcuate nucleus of the hypothalamus. Neuropeptide Y (NPY)/agouti-related protein (AgRP) and proopiomelanocortin (POMC)/cocaine and amphetamine regulated transcript (CART) neurons in the arcuate nucleus project onto cell bodies in other hypothalamic nuclei to affect energy balance through food intake, energy expenditure, and nutrient partitioning. The melanocortin pathway is an integral part of the control of energy homeostasis. α (alpha-melanotropin) is derived from proteolytic processing of POMC and is an agonist (solid arrow) for melanocortin receptor 3 (MC3R)/melanocortin receptor 4 (MC4R) centrally producing catabolic effects on energy homeostasis. AgRP is an inverse agonist (*dashed arrow*) at MC3R/MC4R, producing anabolic effects on energy balance. *Abbreviations*: ATRN, attractin; BBB, blood-brain barrier; CPE, carboxypeptidase E; HCRT, hypocretin/orexin; IR, insulin receptor; Lepr, leptin receptor; MCH, melanin concentrating hormone.

exertion to obtain it, putative intrauterine, and perinatal influences), the median adiposity of the population shifts accordingly. The distribution of adiposities representing the population would not be expected to shift in perfect Gaussian symmetry around this median. That is, as a population is exposed to these environmental "pressures", the tails of the distribution may not change in proportion. Those who are thinnest may show disproportionate resistance to upward pressure by the environment, while those who are fattest may show greater sensitivity to the upward bias imposed by the environment. The opposite responses would characterize these "tails" in the context of environmentally mediated restriction of access to food. There are reasonable evolutionary arguments for such asymmetries in response, based upon the likelihood that strong selective pressure in favor of energy efficiency and proclivity in the acquisition and storage of calories has prevailed. The phenotypic differences among individuals at these extremes of adiposity presumably reflect allelic variation at genes that affect energy intake, expenditure and the chemical form in which excess calories are stored ("partitioning"). The nature of these genes is of obvious interest. The number of "candidate genes"—based upon spontaneous and induced genetic variation in model organisms, and molecular physiology—is now well over 50 (7). While a growing number of association studies have indirectly implicated some of these genes, the molecular genetic basis for human susceptibility to obesity is not well understood.

Genetic factors are currently estimated to account for 40% to 70% of the variance in human adiposity (4). In most individuals, the genetic basis for obesity is complex and likely to involve the interaction of multiple genes as well as gene-by-environment interactions. As with other complex phenotypes, there are rare examples of mono/oligogenic causes for obesity that serve as models for understanding the complex hormonal and neural networks that regulate adiposity, and provide insight to pathways that may account for more common causes of obesity as well as provide targets for therapeutic intervention. Some of them are detailed in Chapters 5.2–5.6. In this chapter we review the important genetic and physiological insights provided by the study of these relatively rare forms of obesity and provide comparisons between animal models and human cases. More details on specific nonsyndromic and syndromic forms of obesity are provided in Chapters 5.2–5.5.

NONSYNDROMIC MONOGENIC OBESITY

The understanding of body weight regulation in humans has been tremendously aided by the study of monogenic rodent models of obesity (Table 1).

Leptin Deficiency

Leptin was identified as a cytokine-like hormone secreted almost exclusively by adipocytes and deficient in the *obese* (Lep^{ob}/Lep^{ob}) mouse (8). Two alleles of *Lep* have been identified in the mouse both of which result in no detectable leptin production. Lep^{ob} is due to a nonsense mutation that results in the synthesis of a truncated protein that is apparently degraded in the adipocyte (8), while Lep^{ob2j} is due to an insertion of a retroviral-like transposon in the first intron of *Lep* that leads to the production of chimeric RNAs in which the first exon is spliced to sequences in the transposon (Chapter 3.1) (9). By screening obese subjects for serum leptin concentrations, Montague et al. were able to identify a single family with two children with undetectable levels of leptin in plasma (10). As in the mouse, human congenital leptin deficiency is inherited in an autosomal recessive manner and produces extreme, earlyonset obesity associated with intense hyperphagia (10), and is discussed in greater detail in chapter 5.4. Five individuals were found to be homozygous for the frameshift mutation ΔG133, producing a truncated protein that is not secreted (11). In addition, a large consanguineous Turkish family has been identified with three family members who are homozygous for the missense Arg105Trp mutation (12). Congenital leptin deficiency in humans is associated with hyperphagia but normal resting and free living energy expenditure, hypogonadotrophic hypogonadism with delayed but spontaneous pubertal development, and abnormalities of T-cell number and function (13) similar to findings in obese mice. Unlike the phenotype in mice, human leptin deficiency is

TABLE 1 Nonsyndromic Monogenic Forms of Obesity in Rodents and Humans

Gene	Murine mutation	Murine phenotype	Human mutation	Human phenotype
Leptin	Obese Lep^ob Lep^ob2j	Extreme, early onset obesity, decreased length, hyperphagia, hypogonadotrophic hypogonadism, cold intolerance, hypercosticosteronemia, T cell abnormalities	ΔG133 Arg105Trp	Extreme, early onset obesity, hyperphagia, delayed puberty, T cell abnormalities
Leptin receptor	Diabetes Lepr^db	Extreme, early-onset obesity, decreased length hyperphagia, hypogonadotrophic hypogonadism, cold intolerance, hypercortisolemia, T cell abnormalities	Exon 16 splice donor G → A	Extreme, early onset obesity, short stature, hyperphagia, delayed puberty
Pro-opiomelanocortin	Induced deletion of POMC	Later onset obesity, slightly increased length, adrenal agenesis, yellow coat color	G7013T, 7133delC, C3804A A6851T 6906delC 6996del 7100insGG 7134delG	Early onset obesity, adrenal insufficiency, red hair
Agouti signaling peptide	A^y	Later onset obesity, increased length, yellow coat color	none	
Carboxypeptidase E	Cpe^fat	Late onset obesity, hyperproinsulinemia	none	
Proconvertase 1	Induced deletion of PC1	Dwarf with low GHRH, normal weight, elevated proinsulin, normal corticosterone	Gly483Arg, A → C + 4 intron 5 donor splice site, Glu250Stop, Del213Ala	Childhood onset obesity, elevated proinsulin, hypocortisolemia, depressed POMC, reactive hypoglycemia, hypogonadotrophic hypogonadism
Tubby	tub	Late onset obesity, retinal degeneration, sensorineural hearing loss	none	
Melanocortin 4 receptor	Induced deletion of Mc4r	Early onset obesity, hyperphagia, increased fat mass, increased lean mass, increased linear growth, and hyperinsulinemia	Numerous	Early onset obesity, hyperphagia, increased fat mass, increased lean mass, increased bone mineral density and bone mineral content, increased linear growth, and hyperinsulinemia

not associated with somatic growth retardation (growth hormone and thyroid hormone axes are normal) or elevated plasma cortisol. Injected leptin replacement in three of these children produced normalization of hyperphagia without demonstrable effects on basal metabolic rate or free living energy expenditure even within the setting of weight loss (13), suggesting that the greatest effect of leptin deficiency is on food intake, but that energy expenditure was raised above that expected in a weight-losing subject. Earlier studies in *obese* mice by Coleman demonstrated that the greatest metabolic effect of the mutation was on food intake (14).

Although obesity is clearly most marked in mice homozygous for the Lep^{ob} mutation, we found a 27% increase in fat mass and 23% increase in percentage body fat in heterozygous $Lep^{ob/+}$ mice (15). Heterozygous leptin deficient humans also have a higher prevalence of obesity and increased percentage body fat than predicted for height and weight and have lower levels of serum leptin than would be predicted for percentage body fat (16). These data suggest that the leptin-related regulatory system is sensitive to haploinsufficiency or decreased production of leptin and can respond by increasing adiposity to achieve a critical lower threshold for circulating leptin. Teleologically, this response may be a safeguard against starvation and loss of reproductive integrity. This observation is consistent with the hypothesis that fat mass is more critically regulated at the low end than at the high end and that counterregulatory measures are stronger to protect against starvation than against excessive adiposity (17,18). Although clearly homozygous loss-of-function *LEP* mutations are rare in the general population, heterozygous mutations, or more subtle regulatory variants, may contribute to more common forms of obesity. Mice that are heterozygous for both Lep^{ob} and $Lepr^{db}$ mutations demonstrate increased adiposity *versus* single heterozygotes at Lep^{ob} or $Lepr^{db}$, suggesting that there are additive interactions on adiposity within this pathway (15). Leptin plays an important role in reproduction by signaling the availability of minimal fat stores necessary for reproductive success. Leptin-deficient C57BL/6J mice generally display hypogo-nadotrophic hypogonadism although this phenotype is clearly dependent upon modifier genes as evidenced by the reduced obesity and increased fertility of Lep^{ob}/Lep^{ob} mice on a Balb/cJ genetic background in contrast to the extreme obesity and infertility on a C57BL/6J background (19). Leptin deficient humans do progress through spontaneous yet delayed puberty, but no leptin deficient human has yet demonstrated fertility (13).

Leptin Receptor Deficiency

Based upon the early parabiosis experiments by Coleman, the *obese* mouse was predicted to produce a circulating factor to which the diabetes mouse was unable to respond (20). Diabetes mice have a phenotype virtually indistinguishable from *obese* mice when maintained on the same genetic background (Chaps. 3.1 and 3.2). Like *obese* mice, diabetes mice are characterized by extreme, early onset obesity with hyperphagia, reduced body length, cold intolerance, infertility, hypercorticosteronemia, and T cell abnormalities (21). Soon after *Lep* was identi-fied, the *leptin receptor (Lepr)* was discovered and loss-of-function mutations were identified in the *diabetes* mouse allelic series (22–24) as well as the *fatty* rat (25,26). Lepr is a member of the cytokine receptor family and mediates leptin signaling through phosphatidylinositol 3-kinase and signal transducer and activa-tor of transcription-3 (STAT3), predominantly in hypothalamic neurons (27). STAT3 signaling is crucial for the regulation of food intake, but not critical for the regulation of reproduction and growth. By screening *obese* human subjects for elevated serum leptin concentrations, a consanguineous family was identified in which three members showed extreme earlyonset obesity associated with statural growth retardation caused by impaired growth hormone secretion (28). All three subjects were homozygous for a splice site mutation in exon 16 that truncates the receptor before the transmembrane domain, rendering all cells incapable of transmitting an intracellular signal. Similar to the *diabetes* mouse, human leptin receptor deficiency produces extreme obesity in an autosomal recessive manner, and is discussed in greater detail in Chapter 5.4. Human leptin receptor–deficient subjects have normal basal temperature, resting metabolic rates, spontaneous but delayed puberty, and normal plasma cortisol concentrations (28). While *obese* and *diabetes* mice on the same genetic background are phenotypically indistinguishable, there are some important phenotypic differences between human leptin and leptin receptor–deficient subjects. Leptin receptor–deficient subjects have unique neuroendocrine features including mild growth retardation in early childhood, impaired basal and stimulated growth hormone secretion, and hypothalamic hypothyroidism. These data suggest that the Lepr has some leptin-independent effects on neuroendocrine function. However, the number of subjects is quite small and could also be related to the effects of other modifying genes.

Proopiomelancocortin Deficiency

Agouti (*Yellow*) was the first murine gene related to monogenic obesity to be positionally cloned (29) (see Chapter 3.1). The autosomal dominant agouti promoter mutation A^y results in ubiquitous ectopic overexpression of agouti signaling protein (ASP) throughout the body, producing the characteristic yellow coat color when it antagonizes the binding of α melanocortin stimulating hormone (α-MSH) at melanocortin 1 receptors (MC1R) in the skin, and producing increased length as well as body mass through antagonism of the MC3R and MC4R in the hypothalamus (30). The natural agonist of the melanocortin receptors, α-MSH, suppresses food intake and increases energy expenditure by actions at MC4R. The physiological antagonist (and inverse agonist) at MC4R was later identified as AgRP. α-MSH and ACTH are both derived from POMC by sequential cleavage by prohormone convertases and other processing enzymes in the arcuate nucleus of the hypothalamus. Many of the POMC neurons in the arcuate nucleus also express the Lepr, and POMC expression is positively correlated with ambient leptin (31). Targeted disruption of *Mc4r* and to a lesser extent *Mc3r* in mice produces obesity and increased linear growth similar to the *Ay* mice except for the expected lack of effect on coat color (32). Mice deficient in AgRP have no discernible abnormalities of body weight or composition in the basal state, with food deprivation, or with overfeeding (33), suggesting that there are powerfully redundant mechanisms for orexigenic signaling (this phenotype is described in detail in Chapter 3.2).

Autosomal recessive *POMC* deficiency is discussed in greater detail in Chapter 5.5 and is due to compound heterozygosity or homozygosity for loss-of-function mutations in a small number of human subjects produces severe, earlyonset obesity associated with hyperphagia (34,35) due to lack of α acting centrally at MC3R and MC4R. Because of a lack of peripheral MSH action, the children also demonstrated pale skin color and red hair due to lack of peripheral agonism at MC1R. The five children initially presented with undetectable levels of cortisol and ACTH early in infancy, consistent with the absence of ACTH ligand for the adrenal cortical MC2R. Heterozygous individuals have been found to have intermediate increases in body weight, suggesting a gene dosage effect for *POMC* (35–37). Mice with an induced deletion for the coding regions of all the *POMC*-derived peptides develop, later onset obesity associated with slightly increased length, adrenal agenesis with undetectable corticosterone and aldosterone, and yellow pelage (38) similar to the human counterparts. Recently, a heterozygous missense mutation (Arg236Gly) in *POMC* has been reported that disrupts the dibasic cleavage of beta MSH and beta-endorphin (39). In vitro studies indicate that this mutation produces an aberrant fusion protein of beta MSH and beta-endorphin that binds to MC4R but has reduced ability to activate the receptor. This Arg236Gly missense mutation has been identified in the heterozygous state in 0.9% of patients with severe earlyonset obesity with normal adrenal function and hair and skin pigmentation (39).

Mahogany and Mahoganoid

Mahogany ($Atrn^{mg}$) and *mahoganoid* ($Mgrn1^{md}$) are mutations in unlinked genes that have similar pleiotropic effects on coat color and energy expenditure in A^y mice. Both mutations are uniquely able to act epistatically to A^y to suppress both the yellow coat color and *obese* phenotypes caused by ectopic overexpression of *ASP*. Both mutations also cause variable degrees of spongiform degeneration of the brain. (40,41). The $Atrn^{mg}$ mutation does not suppress the obesity caused by other rodent genetic models of obesity including $Mc4r$, $Lepr^{db}$, Lep^{ob}, tub, or Cp^{efat} (42,43). Attractin ($Atrn$) encodes a single-pass transmembrane protein. Binding of ASP, but not AgRP, to ATRN in transgenic, biochemical, and genetic-interaction experiments demonstrates that attractin is a low affinity receptor for ASP, but not for AgRP, in vitro and in vivo (40,41). These experiments support the hypothesis that ATRN acts as a low affinity receptor for ASP to co-localize ASP to MC1R and to thereby inversely agonize MC1R in the hair follicle, producing a darker coat color. Only under circumstances of Asp overexpression in the A^y mouse, does ATRN act to co-localize ASP (which is not normally expressed in the brain) to MC3R/MC4R in the hypothalamus. ATRN does not similarly bind AgRP to bring AgRP into proximity to MC3R/MC4R. Therefore, $Atrn^{mg}/Atrn^{mg}$ A^y mice lacking ATRN are unable to co-localize the overexpressed ASP to MC3R/MC4R, and consequently are not *obese* (44).

The mouse coat color mutant *mahoganoid* ($Mgrn1^{md}$) has effects on pigmentation and energy metabolism that are similar to *mahogany* ($Atrn^{mg}$) in that mahoganoid specifically suppresses Ay-induced yellow pigmentation and obesity (45). Mahogunin also has effect on insulin resistance sensitivity separate from its effects on adiposity (46). The gene mutated in *mahoganoid* mice, named *Mahogunin* (*Mgrn1*), encodes an intracellular protein with a C3HC4 RING domain that functions as an E3 ubiquitin ligase (41,47). Mahogunin may ubiquitinate MC3R/MC4R or a MC3R/MC4R-associated proteins (e.g., POMC, α-MSH) to influence the physical proximity or binding of ASP or AgRP to their melanocortin receptors, increase binding of ATRN to ASP, or decrease the amount of α-MSH available to MC1R or MC3R/MC4R through sequestration or turnover of α-MSH. Inactivating mutations of this gene would be expected to increase access of α-MSH to its receptors, darkening coat and reducing food intake. Identification of the molecular targets of MGRN1 should further elucidate the mechanism of action. Situs inversus and a variety of types of congenital heart disease have been observed in embryos and adult *Mgrn1^{md}* mutant mice, suggesting that Mahogunin is critical to establishment and/or maintenance of the left-right axis during development (48). Interestingly, this phenotype of situs inversus is shared with some individuals with Bardet-Biedl syndrome (BBS). and may suggest a critical role for correct function of cilia and establishment of the left-right axis for proper neural development of regions of the brain critical for energy homeostasis.

Mutations in *ATRN* and *MGRN1* genes have not yet been identified in humans either in lean individuals or in subjects with neurodegenerative conditions; but, neither of these genes has been studied extensively in humans. However, the interactions of these genes within a single pathway demonstrate the complex epistatic interactions that may similarly underlie the genetics of obesity in humans.

Prohormone Convertase 1 Deficiency

Like the *POMC* knockout mouse, the *fat* mouse is an example of *autosomal* recessive obesity of later onset and reduced severity relative to the *obese* and *diabetes* mice. Observation of increased levels of circulating proinsulin in these mice led to the identification of the Ser202Pro mutation in the positional candidate gene *carboxypeptidase E* (*Cpe*) that is responsible for prohormone cleavage of C-terminal basic residues from prohormones and proneuropeptides such as proinsulin, proneuropeptide Y, progonadotropin, and POMC (49). Realizing that aberrant prohormone processing could produce obesity, Jackson et al. identified two subjects with compound heterozygous mutations in *prohormone convertase 1* (*PC1*), an enzyme that cleaves prohormones at dibasic amino acids in the step immediately prior to CPE processing (50). Both subjects have been described as having childhood onset obesity, elevated proinsulin, hypocortisolemia with elevated POMC, reactive hypoglycemia, and hypogonadotropic hypogonadism (50,51). Further details about PC1 deficiency are described in Chapter 5.5. The subjects' obesity phenotype is likely due to aberrant POMC and other prohormone processing, and the phenotype of the human subjects recapitulates that of the fat mouse. However, unlike the *fat* mouse, the second PC1-deficient subject described also had severe, malabsorptive diarrhea as a neonate, and the first PC1-deficient subject, in retrospect, also has clinically asymptomatic intestinal malabsorption (50). Therefore, PC1 may also have a role in prohormone processing in enteroendocrine cells that is essential for normal gastrointestinal function, including absorption. Interestingly, the induced homologous recombinant mouse that is deficient for PC1 is growth retarded due to impaired processing of growth hormone releasing hormone (52), and not *obese* or adrenally insufficient even though POMC processing is impaired (52). This animal highlights one of the few examples of a striking divergence in phenotypes between human and murine mutations.

Melanocortin 4 Receptor Deficiency

The most common monogenic form of obesity in humans is due to mutations in *MC4R* and this topic is covered in more detail in Chapter 5.6. The mutations are generally inherited in a co-dominant manner, and homozygous loss-of-function mutations have been identified and result in more severe obesity than in the heterozygous state (53). The penetrance of heterozygous *MC4R* mutations is, however, incomplete for both partially active and inactive *MC4R* mutations, especially in males (53,54). The prevalence of mutations in *MC4R* appears to vary between <1% and 6% of cases of severe obesity (53–56) depending on the age of onset and severity of obesity in each study population. Notably, most of the mutations identified have been missense mutations and almost all are unique and found in single families (53,57). There is no evidence to date of common founder mutations that would account for a significant fraction of the variance in obesity. If this distribution of mutations is representative of genetic variation in other genes increasing adiposity, it will be difficult to identify genes for obesity by traditional association methods unless highly inbred or isolated populations are used. Phenotypically, carriers of *MC4R* mutations have early onset hyperphagia, increased fat mass, increased lean mass, increased bone mineral density and bone mineral content, increased linear growth, and hyperinsulinemia relative to fat mass (53), findings similar to those of the *Mc4r* knockout mouse. Unlike subjects with mutations in *LEP* or *LEPR*, carriers of *MC4R* mutations tend to have amelioration of their obesity and hyperinsulinemia over time (58). Binge eating has not been consistently demonstrated to be associated with mutations in *MC4R* (59–63). The V103I polymorphism in *MC4R* has no observable functional effect but has been associated with a modest protective effect on BMI in several studies (See Chapter 6.3) (64,65).

Tub

A final example of monogenic obesity in the mouse is the autosomal recessive *tubby* mutation that produces mild, late onset obesity in association with cochlear and retinal degeneration due to deficiency of one of a family of tubby-like proteins (TULPs) that encode heterotrimeric-G-protein-responsive intracellular signaling molecules important in neuronal preservation (66–68). Although the phenotype of the mice resembles both BBS and Alström syndrome (see below), mutations in *TUB* have not yet been identified in humans. However, *tubby* mice may indicate that loss of specific populations of neurons, possibly in the hypothalamus, can lead to altered energy homeostasis and that loss of these neurons by other mechanisms could also lead to altered weight regulation. Mutations in a related gene, *TULP1*, have been associated with nonsyndromic autosomal recessive retinitis pigmentosa (RP14) without obesity in humans (69,70).

Lessons to be Learned from Nonsyndromic Obesity

Monogenic forms of nonsyndromic obesity have elegantly demonstrated the utility of animal models in identifying key molecular components in the control of food intake and energy expenditure. Most of the recent advances in this field have been based upon the identification of genes and metabolic pathways originally detected and elucidated in rodent models. Furthermore, with the exception of mutations in *MC4R*, humans with other monogenic forms of nonsyndromic obesity were identified only after defining a specific sub-phenotype (high or low leptin, hyperproinsulinemia, hypocortisolemia, unusual skin, and hair pigmentation) implicating a defect in a particular molecular pathway. This experience under-scores the need—when possible—to collect subphenotypic data when attempting to determine the genetic basis for nonsyndromic obesity. Additionally, it should be noted that in most cases of nonsyndromic obesity in humans, the largest contribution to positive energy balance is, apparently, excess caloric intake. This characteristic may also be more generally applicable to common forms of obesity and suggests that a significant portion of intervention and prevention strategies should be focused on controlling food intake. We are also beginning to appreciate the complex metabolic and neural pathways in which the genes controlling adiposity interact. It is becoming increasingly apparent that in many cases there are gene dosage effects in heterozygotes. In addition, there are interactions of different genes within the same pathway. It is, therefore, possible that quantitative differences in expression or function of these same genes, either alone or in combination with one another, may underlie the more common and genetically complex forms of human obesity. However, to detect genes of small effect size— or that require interactions with other genes—will require much larger study populations than have been previously examined. Again, access to detailed characterization of sub-phenotypes (energy expenditure, appetitive behaviors, body composition, endocrine, neuroendocrine, and autonomic phenotypes that may contribute to or reflect special aspects of obesity as a convergent phenotype) may be helpful in identifying subgroups of human subjects in whom to analyze specific genes.

SYNDROMIC OBESITY

Syndromic obesity is obesity occurring in the clinical context of a distinct set of associated clinical phenotypes. Over 25 syndromic forms of obesity have been identified (http://www.obesitygene.pbrc.edu). Recently, the genetic bases for some of these syndromes have been elucidated, and are beginning to provide insights into the pathogenesis of the derangements of energy homeostasis. Interestingly, although clinically well-defined, there is increasing evidence of genetic heterogeneity for some of these conditions with multiple genes within the same pathway producing identical phenotypes. This finding suggests that for more common polygenetic forms of nonsyndromic obesity, multiple allelic variants within the same molecular pathway may interact in either additive or synergistic ways to produce increasing adiposity. Presented below are a few of the most common syndromic forms of obesity for which the genetic basis has been partially or completely elucidated (Table 2).

Prader-Willi Syndrome

Prader-Willi syndrome (PWS) is the most common syndromic form of obesity, with an incidence of approximately one in 15,000–25,000 live births and is discussed further in Chapter 5.2. PWS is the result of loss of expression of paternal genes on the imprinted region of 15q11-13. Loss of maternal expression of genes in the same region produces Angelman syndrome, a very different symptom complex characterized by severe mental retardation, ataxia, and epilepsy. PWS is characterized by intrauterine and neonatal hypotonia, poor feeding, and failure to thrive that evolves into extreme hyperphagia and central obesity at one to six years of age if caloric restriction is not imposed. PWS is associated with decreased lean body mass, increased adiposity, short stature, and growth hormone deficiency, all of which are partially corrected by growth hormone replacement. Total energy expenditure was 20–47% lower in subjects with PWS compared to *obese* counterparts, and largely accounted for by the reduced lean body mass (71,72).

TABLE 2 Syndromic Forms of Human Obesity

Syndrome	Gene	Mode of inheritance	Phenotype
Prader-Willi syndrome	Contiguous gene disorder	Imprinting defect with loss of paternally expressed genes on 15q11–13	Neonatal hypotonia, poor feeding, evolving into extreme hyperphagia, central obesity, decreased lean body mass, short stature, hypothalamic hypogonadism, mild mental retardation, obsessive compulsive behavior
SIM1 deficiency	*SIM1*	Translocation of 1p22.1 and 6q16.2; interstitial deletion of 6q16	Early onset obesity associated with increased linear growth and hyperphagia
Bardet-Biedl syndrome	At least 12 loci (*BBS1-BBS12*) 12 genes identified	Oligogenic: either autosomal recessive or tri-tetra allelic	Progressive rod-cone dystrophy, postaxial polydactyly, renal cysts, progressive renal disease, dyslexia, learning disabilities, hypogonadism, occasional congenital heart disease, and progressive late-childhood obesity
Alström syndrome	*ALMS1*	Autosomal recessive	Mild truncal obesity, short stature, type 2 diabetes, retinopathy, sensorineural hearing loss, ephropathy, dilated cardiomyopathy
Cohen syndrome	*COH1*	Autosomal recessive	Mild truncal obesity, thin extremities, short stature, mild mental retardation, microcephaly, dysmorphic features, hypotonia, joint laxity, intermittent neutropenia, retinochoroidal dystrophy
Borjeson-Forssman-Lehmann syndrome	*PHF6*	X-linked dominant	Late-childhood truncal obesity, short stature, gynecomastia, hypotonia, poor feeding, large ears, small genitalia, mental retardation, microcephaly, epilepsy

Physical activity is reduced and associated with hypotonia further decreasing energy expenditure (73). Hypothalamic hypogonadism and hypogenitalism are both characteristic, although there have been instances of successful pregnancies in females with PWS that can give rise to children with Angelman syndrome (due to maternally transmitted deletions of 15q11-13) (74). In addition to the endocrinological abnormalities, there are specific dysmorphisms including almond shaped palpebral fissures and small hands and feet. Individuals with PWS characteristically show mild-to-moderate mental retardation with a mean IQ of 60 accompanied by specific obsessive-compulsive and ritualistic behaviors (including severe skin picking) and an increased incidence of psychosis in individuals with maternal uniparental disomy (75). Genetically, PWS can have several etiologies but is always associated with loss of expression of paternally transmitted genes on 15q11-q13. Seventy-five percent of cases are due to paternal deletions of

15q11-q13, 22% are due to maternal uniparental disomy, less than 3% are due to imprinting errors caused by microdeletions of the imprinting center at the *SNURF-SNRPN* (SNRPN upstream reading frame) gene locus, and less than 1% are due to paternal translocations (76). Regardless of the type of mutation, all patients with PWS share the same basic clinical features. Subjects with the paternal deletion have a higher frequency of hypopigmentation of the skin, hair, and eyes due to a contiguous deletion involving the P gene that causes oculocutaneous albinism (77). Notably, there are no known cases of classic PWS or isolated obesity associated with aberrations in a single gene within the 15q11-q13 critical region (76), suggesting that deficiencies of several genes may be necessary to produce the phenotype. Many of the genes in the PWS critical region are expressed within the hypothalamus (78) consistent with an obesity phenotype that appears to be central in origin. The heritable deletion of the mouse orthologous region on mouse chromosome 7 that is similarly imprinted has provided a useful mouse model for PWS (79), although these studies have been hampered by early neonatal mortality due to respiratory distress and poor feeding (80) as often characterizes human neonates with PWS. Hopefully, these mouse models will provide further insight into the underlying molecular etiology in the future.

The molecular pathophysiology of PWS has not yet been completely elucidated. PWS clearly involves all three possible mechanisms for increased adiposity (see Chapter 5.2), but in most individuals hyperphagia apparently contributes more significantly than decreased energy expenditure or increased partitioning of calories to fat. Based upon the associated growth hormone deficiency and hypogonadism, and pattern of expression of genes in the critical genetic interval, a hypothalamic defect is likely to be the primary etiology for the obesity associated with PWS. A defect in hypothalamic development could readily account for the characteristic derangements in energy balance, and there is evidence for reduction in the total number of cells in the paraventricular nucleus from five adults with PWS (81). Whole genome microarray expression studies in whole brain in the PWS mouse model show that *Pomc* expression is significantly increased in the neonatal period and could account for the decreased food intake observed at the beginning of life (82). Additionally, peripheral factors may exacerbate the hyperphagia. Recently, PWS patients have been found to have increased circulating levels of ghrelin, an orexigenic hormone released from the stomach that serves as an endogenous ligand for the growth hormone secretagogue receptor (GHRHR) (1). Ghrelin stimulates food intake in humans (83), and prolonged elevation may be the mechanism for reduced growth hormone secretion in PWS through desensitization of the GHRHR in the pituitary gland (84).

Sim1

A single case of early onset obesity associated with increased linear growth and hyperphagia has been associated with a de novo balanced translocation between 1p22.1 and 6q16.2, disrupting the *single-minded* (*SIM1*) gene, separating the 5′ flanking promoter region from the rest of the downstream coding exons (85). Five additional cases of interstitial deletions of 6p16.2 including *SIM1* have been described and associated with hypotonia, obesity, short extremities, and developmental delay (86–90). SIM1 is a member of the bHLH-PAS (basic helix loop helix + period aryl hydrocarbon receptor single-minded) gene family that is expressed in the supraoptic and paraventricular nuclei of the hypothalamus and acts as a transcription factor involved in midline neurogenesis. *Sim1* deficient mice have hypocellular paraventricular nuclei and are *obese* and hyperphagic (91). Although the downstream targets of *SIM1* have not yet been defined, it is intriguing that it is continually expressed in the paraventricular nucleus of the hypothalamus that integrates food intake and energy expenditure, and in which destructive lesions can cause obesity (92). The phenotype of *SIM1* haploinsufficiency resembles closely the phenotype of the human subjects with *MC4R* mutations; and paraventricular neurons express *MC4R* as well neuropeptide Y receptors Y1 and Y5, orexin 2 receptors, and corticotrophin releasing factor and its receptors (93). Interstitial deletions involving 6q16 are also associated with obesity and share some features of PWS including hypotonia, feeding problems in infancy, and hypogonadism (87) that may point to dysfunction of the paraventricular nucleus of the hypothalamus as part of the etiology for the obesity observed in PWS. Haploinsufficiency of *SIM1* can cause increased weight gain and linear growth, suggesting that transcription factors may play important roles in regulation of human adiposity in a manner analogous to the role of transcription factors for maturity onset diabetes of youth (MODY) (94). To date, no human subjects have been identified with mutations in *SIM1* that segregate with obesity although two common polymorphisms, P352T and A371V have been weakly associated with BMI (95).

Bardet-Biedl Syndrome

BBS is a rare syndromic form of obesity with an estimated incidence of 1 in 150,000 live births in North America and Europe (96), and a higher incidence in isolated populations of Newfoundland (97) and Arab Bedouins (98). BBS is covered in greater detail in Chapter 5.3. Although the populations in Newfoundland and Kuwait are relatively small and isolated, surprisingly, multiple BBS genes contribute to the occurrence of the syndrome in both populations (99). BBS is associated with progressive rod-cone dystrophy, postaxial polydactyly, renal cysts and progressive renal disease, dyslexia, learning disabilities, blunted affect, hypogonadism, occasional congenital heart disease; progressive late childhood obesity with a BMI > 30 is observed in approximately half of subjects with BBS (100). Obesity in BBS is associated with hyperphagia and reduced spontaneous physical activity beyond that of comparably *obese* individuals.

The genetics of BBS before the discovery of the underlying genes was thought to be classical autosomal recessive. Although the resulting phenotypes are essentially indistinguishable, twelve different genes have now been identified as causing BBS. The disease segregates in families as both a classical autosomal recessive trait as well as a digenetic trait in which three or even four alleles interact to determine the penetrance of BBS or to modify the severity and age of onset of disease manifestations (101). All of the common forms of BBS have been associated with tri- or tetra-allelic inheritance (102). BBS2 and BBS6 are especially likely to show oligogenic inheritance (100). Notably, all but one example of oligogenic inheritance have included missense alleles; ultimately, functional assays will be required to determine which of these alleles are pathogenic. Although great progress has been made in identifying the genes for BBS, in ~30% of families the genetic basis has not yet been determined, leaving open the possibility of several additional BBS genes (103). *BBS1* is the most common gene involved in BBS and accounts for approximately 20% to 25% of all cases; a common founder European/North American M390R allele accounts for 80% of all *BBS1* mutations

(104). The high prevalence of this ancient mutation could be due to a selective advantage for carriers. However, the M390R mutation has not been associated with nonsyndromic obesity in the general population of Newfoundland where it is common and implies that it causes only syndromic obesity and/or that studies have not had sufficient power to detect the effect in heterozygous carriers in whom it may interact with other unidentified genes (105). Mutations in the gene for *BBS1* also cause the McCusick Kaufman Syndrome that consists of hydrometrocolpos, postaxial polydactyly, and congenital heart disease, and overlaps phenotypically with BBS. McCusick Kaufman Syndrome is found most commonly in the Amish population (106), and is not associated with obesity. The difference in the phenotypes is likely related to the specific mutation in *BBS1* and/or mutations at other interacting loci that produce BBS. Although still in the early stages of study, genes for BBS are being investigated for association with nonsyndromic pediatric and adult onset obesity. Genetics variants in *BBS2*, *BBS4*, and *BBS6* have been associated with obesity in Caucasians (107).

Identification of the *BBS8* gene encoding a protein involved in pilus formation and twitching mobility that localizes to the basal bodies and centrosome in physical juxtaposition to BBS4 suggests that these proteins play a role in the function of the pericentriolar region of ciliated cells (102). It is, therefore, possible that the underlying pathogenic mechanism for BBS involves dysfunction of the basal body in ciliated cells (102). *C. elegans* orthologs of *BBS1*, *BBS2*, *BBS7*, and *BBS8* are also expressed in the ciliated dendritic endings of neurons. Developmental brain abnormalities resulting from aberrant basal body performance could account for the learning disabilities, behavioral problems, and hyperphagia seen in BBS patients. Defective protein transport across photoreceptor-connecting cilium can cause retinal dystrophy (108), and aberrant mechanosensation at the primary cilium of renal tubular cells can lead to polycystic kidney disease (109). Nodal cilium dysfunction can also cause situs inversus and associated congenital heart disease (110), rare manifestations in some BBS families. Anosmia has also been demonstrated in subjects with BBS and is likely due to defects in the olfactory ciliary structure and function (111). Therefore, the multiple genes causing BBS may be components of a molecular complex or act sequentially in the same cellular process(es) to cause progressively more severe dysfunction as mutations are added in genes in the same "pathway." This model of multiple "hits" within the same pathway may also be more broadly applicable to the much more common polygenic forms of common obesity. The genetic complexity of this very distinct phenotype of BBS may also be a clue to the genetic complexity of polygenic obesity, and to strategies for unraveling it by close attention to gene–gene interactions in putative biochemical, structural and functional "pathways."

Alström Syndrome

Alström syndrome is a rare autosomal recessive, genetically homogeneous disorder characterized by mild truncal obesity that usually begins within the first year of life and continues throughout life unless caloric restriction is imposed (112). It is particularly common among the French Acadians in Nova Scotia and Louisiana, as well as other consanguineous populations. Alström syndrome is associated with short stature that is usually not apparent until after puberty (113), hyperinsulinemia that is out of proportion to the degree of adiposity, and, ultimately, type 2 diabetes. Other consistently associated clinical findings are retinopathy with cone-rod degeneration often presenting as nystagmus and photodysphoria within the first year of life and ultimately resulting in blindness, progressive sensorineural hearing loss, and progressive chronic nephropathy in the second to third decade of life ultimately resulting in renal failure which is the most frequent cause of death. Other more variable manifestations include dilated cardiomyopathy that may present in infancy and remit and recur with time, hepatic dysfunction secondary to hepatic fibrosis, hypothyroidism, primary gonadal failure, and psychomotor developmental delay. Unlike BBS, Alström syndrome is not associated with polydactyly (113). The gene for Alström syndrome, *ALMS1*, was identified simultaneously by two groups and encodes a gene of unknown function expressed ubiquitously at low levels and containing a predicted leucine zipper motif, serine-rich region, potential nuclear localization signal, and histidine-rich region, and large tandem repeat domain comprising 34 imperfect repetitions of 47 amino acids (114,115). Gene disruption due to a balanced translocation of 2p13 and small numbers of nonsense and frameshift mutations have been reported in Alström patients (114,115). Ubiquitous expression of the *ALMS1* gene suggests a reason for the protean clinical manifestations. However, the mechanism by which loss-of-function mutations in this gene produce obesity or any of the other associated phenotypes is still unknown. Polymorphisms in *ALMS1* have been found not to be associated with type 2 diabetes in Caucasians (116).

Cohen Syndrome

Cohen syndrome is a rare autosomal recessive condition overrepresented in the Finnish population. The syndrome is characterized by mild truncal obesity, thin extremities, and short stature starting in mid childhood (117). Cohen syndrome is associated with nonprogressive global developmental delay, mild-to-moderate mental retardation, microcephaly, characteristic facial features (downslanting and wave-shaped palpebral fissures, prominent nasal root, short philtrum, prominent central incisors, and thick hair), hypotonia, joint laxity, intermittent neutropenia, and progressive myopia often associated with retinochoroidal dystrophy (117,118). The clinical findings are not all apparent within the first few years of life, and can be variable among individuals of different ethnicities (119). The gene for Cohen syndrome, *COH1*, was positionally identified and 28 frameshift, premature termination, and missense mutations have been identified in this ubiquitously expressed putative transmembrane protein with a complex domain structure (120). Homology to the Saccharomyces cerevisiae VPS13 proteins suggests that it may be involved in vesicle mediated sorting and transport of proteins within the cell (120). Which protein targets may be aberrantly sorted as a result of mutations in *COH1*, and how they relate to obesity, have not yet been identified.

Borjeson-Forssman-Lehmann Syndrome

Borjeson-Forssman-Lehmann syndrome is a rare X-linked dominant condition associated with late childhood truncal obesity, short stature, and gynecomastia (121,122). Male infants generally display hypotonia, poor feeding, large ears, and small genitalia, similar to infants with PWS with the exception of the large ears. As males get older, they show moderate mental retardation, microcephaly, epilepsy, tapering fingers with lax interphalangeal joints, shortened toes, gynecomastia in adolescence, and progressively coarse facial features with deep set eyes. Many carrier females have no clinical phenotype due to complete X inactivation skewing, although females with incomplete X inactivation skewing have a milder phenotype similar to males. The gene for Borjeson-Forssman-Lehmann syndrome is a novel, widely expressed zinc finger gene plant homeodomain-like finger (*PHF6*) that accumulates in the nucleolus and may have a role in transcription (123). The molecular targets of *PHF6* have not yet been identified nor has the metabolic basis for the obesity in subjects with Borjeson-Forssman-Lehmann syndrome been investigated due to the small number of subjects affected.

Lessons to be Learned from Syndromic Obesity

Most syndromic forms of obesity are associated with mild to severe cognitive deficits and unusual behaviors. While many other syndromes affecting cognition such as Down syndrome are also associated with a higher incidence of obesity (124), the syndromic forms of obesity described above appear to have specific effects on food intake. These data suggest that there may be specific neuroanatomic or functional deficits, particularly in the hypothalamus, that lead to increased energy intake. The development of new techniques including functional imaging of the brain should permit noninvasive determination of which parts of the brain function aberrantly in the context of food intake in each of the syndromic forms of obesity. With few exceptions, although genes for several forms of syndromic obesity have been identified, their function, relevant cells, and their targets have yet to be identified. As additional genomic and informatics capabilities emerge, these questions should be more readily answered and should provide additional insight into the pathophysiology of obesity. To date, mutations in the genes causing syndromic obesity have not been shown to have mutations or to be linked or associated with nonsyndromic obesity; however, this point has not been fully investigated. Other molecules in the pathways identified for syndromic obesity may be more directly relevant to the more common forms of obesity.

CONCLUSION

Like the monogenic mouse obesities, the human syndromic obesities will probably have most heuristic significance for the new molecules and pathways that they reveal in the complex regulatory system that controls body weight. The relevance of these genes and pathways in the genetics that clearly underlies susceptibility to obesity in humans will require the same sort of large scale analyses that will be needed for other putative molecular players in the relevant processes. Fundamentally, this will require the simultaneous consideration of several alleles of many genes in very large numbers of well-phenotyped subjects. Awareness of the relationships among specific candidate molecules—gleaned from model organisms, and syndromic or sporadic severe obesities in humans—will help to rationalize the selection of genes for any specific analysis, and permit explicit mechanistic hypothesis testing, thereby enhancing statistical power. Further refinement can be achieved by selection of subjects based upon specific subphenotypes.

ACKNOWLEDGMENTS

We appreciate the assistance of Roberto Almazan and Margo Weiss with manuscript preparation. This work has been supported in part by NIH DK52431.

REFERENCES

1. Cummings DE, Clement K, Purnell JQ, et al. Elevated plasma ghrelin levels in Prader-Willi syndrome. Nat Med 2002; 8:643–4.
2. Rosenbaum M, Nicolson M, Hirsch J, et al. Effects of weight change on plasma leptin concentrations and energy expenditure. J Clin Endocrinol Metab 1997; 82:3647–54.
3. Woods SC, Seeley RJ, Porte D, Jr., et al. Signals that regulate food intake and energy homeostasis. Science 1998; 280:1378–83.
4. Allison DB, Faith MS, Nathan JS. Risch's lambda values for human obesity. Int J Obes Relat Metab Disord 1996; 20:990–9.
5. Stunkard AJ, Hrubec Z. A twin study of human obesity. JAMA 1986; 256:51–4.
6. Stunkard AJ, Pederson NL, McClearn GE. The body-mass index of twins who have been reared apart. N Engl J Med 1990; 322:1483–7.
7. Rankinen T, Zuberi A, Chagnon YC, et al. The human obesity gene map: the 2005 update. Obesity 2006; 14(4):529–644.
8. Zhang Y, Proenca R, Maffei M, et al. Positional cloning of the mouse obese gene and its human homologue. Nature 1994; 372:425–32.
9. Moon BC. The molecular basis of the obese mutation in ob2J mice. Genomics 1997; 42:152–6.
10. Montague CT, Whitehead JP, Soos MA, et al. Congenital leptin deficiency is associated with severe earlyonset obesity in humans. Nature 1997; 387:903–8.
11. Rau H, O'Rahilly S, Whitehead JP. Truncated human leptin (delta133) associated with extreme obesity undergoes proteasomal degradation after defective intracellular transport. Endocrinology 1999; 140:1718–23.
12. Strobel A, Camoin L, Ozata M, et al. A leptin missense mutation associated with hypogonadism and morbid obesity. Nature Genet 1998; 18:213–5.
13. Farooqi IS, Lord GM, Keogh JM, et al. Beneficial effects of leptin on obesity, T cell hyporesponsiveness, and neuroendocrine/metabolic dysfunction of human congenital leptin deficiency. J Clin Invest 2002; 110;1093–103.
14. Coleman DL. Increased metabolic efficiency in obese mutant mice. Int J Obes 1985; 9(Suppl 2):69–73.
15. Chung WK, Chua M, Wiley J, et al. Heterozygosity for Lep(ob) or Lep(rdb) affects body composition and leptin homeostasis in adult mice. Am J Physiol 1998; 274; R985–90.
16. Farooqi IS, Kamath S, Jones S, et al. Partial leptin deficiency and human adiposity. Nature 2001; 414;34–5.
17. Leibel RL. The role of leptin in the control of body weight. Nutr Rev 2002; 60;S15–19.
18. Rosenbaum M, Heymsfield SB, Matthews DE, et al. Low dose leptin administration reverses effects of sustained weight-reduction on energy expenditure and circulating concentrations of thyroid hormones. J Clin Endocrinol Metab 2002; 87;2391–4.
19. Chehab FF, Mounzih K, Ewart-Toland A, et al. Leptin and reproduction. Nutr Rev 2002; 60:S39–46.
20. Coleman D. Effects of paraboisis of obese with diabetes and normal mice. Diabetologia 1973; 9:294–8.
21. Coleman DL. Diabetes-obesity syndromes in mice. Diabetes 1982; 31:1–6.
22. Chua SC Jr, Chung WK, Wu-Peng XS, et al. Phenotypes of mouse diabetes and rat fatty due to mutations in the OB (leptin) receptor. Science 1996; 271:994–6.
23. Lee GH, Proenca R, Montez JM, et al. Abnormal splicing of the leptin receptor in diabetic mice. Nature 1996; 379:632–5.
24. Tartaglia LA, Dembski M, Weng W, et al. Identification and expression cloning of a leptin receptor, OB-R. Cell 1995; 83:1263–71.
25. Wu-Peng XS, Okada N, Liu SM, et al. Phenotype of the obese Koletsky (f) rat due to Tyr763Stop mutation in the extracellular domain of the leptin receptor (Lepr): evidence for deficient plasma-to-CSF transport of leptin in both the Zucker and koletsky obese rat. Diabetes 1997; 46:513–8.
26. Phillips MS, Liu Q, Hammond HA, et al. Leptin receptor missense mutation in the fatty Zucker rat. Nat Genet 1996; 13:18–9.

27. Bates SH, Myers MG. The role of leptin receptor signaling in feeding and neuroendocrine function. Trends Endocrinol Metab 2003; 14:447–52.
28. Clement K, Vaisse C, Lahlou N, et al. A mutation in the human leptin receptor gene causes obesity and pituitary dysfunction. Nature 1998; 392:398–401.
29. Bultman SJ, Michaud EJ, Woychik RP. Molecular characterization of the mouse agouti locus. Cell 1992; 71:1195–204.
30. Rossi M, Morgan DGA, Small CJ, et al. A C-Terminal fragment of agouti-related protein increases feeding and antagonizes the effect of alpha-melanocyte stimulating hormone in vivo. Endocrinology 1998; 139:4428–31.
31. Cheung CC, Steiner RA. Proopiomelanocortin neurons are direct targets for leptin in the hypothalamus. Endocrinology 1997; 138:4489–92.
32. Huszar D, Fairchild-Huntress V, Dunmore JH, et al. Targeted disruption of the Melanocortin-4 Receptor results in obesity in mice. Cell 1997; 88:131–41.
33. Qian S, Weingarth D, Trumbauer ME, et al. Neither agouti-related protein nor Neuropeptide Y is critically required for the regulation of energy homeostasis in mice. Mol Cell Biol 2002; 22:5027–35.
34. Krude H, Luck W, Horn R, et al. Severe earlyonset obesity, adrenal insufficiency and red hair pigmentation caused by POMC mutations in humans. Nat Genet 1998; 19:155–7.
35. Krude H, Schnabel D, Tansek MZ, et al. Obesity due to proopiomelanocortin deficiency: three new cases and treatment trials with thyroid hormone and ACTH4–10. J Clin Endocrinol Metab 2003; 88:4633–40.
36. Buono P, Pasanisi F, Nardelli C, et al. Six novel mutations in the proopiomelanocortin and melanocortin receptor 4 genes in severely obese adults living in southern Italy. Clin Chem 2005; 51:1358–64.
37. Farooqi IS, Drop S, Clements A, et al. Heterozygosity for a POMC-null mutation and increased obesity risk in humans. Diabetes 2006; 55:2549–53.
38. Yaswen L, Brennan MB, Hochgeschwender U. Obesity in the mouse model of proopiomelanocortin deficiency responds to peripheral melanocortin. Nat Med 1999; 5:1066–70.
39. Challis BG, Creemers JWM, Delplanque J, et al. A missense mutation disrupting a dibasic prohormone processing site in proopiomelanocortin (POMC) increases susceptibility to earlyonset obesity through a novel molecular mechanism. Hum Mol Genet 2002; 11:1997–2004.
40. Gunn TM, Kitada K, Ito S, et al. Molecular and phenotypic analysis of attractin mutant mice. Genetics 2001; 158:1683–95.
41. He L, Jolly AF, Eldridge AG, et al. Spongiform degeneration in mahoganoid mutant mice. Science 2003; 299:710–2.
42. Nagle DL, Vitale J, Woolf EA, et al. The mahogany protein is a receptor involved in suppression of obesity. Nature 1999; 398:148–52.
43. Dinulescu DM, Boston BA, McCall K, et al. Mahogany (mg) stimulates feeding and increases basal metabolic rate independent of its suppression of agouti. PNAS 1998; 95:12707–12.
44. He L, Gunn TM, Bouley DM, et al. A biochemical function for attractin in agouti-induced pigmentation and obesity. Nat Genet 2001; 27:40–7.
45. Miller KA, Carrasquillo MM, Lamoreux ML, et al. Genetic Studies of the mouse mutations mahogany and mahoganoid. Genetics 1997; 146:1407–15.
46. Phan LK, Chung WK, Leibel RL. The mahoganoid mutation (Mgrn1md) improves insulin sensitivity in mice with mutations in the melanocortin signaling pathway independently of effects on adiposity. Am J Physiol Endocrinol Metab 2006; 291: E611–20.
47. Phan LK, LeDuc CA, Chung WK, et al. The mouse mahoganoid coat color mutation disrupts a novel C3HC4 RING domian protein. J Clin Invest 2002; 110:1449–59.
48. Cota CD, Bagher P, Pelc P, et al. Mice with mutations in Mahogunin ring finger-1 (Mgrn1) exhibit abnormal patterning of the left-right axis. Dev Dyn 2006; 235:3438–47.
49. Naggert JK, Varlamov O, Nishina PM, et al. Hyperproinsulinaemia in obese fat/fat mice associated with a carboxypeptidase E mutation which reduces enzyme activity. Nat Genet 1995; 10:135–42.

50. Jackson RS, Farooqi IS, Raffin-Sanson ML, et al. Small-intestinal dysfunction accompanies the complex endocrinopathy of human proprotein convertase 1 deficiency. J Clin Invest 2003; 112:1550–60.
51. Jackson RS, Ohagi S, Raffin-Sanson ML, et al. Obesity and impaired prohormone processing associated with mutations in the human prohormone convertase 1 gene. Nat Genet 1997; 16:303–6.
52. Zhu X, Dey A, Norrbom C, et al. Disruption of PC1/3 expression in mice causes dwarfism and multiple neuroendocrine peptide processing defects. PNAS 2002; 99:10293-8.
53. Farooqi IS, Keogh JM, Yeo GSH, et al. Clinical spectrum of obesity and mutations in the Melanocortin 4 Receptor gene. N Engl J Med 2003; 348:1085–95.
54. Vaisse C, Durand E, Hercberg S, et al. Melanocortin-4 receptor mutations are a frequent and heterogeneous cause of morbid obesity. J Clin Invest 2000; 106:253–62.
55. Farooqi IS, Keogh JM, Aminian S, et al. Dominant and recessive inheritance of morbid obesity associated with melanocortin 4 receptor deficiency. J Clin Invest 2000; 106:271–9.
56. Hinney A, Nottebom K, Heibült O, et al. Several mutations in the Melanocortin-4 receptor gene including a nonsense and a frameshift mutation associated with dominantly inherited obesity in humans. J Clin Endocrinol Metab 1999; 84:1483–6.
57. Lubrano-Berthelier C, Dubern B, Shapiro A, et al. Molecular genetics of human obesity-associated MC4R mutations. Ann NY Acad Sci 2003; 994:49–57.
58. O'Rahilly S, Yeo GSH, Challis BG. Minireview: human obesity-lessons from monogenic disorders. Endocrinology 2003; 144:3757–64.
59. Branson R, Kral JG, Lentes KU, et al. Binge eating as a major phenotype of melanocortin 4 receptor gene mutations. N Engl J Med 2003; 348:1096–103.
60. Farooqi IS, O'Rahilly S. Binge eating as a phenotype of melanocortin 4 receptor gene mutations. N Engl J Med 2003; 349:606–9.
61. Gotoda T. Binge eating as a phenotype of melanocortin 4 receptor gene mutations. N Engl J Med 2003; 349:606–9.
62. Herpertz S, Hebebrand J. Binge eating as a phenotype of melancortin 4 receptor gene mutations. N Engl J Med 2003; 349:606–9.
63. List JF, Habener JF. Defective melanocortin 4 receptors in hyperphagia and morbid obesity. N Engl J Med 2003; 348(12):1160–3.
64. Geller F, Reichwald K, Dempfle A, et al. Melanocortin-4 receptor gene variant I103 is negatively associated with obesity. Am J Hum Genet 2004; 74:572–81.
65. Heid IM, Vollmert C, Hinney A, et al. Association of the 103I MC4R allele with decreased body mass in 7937 participants of two population based surveys. J Med Genet 2005; 42:e21.
66. Santagata S, Baird CL, Gomez CA, et al. G-protein signaling through tubby proteins. Science 2001; 292:2041–50.
67. Noben-Trauth K, North MA, Nishina PM. A candidate gene for the mouse mutation tubby. Nature 1996; 380:534–8.
68. Kleyn PW, Kovats SG, Lee JJ, et al. Identification and characterization of the mouse obesity gene tubby: a member of a novel gene family. Cell 1996; 85:281–90.
69. Banerjee P, Knowles JA, Lewis CA, et al. TULP1 mutation in two extended Dominican kindreds with autosomal recessive Retinitis pigmentosa. Nat Genet 1998; 18:177–9.
70. Hagstrom SA, Nishina PL, Berson EL, et al. Recessive mutations in the gene encoding the tubby-like protein TULP1 in patients with retinitis pigmentosa. Nat Genet 1998; 18:174–6.
71. Schoeller DA, Bandani LG, Dietz WW, et al. Energy expenditure and body composition in Prader-Willi syndrome. Metabolism 1988; 37:115–20.
72. Butler MG, Theodoro MF, Bittel DC, et al. Energy expenditure and physical activity in Prader-Willi syndrome: comparison with obese subjects. Am J Med Genet A 2007; 143:449–59.
73. van Mil EG, Kester AD, Curfs LM, et al. Activity related energy expenditure in children and adolescents with Prader-Willi syndrome. Int J Obes Relat Metab Disord 2000; 24:429–34.

74. Schulz A, Hamborg-Peterson B, Graem N, et al. Fertility in Prader-Willi syndrome: a case report with Angelman syndrome in the offspring. Acta Pediatr 2001; 90:455–9.
75. Boer H, Whittington J, Butler J, et al. Psychotic illness in people with Prader-Willi syndrome due to chromosome 15 maternal unipaternal disomy. Lancet 2002; 359:135–6.
76. Nicholls RD. Genome organization, function, and imprinting in Prader-Willi and Angelman syndrome. Annu Rev Genomics Hum Genet 2001; 2:153–75.
77. Gillessen-Kaesbach G, Lohmann D, Kaya-Westerloh S, et al. Genotype–phenotype correlation in a series of 167 deletion and non-deletion patients with Prader-Willi syndrome. Hum Genet. 1995; 96:638–43.
78. Lee S, Wevrick R. Prader-Willi syndrome transcript are expressed in phenotypically significant regions of the developing mouse brain. Gene Express Patterns 2003; 3: 599–609.
79. Gabriel JM, Ohta T, Ji Y, et al. A transgene insertion creating a heritable chromosome deletion mouse model of Prader-Willi and Angelman syndromes. PNAS 1999; 96:9258–63.
80. Nicholls RD, Ji H, et al. Mouse models for Prader-Willi and Angelman syndromes offer insights into novel obesity mechanisms. Progr Obesity Res 2003; 9:313–9.
81. Swaab DF, Hofman MA. Alterations in the hypothalamic paraventricular nucleus and its oxytocin neurons (putative satiety cells) in Prader-Willi syndrome: a study of five cases. J Clin Endocrinol Metab 1995; 80:573–9.
82. Bittel DC, Kibiryeva N, McNulty SG, et al. Whole genome microarray analysis of gene expression in an imprinting center deletion mouse model of Prader-Willi syndrome. Am J Med Genet A 2007; 143(5):422–9.
83. Kojima M. Ghrelin, an orexigenic signaling molecule from the gastrointestinal tract. Curr Opin Pharmacol 2002; 2:665–8.
84. Date Y, Murakami N, Kojima M, et al. Central effects of a novel acylated peptide, ghrelin, on growth hormone release in rats. Biochem Biophys Res Commun 2000; 275:477–80.
85. Holder JL, Butte NF. Profound obesity associated with a balanced translocation that disrupts the SIM1 gene. Human Mol Genet 2000; 9:101–8.
86. Varela MC, Simoes-Sato AY, Kim CA, et al. A new case of interstitial 6q16.2 deletion in a patient with Prader-Willi-like phenotype and investigation of SIM1 gene deletion in 87 patients with syndromic obesity. Eur J Med Genet 2006; 49:298–305.
87. Faivre L, Cormier-Daire V, Lapierre JM, et al. Deletion of the SIM1 gene (6q16.2) in a patient with a Prader-Willi-like phenotype. J Med Genet 2002; 39:594–6.
88. Gilhuis HJ, van Ravenswaaij CM, Hamel BJ, et al. Interstitial 6q deletion with a Prader-Willi-like phenotype: a new case and review of the literature. Eur J Paediatr Neurol 2000; 4:39–43.
89. Turleau C, Demay G, Cabanis MO, et al. 6q1 monosomy: a distinctive syndrome. Clin Genet 1988; 34:38–42.
90. Villa A, Urioste M, Bofarull JM, et al. De novo interstitial deletion q16.2q21 on chromosome 6. Am J Med Genet 1995; 55:379–83.
91. Michaud JL, Boucher F, Melnyk A, et al. Sim1 haploinsufficiency causes hyperphagia, obesity and reduction of the paraventricular nucleus of the hypothalamus. Hum Mol Genet 2001; 10:1465–73.
92. Kirchgessner AL. PVN-hindbrain pathway involved in the hypothalamic hyperphagia-obesity syndrome. Physiol Behav 1988; 42:517–28.
93. Schwartz MW, Purnell JQ, Vaisse C, et al. Elevated plasma ghrelin levels in Prader-Willi syndrome. Nat Med 2002; 8:643–4.
94. Yamagata K. Regulation of pancreatic betra-cell function by the HNF transcription network: lessons from maturity-onset diabetes of the young (MODY). Endocrine J 2003; 50:491–9.
95. Hung CC, Luan J, Sims S, et al. Studies of the SIM1 gene in relation to human obesity and obesity-related traits. Int J Obes (Lond) 2007; 31:429–34.
96. Klein DA. The syndrome of Laurence–Moon–Bardet–Biedl and allied diseases in Switzerland. Clinical, genetic and epidemiological studies. J Neuro Sci 1969; 9:479–513.

97. Green JS, Harnett JD, Farid NR, et al. The cardinal manifestations of Bardet-Biedl syndrome, a form of Laurence–Moon–Biedl syndrome. N Engl J Med 1989; 321: 1002–9.

98. Farang TI. High incidence of Bardet–Biedl syndrome among Bedouin. Clin Genet 1989; 36:463–4.

99. Woods MO, Parfrey PS, Hefferton D, et al. Genetic Heterogeneity of Bardet–Biedl syndrome in a distinct Canadian population: evidence for a fifth locus. Genomics 1999; 55:2–9.

100. Beales PL, Ross AJ, Ansley SJ, et al. Genetic interaction of BBS1 mutations with alleles at other BBS loci can result in non-Mendelian Bardet–Biedl syndrome. Am J Hum Genet 2003; 72:1187–99.

101. Badano JL, Hoskins BE, Lewis RA, et al. Heterozygous mutations in BBS1, BBS2 and BBS6 have a potential epistatic effect on Bardet–Biedl patients with two mutations at a second BBS locus. Hum Mol Genet 2003; 12:1651–9.

102. Ansley SJ, Blacque OE, Hill J, et al. Basal body dysfunction is a likely cause of pleiotropic Bardet-;Biedl syndrome. Nature 2003; 425:628–33.

103. Katsanis N. The oligogenic properties of Bardet-Biedl syndrome. Human Mol Genet 2004; 13:R65–R71.

104. Mykytyn K, Searby CC, Beck G, et al. Evaluation of complex inheritance involving the most common Bardet-Biedl Syndrome Locus (BBS1). Am J Hum Genet 2003; 72: 429–37.

105. Fan Y, Peddle L, Hefferton D, et al. Bardet-Biedl syndrome 1 genotype and obesity in the Newfoundland population. Intl J Obesity 2004; 28:680–4.

106. Stone DL, Bouffard GG, Banerjee-Basu S, et al. Mutation of a gene encoding a putative chaperonin causes McKusick–Kaufman syndrome. Nat Genet 2000; 25:79–82.

107. Benzinou M, Walley A, Lobbens S, et al. Bardet-Biedl syndrome gene variants are associated with both childhood and adult common obesity in French Caucasians. Diabetes 2006; 55:2876–82.

108. Pazour GJ, Deane JA, Cole DG, et al. The intraflagellar transport protein, IFT88, is essential for vertebrate photoreceptor assembly and maintenance. J Cell Biol 2002; 157:103–14.

109. Nauli SM, Luo Y, Williams E, et al. Polycystins 1 and 2 mediate mechanosensation in the primary cilium of kidney cells. Nat Genet 2003; 33:129–37.

110. Nonaka S, Okada Y, Takeda S, et al. Randomization of Left–Right asymmetry due to loss of Nodal Cilia Generating leftward flow of extraembryonic fluid in mice lacking KIF3B motor protein. Cell 1998; 95:829–37.

111. Kulaga H, Eichers E, Badano J, et al. Loss of BBS proteins causes anosmia in humans and defects in olfactory cilia structure and function in the mouse. Nat Genet 2004; 36:994–8.

112. Alström CH, Nilsson LB, Asander H. Retinal degeneratin combined with obesity, diabetes mellitus and neurogenous deafness: a specific syndrome (not hitherto described) distinct from Laurence–Moon–Biedl syndrome. A clinical endocrinological and genetic examination based on large pedigree. Acta Psychiat 1959; 34:1–35.

113. Marshall JD, Shea SE, Salisbury SR, et al. Genealogy, natural history, and phenotype of Alström syndrome in a large acadian kindred and three additional families. Am J Med Genet 1997; 73:160–1.

114. Hearn T, Spalluto C, Hanley NA, et al. Mutations of ALMS1, a large gene with tandem repeat encodin 47 amino acids, causes Alström syndrome. Nat Genet 2002; 31:79–83.

115. Collin GB, Ikeda A, So WV, et al. Mutations in ALMS1 cause obesity, type 2 diabetes and neurosensory degeneration in Alström syndrome. Nat Genet 2002; 31:74–8.

116. Patel S, Minton JA, Weedon MN, et al. Common variations in the ALMS1 gene do not contribute to susceptibility to type 2 diabetes in a large white UK population. Diabetologia 2006; 49:1209–13.

117. Cohen MM, Smith DW, Graham CB, et al. A new syndrome with hypotonia, obesity, mental deficiency, and facial, oral, ocular, and limb anomalies. J Pediatr 1973; 83: 280–4.

118. Chandler KE, Al-Gazali L, Kolehmainen J, et al. Diagnostic criteria, clinical character-istics and natural history of Cohen syndrome. J Med Genet 2003; 40:233–41.

119. Hennies HC, Seifert W, Schumi C, et al. Allelic Heterogenity in the COH1 gene explains clinical variability in cohen syndrome. Am J Hum Genet 2004; 75:138–45.

120. Kolehmainen J, Saarinen A, Chandler K, et al. Cohen syndrome is caused by mutations in a novel gene, COH1, encoding a transmembrane protein with a pre-sumed role in vesicle-mediated sorting and intracellular protein transport. Am J Hum Genet 2003; 72:1359–69.

121. Börjeson M, Lehmann O. An X-linked recessively inherited syndrome characterised by grave mental deficiency, epilepsy and endocrine disorder. Acta Med Scand 1962; 171:13–21.

122. Turner G, White SM, Delatycki M, et al. The clinical picture of the Börjeson–Forssman–Lehman syndrome in males and heterozygous females with PHF6 muta-tions. Clin Genet 2004; 65:226–32.

123. Lower KM, Kerr BA, Matthews KD, et al. Mutations in PHF6 are associated with Börjeson–Frossman–Lehman Syndrome. Nat Genet 2002; 32:661–5.

124. Bell AJ. Prevalence of overweight and obesity in Down syndrome and other mentally handicapped adults living in the community. J Intel Disab Res 1992; 36:359–64.

Prader-Willi Syndrome

Oenone Dudley and Françoise Muscatelli

Institut de Biologie du Développement de Marseille Luminy, Marseille, France

Obesity is a feature of several congenital syndromes associated with a learning disability including Prader-Willi syndrome (PWS), Bardet-Biedl syndrome, Cohen syndrome, Albright hereditary osteodystrophy, Borjeson-Forssman-Lehmann syndrome, and some rarer disorders (Introduction) (1). Of these, PWS is the most common form of syndromal obesity, with an estimated incidence of 1:25,000 (2) and prevalence of 1:52,000 (3,4). In this chapter we describe the clinical phenotype and the genetic basis and review underlying mechanisms and behavior patterns that influence the hyperphagia and obesity found in PWS.

THE PRADER-WILLI PHENOTYPE

PWS is a genetically imprinted neurodevelopmental disorder first identified by Prader et al. in 1956 (5). The clinical criteria were refined by Holm in 1993 (6), and later by Gunay-Aygun in 2001 as a result of improved genetic diagnosis (7). It is a complex disorder which evolves with age. Holm details the complexity of the disorder, which is variable across individuals, whereas Gunay-Aygun characterizes the developmental phases (Table 1). The essential clinical diagnostic criteria include neonatal hypotonia and poor suck (0–2 years), global developmental delay (2–6 years), hyperphagia and propensity to obesity (6–12 years), mild learning difficulties, hyperphagia, hypogonadism, and behavior problems such as temper tantrums and obsessive compulsive symptoms (13 years through adulthood). There is a primary underlying metabolic disturbance involving growth hormone deficiency (8) which, together with hyperphagia due to the absence of normal satiety mechanisms, (9) results in both short stature and obesity. Diabetes mellitus and cardiac problems are frequent complications (10). Respiratory problems and sleep apnoea of a primary and secondary nature also affect many individuals with PWS (11,12). A characteristic facial appearance, small hands and feet, Hypogonadism, and abnormal menses in female adults are also well documented (6). The paradox of PWS concerns the presence of two distinct phenotypes: that of the newborn infant who is under weight, has difficulty feeding, and fails to thrive, and that of the older child or adult who is constantly hungry, who will overeat at every opportunity and who will become severely obese in the absence of intervention. Thus, at birth, nasogastric tube feeding is almost universal, feeding duration is lengthy, and weight gain is slow (2,13). Once hyperphagia develops, weight gain is more rapid than normal, and restrictive measures involving a low calorie diet and limiting access to food to the extent of locking food cupboards and padlocking fridges usually become necessary (14). People with PWS eat three times more than the normal caloric intake and have shorter periods of satiety (9). They also rarely vomit. The compulsion to seek food may extend to raiding dustbins, shoplifting, and stealing money to buy food (15). As adults, none are able to live independently because the hyperphagia becomes uncontrollable and the resulting obesity becomes life-threatening. The transition from

TABLE 1   Evolution of Diagnostic Criteria for PWS

Holm et al. (6)	Gunay-aygun et al. (7)
Major criteria (abbreviated)	*Features sufficient to prompt DNA testing*
Neonatal hypotonia and infantile central hypotonia with poor suck	Birth to 2 years: hypotonia with poor suck
Feeding problems in infancy	2–6 years: Hypotonia with history of poor suck; global developmental delay
Excessive or rapid weight gain after 12 months but before 6 years of age; central obesity in the absence of intervention	6–12 years: History of hypotonia with poor suck; global developmental delay; excessive eating (hyperphagia; obsession with food) with central obesity if uncontrolled
Characteristic facial features	
Global developmental delay	
Hyperphagia/food foraging/obsession with food	
Hypogonadism, genital hypoplasia, cryptorchidism, small penis, and/or testes in males; absence or severe hypoplasia of labia minora and/or clitoris in females, delayed puberty	13 years–adult: Cognitive impairment, usually mild mental retardation; excessive eating; hypothalamic hypogonadism and/or typical behavior problem (including temper tantrums and obsessive/compulsive features)
Deletion 15q11-13 or other ytogenetic/molecular abnormality of the Prader-Willi chromosome region, including maternal disomy	
Minor criteria	
Decreased fetal movement or infantile lethargy or weak cry in infancy, improving with age	
Behavior problems—temper tantrums, violent outbursts and obsessive/compulsive behavior, tendency to be argumentative, oppositional, rigid, manipulative, possessive, and stubborn; perseverating, stealing, and lying	
Sleep disturbance or sleep apnoea	
Short stature for genetic background by age 15 (in the absence of growth hormone intervention)	
Hypopigmentation—fair skin and hair compared to family	
Small hands (< 25th percentile) and/or feet (<10th percentile) for height/age	
Narrow hands with straight ulnar border	
Eye abnormalities (esotropia, myopia)	
Thick, viscous saliva with crusting at the corners of the mouth	
Speech articulation defects	
Skin picking	
Supportive findings (increase the certainty of diagnosis but are not scored)	
High pain threshold	
Decreased vomiting	
Temperature instability in infancy or altered temperature sensitivity in older children and adults	
Scoliosis and/or kyphosis	
Early adrenarche	
Osteoporosis	
Unusual skill with jigsaw puzzles	
Normal neuromuscular studies	
Scoring 1 point for major criteria; half point for minor criteria. <3 years, five points required, including 4 major criteria; >2 years, eight points required, including five major criteria	

an infant who fails to thrive into an overeating child can occur at any point between the age of one and six years. The cause of this transformation remains unexplained.

PWS IS A COMPLEX MULTIGENIC GENETIC DISORDER INVOLVING IMPRINTED GENES

In the early 1980s, cytogenetic analysis revealed chromosomal 15q deletions in some PW patients (16,17). In 1986, Butler et al. (18) studied the parental origin of such deletions and showed that the del[15q] was paternal in origin, although chromosomes of both parents were normal. Finally in 1989, Nicholls et al. demonstrated maternal uniparental disomy (mUPD) in some PWS patients in which no deletion was cytogenetically evident: two maternal chromosome 15 were present but there was an absence of paternal genes from the 15q11-q13 segment. Currently it is estimated that approximately 70% to 75% of patients with PWS have a paternal deletion and 25% to 30% have a mUPD. Both types of mutations are sporadic, they are not inherited. The percentage of mUPD mutations is positively correlated with the age of the mother and increasing maternal age at conception is likely to increase the number of mUPD births (19). Genomic imprinting is an epigenetic process by which a subset of autosomal genes is differentially expressed, depending on parent-of-origin (20). PWS results from the absence of expression of genes which are normally expressed by the paternal allele only, the maternal allele being silenced. Thus, PWS is a classic example of a human disease that involves genomic imprinting (21,22). Approximately 1% of PWS patients present imprinting defects: in these patients, the disease is due to aberrant imprinting and results in silencing of the paternal genes that are normally expressed. In approximately 10% of cases, the imprinting defects are caused by a microdeletion affecting the 5′ end of the SNURF-SNRPN locus. These deletions define the 15q imprinting center (IC), which regulates imprinting in the whole domain. In the majority of patients with an imprinting defect, the incorrect imprint has arisen without a DNA sequence change, possibly as the result of stochastic errors of the imprinting process or the effect of exogenous factors. Imprinting mutations may be inherited and de novo IC deletions can have an increased recurrence risk (23).

PWS results from the lack of expression of the paternal imprinted genes located in the 15q11-q13 region and there is no reported PWS patient with a normal paternal copy of 15q11-q13. These data imply that PWS is a multigenic syndrome, involving more than one mutated gene.

The identification of genes responsible for specific PWS symptoms is a difficult task, and requires the isolation of candidate genes among all the paternally expressed sequences in a large physical interval (2–3 megabases). One approach is to characterize all the human candidates in the region and to clone their mouse orthologues. This allows the creation of animal models, in order to determine the role of each gene in the etiology of PWS (22) (see below). Regardless of genotype, the main phenotypic characteristics are similar. However, some genotype-phenotype correlations in PWS indicate certain behavioral differences between patients with deletion or mUPD (24,31). Deletion type has been further subdivided into Type I (larger) and Type II (smaller) (32) and there is evidence to suggest that deletion size has a bearing on severity of phenotype (33). However, there is no evidence to suggest that genotype has any impact on levels of hyperphagia and obesity in PWS. Thus, although there is no doubt that the cause of hyperphagia and obesity is genetic, the gene responsible is still unknown.

There has been one report, from a genome wide scan analysis, of a linkage between three loci and childhood-onset severe obesity in some French Caucasian families, one of which was a locus on chromosome 15q (34). However, there have been no further reports of linkage analysis associating the 15q11-q13 locus to obese non-PWS patients. We therefore hypothesize that obesity and hyperphagia in PWS results from the inactivation of at least two paternal imprinted genes.

Mouse Models of PWS

The mouse 7C chromosomal region has conserved synteny with the human 15q11-q13 region. Nearly all the content of genes is conserved, their order and their imprinted regulation (35). Four potential mouse models, with a global deficiency of paternal gene expression in the 7C chromosome, have been reported. Prader-Willi syndrome models include those with mUPD (36), an imprinting defect (37), a transgenic deletion model with a chromosome deletion of the same apparent size and gene content as in human (38), and a more specific deletion between *Snrpn* and *Ube3a* (39). The postnatal phenotype of these PWS mouse models appears to be equivalent to that of PWS infants at birth. In all cases, the main feature of the observed phenotype is lethality (depending on the genetic background) during the first post-natal week, associated with various degrees of poor feeding, respiratory distress, hypotonia, and growth retardation. These observations are consistent with the feeding difficulties and failure to thrive that characterize PWS infants. Neonatal mice with a transgenic deletion PWS have severe hypoglycemia at post-natal day 2 as the probable cause of death (40). Reduced concentrations of *Agrp* and increased concentrations of *Pomc* could also contribute to their failure to thrive (41). Furthermore, concerning specific genetic background, the mouse models with transgenic deletion PWS or imprinting mutation survive but do not become obese (A.P. Goldstone, personal communication) (42). However, such models do not allow us to determine the role of each gene in the PWS phenotype, and it is not possible to exclude the possibility that the mice that died may have developed obesity later if they had survived. Several knockout mouse models of individual candidate genes for PWS have also been created. No abnormal phenotype has been reported for the small nuclear ribonucleoprotein polypeptide N (*Snrpn*) knockout model, the *Snurf* knockout mouse, or the *Mknr3* knockout model. Only the inactivation of the Necdin (*Dnd*) gene appears to replicate a number of symptoms of PWS such as early post-natal lethality. The penetrance of lethality is dependent on genetic background and is due to respiratory problems. Sensory-motor defects, skin scraping, high pain threshold and superior visuospatial learning have also been reported in Necdin deficient mice (43–48). However, none of these models replicate the hyperphagia and obesity found in humans with PWS. Either this is due to the fact that the mouse and human phenotype are not identical, or that there are other genes, as yet to be identified, either within or outside the PWS critical region which interact with genes within the region (Fig. 1) (49).

ETIOLOGY OF OBESITY IN PWS

Obesity in PWS is the outcome of two principal factors: one is the underlying metabolic disturbance predisposing to excessive weight gain; the second is a compulsive urge to overeat (hyperphagia). Research into the underlying pathophysiology of obesity in PWS encompasses metabolic studies, studies of neuroendocrine function, neuroanatomical studies, and behavioral research. While these

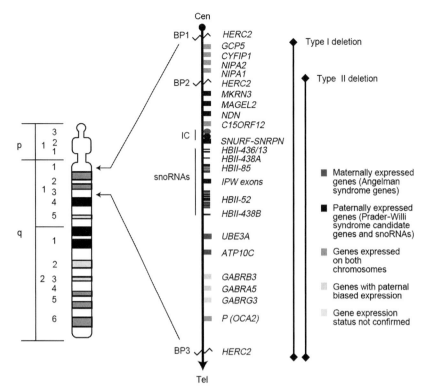

Ideogram of chromosome 15, showing genes located in the typical deletion
region of Prader-Willi syndrome

FIGURE 1 (*See color insert.*) Physical map of Prader-Willi syndrome genes. *Source*: Adapted
from Ref. 59.

areas are considered separately here for purposes of presentation, it is understood
that metabolic functioning, neurological mechanisms, and behavior are in fact
intricately interrelated.

Metabolic Studies

Propensity to weight gain in PWS is promoted by a body composition which,
from birth, has an elevated fat mass, and a reduced lean mass (8,50). This is
further compounded by a growth hormone/insulin growth factor axis deficiency
(51,52). In consequence, calorie intake must be restricted compared to a normal diet
(53), and the capacity for energy expenditure through physical exercise is compromised (54).

Fat distribution appears to be different in PWS: compared to non-PWS obese
individuals, people with PWS have less lean mass on the trunk, arms, and legs
(55). The nature of adipose tissue is also different in PWS compared to non-PWS
obese individuals. People with PWS have more subcutaneous, and less visceral,
adipose tissue (56).

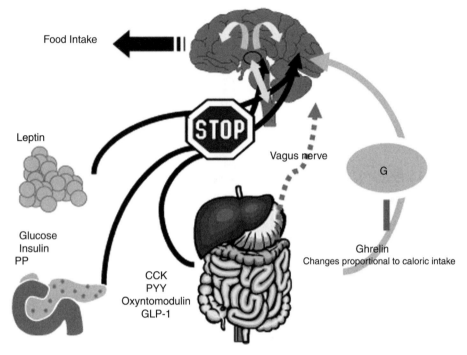

FIGURE 2   Peripheral satiety signals. *Source*: From Ref. 49.

Neuroendocrinological Investigations

Attempts to understand the pathophysiological basis of obesity and hyperphagia in PWS have resulted in a considerable body of research focussing on the role of appetite regulatory peptides which are generated in the gastrointestinal system or body tissues and linked to receptors in the hypothalamus (57,58).

Peptides such as ghrelin produced in the stomach, and Neuropeptide Y (NPY) produced in the hypothalamus, are postulated to stimulate appetite and food intake, whereas other intestinal peptides such as cholecystokinin (CCK), peptide YY (PYY), oxyntomodulin, glucagon-like peptide-1 (GLP1) and obestatin suppress hunger (Fig. 2) (59). Leptin is produced by adipose issue and inhibits eating and stimulates energy expenditure. Pancreatic hormones, such as insulin, glucagons, and somatostatin interact with other hormones to regulate glucose levels and appetite.

To date no comprehensive pathophysiological mechanisms have been identified. However, it is clear that neuroendocrine function in PWS is atypical compared with both normal weight and obese people without PWS.

Cholecystokinin is thought to be responsible for initiating satiety during a meal (60). It is produced in the endocrine I cells in the duodenum and jejunum in response to fat, amino acids and gastric acid, and it delays gastric emptying and inhibits release of gastric acid. Cholecystokinin levels are normal in PWS, but in contrast to non-PWS obese controls, fasting levels are not correlated with free fatty acid levels (61).

Pancreatic polypeptide (PP) secretion which normally suppresses appetite has been reported to be deficient in PWS, but short-term infusion of PP has no effect (62). Anorexigenic PYY levels are low in non-PWS obese individuals and they are also low in individuals with PWS (63). Orexigenic NPY neurons in the hypothalamus are normal in PWS (10), although serum levels of NPY are low-normal in adults with PWS (64). AgRP which stimulates food intake through inhibiting the action of melanocortin, an anorexigenic peptide, appears to be normal in adults with PWS (10). Opioids have been reported to increase appetite particularly for sweet food but studies of serum levels of betaendorphins have been found to be normal in children with PWS (65). Leptin deficiency is associated with obesity (66). However, leptin appears to be normally regulated in PWS (67,68).

Ghrelin is primarily produced in the stomach and increases food intake in individuals with anorexia and chronic illness (69–71). Ghrelin is an endogenous ligand of the growth hormone secretagogue receptor (GHSR) located in the hypothalamus and pituitary, which stimulates secretion of growth-releasing hormone (GHRH) and GH (72) and food intake (73,74). It activates orexigenic NPY and AGRP neurons, and inhibits anorexigenic proopiomelanocortin (POMC) neurons. Chronic administration of ghrelin to rodents results in obesity (75). Fasting ghrelin levels relative to level of obesity have been found to be higher in children and adults with PWS compared to obese and normal weight controls (76). Normally ghrelin levels are inversely correlated with weight but in PWS levels are abnormally elevated and do not fall as weight increases. In addition, normalization of ghrelin levels in individuals with PWS does not reduce their appetite (77). Obestatin is a hormone produced in the small intestine which encodes for the same gene as ghrelin. Studies of mice suggest that it has a counter effect to ghrelin by suppressing appetite (78). However, although ghrelin levels are elevated in PWS compared to non-PWS obese controls, obestatin levels are appropriate for body mass index (BMI) in PWS compared to obese controls (79). Adiponectin, a protein secreted from adipose tissue, which is decreased in non-PWS obese individuals, is higher in adults with PWS although lower than normal weight adults suggesting that they are more protected from developing type 2 diabetes compared to non-PWS obese adults (80). The lack of consistent therapeutic response to PP infusion, and the persistence of hyperphagia despite correction of ghrelin levels suggests that hormonal defects alone cannot explain the eating disorder in PWS, and that brain defects may play a more crucial role.

Neuroanatomical Investigations

Much of the phenotype of PWS is compatible with a hypothalamic defect. Concerning the eating disorder in particular, the paraventricular nucleus (PVN) within the hypothalamus is the centre for appetite regulation. The PVN produces neuropeptide hormones, oxytocin, and vasopressin. Oxytocin-expressing neurons, in particular, are depressed in PWS (64,81) and may underlie the faulty satiety mechanisms. However, other parts of the brain are also involved in appetite regulation. Appetite itself is not a unitary phenomenon: it involves the incentive to eat (hunger), the feeling of fullness (satiation), and the duration of feeling full (satiety). Different parts of the brain are activated in relation to these different processes (82). People with PWS show disturbance in all three domains: they feel more hungry, eat three times as much, eat for longer, and feel hungry again sooner than non-PWS controls (9,83).

Using functional magnetic resonance imaging (fMRI) techniques, Shapira and colleagues found delayed activation in areas of the brain associated with satiety in the hypothalamus, insula, ventromedial prefrontal cortex, and nucleus accumbens (84). Positron emission tomography (PET scans) of areas of the brain activated after fasting and during low calorie and high calorie breakfast show similar patterns between non-PWS and PWS individuals and include neural activation patterns associated with hunger in the hypothalamus, amygdala, basal ganglia, thalamus and anterior cingulate, and with satiation and satiety in the orbitofrontal, temporal, and prefrontal cortices. Different areas of neural activation occur depending on the number of calories consumed, thus a low calorie meal produces more activation in the lateral orbitofrontal cortex and a high calorie meal produces greater activation in the medial orbitofrontal cortex. It is postulated that a low calorie meal is experienced as more unsatisfying, therefore more punitive than a high calorie meal. This is consistent with research demonstrating a link between punishment and lateral orbitofrontal cortex activation; and reward with medial orbitofrontal cortex activation (85). A further study using fMRI techniques to examine responses to visual food stimuli before and after eating showed that people with PWS differ from healthy weight controls in levels and areas of preprandial and postprandial brain activation. Healthy weight adolescents show greater activation prior to a meal, whereas adolescents with PWS show greater activation after the meal. The amygdala, orbitofrontal cortex, medial prefrontal cortex, and frontal operculum are activated in healthy weight adolescents. The orbitofrontal, medial prefrontal cortex, insula, hippocampus, and parahippocampal gyrus are activated in PWS (86).

Behavioral Studies

Compulsive symptoms including repetitive behavior, ordering, hoarding, insistence on routines are well documented in PWS (87–89) and there is some evidence that hyperphagia in children increases in proportion to the degree of compulsive behavior (90). Indeed Clarke et al. (86) excluded preoccupation with food from their assessment of compulsive behavior on the basis that this was virtually a constant phenomenon. Thus hyperphagia may be due not only to lack of satiety, but also to a tendency towards ritualistic, repetitive behavior, which is found in general in people with PWS. There is some evidence to show that compulsivity and therefore, hyperphagia, peaks in young adulthood (20–30 years) and diminishes in middle age in PWS (91). However, the degree of obesity also appears to play a role: lower BMI has been found to be associated with greater levels of compulsivity, suggesting that hyperphagia diminishes with increasing levels of obesity in PWS. The proposed explanation for this is that restriction of food intake while reducing BMI, results in less satiety and therefore greater distress, leading to more compulsivity. Another study found no relationship between compulsivity scores and eating behavior in PWS, but did find that younger people with PWS with lower BMI spent more time seeking and covertly eating food (92). Other studies have explored food preferences in PWS. Although it is the case that people with PWS will eat any food, they also do express preferences for certain foods, in particular high carbohydrate and sweet foods (85,93). Choice of food depends not only on food preference, but also quantity. Hence, when a favorite food is available an individual with PWS will choose this over a larger quantity of less preferred food. However, if the choice consists of a mixture of preferred and less preferred foods, quantity becomes the determining factor in food selection (94).

A NEW MODEL OF PWS: A SYNDROME OF STARVATION

Experiments indicating faulty satiety mechanisms, and the early phenotype of the infant who fails to thrive have led to a reconceptualisation of PWS as a syndrome of "starvation" rather than one of obesity (95). The hypothesis proposes that the genetic defect causes a disruption of the transfer of resources between placenta and foetus. This results in foetal malnutrition which impedes the development of the brain and normal hypothalamic-pituitary-adrenal (HPA) function. This in turn leads to a reprogramming of the body's metabolism so that it continues to behave as though it is in a state of starvation even when this is no longer the case. The proposition that foetal malnourishment leads to obesity and metabolic reprogramming derives support from studies showing an association between foetal malnutrition and adult cardiovascular and metabolic disorders in general (96,99) although some do not support such a link (100). The hypothesis postulates that an adverse intrauterine environment alters the foetal metabolic and hormonal composition to ensure foetal survival (101) which predisposes towards the development of obesity (102). The link between foetal malnourishment and subsequent obesity is supported by evidence of increased risk of adult obesity in the offspring of mothers subjected to famine during mid to late pregnancy (103).

Regarding PWS, low birth weight is characteristic of the neonatal phenotype (25,104,105) and clinical data regarding significant intrauterine disturbance in PWS has been reported (106). In particular, rates of polyhydramnios are high. Polyhydramnios is associated with both gestational diabetes and congenital defects, and may be an indicator of genetic metabolic reprogramming.

Further evidence of metabolic reprogramming in PWS, is provided by a study showing increased fat mass and elevated BMI-adjusted leptin levels even in underweight infants with PWS long before they become obese (107).

Once the metabolism is programmed to extract maximum resources from limited nutrient supply, then exposure to a food rich environment results in more rapid than normal weight gain, thus rapid catch-up growth in the first two years of underweight infants has been found to be linked to the development of obesity in general (108). Such rapid catch-up growth is typically a feature of PWS. Reprogramming of the HPA axis as a result of foetal malnutrition has also been linked to increased cortisol secretion, which in turn is linked to raised levels of stress and emotional problems (109), and also increases hyperphagia. Anecdotal evidence indeed suggests that weight gain in people with PWS, as in other people, is particularly exacerbated during periods of stress.

CLINICAL MANAGEMENT

The fact that PWS is a genetic disorder has led to an emphasis on exploring biological factors, and a relative neglect of environmental factors. Nonetheless, individual variability in PWS is large. Can this be explained solely in terms of the extent of the genetic defect, for example, deletion size, or do social factors play a role? Knowledge of environmental factors which influence the progression of PWS is not only important for understanding the nature of obesity in PWS, but also for determining appropriate clinical management.

For example, early diagnosis appears to play an important role in reducing obesity in children and adults with PWS (110) presumably because it leads to earlier intervention and closer supervision.

Lower levels of obesity and reduced behavioral disturbance have been associated with living in out-of-home placements for adults in the USA (91,111). Lower preoccupation with food in residential homes compared to living in the community has also been reported in a UK study (112). However, as has already been noted, degree of obesity may have an impact on degree of preoccupation with food (91).

Anorectic medication used in the treatment of other forms of obesity appears to have no impact (113). Surgery is not recommended because it does not diminish the problem of hyperphagia, and the ensuing medical complications are even more severe (114). To date, the most successful medical intervention has been growth hormone therapy which increases lean mass and height, and thereby reduces obesity (115,117). There is some data to suggest that it may also have positive psychological and educational benefits (118). On the other hand concerns regarding deleterious effects such as onset or aggravation of scoliosis, respiratory complications and even mortality have been raised by some clinicians (119,120). The availability of growth hormone therapy in the treatment of PWS is a recent phenomenon (since 2000 in the United States). In Europe treatment generally stops when full bone growth has been achieved. Long-term follow-up is required to fully assess the risks and the benefits, as well as optimum age of onset and duration of treatment.

CONCLUSION

The eating disorder and obesity in PWS are atypical compared to other forms of obesity and much remains to be understood concerning the pathophysiology of the disorder. Nonetheless, there has been significant progress over the past 10 years. The challenge for the future is to understand the links between genetic, metabolic, neuroanatomical, behavioral, and environmental aspects which will not only advance understanding and care of PWS, but may also provide insights into the nature of hyperphagia and obesity in general.

REFERENCES

1. Gunay-Aygun M, Cassidy SB, Nicholls RD. Prader-Willi and other syndromes associated with obesity and mental retardation. Behav Genet 1997; 27(4):307–24.
2. Butler MG. Prader-Willi syndrome: current understanding of cause and diagnosis. Am J Med Genet 1990; 35(3):319–32.
3. Whittington JE, Holland AJ, Webb T, et al. Population prevalence and estimated birth incidence and mortality rate for people with Prader-Willi syndrome in one UK Health Region. J Med Genet 2001; 38(11):792–8.
4. Smith A, Egan J, Ridley G, et al. Birth prevalence of Prader-Willi syndrome in Australia. Arch Dis Child 2003; 88(3):263–4.
5. Prader A, Labhart A, Willi H. Ein Syndro von Adipositas, Kryptorchismus und Oligophrenie nach myatonieartigem Zustand in Neugeborenenamter. Schweizeische Medizinishe Wochenschrift 1956; 86:1260–1.
6. Holm V, Cassidy S, Butler M, et al. Prader-Willi syndrome: consensus diagnostic criteria. Pediatrics 1993; 91:398–402.
7. Gunay-Aygun M, Schwartz S, Heeger S, et al. The changing purpose of Prader-Willi syndrome clinical diagnostic criteria and proposed revised criteria. Pediatrics 2001; 108(5):E92.
8. Goldstone AP, Brynes AE, Thomas EL, et al. Resting metabolic rate, plasma leptin concentrations, leptin receptor expression, and adipose tissue measured by whole-body magnetic resonance imaging in women with Prader-Willi syndrome. Am J Clin Nutr 2002; 75(3):468–75.

9. Holland AJ, Treasure J, Coskeran P, et al. Measurement of excessive appetite and metabolic changes in Prader-Willi syndrome. Int J Obes Relat Metab Disord 1993; 17(9):527–32.

10. Butler JV, Whittington JE, Holland AJ, et al. Prevalence of, and risk factors for, physical ill-health in people with Prader-Willi syndrome: a population-based study. Dev Med Child Neurol 2002; 44(4):248–55.

11. Nixon GM, Brouillette RT. Sleep and breathing in Prader-Willi syndrome. Pediatr Pulmonol 2002; 34(3):209–17.

12. Festen DA, de Weerd AW, van den Bossche RA, et al. Sleep-related breathing disorders in pre-pubertal children with Prader-Willi Syndrome and effects of growth hormone treatment. J Clin Endocrinol Metab 2006.

13. LR G, RC A. Management of Prader-Willi syndrome. 1995, New York: Springer-Verlag.

14. K. WBaJ. Tools for psychological and behavioural management. 3rd ed: Management of Prader-Willi syndrome. ed. 2006, USA: Springer. 317-343.

15. Hoffman CJ, Aultman D, Pipes P. A nutrition survey of and recommendations for individuals with Prader-Willi syndrome who live in group homes. J Am Diet Assoc 1992; 92(7):823–30, 33.

16. Ledbetter DH, Riccardi VM, Airhart SD, et al. Deletions of chromosome 15 as a cause of the Prader-Willi syndrome. N Engl J Med 1981; 304(6):325–9.

17. Mattei MG, Souiah N, Mattei JF. Chromosome 15 anomalies and the Prader-Willi syndrome: cytogenetic analysis. Hum Genet 1984; 66(4):313–34.

18. Butler MG, Meaney FJ, Palmer CG. Clinical and cytogenetic survey of 39 individuals with Prader–Labhart–Willi syndrome. Am J Med Genet 1986; 23(3):793–809.

19. Whittington JE, Butler JV, Holland AJ. Changing rates of genetic subtypes of Prader-Willi syndrome in the UK. Eur J Hum Genet 2006.

20. Reik W, Walter J. Imprinting mechanisms in mammals. Curr Opin Genet Dev 1998; 8(2):154–64.

21. Lalande M. Parental imprinting and human disease. Annu Rev Genet 1997; 30:73–195.

22. Nicholls RD. Incriminating gene suspects, Prader-Willi style. Nat Genet 1999; 23(2):132–4.

23. Horsthemke B, Buiting K. Imprinting defects on human chromosome 15. Cytogenet Genome Res 2006; 113(1–4):292–9.

24. Whittington J, Holland A, Webb T, et al. Cognitive abilities and genotype in a population-based sample of people with Prader-Willi syndrome. J Intellect Disabil Res 2004; 48(2):172–87.

25. Gunay-Aygun M, Heeger S, Schwartz S, et al. Delayed diagnosis in patients with Prader-Willi syndrome due to maternal uniparental disomy 15. Am J Med Genet 1997; 71(1):106–10.

26. Roof E, Stone W, MacLean W, et al. Intellectual characteristics of Prader-Willi syndrome: comparison of genetic subtypes. J Intellect Disabil Res 2000; 44:25–30.

27. Veltman MW, Thompson RJ, Roberts SE, et al. Prader-Willi syndrome—a study comparing deletion and uniparental disomy cases with reference to autism spectrum disorders. Eur Child Adolesc Psychiatry 2004; 13(1):42–50.

28. Boer H, Holland A, Whittington J, et al. Psychotic illness in people with Prader-Willi syndrome due to chromosome 15 maternal uniparental disomy. Lancet 2002; 359(9301):135–6.

29. Vogels A, Matthijs G, Legius E, et al. Chromosome 15 maternal uniparental disomy and psychosis in Prader-Willi syndrome. J Med Genet 2003; 40(1):72–3.

30. Dykens EM. Are jigsaw puzzle skills 'spared' in persons with Prader-Willi syndrome? J Child Psychol Psychiatry 2002; 43(3):343–52.

31. Cassidy SB, Forsythe M, Heeger S, et al. Comparison of phenotype between patients with Prader-Willi syndrome due to deletion 15q and uniparental disomy 15. Am J Med Genet 1997; 68(4):433–40.

32. Christian SL, Robinson WP, Huang B, et al. Molecular characterization of two proximal deletion breakpoint regions in both Prader-Willi and Angelman syndrome patients. Am J Hum Genet 1995; 57(1):40–8.

33. Butler MG, Bittel DC, Kibiryeva N, et al. Behavioral differences among subjects with Prader-Willi syndrome and type I or type II deletion and maternal disomy. Pediatrics 2004; 113(3):565–73.

34. Meyre DDJ, Francke S, Lecoeur C, et al. First genome wide search for young-onset obesity susceptibility genes shows 3 loci on 6q, 15q and 16q. Presented at American Diabetes Association's 62nd., San Fransisco, USA, 2002.

35. Nicholls RD, Knepper JL. Genome organization, function, and imprinting in Prader-Willi and Angelman syndromes. Annu Rev Genomics Hum Genet 2001; 2:153–75.

36. Cattanach BM, Barr JA, Evans EP, et al. A candidate mouse model for Prader-Willi syndrome which shows an absence of Snrpn expression. Nat Genet 1992; 2(4):270–4.

37. Yang T, Adamson TE, Resnick JL, et al. A mouse model for Prader-Willi syndrome imprinting-centre mutations. Nat Genet 1998; 19(1):25–31.

38. Gabriel JM, Merchant M, Ohta T, et al. A transgene insertion creating a heritable chromosome deletion mouse model of Prader-Willi and angelman syndromes [In Process Citation]. Proc Natl Acad Sci USA 1999; 96(16):9258–63.

39. Tsai TF, Jiang YH, Bressler J, et al. Paternal deletion from Snrpn to Ube3a in the mouse causes hypotonia, growth retardation and partial lethality and provides evidence for a gene contributing to Prader-Willi syndrome. Hum Mol Genet 1999; 8(8):1357–64.

40. Stefan M, Claiborn KC, Stasiek E, et al. Genetic mapping of putative Chrna7 and Luzp2 neuronal transcriptional enhancers due to impact of a transgene-insertion and 6.8 Mb deletion in a mouse model of Prader-Willi and Angelman syndromes. BMC Genom 2005; 6:157.

41. Ge YL, Ohta T, Driscoll DJ, et al. Anorexigenic melanocortin signaling in the hypothalamus is augmented in association with failure-to-thrive in a transgenic mouse model for Prader-Willi syndrome. Brain Res 2002; 957(1):42–5.

42. Chamberlain SJ, Johnstone KA, DuBose AJ, et al. Evidence for genetic modifiers of postnatal lethality in PWS-IC deletion mice. Hum Mol Genet 2004; 13(23):2971–7.

43. Gerard M, Hernandez L, Wevrick R, et al. Disruption of the mouse necdin gene results in early post-natal lethality. Nat Genet 1999; 23(2):199–202.

44. Muscatelli F, Abrous DN, Massacrier A, et al. Disruption of the mouse necdin gene results in hypothalamic and behavioral alterations reminiscent of the human prader-willi syndrome [In Process Citation]. Hum Mol Genet 2000; 9(20):3101–10.

45. Tsai TF, Armstrong D, Beaudet AL. Necdin-deficient mice do not show lethality or the obesity and infertility of Prader-Willi syndrome [letter]. Nat Genet 1999; 22(1):15–6.

46. Ren J, Lee S, Pagliardini S, et al. Absence of Ndn, encoding the Prader-Willi syndrome-deleted gene necdin, results in congenital deficiency of central respiratory drive in neonatal mice. J Neurosci 2003; 23(5):1569–73.

47. Kuwako K, Hosokawa A, Nishimura I, et al. Disruption of the paternal necdin gene diminishes TrkA signaling for sensory neuron survival. J Neurosci 2005; 25(30):7090–9.

48. Andrieu D, Watrin F, Niinobe M, et al. Expression of the Prader-Willi gene Necdin during mouse nervous system development correlates with neuronal differentiation and p75NTR expression. Gene Expr Patterns 2003; 3(6):761–5.

49. Goldstone AP. Peripheral satiety signals, in second international expert meeting on Prader-Willi Syndrome, 2006. Toulouse, France.

50. Brambilla P, Bosio L, Manzoni P, et al. Peculiar body composition in patients with Prader–Labhart–Willi syndrome. Am J Clin Nutr 1997; 65(5):1369–74.

51. Eiholzer U, Bachmann S, l'Allemand D. Is there growth hormone deficiency in Prader-Willi syndrome? Six arguments to support the presence of hypothalamic growth hormone deficiency in Prader-Willi syndrome. Horm Res 2000; 53(Suppl 3):44–52.

52. Eiholzer U, l'Allemand D, van der Sluis I, et al. Body composition abnormalities in children with Prader-Willi syndrome and long-term effects of growth hormone therapy. Horm Res 2000; 53(4):200–6.

53. Scheimann AO, Lee PD, Ellis KJ. Gastrointestinal System, Obesity and Body Composition. USA: Springer, 2006:153–200.

54. van Mil EG, Westerterp KR, Kester AD, et al. Activity related energy expenditure in children and adolescents with Prader-Willi syndrome. Int J Obes Relat Metab Disord 2000; 24(4):429–34.

55. Theodoro MF, Talebizadeh Z, Butler MG. Body composition and fatness patterns in Prader-Willi syndrome: comparison with simple obesity. Obesity (Silver Spring) 2006; 14(10):1685–90.

56. Goldstone AP, Thomas EL, Brynes AE, et al. Visceral adipose tissue and metabolic complications of obesity are reduced in Prader-Willi syndrome female adults: evidence for novel influences on body fat distribution. J Clin Endocrinol Metab 2001; 86(9):4330–8.

57. Goldstone AP. Prader-Willi syndrome: advances in genetics, pathophysiology and treatment. Trends Endocrinol Metab 2004; 15(1):12–20.

58. Goldstone AP. The hypothalamus, hormones, and hunger: alterations in human obesity and illness. Prog Brain Res 2006; 153:57–73.

59. Bittel DC, Butler MG. Prader-Willi syndrome: clinical genetics, cytogenetics and molecular biology. Expert Rev Mol Med, 2005; 7(14):1-20.

60. Woods SC. Gastrointestinal satiety signals I. An overview of gastrointestinal signals that influence food intake. Am J Physiol Gastrointest Liver Physiol 2004; 286(1):G7–13.

61. Butler MG, Carlson MG, Schmidt DE, et al. Plasma cholecystokinin levels in Prader-Willi syndrome and obese subjects. Am J Med Genet 2000; 95(1):67–70.

62. Zipf WB, O'Dorisio TM, Berntson GG. Short-term infusion of pancreatic polypeptide: effect on children with Prader-Willi syndrome. Am J Clin Nutr 1990; 51(2):162–6.

63. Butler MG, Bittel DC, Talebizadeh Z. Plasma peptide YY and ghrelin levels in infants and children with Prader-Willi syndrome. J Pediatr Endocrinol Metab 2004; 17(9):1177–84.

64. Hoybye C. Endocrine and metabolic aspects of adult Prader-Willi syndrome with special emphasis on the effect of growth hormone treatment. Growth Horm IGF Res 2004; 14(1):1–15.

65. Johnson RD. Opioid involvement in feeding behaviour and the pathogenesis of certain eating disorders. Med Hypotheses 1995; 45(5):491–7.

66. Farooqi IS, O'Rahilly S. Genetics of obesity in humans. Endocr Rev 2006.

67. Butler MG, Moore J, Morawiecki A, et al. Comparison of leptin protein levels in Prader-Willi syndrome and control individuals. Am J Med Genet 1998; 75(1):7–12.

68. Bueno G, Moreno LA, Pineda I, et al. Serum leptin concentrations in children with Prader-Willi syndrome and non-syndromal obesity. J Pediatr Endocrinol Metab 2000; 13(4):425–30.

69. Shimizu Y, Nagaya N, Isobe T, et al. Increased plasma ghrelin level in lung cancer cachexia. Clin Cancer Res 2003; 9(2):774–8.

70. Sturm K, MacIntosh CG, Parker BA, et al. Appetite, food intake, and plasma concentrations of cholecystokinin, ghrelin, and other gastrointestinal hormones in undernourished older women and well-nourished young and older women. J Clin Endocrinol Metab 2003; 88(8):3747–55.

71. Korbonits M, Goldstone AP, Gueorguiev M, et al. Ghrelin—a hormone with multiple functions. Front Neuroendocrinol 2004; 25(1):27–68.

72. Kojima M, Hosoda H, Date Y, et al. Ghrelin is a growth-hormone-releasing acylated peptide from stomach. Nature 1999; 402(6762):656–60.

73. Nagaya N, Uematsu M, Kojima M, et al. Elevated circulating level of ghrelin in cachexia associated with chronic heart failure: relationships between ghrelin and anabolic/catabolic factors. Circulation 2001; 104(17):2034–8.

74. Wren AM, Small CJ, Ward HL, et al. The novel hypothalamic peptide ghrelin stimulates food intake and growth hormone secretion. Endocrinology 2000; 141(11):4325–8.

75. Kojima M, Kangawa K. Ghrelin, an orexigenic signaling molecule from the gastrointestinal tract. Curr Opin Pharmacol 2002; 2(6):665–8.

76. Cummings DE, Clement K, Purnell JQ, et al. Elevated plasma ghrelin levels in Prader-Willi syndrome. Nat Med 2002; 8(7):643–4.

77. Tan TM, Vanderpump M, Khoo B, et al. Somatostatin infusion lowers plasma ghrelin without reducing appetite in adults with Prader-Willi syndrome. J Clin Endocrinol Metab 2004; 89(8):4162–5.

78. Zhang JV, Ren PG, Avsian-Kretchmer O, et al. Obestatin, a peptide encoded by the ghrelin gene, opposes ghrelin's effects on food intake. Science 2005; 310(5750):996–9.

79. Park WH, Oh YJ, Kim GY, et al. Obestatin is not elevated or correlated with insulin in children with Prader-Willi syndrome. J Clin Endocrinol Metab 2006.

80. Hoybye C, Bruun JM, Richelsen B, et al. Serum adiponectin levels in adults with Prader-Willi syndrome are independent of anthropometrical parameters and do not change with GH treatment. Eur J Endocrinol 2004; 151(4):457–61.

81. Swaab DF, Purba JS, Hofman MA. Alterations in the hypothalamic paraventricular nucleus and its oxytocin neurons (putative satiety cells) in Prader-Willi syndrome: a study of five cases. J Clin Endocrinol Metab 1995; 80(2):573–9.

82. Kishi T, Elmquist JK. Body weight is regulated by the brain: a link between feeding and emotion. Mol Psychiatry 2005; 10(2):132–46.

83. Lindgren AC, Barkeling B, Hagg A, et al. Eating behavior in Prader-Willi syndrome, normal weight, and obese control groups. J Pediatr 2000; 137(1):50–5.

84. Shapira NA, Lessig MC, He AG, et al. Satiety dysfunction in Prader-Willi syndrome demonstrated by fMRI. J Neurol Neurosurg Psychiatry 2005; 76(2):260–2.

85. Hinton EC, Holland AJ, Gellatly MS, et al. Neural representations of hunger and satiety in Prader-Willi syndrome. Int J Obes (Lond) 2006; 30(2):313–21.

86. Holsen LM, Zarcone JR, Brooks WM, et al. Neural mechanisms underlying hyperphagia in Prader-Willi syndrome. Obesity (Silver Spring) 2006; 14(6):1028–37.

87. Dykens EM, Cassidy SB. Prader-Willi syndrome: genetic, behavioral, and treatment issues. Child Adol Psych Clinics North Am 1996; 5(4):913–27.

88. Clarke DJ, Boer H, Whittington J, et al. Prader-Willi syndrome, compulsive and ritualistic behaviours: the first population-based survey. Br J Psychiatry 2002; 180:358–62.

89. Wigren M, Hansen S. Rituals and compulsivity in Prader-Willi syndrome: profile and stability. J Intellect Disabil Res 2003; 47:428–38.

90. Dimitropoulos A, Blackford J, Walden T, et al. Compulsive behavior in Prader-Willi syndrome: examining severity in early childhood. Res Dev Disabil 2006; 27(2):190–202.

91. Dykens EM. Maladaptive and compulsive behavior in Prader-Willi syndrome: new insights from older adults. Am J Ment Retard 2004; 109(2):142–53.

92. Young J, Zarcone J, Holsen L, et al. A measure of food seeking in individuals with Prader-Willi syndrome. J Intellect Disabil Res 2006; 50:18–24.

93. Fieldstone A, Zipf WB, Schwartz HC, et al. Food preferences in Prader-Willi syndrome, normal weight and obese controls. Int J Obes Relat Metab Disord 1997; 21(11):1046–52.

94. Glover D, Maltzman I, Williams C. Food preferences among individuals with and without Prader-Willi syndrome. Am J Ment Retard 1996; 101(2):195–205.

95. Holland A, Whittington J, Hinton E. The paradox of Prader-Willi syndrome: a genetic model of starvation. Lancet 2003; 362(9388):989–91.

96. Barker DJ. The fetal and infant origins of disease. Eur J Clin Invest 1995; 25(7):457–63.

97. Lucas A. Role of nutritional programming in determining adult morbidity. Arch Dis Child 1994; 71(4):288–90.

98. Reynolds RM, Phillips DI. Long-term consequences of intrauterine growth retardation. Horm Res 1998; 49(Suppl 2):28–31.

99. Oken E, Gillman MW. Fetal origins of obesity. Obes Res 2003; 11(4):496–506.

100. Parsons TJ, Power C, Manor O. Fetal and early life growth and body mass index from birth to early adulthood in 1958 British cohort: longitudinal study. BMJ 2001; 323(7325):1331–5.

101. Remacle C, Bieswal F, Reusens B. Programming of obesity and cardiovascular disease. Int J Obes Relat Metab Disord 2004; 28(Suppl 3):S46–53.

102. Dietz WH. Critical periods in childhood for the development of obesity. Am J Clin Nutr 1994; 59(5):955–9.

103. Ravelli GP, Stein ZA, Susser MW. Obesity in young men after famine exposure in utero and early infancy. N Engl J Med 1976; 295(7):349–53.

104. Varela MC, Kok F, Setian N, et al. Impact of molecular mechanisms, including deletion size, on Prader-Willi syndrome phenotype: study of 75 patients. Clin Genet 2005; 67(1):47–52.

105. Gillessen-Kaesbach G, Robinson W, Lohmann D, et al. Genotype–phenotype correlation in a series of 167 deletion and non-deletion patients with Prader-Willi syndrome. Hum Genet 1995; 96(6):638–43.

106. Dudley O, Muscatelli F. Clinical evidence of intrauterine disturbance in Prader-Willi syndrome, a genetically imprinted neurodevelopmental disorder. Early Hum Dev 2006.

107. Eiholzer U, Blum WF, Molinari L. Body fat determined by skinfold measurements is elevated despite underweight in infants with Prader–Labhart–Willi syndrome. J Pediatr 1999; 134(2):222–5.

108. Ong KK, Ahmed ML, Emmett PM, et al. Association between postnatal catch-up growth and obesity in childhood: prospective cohort study. BMJ 2000; 320(7240): 967–71.

109. Phillips DI, Jones A. Fetal programming of autonomic and HPA function: do people who were small babies have enhanced stress responses? J Physiol 2006; 572:45–50.

110. Vogels A, Fryns JP. Age at diagnosis, body mass index and physical morbidity in children and adults with the Prader-Willi syndrome. Genet Couns 2004; 15(4): 397–404.

111. Hanchett J, Greenswag L. Health care guidelines for individuals with Prader-Willi syndrome. Presented at Prader-Willi Syndrome Association, USA, 1998.

112. Russell H, Oliver C. The assessment of food-related problems in individuals with Prader-Willi syndrome. Br J Clin Psychol 2003; 42:379–92.

113. Dykens E, Shah B. Psychiatric disorders in Prader-Willi syndrome: epidemiology and management. CNS Drugs 2003; 17(3):167–78.

114. Grugni G, Guzzaloni G, Morabito F. Failure of biliopancreatic diversion in Prader-Willi syndrome. Obes Surg 2000; 10(2):179–81; discussion 182.

115. Lindgren AC, Hagenas L, Muller J, et al. Growth hormone treatment of children with Prader-Willi syndrome affects linear growth and body composition favourably. Acta Paediatr 1998; 87(1):28–31.

116. Carrel AL, Myers SE, Whitman BY, et al. Benefits of long-term GH therapy in Prader-Willi syndrome: a 4-year study. J Clin Endocrinol Metab 2002; 87(4):1581–5.

117. Hoybye C, Hilding A, Jacobsson H, et al. Growth hormone treatment improves body composition in adults with Prader-Willi syndrome. Clin Endocrinol (Oxf) 2003; 58(5):653–61.

118. Whitman BY, Myers S, Carrel A, et al. The behavioral impact of growth hormone treatment for children and adolescents with Prader-Willi syndrome: a 2-year, controlled study. Pediatrics 2002; 109(2):E35.

119. Grugni G, Livieri C, Corrias A, et al. Death during GH therapy in children with Prader-Willi syndrome: description of two new cases. J Endocrinol Invest 2005; 28(6):554–7.

120. Eiholzer U. Deaths in children with Prader-Willi syndrome. A contribution to the debate about the safety of growth hormone treatment in children with PWS. Horm Res 2005; 63(1):33–9.

Bardet-Biedl Syndrome: New Insights into Ciliopathies and Oligogenic Traits

Hélène Dollfus
Laboratoire EA 3949, Faculté de Médecine de Strasbourg, Centre de Référence pour les Affections Genetiques Ophtalmologiques, Hôpitaux Universitaires de Strasbourg, Strasbourg, France

Philip Beales
Molecular Medicine Unit, UCL Institute of Child Health, London, U.K.

Nicholas Katsanis
McKusick-Nathans Institute of Genetic Medicine, Johns Hopkins University, Baltimore, Maryland, U.S.A.

Bardet-Biedl syndrome [(BBS); OMIM 209900] is a clinically pleiotropic disorder transmitted primarily in an autosomal recessive fashion whose hallmarks include obesity, progressive retinal degeneration, polydactyly, hypogenitalism, cognitive impairment, and kidney dysplasia. The incidence of BBS has been estimated to be 1 in 150,000 in European populations but is much higher in some populations with a high level of consanguinity (the Middle East and North Africa, for example) or that are geographically isolated (Newfoundland). Since 1994, the use of homozygosity mapping in consanguineous BBS families has allowed the progressive recognition of a surprisingly high level of nonallelic genetic heterogeneity. Since the identification of the first gene in 2000 (*BBS6*, also called MKKS as it is mutated in the closely related McKusick-Kaufmann syndrome) mutations in BBS patients have been found in a total of 12 genes (*BBS1-12*) (1–5). Recent molecular evidence has revealed an unexpected connection between the BBS proteins and primary cilia (6), microtubule-based structures arising from the basal body that are notably involved as mechanosensors in kidney epithelium, in the organization of photoreceptor cells of the retina, and also in several morphogenetic signaling pathways, such as the planar cell polarity (PCP) noncanonical Wnt signaling pathway (7). This allowed the characterization of BBS as a ciliopathy, an expanding group of clinically distinct but overlapping disorders that includes autosomal dominant polycystic kidney disease, nephronophthisis, Alström syndrome (see Chapter 5.1), orofaciodigital syndrome type 1, and, most recently, Meckel syndrome and Joubert syndrome (8).

CLINICAL MANIFESTATIONS

The condition is characterized by five main features: obesity, polydactyly, retinitis pigmentosa, urogenital anomalies, and cognitive dysfunction. The clinical criteria are summarized on Tables 1 and 2.

Obesity
The overweight appears early in life but usually not prenatally. Although not a constant feature, it remains a hallmark of the disorder, as it is found in >75% of BBS patients (Fig. 1). The mean BMI is $35 \, \text{kg/m}^2$. Morbid obesity (BMI > 40) is

TABLE 1 Criteria for the Diagnosis of BBS

Major criteria	Minor criteria
Retinitis pigmentosa (rod-cone or cone-rod)	Hypertrophy LV/cardiopathy
Postaxial polydactyly	Syndactyly/brachydactyly
Obesity	Ataxia and moderate spasticity
Cognitive impairment	Psychomotor retardation
Large or multicystic kidneys	Langage alteration
Kidney failure	
Hypogenitalism-hydrometrocolpos	Polyuria-polydipsia
	Liver fibrosis
	Glucidic intolerance

Source: Adapted from Ref. 9.

more often found in female patients. The pathophysiology of the obesity remains unknown, it was initially thought to be related to a central origin, however a peripherally cause could be implied. To date, there is no direct understanding of the origin of the obesity. Recent data from some BBS knockout mice have suggested that obesity might be the result of loss of satiety, although some data have also suggested that the obesity phenotype may be part of metabolic syndrome (10,11). Dietary recommendations as well as exercise are strongly advocated as there are no other remedial routes available to date.

Extremities

Most patients present with a postaxial polydactyly, brachydactyly and more rarely syndactylies. The polydactyly (Fig. 2) may be variable involving only one hand for instance or all four extremities. Removal of the extra digits may be performed early in life and as such scarring at the level of the cubital side of hands should be looked for.

TABLE 2 Summary of Genes Identified in Bardet-Biedl Syndrome

Gene	Localization	Exon number	Protein function
BBS1	11q13	17	Ciliary protein: expression pattern compatible identical to *BBS2*, *BBS6* and *BBS4*.
BBS2	16q21	17	Ciliary protein
BBS3	3p13	9	Small protein G-ADP-ribosylation factor-like 6 (ARF-like 6); X-box sequence; implicated in axonemal trasnport.
BBS4	15q22	16	Interaction with pericentriolar protein PCM1.
BBS5	2q31	12	Ciliary protein (identified by homology with other ciliary and flagellar proteins).
BBS6/ MMKS	20p12	6	Type 2 chaperonine related protein
BBS7 (FLJ10715)	4q27	9	Ciliary protein: bidirectional movement along the ciliary axoneme
BBS8	14q32	15	Contains a TPR motif; bidirectional movement along the ciliary axoneme
BBS9	7p14	23	Parathormone related protein.
BBS10	12q21.2	2	Related to type 2 chaperonine protein
BBS11	9q33.1	2	Not confirmed
BBS12	4q27	2	Related to type 2 chaperonine protein

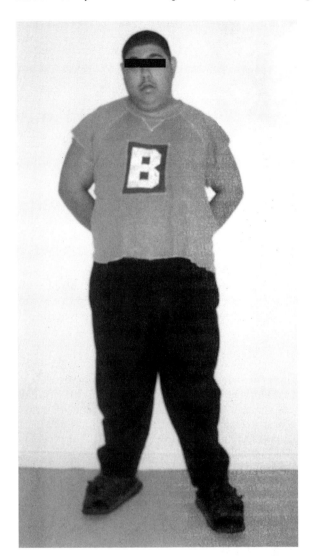

FIGURE 1   General gestalt of an obese patient with Bardet-Biedl syndrome.

Retinitis Pigmentosa

Retinitis pigmentosa occurs early and is usually diagnosed at the age of 5. Electro-retinogram findings occur before the ocular fundus changes that are observed in most of the patients before the age of 10. The condition can alter both rods and cones and according to the cell type predominantly involved affect initially central vision and/or the peripheral fields. Most of the patients experience classical rod-cone dystrophy with progressive narrowing of the visual fields, difficulties in night vision and later a decrease of the central vision. Inversely, the central vision may be initially affected in the cone-rod dystrophy. The visual handicap is usually severe and specialized aids and educations are advocated (Fig. 3).

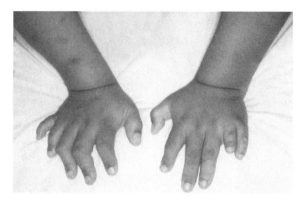

FIGURE 2 Bilateral postaxial polydactyly in a patient with Bardet-Biedl syndrome.

Reproductive Tract

Women with BBS may present with genital tract anomalies such as a hypoplasic vagina or a congenital hydrometrocolpos. Men present with hypogenitalism with small testis and a small penis. There is no specific endocrine anomaly described. Fertility in men is diminished but not abolished, and females can have normal fertility.

Kidney Anomalies

In more then 50% of the cases kidneys are involved. Prenatally, in some cases: large kidneys or more rarely multicystic kidneys are observed. During life, the kidney function may be altered progressively. A deficiency in the urine concentration (polyuria and polydyspsia, nephrogenic insipidious diabetes) is the first biological manifestation of kidney dysfunction. The evolution towards renal failure occurs in at least one-third of the patients (intersticial nephritis–glomerular dysfunction). Ten percent of the patients will need dialysis or renal transplantation.

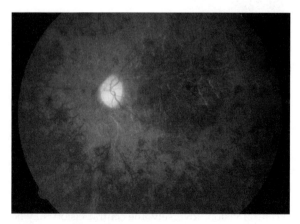

FIGURE 3 (*See color insert.*) Fundus picture of a Bardet-Biedl syndrome patient showing retinitis pigmentosa (pigment migrations cover degenerated retina).

Other Features of BBS

Glucose intolerance and diabetes are observed in 30% to 50% of BBS cases. High blood pressure is also frequent. Hypothyroidy has been reported. A minority of patients have cardiac malformations. Anosmia has been recently reported as a common feature in the syndrome (12). Premature aging of the hearing function is also reported (7). Hirschprungs disease can be associated to the syndrome.

Differential Diagnosis

Other syndromic forms of obesity can be considered as differential diagnosis.

Prader-Willi Syndrome

Neonatal hypotonia is a hallmark of the Prader-Willi syndrome (PWS), no polydactyly or retinal degeneration occurs in PWS. In case of doubt the molecular testing is straight-forward (See Chapter 5.2).

Alström Syndrome

This syndrome associate obesity, transient cardiomyopathy in early infancy, retinal degeneration, progressive deafness, diabetes, kidney, and liver involvement may also occur. There is no polydactyly in this syndrome. This syndrome is due to mutations in the *ALSM1* gene (13,14).

Cohen Syndrome

In Cohen syndrome, cognitive impairment with gynoïd obesity associated with retinal degeneration and myopia is characteristic. The facial and dental gestalt as well as the molecular diagnosis are useful. The gene has been recently identified as *COCH1* (15).

Meckel Syndrome

In utero the discovery of large kidneys and polydactyly may be confusing as Meckel syndrome share these two features with BBS. However, Meckel syndrome is defined by an associated occipital encephalocele and other malfomations and is nonviable. Interestingly, this syndrome is also a ciliopathy and overlap with BBS exists clinically and on molecular terms (Fig.2) (16).

Genetic Counselling

The extensive genetic heterogeneity of BBS has profound implications for diagnostic and genetic counseling applications. Two majors genes, *BBS1* and *BBS10* each account for ~20% of the mutational load in families of European descent, whereas each of the other 10 genes accounts for ≤5% and some of them were found mutated in only few, or even a single family (the latter in the case of *BBS11*). Two recurrent mutations have been described: M390R in *BBS1* and C91fsX95 in *BBS10*. The other genes are implied in less then 1% (*BBS11*) to 8% (*BBS12*) of the cases. Taken together, the 12 known BBS genes account for about 75% of families, suggesting that additional BBS genes remain to be identified (Fig. 4). The number of genes implied implies time-consuming molecular investigations unless the patient bears one of the common mutations or has been investigated through diagnostic chips with previously described mutations. A further complication is the finding that in some cases, inheritance departs from classic autosomal recessive inheritance and involves three mutated alleles in two genes defining oligogenic inheritance, while severity can also be modulated by an allele of a modifier gene.

To date, genetic counselling is performed on the basis of a classical auto-somal recessive condition with a 25% risk of recurrence. Prenatal diagnosis by molecular analysis of chorial villosities can be offered if two pathogenic mutations in one BBS gene are clearly and unambiguously identified. If no mutation is identified, the only way to seek for a recurrence in case of a couple with an affected child is ultrasound detection of polydactyl and/or enlarged kidneys.

BBS GENES AND THE CILIOPATHY CONCEPT
Identifying BBS Genes

The identification of BBS genes is a long-standing story initiated originally by homozygosity mapping in consanguineous families, an efficient strategy for locat-ing the genes implicated in rare recessive diseases, when families available for linkage analysis are limited in number and size. BBS was in fact the first example where linkage and heterogeneity could be demonstrated at the same time by this strategy. Implementation of this strategy awaited the construction of the first whole genome microsatellite map. Very recently, it was shown that SNP micro-arrays provide a faster and much more informative technique. Indeed, it would have been impossible to disentangle the extreme genetic complexity of BBS with-out such an approach, applied to families from the Middle East, Newfoundland, Turkey or Puerto Rico. However, when a single or very few families are used, the candidate region identified by homozygosity mapping is in general very large and contains many genes. This led, in the case of BBS, to use in addition to homo-zygosity mapping comparative genomic approaches. When it became clear that BBS genes code for proteins implicated in cilia assembly or function, comparison of sequenced genomes allowed selection of candidate genes that have orthologs in ciliated organisms (vertebrates, drosophila, *C. elegans*, chlamydia, trypanozoma) but not in nonciliated ones (*arabidopsis*, yeast) or in *Giardia lamblia* (an organism that does not contain well-conserved orthologs to known BBS genes). This

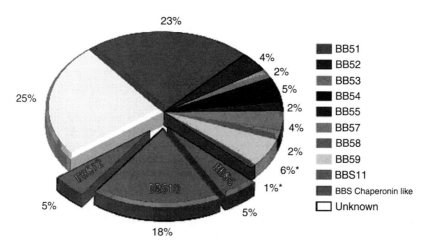

FIGURE 4 (*See color insert.*) Schematic colored representation of the identified Bardet-Biedl syndrome (BBS) genes and their percentage of mutation detected in the BBS patient population.

combination of homozygosity mapping and comparative genomics allowed the identification of *BBS3, BBS5*, and *BBS9* (17).

BBS AND EPISTATIC INETRACTIONS

BBS is the first example in human genetics of oligogenism or triallelism. Indeed, in some patients it appears necessary to carry three mutations: two in a first BBS gene and the third in a second BBS gene (18,19). Therefore, BBS is a model for studying epistatic interactions that have an important role in phenotypic variability. Genetic dissection of this epistatic effect permitted the identification of a novel locus, MGC1203. This gene encodes a pericentriolar protein that interacts and co-localizes with the BBS proteins. Sequencing of this locus in two independent BBS cohorts revealed a significant enrichment of a heterozygous C430T mutation in patients, and a transmission disequilibrium test (TDT) in families showed strong over-transmission of this variant allele. A 430T allele enhances the use of a cryptic splice acceptor site. Moreover, in *zebrafish* a modest suppression of *mgc1203* exerts an epistatic effect on the developmental phenotype of BBS morphants (20).

BBS as a Model Ciliopathy

The physiopathology of the disorder was unveiled in 2003 when Ansley et al. published the identification of BBS8 as a centrosomal or basal body protein involved in primary cilia constitution (6). BBS is now a well recognized ciliopathy (8). Cilia are cylindrical structures made of nine doublets of microtubules constructed on top of the basal body, a centriole-like organelle. Motile cilia have most often a central pair of microtubules $(9+2)$ and nonmotile or primary cilia do not have central microtubules $(9+0)$, although this rule is by no means absolute, since examples of both $9+0$ motile cilia and $9+2$ primary cilia have been reported (21). As opposed to the well-known primary ciliary dyskinesia (Kartagener syndrome $9+2$ cilia affected), BBS is related largely to non-motile cilia usually present as a single copy in numerous cell types of the body (22). Assembly and maintenance of cilia relies on active transport of cilium precursors to the distal tip [Intraflagellar Transport or (IFT)], that is the site of construction. Kinesin II transport complex particles made of at least 18 proteins to the tip where extensive remodelling takes place during construction/modulation of the cilium. A dynein motor brings the modified complex back towards the basal body. IFT was initially discovered in the model organisms *Chlamydomonas* and is remarkably well conserved during evolution, from protists to mammals. Cilia are involved in the exploration of external or internal environment via chemo-, photo-, and mechanosensory functions (23–25). Sensory cilia are found in the retina defining the outer segment of photoreceptor cells, in olfactory epithelia cells and hair cells of the inner ear. In the kidney, cilia are used for sensing fluid flow of the epithelial surface. In addition, cilia act at critical stages in embryonic development (definition of left-right asymmetry) but also in other tissues such as the nervous system. It is now clear that primary cilia play a central biological role in many tissues. In addition to BBS, cilia have been implicated in kidney dysplasia such as polycystic kidney disease (PKD1 and PKD2 loci) and in nephronophtisis including Senior-Loken syndrome (genes: NPHP1 to NPHP5).

Cellular Biology of BBS and Animal Models

A considerable amount of papers have now confirmed that BBS is the result of centrosomal/ciliary dysfunction.

Cell Biology

Recent cell biology studies showed that *BBS4* localizes to the centriolar satellites of centrosomes and basal bodies of primary cilia where it functions as an adaptor of a subunit of the dynein transport machinery to recruit pericentriolar material-1 protein and its associated cargo to the satellites (26). Silencing of *BBS4* induces PCM1 mislocalization and concomitant de-anchoring of centrosomal microtubules, arrest in cell division, and apoptotic cell death. Expression of two truncated forms of BBS4 that are similar to those found in some individuals with BBS had a similar effect on PCM1 and microtubules (26).

C. Elegans Model

Loss-of-function mutations in *BBS7* and *BBS8* of *C. elegans* compromise cilia structure and function (27). *BBS5* inhibits flagellum formation (28,29). Noticeably, all known *C. elegans BBS* genes are expressed exclusively in ciliated neurons, owing to the presence of a ciliary specific DAF-19 RFX transcription factor binding site (X box) in their promoters. Recently, *bbs1* has been shown in *C. elegans* to be implied in the polygenic control of fat storage in this organism underlining the fact that ciliated neurons may be involved in a ancient neuroendocrine axis (Chap. 4.1) (30).

Zebrafish Model

Numerous BBS functional studies were performed in zebrafish using BBS-specific morpholinos (MO). Injection of serial MO concentrations into wild-type embryos yielded dosage-dependent early developmental defects in gastrulation movements based on the recently developed hypothesis implicating the BBS proteins in the PCP pathway. Suppression of maternal *bbs* message causes shortening of the rostrocaudal body axis and dorsal thinning, broadening and kinking of the notochord, elongation of the somites and decreased somitic definition and symmetry. Testing for genetic interaction with other *bbs* genes by injecting sub-effective MO doses for each transcript is an informative way to study interactions between bbs genes (5,20).

Knockout Mice

Knockout mice are useful models to study the phenotype and genetic interactions. The *bbs4*-null mice exhibit common features with the human phenotype and confirm the connection of BBS4 with ciliated cells (31). Likewise, MKKS-null mice (*bbs6-/-*) have a phenotype resembling Bardet-Biedl except for the polydactyly and the vaginal malformations (11). *Bbs2* null mice disclosed also compatible phenotype (32). Recently, mice with mutations in genes involved in BBS have been shown to share phenotypes with PCP mutants including open eyelids, neural tube defects, and disrupted cochlear stereociliary bundles. The evolutionarily conserved (PCP) pathway (or non-canonical Wnt pathway) drives several important cellular processes, including epithelial cell polarization, cell migration and mitotic spindle orientation. In vertebrates, PCP genes have a vital role in polarized convergent extension movements during gastrulation and neurulation underlining the important biological involvement of the BBS genes (7).

BBS GENES AS A GENETIC RISK FACTOR FOR OBESITY

There is a growing interest in the genetically complex common disorders such as obesity. BBS genes have been considered to participate to be a genetic contributor to the determination of common obesity (33).

A first study was on variants of BBS6 in a cohort of 60 Danish patients with juvenile obesity (34). Except for one mutation (A242S) there was no obvious contribution to the pathogenesis of obesity. This is in contrast with a French study in which variants of BBS 1, 2, 4, and 6 were determined in 48 French patients and analyzed on 1943 French Caucasian obese patients and 1299 no obese individual (35). Association by transmission disequilibrium showed a significant association for a BBS4 variant for instance. The authors conclude that this preliminary data suggested that variations at BBS genes are associated with risk of common obesity.

CONCLUSION

The phenotypic consequences of BBS gene alteration are far-reaching in many tissues of the body with important clinical consequences such as retinal degeneration, obesity, or cognitive impairment. Retinal degeneration and obesity are the two most disabling features of the condition and would warrant preventive or curative therapeutics. This is why crucial pathophysiologic investigations remain to be done in order to look toward possible preventive or therapeutic approaches to this devastating disorder.

REFERENCES

1. Beales P. Lifting the lid on Pandora's box: the Bardet-Biedl syndrome. Curr Opin Genet Dev 2005; 15:315–23.
2. Nishimura DY, Swiderski RE, Searby CC, et al. Comparative genomics and gene expression analysis identifies BBS9, a new Bardet-Biedl syndrome gene. Am J Hum Genet 2005; 77(6):1021–33.
3. Stoetzel C, Laurier V, Davis E, et al. BBS10 encodes a vertebrate-specific chaperonin-like protein and is a major BBS locus. Nat Genet 2006; 38(5):521–4.
4. Chiang AP, Beck JS, Yen HJ, et al. Homozygosity mapping with SNP arrays identifies TRIM32, an E3 ubiquitin ligase, as a Bardet-Biedl syndrome gene (BBS11). Proc Natl Acad Sci USA 2006; 103(16):6287–92.
5. Stoetzel C, Laurier V, Muller J, et al. Identification of a Novel BBS Gene (BBS12) highlights the major role of a vertebrate-specific branch of chaperonin-related proteins in Bardet-Biedl syndrome. Am JHum Genet 2007; 80(1):1–11.
6. Ansley SJ, Badano JL, Blacque OE, et al. Basal body dysfunction is a likely cause of pleiotropic Bardet-Biedl syndrome. Nature 2003; 425:628–33.
7. Ross AJ, May-Simera H, Eichers ER, et al. Disruption of Bardet-Biedl syndrome ciliary proteins perturbs planar cell polarity in vertebrates. Nat Genet 2005; 37(10): 1135–40.
8. Badano JL, Mitsuma N, Beales PL, et al. The ciliopathies: an emerging class of human genetic disorders. Annu Rev Genomics Hum Genet 2006; 7:125–48.
9. Beales PL, Elcioglu N, Woolf AS, et al. New criteria for improved diagnosis of Bardet-Biedl syndrome: results of a population survey. J Med Genet 1999; 36:437–46.
10. Eichers ER, Abd-El-Barr MM, Paylor R, et al. Phenotypic characterization of Bbs4 null mice reveals age-dependent penetrance and variable expressivity. Hum Genet 2006; 120(2):211–26.
11. Fath MA, Mullins RF, Searby C, et al. Mkks-null mice have a phenotype resembling Bardet-Biedl syndrome. Hum Mol Genet 2005; 14(9):1109–18.
12. Kulaga HM, Leitch CC, Eichers ER, et al. Loss of BBS proteins causes anosmia in humans and defects in olfactory cilia stracture and function in the mouse. Nat Genet 2004; 36(9):994–8.
13. Hearn T, Renforth GL, Spalluto C, et al. Mutation of ALMS1, a large gene with a tandem repeat encoding 47 amino acids, causes Alstrom syndrome. Nat Genet 2002; 31(1):79–83.

14. Collin GB, Marshall JD, Ikeda A, et al. Mutations in ALMS1 cause obesity, type 2 diabetes and neurosensory degeneration in Alstrom syndrome. Nat Genet 2002; 31(1):74–8.
15. Kolehmainen J, Black GC, Saarinen A, et al. Cohen syndrome is caused by mutations in a novel gene, COH1, encoding a transmembrane protein with a presumed role in vesicle-mediated sorting and intracellular protein transport. Am J Hum Genet 2003; 72(6):1359–69.
16. Karmous-Benailly H, Martinovic J, Gubler MC, et al. Antenatal presentation of Bardet-Biedl syndrome may mimic Meckel syndrome. Am J Hum Genet 2005; 76(3):493–504.
17. Nishimura DY, Swiderski RE, Searby CC, et al. Comparative genomics and gene expression analysis identifies BBS9, a new Bardet-Biedl syndrome gene. Am J Hum Genet 2005; 77(6):1021–33.
18. Katsanis N, Ansley SJ, Badano JL, et al. Triallelic inheritance in Bardet-Biedl syndrome, a mendelian recessive disorder. Science 2001; 293:2256–9.
19. Katsanis N. The oligogenic properties of Bardet-Biedl syndrome. Hum Mol genet 2004; 13(Spec No 1):R65–71.
20. Badano JL, Leitch CC, Ansley SJ, et al. Dissection of epistasis in oligogenic Bardet-Biedl syndrome. Nature 2006; 439(7074):326–30.
21. Davis EE, Brueckner M, Katsanis N. The emerging complexity of the vertebrate cilium: new functional roles for an ancient organelle. Dev Cell 2006; 11(1):9–19.
22. Satir P, Christensen ST. Overview of Structure and Function of Mammalian Cilia. Annu Rev Physiol 2007; 69:377–400.
23. Blacque OE, Leroux MR. Bardet-Biedl syndrome: an emerging pathomechanism of intracellular transport. Cell Mol Life Sci 2006; 63(18):2145–61.
24. Marshall WF, Nonaka S. Cilia: tuning in to the cell's antenna. Curr Biol 2006; 16(15): R604–14.
25. Singla V, Reiter JF. The primary cilium as the cell's antenna: signaling at a sensory organelle. Science 2006; 313(5787):629–33.
26. Kim JC, Badano JL, Sibold S. The Bardet-Biedl protein BBS4 targets cargo to the pericentriolar region and is required for microtubule anchoring and cell cycle progression. Nat Genet 2004; 36(5):462–70.
27. Blacque OE, Reardon MJ, Li C, et al. Loss of C. elegans BBS-7 and BBS-8 protein function results in cilia defects and compromised intraflagellar transport. Genes Dev 2004; 18(13):1630–42.
28. Li JB, Gerdes JM, Haycraft CJ. Comparative genomics identifies a flagellar and basal body proteome that includes the BBS5 human disease gene. Cell. 2004; 117(4):541–52.
29. Yen HJ, Tayeh MK, Mullins RF, et al. Bardet-Biedl syndrome genes are important in retrograde intracellular trafficking and Kupffer's vesicle cilia function. Hum Mol Genet. 2006; 15(5):667–77.
30. Mak HY, Nelson LS, Basson M, et al. Polygenic control of Caenorhabditis elegans fat storage. Nat Genet 2006; 38(3):363–8.
31. Mykytyn K, Mullins RF, Andrews M, et al. Bardet-Biedl syndrome type 4 (BBS4)-null mice implicate Bbs4 in flagella formation but not global cilia assembly. Proc Natl Acad Sci USA 2004; 101(23):8664–9.
32. Nishimura DY, Fath M, Mullins RF, et al. Bbs2-null mice have neurosensory deficits, a defect in social dominance, and retinopathy associated with mislocalization of rhodopsin. Proc Natl Acad Sci USA 2004; 101(47):16588–93.
33. Sheffield VC. Use of isolated populations in the study of a human obesity syndrome, the Bardet-Biedl syndrome. Pediatr Res 2004; 55(6):908–11.
34. Andersen KL, Echwald SM, Larsen LH. Variation of the McKusick-Kaufman gene and studies of relationships with common forms of obesity. J Clin Endocrinol Metab 2005; 90(1):225–30. Epub 2004.
35. Benzinou M, Walley A, Lobbens S, et al. Bardet-Biedl syndrome gene variants are associated with both childhood and adult common obesity in French Caucasians. Diabetes 2006; 55(10):2876–82.

5.4 Leptin and Leptin Receptor Mutations

I. Sadaf Farooqi and Stephen O'Rahilly

Departments of Medicine and Clinical Biochemistry, Addenbrooke's Hospital, Cambridge University Hospitals NHS Foundation Trust, Cambridge, U.K.

With the identification of leptin and its receptor, the physiological circuits controlling energy homeostasis have become increasingly well understood. In 1994, Friedman and colleagues showed that the severely obese Lep^{ob}/Lep^{ob} mice harbored mutations in the *lep* gene resulting in a complete lack of its protein product leptin (1). Administration of recombinant leptin reduced the food intake and body weight of leptin-deficient Lep^{ob}/Lep^{ob} mice and corrected all their neuroendocrine and metabolic abnormalities. Leptin acts through the long isoform of the leptin receptor (LEPRb), a member of the interleukin-6 receptor family of class 1 cytokine receptors. Leptin receptor has intracellular motifs necessary for activation of the Jak-STAT signal transduction pathway and leptin receptor activation ultimately results in phosphorylation of STAT3 which translocates into the nucleus to activate downstream target genes. The signaling form of the leptin receptor is deleted in $lepr^{db}/lepr^{db}$ mice, which are consequently unresponsive to endogenous or exogenous leptin (2).

Leptin, acting via its receptor in the hypothalamus, activates anorexigenic pathways mediated by neurons producing proopiomelanocortin (POMC) and cocaine and amphetamine related transcript (CART) and inhibits orexigenic pathways mediated by neurons expressing neuropeptide Y (NPY) and agouti-related protein (AgRP). These pathways interact with other brain centers to coordinate appetite and modulate efferent signals to the periphery regulating intermediary metabolism and energy expenditure. Leptin administration in Lep^{ob}/Lep^{ob} and wild-type mice showed that leptin acts as an afferent signal in a negative feedback loop regulating adiposity, leading to decreased food intake, increased energy expenditure, and weight loss. Reduced leptin also acts as a signal of nutritional deprivation, with low leptin levels initiating an adaptive response to conserve energy, manifested by increased food intake, decreased energy expenditure, and shutdown of the reproductive and other endocrine axes (3). The identification of humans with mutations in the genes encoding leptin and its receptor and the characterization of the associated phenotypes, have provided insights into the role of leptin in human physiology.

MUTATIONS IN GENES ENCODING LEPTIN AND THE LEPTIN RECEPTOR

In 1997, we reported two severely obese cousins from a highly consanguineous family of Pakistani origin (4). Both children had undetectable levels of serum leptin and were found to be homozygous for a frameshift mutation in the *LEP* gene (ΔG133), which resulted in a truncated protein that was not secreted. We have since identified five further affected individuals from four other families (5,6) (and unpublished observations) who are also homozygous for the same mutation in the leptin gene. All the families are of Pakistani origin but not known to be related over five generations. A large Turkish family in which three adults carry a homozygous missense mutation (C→T substitution at codon 105 resulting in Arg→Trp) in the *LEP* gene have also been described (7). To date, only one mutation in the leptin receptor gene (*LEPR*) has been reported, in three severely obese adult siblings from a consanguineous family of Algerian origin (8). This mutation results in abnormal splicing of leptin receptor transcripts and generates a mutant leptin receptor that lacks both transmembrane and intracellular domains. The mutant receptor circulates at high concentrations bound to leptin, resulting in very elevated serum leptin concentrations.

We recently sequenced the leptin receptor gene in a cohort of patients with severe, early onset obesity in the absence of developmental delay and identified eight unrelated probands with homozygous or compound heterozygous loss of function mutations in the leptin receptor gene. The prevalence of pathogenic leptin receptor mutations in this cohort was 3%. Six of the probands were from consanguineous families but two probands (including a compound heterozygote patient) were U.K. Caucasians whose parents were unrelated. Although the prevalence of leptin and leptin receptor mutations is likely to be higher amongst ethnic groups where consanguinity is common, such mutations should be considered in patients with severe hyperphagic obesity of early onset.

CLINICAL PHENOTYPES ASSOCIATED WITH LEPTIN AND LEPTIN RECEPTOR DEFICIENCY

The clinical phenotypes associated with congenital leptin and leptin receptor deficiencies are similar. Leptin and Leptin receptor deficient subjects are of normal birthweight, but exhibit rapid weight gain in the first few months of life resulting in severe obesity (5). Body composition measurements using dual energy X-ray absorptiometry (DEXA) show that leptin deficiency and leptin receptor deficiency is characterized by the preferential deposition of fat mass giving a distinct clinical appearance (Fig. 1) (5). All patients were hyperinsulinemie consistent with the severity of obesity and some adults have developed type 2 diabetes in the 3rd–4th decade (5). All subjects in these families are characterized by intense hyperphagia with food seeking behavior and aggressive behavior when food was denied (5). Energy intake at an ad libitum meal is markedly elevated in leptin and leptin receptor deficient subjects.

In leptin-deficient humans we found no detectable changes in resting metabolic rate using indirect calorimetry or total energy expenditure using chamber calorimetry (9). Free-living energy expenditure measured using the doubly labelled water method was not significantly different after adjustment for body composition. However, Ozata et al. reported abnormalities of sympathetic nerve function in leptin-deficient adults consistent with defects in the efferent sympathetic limb of thermogenesis (10). Leptin and leptin receptor deficiency are associated with hypothalamic hypothyroidism and hypogonadotropic hypogonadism. Evidence from rodents suggests that leptin is necessary for the normal biosynthesis and secretion of thyrotropin-releasing hormone (TRH) and that complete leptin deficiency is associated with a moderate degree of hypothalamic hypothyroidism characterized by low free thyroxine and high serum thyroid stimulating hormone (TSH) which is bioinactive (11). In leptin-deficient children, plasma free thyroxine concentrations are within the normal range, but four children had significantly elevated TSH levels (5) and the pulsatility of TSH secretion, studied

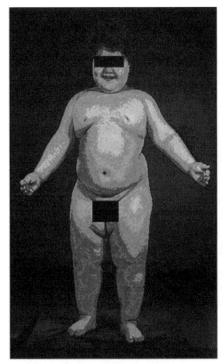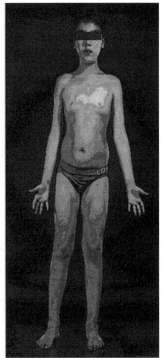

| 3-year-old weighing 42 kg | 7-year-old weighing 32 kg |

FIGURE 1 Effects of recombinant human leptin treatment in leptin deficiency, before (*left*) and after (*right*) treatment.

in a single adult with congenital leptin deficiency, was characterized by a markedly disorganized secretory pattern (12). Two subjects homozygous for a nonsense mutation in the leptin receptor were diagnosed with hypothyroidism in childhood and thyroid hormone replacement therapy commenced (8).

Normal pubertal development does not occur in adults with leptin or leptin receptor deficiency, with biochemical evidence of hypogonadotropic hypogonadism (7,8). However, there is some evidence for the delayed but spontaneous onset of menses in one leptin and three leptin receptor deficient adults (10). Leptin-deficient children have normal linear growth in childhood and normal insulin-like growth factor 1 (IGF-1) levels (5). However, because of the absence of a pubertal growth spurt, the final height of adult subjects is reduced. In the one previously reported leptin receptor deficient family, short stature and abnormal serum levels of GH, IGFBP3 were noted in childhood (8). However, assessment of the GH/IGF axis is difficult in obese children and adults as obesity itself is associated with abnormalities in basal and dynamic tests of the GH/IGF axis. While impaired linear growth has been reported in some cases of LEPR deficiency, this does not appear to be a common characteristic of this disorder. We demonstrated that children with leptin deficiency had profound abnormalities of T cell number and function (5), consistent with high rates of childhood infection and a high-reported rate of childhood mortality from infection in obese Turkish subjects (10). We have made similar observations in leptin receptor deficiency.

COMPARISON WITH RODENT MODELS OF LEPTIN INACTION

Most of these phenotypes closely parallel those seen in murine leptin deficiency (Table 1). However, there are some phenotypes where the parallels between human and mouse are not as clear-cut. Thus, while leptin-deficient mice are stunted, it appears that growth retardation is not a feature of leptin inaction in humans. Lep^{ob}/Lep^{ob} mice have marked activation of the hypothalamic pituitary adrenal axis with very elevated corticosterone levels. In humans, no abnormalities of cortisol secretion have been reported. The contribution of reduced energy expenditure to the obesity of the Lep^{ob}/Lep^{ob} mouse is reasonably well established (13), but measurements of resting and free-living energy expenditure in humans with leptin inaction are not markedly abnormal after adjusting for changes in body composition.

RESPONSE TO LEPTIN ADMINISTRATION IN LEPTIN DEFICIENCY

We have reported the dramatic and beneficial effects of daily subcutaneous injections of recombinant human leptin leading to a reduction in body weight and fat mass in three congenitally leptin-deficient children (5,9). We have recently

TABLE 1   Phenotypes Associated with Leptin Deficiency in Rodents (*ob/ob*) and Humans

Phenotype	OB/OB	Human leptin deficiency
Total body weight	3 × normal	Mean BMI sds = 6.2
Body composition		
Fat mass	Over 50%	Mean 57% of body weight
Lean mass	Decreased	Normal for age
Bone mineral content	Increased	Normal for age
Food intake	Increased meal size	Increased meal size and frequency
Energy expenditure		
Body temperature	Decreased in response to cold	Normal in basal state
Basal metabolic rate	Decreased oxygen consumption	Appropriate for body composition
Physical activity	Reduced	Reduced
SNS activation	Basal decreased and refractory to cold exposure	Reduced in response to cold
Metabolic responses		
Diabetes	Fasting; hyperglycaemia	Normoglycaemia
Hyperinsulinaemia	Severe; resistance to exogenous insulin	Appropriate for degree of obesity
T cell–mediated immunity	Decreased CD4 cells; reduced T cell proliferation	Decreased CD4 cells, reduced T cell proliferation
Neuroendocrine function		
Reproductive	Hypogonadotropic hypogonadism	Hypogonadotropic hypogonadism
Thyroid	Hypothalamic and ? peripheral effects	Mild hypothalamic hypothyroidism
Growth	Stunted	Normal linear growth and IGF-1 levels
Adrenal	Corticosterone excess	Normal cortisol and ACTH levels

Abbreviations: IGF-1, insulin-like growth factor 1; ACTH, adrenocorticotrophic hormone.

commenced therapy in two other children and seen comparably beneficial results (personal observations). All children showed a response to initial leptin doses that were designed to produce plasma leptin levels at only 10% of those predicted by height and weight (i.e., approximately 0.01 mg/kg of lean body mass). The most dramatic example of leptin's effects was with a 3-year old boy, severely disabled by gross obesity (weight 42 kg), who now weighs 32 kg (75th centile for weight) after 48 months of leptin therapy (Fig. 1). Leptin therapy has also been successfully used in the three Turkish leptin-deficient adults (14). The major effect of leptin was on appetite with normalization of hyperphagia. Leptin therapy reduced energy intake during an 18 MJ ad libitum test meal by up to 84% (5 MJ ingested pre-treatment vs. 0.8 MJ post-treatment in the child with the greatest response) (5). Leptin treatment was associated with reduced hunger scores with no change in satiety in adults with leptin deficiency (14). We were unable to demonstrate a major effect of leptin on basal metabolic rate or free-living energy expenditure, but, as weight loss by other means is associated with a decrease in basal metabolic rate, the fact that energy expenditure did not fall in our leptin-deficient subjects is notable. The administration of leptin permitted progression of appropriately timed pubertal development in the single child of appropriate age and did not cause the early onset of puberty in the younger children (5). In adults with leptin deficiency, leptin induced the development of secondary sexual charateristics and pulsatile gonadotrophin secretion. In the three previously reported children small, but sustained, increases in free T_4, free T_3, and TSH occurred within one month of leptin therapy. These observations are fully consistent with an effect of leptin at the hypothalamic level. A fourth patient had substantial elevation of TSH before treatment, such that thyroxine therapy was commenced (6). However, replacement therapy was stopped when thyroid function tests normalized after leptin treatment.

Throughout the trial of leptin administration, weight loss continued in all subjects, albeit with refractory periods which were overcome by increases in leptin dose (5). The families in the UK harbor a mutation which leads to a prematurely truncated form of leptin and thus wild-type leptin is a novel antigen. Thus, all subjects developed anti-leptin antibodies after ~6 weeks of leptin therapy, which interfered with interpretation of serum leptin levels and in some cases were capable of neutralizing leptin in a bioassay (5). These antibodies are the likely cause of refractory periods occurring during therapy. The fluctuating nature of the antibodies probably reflects the complicating factor that leptin deficiency is itself an immuno-deficient state (15) and administration of leptin leads to a change from the secretion of predominantly Th2 to Th1 cytokines, which may directly influence antibody production. Thus far, we have been able to regain control of weight loss by increasing the dose of leptin.

PARTIAL LEPTIN DEFICIENY IN HETEROZYGOTE CARRIERS

The major question with respect to the potential therapeutic use of leptin in more common forms of obesity relates to the shape of the leptin dose response curve. We have clearly shown that at the lower end of plasma leptin levels, raising leptin levels from undetectable to detectable has profound effects on appetite and weight. Heymsfield et al. administered supraphysiological doses (0.1–0.3 mg/kg body weight) of leptin to obese subjects for 28 weeks (16). On average, some subjects lost weight, but the extent of weight loss and the variability between subjects has led many to conclude that the leptin resistance of common obesity cannot be usefully overcome by leptin supplementation, at least when administered peripherally. However, it is of interest that there was a significant effect on weight in some subjects with low serum leptin levels, suggesting that leptin can continue to have a dose/response effect on energy homeostasis across a wide serum concentration range. To test this hypothesis, we studied the heterozygous relatives of our leptin-deficient subjects (17). Serum leptin levels in the heterozygous subjects were found to be significantly lower than expected for percent body fat and they had a higher prevalence of obesity than seen in a control population of similar age, sex, and ethnicity (17). Additionally, % body fat was higher than predicted from their height and weight in the heterozygous subjects compared to control subjects of the same ethnicity (17). These findings closely parallel those in heterozygous ob/– and db/– mice. These data provide further support for the possibility that leptin can produce a graded response in terms of body composition across a broad range of plasma concentrations.

All heterozygous subjects had normal thyroid function and appropriate gonadotropins, normal development of secondary sexual characteristics, normal menstrual cycles and fertility suggesting that low leptin levels are sufficient to preserve these functions (17). This is consistent with the data of Ioffe and colleagues who demonstrated that several of the neuroendocrine features associated with leptin deficiency were abolished in low level leptin transgenic mice, which were fertile with normal corticosterone levels (18). However, these low level leptin transgenic mice still exhibited an abnormal thermoregulation in response to cold exposure and had mildly elevated plasma insulin concentrations, suggesting that there are different thresholds for the various biological responses elicited by changes in serum leptin concentration and that these could be reversed by leptin administration. Heterozygote leptin receptor deficient subjects, although not obese, have an increased fat mass. These findings are consistent with the findings of Chung et al., who demonstrated an increase in fat mass in both heterozygous $Lep^{ob/+}$ and $lepr^{ob/+-}$ (19).

LEPTIN ADMINISTRATION IN COMMON OBESITY

Our findings in the heterozygous individuals have some potential implications for the treatment of common forms of obesity. Whilst serum leptin concentrations correlate positively with fat mass, there is considerable inter-individual variation at any particular fat mass. Leptin is inappropriately low in some obese individuals and the relative hypoleptinemia in these subjects may be actively contributing to their obesity and may be responsive to leptin therapy. Heymsfield et al., found no relationship between baseline plasma leptin levels and therapeutic response, however, study subjects were not preselected for relative hypoleptinemia (16). A therapeutic trial in a subgroup of subjects selected for disproportionately low circulating leptin levels would be of great interest.

CONCLUSION

Several monogenic forms of human obesity have now been identified by searching for mutations homologous to those causing obesity in mice. Although such monogenic obesity syndromes are rare, the characterization of these disorders has provided insights into the role of leptin in human physiology. Importantly, administration of recombinant human leptin in leptin deficiency represents the first rational mechanistically based therapy for obesity and has the potential to provide immense clinical benefits for the patients concerned.

REFERENCES

1. Zhang Y, Proenca R, Maffei M, et al. Positional cloning of the mouse obese gene and its human homologue. Nature 1994; 372:425–32.
2. Tartaglia LA. The leptin receptor. J Biol Chem 1997; 272:6093–6.
3. Flier JS. Clinical review 94: What's in a name? In search of leptin's physiologic role. J Clin Endocrinol Metab 1998; 83:1407–13.
4. Montague CT, Farooqi IS, Whitehead JP, et al. Congenital leptin deficiency is associated with severe earlyonset obesity in humans. Nature 1997; 387:903–8.
5. Farooqi IS, Matarese G, Lord GM, et al. Beneficial effects of leptin on obesity, T cell hyporesponsiveness, and neuroendocrine/metabolic dysfunction of human congenital leptin deficiency. J Clin Invest 2002; 110:1093–103.
6. Gibson WT, Farooqi IS, Moreau M, et al. Congenital leptin deficiency due to homozygosity for the Delta133G mutation: report of another case and evaluation of response to four years of leptin therapy. J Clin Endocrinol Metab 2004; 89:4821–6.
7. Strobel A, Issad T, Camoin L, et al. A leptin missense mutation associated with hypogonadism and morbid obesity. Nat Genet 1998; 18:213–5.
8. Clement K, Vaisse C, Lahlou N, et al. A mutation in the human leptin receptor gene causes obesity and pituitary dysfunction. Nature 1998; 392:398–401.
9. Farooqi IS, Jebb SA, Langmack G, et al. Effects of recombinant leptin therapy in a child with congenital leptin deficiency. N Engl J Med 1999; 341:879–84.
10. Ozata M, Ozdemir IC, Licinio J. Human leptin deficiency caused by a missense mutation: multiple endocrine defects, decreased sympathetic tone, and immune system dysfunction indicate new targets for leptin action, greater central than peripheral resistance to the effects of leptin, and spontaneous correction of leptin-mediated defects. J Clin Endocrinol Metab 1999; 84:3686–95.
11. Flier JS, Harris M, Hollenberg AN. Leptin, nutrition, and the thyroid: the why, the wherefore, and the wiring. J Clin Invest 2000; 105:859–61.
12. Mantzoros CS, Ozata M, Negrao AB, et al. Synchronicity of frequently sampled thyrotropin (TSH) and leptin concentrations in healthy adults and leptin-deficient subjects: evidence for possible partial TSH regulation by leptin in humans. J Clin Endocrinol Metab 2001; 86:3284–91.
13. Trayhurn P, Thurlby PL, James WPT. Thermogenic defect in pre-obese ob/ob mice. Nature 1977; 266:60–2.
14. Licinio J, Caglayan S, Ozata M, et al. Phenotypic effects of leptin replacement on morbid obesity, diabetes mellitus, hypogonadism, and behavior in leptin-deficient adults. Proc Natl Acad Sci USA 2004; 101:4531–6.
15. Lord GM, Matarese G, Howard JK, et al. Leptin modulates the T-cell immune response and reverses starvation-induced immunosuppression. Nature 1998; 394:897–901.
16. Heymsfield SB, Greenberg AS, Fujioka K, et al. Recombinant leptin for weight loss in obese and lean adults: a randomized, controlled, dose-escalation trial. JAMA 1999; 282:1568–75.
17. Farooqi IS, Keogh JM, Kamath S, et al. Partial leptin deficiency and human adiposity. Nature 2001; 414:34–5.
18. Ioffe E, Moon B, Connolly E, et al. Abnormal regulation of the leptin gene in the pathogenesis of obesity. Proc Natl Acad Sci USA 1998; 95:11852–7.
19. Chung WK, Belfi K, Chua M, et al. Heterozygosity for Lep(ob) or Lep(rdb) affects body composition and leptin homeostasis in adult mice. Am J Physiol 1998; 274:R985–90.

POMC and PC1 Mutations

I. Sadaf Farooqi and Stephen O'Rahilly

*Departments of Medicine and Clinical Biochemistry, Addenbrooke's Hospital,
Cambridge University Hospitals NHS Foundation Trust, Cambridge, U.K.*

Considerable attention has focused on deciphering the hypothalamic pathways that mediate the behavioral and metabolic effects of leptin. Leptin stimulates the expression of proopiomelanocortin (POMC) which is sequentially cleaved by pro-hormone convertases to yield the melanocortin peptides. In this chapter, we here review genetic defects impairing the synthesis and processing of POMC which have clearly established that the melanocortin system plays a critical role in energy homeostasis in humans.

The first-order neuronal targets of leptin action in the brain are anorectic POMC and orexigenic Neuropeptide-Y/Agouti-related protein (NPY/AgRP) neurons in the hypothalamic arcuate nucleus, where the signaling isoform of the leptin receptor is highly expressed (1). Over 40% of POMC neurons in the arcuate nucleus express the mRNA for the long form of the leptin receptor and POMC expression is regulated positively by leptin. Proopiomelanocortin undergoes extensive and tissue-specific post-translational processing by pro-protein convertases (PCs) to yield a range of biologically active peptides (2). The expression of pro-hormone convertase 2 (PC2) within the hypothalamus leads to the production of alpha-, beta- and gamma-MSH (α-, β-, and γ-MSH, the melanocortins) but not adrenocorticotrophic hormone (ACTH) whereas in the pituitary corticotrophs, expression of pro-hormone convertase 1 (PC1), but not PC2, results in the production of N-terminal peptide, joining peptide, ACTH, and β-lipotropin (3,4). The melanocortins mediate their effects through a family of five related G protein-coupled receptors, two of which, MC3R and MC4R, are highly expressed within the central nervous system. Of the two centrally expressed melanocortin receptors, the MC4R is the one most closely linked to energy homeostasis (5). Thus, humans and mice lacking the MC4R are markedly obese and hyperphagic as well as showing increased linear growth and severe hyperinsulinaemia from a young age (6–8) (chap. 5.6). Mice lacking the MC3R have subtle abnormalities of body composition, which occur later in life (9,10), although no MC3R mutations convincingly linked to monogenic human obesity have been described.

CLINICAL PHENOTYPE OF COMPLETE POMC DEFICIENCY

In 1998, Krude et al. provided the first description of humans congenitally lacking *POMC* gene products (11). One proband was a compound heterozygote for two nonsense mutations and a second patient was homozygous for a mutation in the 5'-untranslated region that introduced an additional out-of-frame start site, thus interfering with *POMC* translational initiation (Fig. 1). Subsequently, Krude and Gruters have reported three additional unrelated European children with congenital POMC deficiency who were either homozygous or compound heterozygous for *POMC* mutations (Fig. 1) (12). We have recently identified a sixth patient with complete POMC deficiency, being homozygous for a complete loss of function

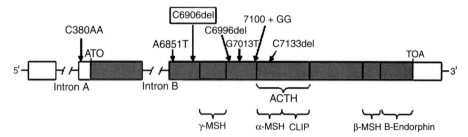

FIGURE 1 *POMC* gene structure with mutations resulting in complete deficiency. Structure of the *POMC* gene and location of all homozygous and compound heterozygous mutations identified to date. Untranslated (*white*) and translated regions (*filled*) indicated. Proband 1, compound heterozygote for G7013T and C7133del; proband 2, C3804A (homozygous); proband 3, compound heterozygote for A6851T and 6996del; proband 4, C3804A (homozygous); proband 5, compound heterozygote for 7100 + GG and C3804A; proband 6 (reported here and outlined), C6906del (homozygous). *Abbreviations*: ACTH, adrenocorticotrophic hormone; α-MSH, alpha-melano stimulating hormone; β-MSH, beta-melano stimulating hormone; γ-MSH, gamma-melano stimulating hormone; POMC, proopiomelanocortin.

mutation which results in the loss of all POMC-derived peptides (personal observations). These patients all presented in early life with features of hypocortisolaemia secondary to ACTH deficiency, leading to hypoglycemia, prolonged jaundice, susceptibility to the effects of infection and in one case, neonatal death (12). The children responded well to physiological replacement with glucocorticoids, but all subsequently developed marked obesity in association with hyperphagia. Birth weights have been unremarkable in all children reported to date, including our patient, indicating that the effects on growth and weight are exclusively post-natal. In this disorder, in both humans and murine models, obesity occurs despite profound glucocorticoid deficiency, a condition normally associated with severe weight loss. Notably, in *Pomc* null mice, restoration of relatively normal glucocorticoid levels results in a marked worsening of the obesity and insulin resistance (13), suggesting that the glucocorticoid deficiency modulates the severity of the metabolic phenotype.

Notably, all children thus far reported have pale skin and red hair, features consistent with the known role of POMC-derived peptides in the determination of the phaeomelanin to eumelanin ratio in melanocytes. The Turkish proband is the first reported patient with POMC deficiency who does not have red hair. It is likely this can be explained by his differing genetic background as the other reported patients were all white Caucasian subjects. The retention of dark hair in this child and his similarly affected deceased sibling indicates that the synthesis of eumelanin in humans is not absolutely dependent on the presence of melanocortin peptides. It can be assumed, that in ethnic groups that are predominantly characterized by dark hair, other genetic variants maintain eumelanin synthesis in the absence of POMC-derived ligand, while in Northern European races, such eumelanin synthesis is more critically dependent on the presence of such ligands (14). Thus, the cardinal features of congenital POMC deficiency are isolated ACTH deficiency, hyperphagia and severe early onset obesity. Although red hair may be an important diagnostic clue in patients of Caucasian origin, its absence in patients originating from other ethnic groups should not result in this diagnostic consideration being excluded.

POMC HAPLOINSUFFICIENCY

Krude et al. have previously attempted to assess the impact of loss of one *POMC* allele in the parents and heterozygous relatives of their probands (12). They estimated the maximum lifetime BMI SDS in adult *POMC* heterozygotes and suggested that most had a maximum lifetime BMI SDS of 1, which is at the upper end of the normal range (12). We had the opportunity to study the large Turkish consanguineous pedigree with 12 heterozygote carriers and seven wild-type subjects. The significantly higher prevalence of obesity/overweight in the carriers provides compelling support for the idea that loss of one copy of *POMC* is sufficient to markedly predispose to obesity (personal observations). This is particularly relevant as we and others have described a variety of heterozygous point mutations in *POMC*, including mutations in α- and β-MSH, which significantly increase obesity risk but are not invariably associated with obesity (15–17).

POMC MUTATIONS AFFECTING SPECIFIC MELANOCORTIN PEPTIDES

In order to determine whether missense/nonsense mutations within the melanocortin peptides might predispose to obesity, we screened the coding region of the POMC gene for mutations in over 600 U.K. Caucasian subjects with severe earlyonset obesity (16). We identified a number of sequence variants in *POMC* in severely obese children. Three of these missense mutations directly affect regions of the POMC gene that encode melanocortin peptides (Fig. 2). R236G was identified in three patients but also two controls. We have previously shown that this mutation disrupts a di-basic cleavage site between β-MSH and β-endorphin, resulting in a β-MSH/β-endorphin fusion protein that binds to MC4R, but has reduced ability to activate the receptor (15). Its presence in both obese probands and controls reflects previous studies that show that this is not a highly penetrant cause of inherited obesity but may increase the risk of obesity in carriers (15). We identified five unrelated probands who were heterozygous for a rare missense variant in the region encoding β-MSH, Tyr221Cys (16). This frequency was significantly increased ($p < 0.001$) compared to the general U.K. Caucasian population and the variant cosegregated with obesity/overweight in affected family

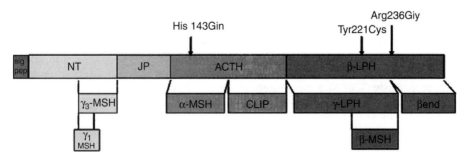

FIGURE 2 POMC processing and point mutations in melanocortin peptides. *Abbreviations*: ACTH, adrenocorticotrophic hormone; α-MSH, alpha melano-stimulating hormone; β-LPH, beta-lipotropic hormone; β-MSH, β-melano stimulating hormone; γ-MSH, γ-melano stimulating hormone.

members. The overrepresentation of this mutation in obese subjects is supported by independent studies in a German population (17). Compared to wild-type β-MSH, the variant peptide was impaired in its ability to bind to and activate signaling from the MC4R (16). Obese children carrying the Tyr221Cys variant were hyperphagic and showed increased linear growth, both of which are features of MC4R deficiency (16). These studies support a role for β-MSH in the control of human energy homeostasis. Interestingly, we found a missense mutation in α-MSH in a single proband, which had a major deleterious effect on its function (16). However, this variant was found in one lean family member and one lean unrelated control. While it is likely that this variant is contributing to the obesity of the proband, it is notable that our studies provide more compelling evidence for a specific role for β-MSH than α-MSH in the control of human energy balance. It is possible that an important role for β-MSH in the control of energy balance has been overlooked as attention has been principally focused on α-MSH as the probable endogenous ligand in rodents (18). This is largely because rodents lack the proximal di-basic site that is necessary for the proteolytic cleavage event that produces β-MSH in humans.

GENETIC VARIATION AT THE POMC LOCUS AND COMMON OBESITY

It is notable that a number of genetic linkage studies have identified chromosome 2p22 (a region encompassing the *POMC* gene) as the site of a gene or genes influencing common obesity and obesity-related traits. The strongest evidence for a quantitative trait locus (QTL) influencing obesity-related phenotypes comes from the San Antonio Family Heart Study undertaken in Mexican American extended families, with a log odds ratio (LOD) score of 7.5 for serum leptin levels on chromosome 2p22 (19). Strong evidence for linkage of plasma leptin levels, one of the most robust markers of fat mass, to this region of chromosome 2 was also seen in a genome wide scan performed in French obese sibling pairs (20). Other studies have suggested a role for genes in this region in phenotypes such as serum triglycerides (21), blood pressure (22), physical inactivity (23), and Type 2 diabetes (24). Association studies of the *POMC* gene and indices of adiposity have been inconsistent (25,26), but most have been underpowered. The extent to which these effects are the consequence of variation in or around the *POMC* locus itself has yet to be determined but the knowledge that the control of human energy balance is sensitive to *POMC* gene dose strengthens the candidacy of *POMC* as a site where variants affecting expression could influence body weight. It is plausible that genetic variation around the *POMC* locus might confer a risk of obesity through a gene-environment interaction. We recently reported that 129 mice heterozygous for a null mutation in the *pomc* gene become significantly hyperphagic and obese on a high-fat diet but not on normal chow (27). Interestingly, in a recent genome wide scan analysis in Mexican American families, suggestive evidence of linkage with saturated fat intake was found on chromosome 2p22 (28).

MUTATIONS IN PROHORMONE CONVERTASE 1

Many biologically inactive prohormones and neuropeptides are cleaved by serine endoproteases to release biologically active peptides. The prohormone convertases (PC1 and 2) are expressed in neuroendocrine tissues and act upon a range of substrates including proinsulin, proglucagon and POMC (2). Prohormone convertase 1 is itself synthesized as an inactive precursor, then undergoes two autocatalytic events, firstly within the endoplasmic reticulum and then within the secretory vesicles of the regulated secretory pathway to generate a fully active 66 kDa isoform that is stored in mature secretory granules.

We have previously reported an adult female with severe earlyonset obesity, hypogonadotropic hypogonadism, postprandial hypoglycemia, hypocortisolemia, and evidence of impaired processing of POMC and proinsulin (29). She was found to be a compound heterozygote for *PC1* mutations: Gly593Ag, which causes failure of maturation of the inactive propeptide form of PC1 (pro-PC1) and its retention in the endoplasmic reticulum, and A → C^{+4} in the donor splice site of intron 5, resulting in exon skipping, a frameshift, and a premature stop codon in the catalytic domain (30). We have described the second case of congenital PC1 deficiency, in a patient who was a compound heterozygote for two loss of function mutations: Glu250stop, which is predicted to truncate the PC1 protein within the catalytic domain, and Ala213del, which deletes a highly conserved alanine residue near the catalytically essential His208 residue (31). Intriguingly, this patient suffered from severe small intestinal absorptive dysfunction as well as the characteristic severe earlyonset obesity, impaired pro-hormone processing, and hypocortisolemia (Table 1). We hypothesized that the small intestinal dysfunction seen in this patient and, to a lesser extent, in the first patient we described may be the result of a failure of maturation of propeptides within the enteroendocrine cells and nerves that express PC1 throughout the gut. The finding of elevated levels of progastrin and proglucagon provided in vivo evidence that pro-hormone processing in enteroendocrine cells was abnormal (31).

PC1 deficiency has been described in two independent mouse models with notable differences in phenotype. In one mouse model, about 40% of *Pc1* null embryos die before birth, and another 40% within 6 days. The remaining pups appear normal at birth but are only 60% of the size of heterozygous or wild-type littermates with reduced growth associated with decreased levels of growth hormone (GH) mRNA and decreased circulating GH (32). They suffer from chronic mild diarrhea associated with bulky moist stools. Blood glucose levels are normal despite a severe impairment in proinsulin processing, which results in accumulation of immature secretory granules in the pancreatic beta cells. However, these *Pc1* null mice were not reported to be obese, leading to the suggestion that PC1 may serve different functions in rodents compared to humans. Recently, a second mouse model of Pc1 deficiency has been generated spontaneously by ENU mutagenesis resulting in a homozygous missense mutation (N222D) in the catalytic domain (33). These *Pc1* knockouts are hyperproinsulinaemic, are 30% heavier than wild-type littermates with an increase in food intake.

TABLE 1 PC1 Deficiency—Clinical Features and Affected Prohormone Conversion

Obesity	POMC–MSH
Hypogonadotropic hypogonadism	ProGnRH–GnRH
Hypoadrenalism	POMC–ACTH
Reactive hypoglycemia/impaired glucose tolerance	Proinsulin–insulin
Intestinal malabsorption	Proglucagon–GLP1 and GLP2

Abbreviations: ACTH, adrenocorticotrophic hormone; GnRH, gonadotroophin-releasing hormone; MSH, melano stimulating hormone; POMC, proopiomelanocortin.

An important caveat regarding pro-hormone processing disorders is that it is very difficult to state with certainty which altered phenotypes are due to which altered processing events. This uncertainty derives from the fact that these enzymes act on multiple precursors, some of which may not as yet be fully characterized.

CONCLUSION

POMC undergoes extensive and tissue specific post-translational processing to yield a range of biologically active peptides. Historically, the most clearly defined roles of these peptides are in the control of adrenal steroidogenesis by cortico-troph-derived ACTH and skin pigmentation by α-MSH. However, a rapidly expanding body of work has established that POMC-derived peptides synthesized in neurons of the hypothalamus play a central role in the control of energy homeostasis. Inherited abnormalities in POMC synthesis and processing and defects in the action of POMC-derived peptides in both humans and mice have helped shape our current understanding of the importance of the melanocortin system in human energy balance.

REFERENCES

1. Schwartz MW, Woods SC, Porte D, et al. Central nervous system control of food intake. Nature 2000; 404(6778):661–71.
2. Bertagna X. Proopiomelanocortin-derived peptides. Endocrinol Metab Clin North Am 1994; 23(3):467–85.
3. Hadley ME, Haskell-Luevano C. The proopiomelanocortin system. Ann NY Acad Sci 1999; 885:1–21.
4. Pritchard LE, Turnbull AV, White A. Pro-opiomelanocortin processing in the hypothalamus: impact on melanocortin signalling and obesity. J Endocrinol 2002; 172(3):411–21.
5. Cone RD. The central melanocortin system and energy homeostasis. Trends Endocrinol Metab 1999; 10(6):211–6.
6. Huszar D, Lynch CA, Fairchild-Huntress V, et al. Targeted disruption of the melano-cortin-4 receptor results in obesity in mice. Cell 1997; 88(1):131–41.
7. Farooqi IS, Yeo GS, Keogh JM, et al. Dominant and recessive inheritance of morbid obesity associated with melanocortin 4 receptor deficiency. J Clin Invest 2000; 106(2):271–9.
8. Farooqi IS, Keogh JM, Yeo GS, et al. Clinical spectrum of obesity and mutations in the melanocortin 4 receptor gene. N Engl J Med 2003; 348(12):1085–95.
9. Butler AA, Kesterson RA, Khong K, et al. A unique metabolic syndrome causes obesity in the melanocortin-3 receptor-deficient mouse. Endocrinology 2000; 141(9):3518–21.
10. Chen AS, Marsh DJ, Trumbauer ME, et al. Inactivation of the mouse melanocortin-3 receptor results in increased fat mass and reduced lean body mass. Nat Genet 2000; 26(1):97–102.
11. Krude H, Biebermann H, Luck W, et al. Severe earlyonset obesity, adrenal insufficiency and red hair pigmentation caused by POMC mutations in humans. Nat Genet 1998; 19(2):155–7.
12. Krude H, Biebermann H, Schnabel D, et al. Obesity due to proopiomelanocortin deficiency: three new cases and treatment trials with thyroid hormone and ACTH4-10. J Clin Endocrinol Metab 2003; 88(10):4633–40.
13. Coll AP, Challis BG, Lopez M, et al. Proopiomelanocortin-deficient mice are hypersensitive to the adverse metabolic effects of glucocorticoids. Diabetes 2005; 54(8):2269–76.
14. Barsh GS. The genetics of pigmentation: from fancy genes to complex traits. Trends Genet 1996; 12(8):299–305.

15. Challis BG, Pritchard LE, Creemers JW, et al. A missense mutation disrupting a dibasic prohormone processing site in proopiomelanocortin (POMC) increases susceptibility to earlyonset obesity through a novel molecular mechanism. Hum Mol Genet 2002; 11(17):1997–2004.

16. Lee YS, Challis BG, Thompson DA, et al. A POMC variant implicates beta-melanocyte-stimulating hormone in the control of human energy balance. Cell Metab 2006; 3(2):135–40.

17. Biebermann H, Castaneda TR, Van Landeghem F, et al. A role for beta-melanocyte-stimulating hormone in human body-weight regulation. Cell Metab 2006; 3(2):141–6.

18. Mountjoy KG, Wong J. Obesity, diabetes and functions for proopiomelanocortin-derived peptides. Mol Cell Endocrinol 1997; 128(1–2):171–7.

19. Comuzzie AG, Hixson JE, Almasy L, et al. A major quantitative trait locus determining serum leptin levels and fat mass is located on human chromosome 2. Nat Genet 1997; 15(3):273–6.

20. Delplanque J, Barat-Houari M, Dina C, et al. Linkage and association studies between the proopiomelanocortin (POMC) gene and obesity in caucasian families. Diabetologia 2000; 43(12):1554–7.

21. Imperatore G, Knowler WC, Pettitt DJ, et al. A locus influencing total serum cholesterol on chromosome 19p: results from an autosomal genomic scan of serum lipid concentrations in Pima Indians. Arterioscler Thromb Vasc Biol 2000; 20(12):2651–6.

22. Rankinen T, An P, Rice T, et al. Genomic scan for exercise blood pressure in the Health, Risk Factors, Exercise Training and Genetics (HERITAGE) Family Study. Hypertension 2001; 38(1):30–7.

23. Simonen RL, Rankinen T, Perusse L, et al. Genome-wide linkage scan for physical activity levels in the Quebec Family study. Med Sci Sports Exerc 2003; 35(8):1355–9.

24. Demenais F, Kanninen T, Lindgren CM, et al. A meta-analysis of four European genome screens (GIFT Consortium) shows evidence for a novel region on chromosome 17p11.2-q22 linked to type 2 diabetes. Hum Mol Genet 2003; 12(15):1865–73.

25. Baker M, Gaukrodger N, Mayosi BM, et al. Association between common polymorphisms of the proopiomelanocortin gene and body fat distribution: a family study. Diabetes 2005; 54(8):2492–6.

26. Hixson JEAL, Cole S, Birnbaum S, et al. Normal variation in leptin levels in associated with polymorphisms in the proopiomelanocortin gene, POMC. Clin Endocrinol Metab 1999; 84(9):3187–91.

27. Challis BG, Coll AP, Yeo GS, et al. Mice lacking proopiomelanocortin are sensitive to high-fat feeding but respond normally to the acute anorectic effects of peptide-YY (3-36). Proc Natl Acad Sci USA 2004; 101(13):4695–700.

28. Cai G, Cole SA, Bastarrachea-Sosa RA, et al. Quantitative trait locus determining dietary macronutrient intakes is located on human chromosome 2p22. Am J Clin Nutr 2004; 80(5):1410–4.

29. O'Rahilly S, Gray H, Humphreys PJ, et al. Brief report: impaired processing of prohormones associated with abnormalities of glucose homeostasis and adrenal function. N Engl J Med 1995; 333(21):1386–90.

30. Jackson RS, Creemers JW, Ohagi S, et al. Obesity and impaired prohormone processing associated with mutations in the human prohormone convertase 1 gene. Nat Genet 1997; 16(3):303–6.

31. Jackson RS, Creemers JW, Farooqi IS, et al. Small-intestinal dysfunction accompanies the complex endocrinopathy of human proprotein convertase 1 deficiency. J Clin Invest 2003; 112(10):1550–60.

32. Zhu X, Zhou A, Dey A, et al. Disruption of PC1/3 expression in mice causes dwarfism and multiple neuroendocrine peptide processing defects. Proc Natl Acad Sci USA 2002; 99(16):10293–8.

33. Lloyd DJ, Bohan S, Gekakis N. Obesity, hyperphagia and increased metabolic efficiency in Pc1 mutant mice. Hum Mol Genet 2006; 15(11):1884–93.

5.6 MC4R Mutations

Cécile Lubrano-Berthelier
INSERM, U872, Nutriomique, Centre de Recherche des Cordeliers, Université Pierre et Marie Curie-Paris6, Paris, France

Christian Vaisse
Diabetes Center and Department of Medicine, University of California, San Francisco, San Francisco, California, U.S.A.

Leptin acts on the arcuate nucleus of the hypothalamus by modulating the expression of anorexigenic melanocortins derived from proopiomelanocortin (POMC) as well as the expression of the orexigenic neuropeptide AgRP. These peptides modulate food intake and energy expenditure by acting on a common receptor, expressed on second order neurons in the para-ventricular nucleus of the hypothalamus, the melanocortin-4 receptor (MC4R). The use of pharmacological agonists of MC4R in rodents reduces food intake, while antagonists of this receptor increase it (1,2).

Mice with a genetic invalidation of MC4R (*Mc4R−/−*mice) develop obesity and increased linear growth but are otherwise normal. These mice are hyperphagic and have decreased energy expenditure. Mice heterozygous for this invalidation of MC4R (*Mc4R+/−*mice) present an intermediate, background dependent, and level of obesity (3). These observations suggest that both alleles of MC4R are required for adequate regulation of long term energy homeostasis in rodents (for details see Chapter 3.1 and 3.2).

The human MC4R is a 332 amino acid protein encoded by a single exon genelocalized on chromosome 18q22 (4,5). In 1998, the first human obesity associated MC4R mutations were reported in the U.K. (6) and in France (7). Both mutations (two frameshift mutations: Ins GATT codon 244 and Del CTCT codon 211) resulted in a truncation of the MC4R protein. The severely obese carriers were heterozygous for these mutations, which cosegregated with obesity in the family of the probands. These reports were the initial demonstration of a role for MC4R mutations in human obesity.

PREVALENCE OF MC4R MUTATIONS IN HUMAN OBESITY

Since these initial reports, a large number of studies have examined the prevalence of MC4R mutations in various cohorts of obese children and adults (Table 1). In most of these studies, the *MC4R* gene was screened for mutations by direct sequencing although other methods have also been used, in particular for the population based studies.

Results from these studies can be summarized as follows: The frequency of heterozygous carriers of rare missense, nonsense, and frameshift MC4R mutations in cohorts of patients with severe or early onset obesity varies from 1% to 6% with an average of 2.5% in adult patients with severe obesity (body mass index, BMI > 35) or children with early onset obesity (BMI > 97 percentile). This

TABLE 1 Frequency of MC4R Mutations in Human Obesity

Obesity onset, original population	Obese subjects	Control subjects	Obese mutant carriers	Control mutant carriers	References
Early and late, U.S.	140	50	1	0	(8)
Late, U.S.	237		1		(9)
Early, France	172		3	0	(10)
Early, France	266		4	0	(11)
Late, U.S.	165		6	0	(11)
Early, France	109		3	0	(12)
Late, Switzerland	469	25	5	0	(13)
Early, Germany	808	327	20	0	(14)
Early, France	63	283	4	0	(15)
Early, Denmark	750	706	21	0	(16)
Not specified, U.K.	230	142	0	0	(17)
Early and late, Italy	120	60	2	0	(18)
Late, Sweden and African-American, U.S.	264	264	2	2	(19)
Early, Italy	208	0	1	0	(20)
Late, Pimas	300	126	14	0	(21)
Late, Spain	159	154	1	1	(22)
Early, Turkey	40		1		(23)
Early, U.K.	500	54	26	0	(24)
Adult, Italy	196	100	5	0	(45)
Early, Finland	56		1	0	(26)
Late, Finland	252	321	1	3	(26)
Early and late, France	769	811	19	1	(27,28)
Late, Belgium	95		0	0	(29)
Early, Belgium	123		0	0	(29)
Total	6491	3423	141	7	
Frequency			2.17%	0.20%	
CI 95%			[1.82;2.53]	[0.05;0.36]	

Note: Only carriers of rare nonsynonymous variants are considered; carriers of the Val103Ile variant, which is present in 1–2% of obese and controls, are not included.

frequency is higher in cohorts selected for the highest level of obesity. The frequency of such heterozygous carriers in non-obese controls or in the general population is about 10-fold lower than in the cohorts of obese patients. Together these observations suggest that MC4R mutations are the cause of approximately 2.5% of earlyonset and/or severe adult obesity cases. It should be emphasized that this prevalence reflects the pooling of different mutations, as most MC4R mutations are carried only by a single individual. When available, family studies confirm the autosomal dominant transmission of obesity associated with MC4R mutations. Penetrance is incomplete and the clinical expression associated with heterozygous MC4R mutations varies underlying the role of the environment and other potentially modulating genetic factors (27).

Homozygous or compound heterozygous carriers of MC4R mutations are very rare. Three carriers of homozygous null mutations in the MC4R have been detected in these screenings (12,24). As expected from a dominant condition, such patients have a very early onset of more severe obesity, than heterozygous carriers, but do not display any additional unrelated phenotypes.

MOLECULAR AND FUNCTIONAL ASPECTS OF HUMAN OBESITY ASSOCIATED MC4R MUTATIONS

Most MC4R mutations are carried only by a single individual, and over 90 obesity-associated MC4R mutations have been described. Most of these mutations are missense mutations that do not truncate the receptor. Evidence for their effect on MC4R function has been provided by in vitro studies (Fig. 1). In addition to supporting the pathogenicity of these mutations, these studies have also provided novel insights into the function of MC4R (24) and for review see references 28, 30, 31.

MC4R is a member of the A family (rhodopsin-like) of G-protein coupled receptor (32,33). MC4R transduces signal by coupling to heterotrimeric Gs proteins resulting in the activation of adenylate cyclase and an increase in intracellular cAMP. The function most commonly assayed in MC4R obesity-associated mutants is their response to melanocortin agonists following expression in cell lines, and many display an impaired response in such an assay (Fig. 2).

Further studies have demonstrated that in a majority of cases, this decreased response to agonist stimulation resulted from intracellular retention of the mutated receptor (10). MC4R also exhibits a constitutive activity on which the antagonist AgRP acts as an inverse agonist (34,35). This seems to have a relevant anorexigenic role as a subset of mutations, in particular localized in the N-terminal domain of the receptor, have been found to exhibit an isolated reduction in this constitutive activity (36). On the basis of these in vitro findings, delineating three types of functional alterations in obesity-associated mutant MC4R, a functional classification of these mutations has been proposed (Table 2).

CLINICAL FEATURES OF MC4R MUTATION CARRIERS

Homozygous MC4R mutations cause very severe early onset obesity. In heterozygous MC4R mutations carriers the onset and the severity of the obesity varies and is related to the severity of the functional alteration caused by the mutation.

In addition to obesity, are there clinical or biochemical clues that can differentiate MC4R mutations carriers from other obese patients? MC4R mutations carriers display increased linear growth, in particular in the first five years of life (24) but do not appear to be taller as adults (27). This trend is often observed in overweight and obese children. Assessment of body composition in these patients demonstrates increase in both fat and lean mass (31). Studies performed in U.K. children, has suggested that bone mineral density is increased in MC4R mutation carriers (24,31). This increased bone density may be caused, at least in part, by a decrease in bone resorption as a decrease of bone resorption markers has been observed in patients with homozygous MC4R mutations (37).

Obese children carrying MC4R mutations have a marked hyperphagia that decreases with age, when compared to their siblings (31), while in both children and adults, no evidence has been found for a decreased metabolic rate in these patients. In one study of severely obese adults, carriers of MC4R mutations as well as non-obesity associated MC4R polymorphisms were found to all present with binge eating disorder (13). The genetic approach used in this study appeared controversial (38–40,24) and the finding has not been confirmed in other studies (41,42).

MC4R variant reported in human obesity

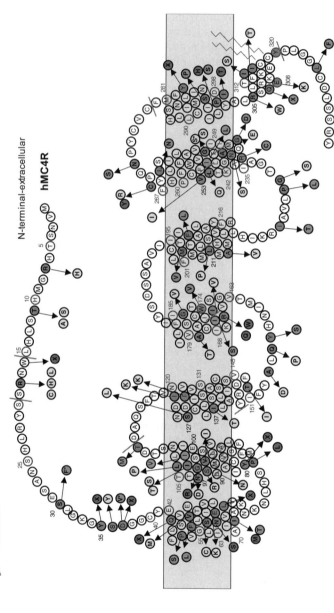

FIGURE 1 (*See color insert.*) Schematic representation of MC4R and the sequence variants detected in human obesity. The positions of the sequence variants are indicated on the secondary structure of MC4R. Amino acids are indicated as circles in single-letter code. Amino acids affected by a mutation are indicated in purple circles. S30F*/G252S* and Y35STOP**/D37V** are double mutants. Note that the mutations are not clustered in a specific functional domain of the protein.

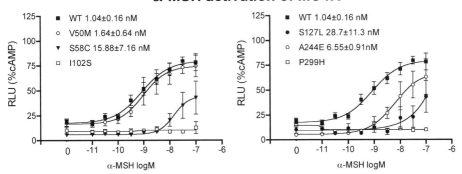

FIGURE 2 Example of α-MSH activation of obesity-associated MC4R mutants. Activity of the receptors was assayed by analyzing their ability to activate the expression of a cAMP-induced luciferase reporter gene. WT and mutant MC4R are transiently transfected in a stable HEK 293 cell line expressing pCRE-luciferase. Data points represent Mean ± SEM of at least three independent experiments performed in triplicates. Mean ± SEM of the EC50 (nM) is indicated for each variant. The WT receptor activation curve is shown on all graphs for comparison with mutated receptors. *Abbreviations*: α-MSH, alpha melanocyte stimulating hormone; WT, wild type.

Adult MC4R mutation carriers do not have an increased prevalence of diabetes or other obesity complications (42). In U.K. children, fasting insulinemia was found to be significantly elevated in MC4R mutation carriers, particularly before the age of 10 years when compared to age, sex, and BMI-matched control (24). This hyperinsulinemia has not consistently been observed in children (12) and in adults (42,23).

Finally, with respect to endocrine function, HPA and, reproductive axis (12,24,27) as well as thyroid function are normal in MC4R mutation carriers.

In summary, there are currently no evident clinical biochemical markers that can unambiguously differentiate MC4R mutations carriers from other obese patients.

CONCLUSION

Genetic and functional studies of the association of MC4R mutations and obesity have validated the critical role of MC4R in human body weight regulation. However, they also suggest that, in a clinical context, no specific phenotype can be

TABLE 2 Functional Classification of Human Obesity-Associated MC4R Mutations

		Membrane expression	Melanocortin activation	Basal activity
Class 1—severe (includes truncations)		None or reduced	Decreased or absent	Decreased or absent
Class 2—intermediate	A	Normal	Normal	Decreased
	B	Normal	Decreased	Normal
	C	Normal	Decreased	Decreased
Class 3—other		Includes mutations with a yet unclear pathogenic role (Example: increased basal activity)		

used to predict the presence of an MC4R mutation in obese subjects. This form of obesity which resembles common forms of early onset obesity is therefore a non-syndromic, oligogenic obesity that can be placed between the exceptional forms of monogenic obesity with complete penetrance and the polygenic forms of common obesity.

It is possible that other phenotypes not studied yet might permit this differentiation and it is important to pursue the precise functional and phenotype characterization of naturally occurring MC4R mutation carried by obese subjects. In view of therapeutic intervention aiming at improving melanocortin action in the control of body weight homeostasis, these studies place the MC4R in a pathway that could serve as a potential control point for therapeutic targeting of human obesity. Several pharmaceutical companies have programs to develop selective MC4R agonists (43). They have to face normal concerns of targeting GPCRs (31) and specific difficulties of possible side effects due to the widespread expression of MC4R in the brain and the already demonstrated role of MC4R in erectile function (44). This type of treatment should also be evaluated in patients heterozygous for MC4R mutations in specific clinical investigation protocols. Regardless, it is likely that, in the near future, MC4R agonist drugs will be successfully developed to provide effective antiobesity treatment probably in combination with other approaches such as well-balanced diet and physical activity.

REFERENCES

1. Fan W, Boston BA, Kesterson RA, et al. Role of melanocortinergic neurons in feeding and the agouti obesity syndrome. Nature 1997; 385(6612): 165–8.
2. Thiele TE, Van Dijk G, Yagaloff KA, et al. Central infusion of melanocortin agonist MTII in rats: assessment of c-Fos expression and taste aversion. Am J Physiol 1998; 274(1): R248–54.
3. Huszar D, Lynch CA, Fairchild-Huntress V, et al. Targeted disruption of the melanocortin-4 receptor results in obesity in mice. Cell 1997; 88(1): 131–141.
4. Gantz I, Miwa H, Konda Y, et al. Molecular cloning, expression, and gene localization of a fourth melanocortin receptor. J Biol Chem 1993; 268(20): 15174–9.
5. Sundaramurthy D, Campbell DA, Leek JP, et al. Assignment of the melanocortin 4 receptor (MC4R) gene to human chromosome band 18q22 by in situ hybridisation and radiation hybrid mapping. Cytogenet Cell Genet 1998; 82(1–2): 97–8.
6. Yeo GS, Farooqi IS, Aminian S, et al. A frameshift mutation in MC4R associated with dominantly inherited human obesity. Nat Genet 1998; 20(2): 111–2.
7. Vaisse C, Clement K, Guy-Grand B, et al. A frameshift mutation in human MC4R is associated with a dominant form of obesity. Nat Genet 1998; 20(2): 113–4.
8. Gu W, Tu Z, Kleyn PW, et al. Identification and functional analysis of novel human melanocortin-4 receptor variants. Diabetes 1999; 48(3): 635–9.
9. Donohoue PA, Tao YX, Collins M, et al. Deletion of codons 88-92 of the melanocortin-4 receptor gene: a novel deleterious mutation in an obese female. J Clin Endocrinol Metab 2003; 88(12): 5841–5.
10. Lubrano-Berthelier C, Durand E, Dubern B, et al. Intracellular retention is a common characteristic of childhood obesity-associated MC4R mutations. Hum Mol Genet 2003; 12(2): 145–53.
11. Lubrano-Berthelier C, Cavazos M, Le Stunff C, et al. The Human MC4R Promoter: characterization and role in obesity. Diabetes 2003; 52(12): 2996–3000.
12. Lubrano-Berthelier C, Le Stunff C, Bougnères P, et al. A homozygous null mutation delineates the role of the melanocortin-4 receptor in humans. JCEM 2004; 89(5): 2028–32.
13. Branson R, Potoczna N, Kral JG, et al. Binge eating as a major phenotype of melanocortin 4 receptor gene mutations. N Engl J Med 2003; 348(12): 1096–103.

14. Hinney A, Hohmann S, Geller F, et al. Melanocortin-4 receptor gene: case-control study and transmission disequilibrium test confirm that functionally relevant mutations are compatible with a major gene effect for extreme obesity. J Clin Endocrinol Metab 2003; 88(9): 4258–67.

15. Dubern B, Clement K, Pelloux V, et al. Mutational analysis of melanocortin-4 receptor, agouti-related protein, and alpha-melanocyte-stimulating hormone genes in severely obese children. J Pediatr 2001; 139(2): 204–9.

16. Larsen LH, Echwald SM, Sørensen TIA, et al. Prevalence of mutations and functional analyses of Melanocortin 4 Receptor variants identified among 750 men with juvenile-onset obesity. J Clin Endocrinol Metab 2005; 90(1): 219–24.

17. Gotoda T, Scott J, Aitman TJ. Molecular screening of the human melanocortin-4 receptor gene: identification of a missense variant showing no association with obesity, plasma glucose, or insulin. Diabetologia 1997; 40(8): 976–9.

18. Santini F, Maffei M, Ceccarini G, et al. Genetic screening for melanocortin-4 receptor mutations in a cohort of Italian obese patients: description and functional characterization of a novel mutation. J Clin Endocrinol Metab 2004; 89(2): 904–8.

19. Jacobson P, Ukkola O, Rankinen T, et al. Melanocortin 4 receptor sequence variations are seldom a cause of human obesity: the Swedish Obese Subjects, the HERITAGE Family Study, and a Memphis cohort. J Clin Endocrinol Metab 2002; 87(10): 4442–6.

20. Miraglia Del Giudice E, Cirillo G, Nigro V, et al. Low frequency of melanocortin-4 receptor (MC4R) mutations in a Mediterranean population with earlyonset obesity. Int J Obes Relat Metab Disord 2002; 26(5): 647–51.

21. Ma L, Tataranni PA, Bogardus C, et al. Melanocortin 4 receptor gene variation is associated with severe obesity in Pima Indians. Diabetes 2004; 53(10): 2696–9.

22. Marti A, Corbalan MS, Forga L, et al. A novel nonsense mutation in the melanocortin-4 receptor associated with obesity in a Spanish population. Int J Obes Relat Metab Disord 2003; 27(3): 385–8.

23. Mergen M, Mergen H, Ozata M, et al. A novel melanocortin-4 receptor (MC4R) gene mutation associated with morbid obesity. J Clin Endocrinol Metab 2001; 86(7): 3448–51.

24. Farooqi IS, Keogh JM, Yeo GS, et al. Clinical spectrum of obesity and mutations in the melanocortin 4 receptor gene. N Engl J Med 2003; 348(12): 1085–95.

25. Buono P, Pasanisi F, Nardelli C, et al. Six novel mutations in the proopiomelanocortin and melanocortin receptor 4 genes in severely obese adults living in southern Italy. Clin Chem 2005; 51(8): 1358–64.

26. Valli-Jaakola K, Lipsanen-Nyman M, Oksanen L, et al. Identification and characterization of melanocortin-4 receptor gene mutations in morbidly obese finnish children and adults. J Clin Endocrinol Metab 2004; 89(2): 940–5.

27. Vaisse C, Clement K, Durand E, et al. Melanocortin-4 receptor mutations are a frequent and heterogeneous cause of morbid obesity. J Clin Invest 2000; 106(2): 253–62.

28. Lubrano-Berthelier C, Cavazos M, Dubern B, et al. Molecular genetics of human obesity-associated MC4R mutations. Ann NY Acad Sci 2003; 994:49–57.

29. Beckers S, Mertens I, Peeters A, et al. Screening for melanocortin-4 receptor mutations in a cohort of Belgian morbidly obese adults and children. Int J Obes (Lond) 2006; 30(2): 221–5.

30. Govaerts C, Srinivasan S, Shapiro A, et al. Obesity-associated mutations in the melanocortin 4 receptor provide novel insights into its function. Peptides 2005; 26(10): 1909–19.

31. Mackenzie RG. Obesity-associated mutations in the human melanocortin-4 receptor gene. Peptides 2006; 27(2):395–403.

32. Gether U. Uncovering molecular mechanisms involved in activation of G protein-coupled receptors. Endocr Rev 2000; 21(1): 90–113.

33. Fredriksson R, Lagerstrom MC, Lundin LG, et al. The G-protein-coupled receptors in the human genome form five main families. Phylogenetic analysis, paralogon groups, and fingerprints. Mol Pharmacol 2003; 63(6): 1256–72.

34. Nijenhuis WA, Oosterom J, Adan RA. AgRP(83–132) acts as an inverse agonist on the human-melanocortin-4 receptor. Mol Endocrinol 2001; 15(1): 164–71.

35. Haskell-Luevano C, Monck EK. Agouti-related protein functions as an inverse agonist at a constitutively active brain melanocortin-4 receptor. Regul Pept 2001; 99(1): 1–7.
36. Srinivasan S, Lubrano-Berthelier C, Govaerts C, et al. Constitutive activity of the melanocortin-4 receptor is maintained by its N-terminal domain and plays a role in energy homeostasis in humans. J Clin Invest 2004; 114(8): 1158–64.
37. Elefteriou F, Ahn JD, Takeda S, et al. Leptin regulation of bone resorption by the sympathetic nervous system and CART. Nature 2005; 434(7032): 514–20.
38. Herpertz S, Siffert W, Hebebrand J. Binge eating as a phenotype of melanocortin 4 receptor gene mutations. N Engl J Med 2003; 349(6): 606–9.
39. Gotoda T. Binge eating as a phenotype of melanocortin 4 receptor gene mutations. N Engl J Med 2003; 349(6): 606–9.
40. Farooqi IS, Yeo GS, O'Rahilly S. Binge eating as a phenotype of melanocortin 4 receptor gene mutations. N Engl J Med 2003; 349(6): 606–9.
41. Hebebrand J, Geller F, Dempfle A, et al. Binge-eating episodes are not characteristic of carriers of melanocortin-4 receptor gene mutations. Mol Psychiatry 2004; 9(8): 796–800.
42. Lubrano-Berthelier C, Dubern B, Lacorte JM, et al. Melanocortin 4 receptor mutations in a large cohort of severely obese adults: prevalence, functional classification, genotype–phenotype relationship, and lack of association with binge eating. J Clin Endocrinol Metab 2006; 91(5): 1811–8.
43. Arbeeny CM. Addressing the unmet medical need for safe and effective weight loss therapies. Obes Res 2004; 12(8): 1191–6.
44. Martin WJ, MacIntyre DE. Melanocortin receptors and erectile function. Eur Urol 2004; 45(6): 706–13.

6.1 Overview of Genetic Studies in Polygenic Obesity and Methodological Challenges

David T. Redden, Jasmin Divers, Laura K. Vaughan, Miguel Padilla, Solomon Musani, Hemant K. Tiwari, and David B. Allison
Section on Statistical Genetics, Department of Biostatistics, University of Alabama at Birmingham, Birmingham, Alabama, U.S.A.

With ever better versions of the human genome map and other genetic technologies available, greater opportunities to study causative genetic factors for complex diseases and traits such as obesity and obesity-related phenotypes continue to emerge. Researchers have and continue to devote substantial effort in an attempt to isolate genetic markers associated with obesity. Such investigators have many opportunities to advance obesity research yet also face numerous methodological challenges. This chapter presents a brief overview of the ongoing research and reviews the current approaches, techniques, and challenges in genetic research of obesity and obesity-related phenotypes.

BRIEF REVIEW OF OBESITY-RELATED GENETIC STUDIES

The twelfth update of the Human Obesity Gene Map provides a detailed listing of many published results through October 2005 (1). As of 2005, over 600 genes, markers, and chromosomal regions have been associated or linked with human obesity phenotypes. In 2005, there were 426 reported statistically significant associations between obesity-related phenotypes and DNA sequence variations in 127 candidate genes. Some of the genes identified are related to energy metabolism control, control of food intake and or metabolic pathways, while the function of others genes has yet to be elucidated (2). Of the 127 genes, 22 genes were supported by replication from at least five positive studies, with twelve replicating in at least 10 studies—adiponectin (*ADIPOQ*), adrenergic, beta-3-, receptor (*ADRB3*), 5-hydroxytryptamine (serotonin) receptor 2C (*HTR2C*), guanine nucleotide binding (*GNB*) protein (G protein), beta polypeptide, Leptin (*LEP*), leptin receptor (*LEPR*), glucocorticoid receptor (*NR3C1*), peroxisome proliferator-activated receptor gamma (*PPARG*), uncoupling protein 1,2,3 (*UCP1, UCP2,* and *UCP3*). A study was considered replicated if an independent study identified a statistically significant association with the same polymorphism ($P < 0.05$). Additionally, there were 92 studies with 58 candidate genes that showed no statistically significant evidence of association with obesity-related phenotypes, including four genes that showed no compelling association in four or more studies—*ADIPOQ, PPARG, ADRB3,* and interleukin (*IL6*). Note that by the definition the authors of the Obesity Gene Map employed, a gene can show up on both the list of replicated genes and the list of genes showing no evidence (e.g. *ADRB3, PPARG, LEPR, GNB3, UCP2*). Indeed, a gene is likely to do so if there are many separate reports investigating its association with obesity-related phenotypes. This highlights the need for careful consideration of the definition of replication. We will discuss potential issues dealing with non-replication of genetic studies of obesity later in this chapter (Table 1).

The vast majority of association studies have been conducted on candidate genes identified either through linkage studies or based on biochemical knowledge or animal studies. Recently, genome-wide association (GWA) studies have been made possible through advances in the identification and mass genotyping of molecular variants, in particular single nucleotide polymorphisms (SNPs). With the advent of GWA studies, new statistical tools are needed to address the issue of utilizing the massive number of markers available (3).

TESTING GENOTYPIC VS. ALLELIC EFFECTS

Genetic association studies aim to correlate disease frequency or trait levels with genotype. The measurement scale of the phenotypic variable (nominal, ordinal, or continuous) under consideration influences the manner in which the association test is conducted. A common point of confusion is whether to test for association with genotypes or alleles. For simplicity, we begin by illustrating this issue with the example of a dichotomous trait (e.g. obese vs. not obese). Given that each individual carries two alleles at autosomal loci, the data collected in a case-control study testing the association between a dichotomous phenotype (e.g. "case" and "control") and a specific genetic marker can be represented either by a 2×2 or a 2×3 table. The difference between these two tables reflects the investigator's choice to investigate either an allelic (2×2 tables) or a genotypic effect (2×3 tables). For SNP data for example, this two tables are similar to those shown in Figure 1.

The allelic formulation is valid (in terms of significance testing) *if and only if* Hardy-Weinberg equilibrium (HWE) holds in the combined case-control population (4) and the two methods are asymptotically equivalent in terms of effect size estimation if and only if the mode of inheritance at the locus under study is strictly additive. Note that the equilibrium within each (case and control) population separately is not sufficient to guarantee equivalence between the allelic and genotypic tests. When this assumption fails, the chi-square test statistic obtained using the allelic formulation is not valid since the assumption that the two alleles are transmitted independently from each other is violated. The genotypic formulation of the case-control test is more flexible in testing for nonadditive effects (e.g. dominant, recessive, or overdominant effects) and does not require the assumption of HWE. Therefore, we concur with Sasieni (4) that it is not appropriate to treat each allele a person has as independent in the test of association between alleles and phenotypes. Instead, one should test for association between genotypes and phenotypes.

POPULATION STRATIFICATION AND STATISTICAL METHODS

Population stratification can be defined as the presence of subgroups within a population with different allele frequencies that are attributable to differences in ancestry. An often cited cause of population stratification is the admixture process, the event of two populations with different allele frequencies intermating and producing an admixed population. If the prevalence of disease or the mean phenotypic values differ between the subgroups, an association between a genetic marker and a phenotype may exist and yet the marker may not cause changes in

TABLE 1 Genes Showing Positive Evidence for Association Between Markers of Candidate Genes with Obesity-Related Phenotypes in at Least 10 Studies

Gene	No. positive replications	No. negative replications	Phenotypes
ADIPOQ	12	4	BMI, waist circumference, abdominal visceral fat, weight change during acarbose trial, waist-to-hip ratio, obesity, body weight, waist circumference, sagittal abdominal diameter
ADRB2	20	1	BMI, waist-to-hip ratio, body-weight increase, catecholamine-induced lipolysis in adipocytes, fat mass, body fat, skinfolds, lipolysis, abdominal visceral fat, waist circumference, hip circumference, leptin
ADRB3	31	4	BMI, obesity, fat mass, waist-to-hip ratio, hip circumference, body-weight increase (5, 20, and 25 years), abnormal subcutaneous fat, abdominal visceral & subcutaneous fat, body weight in obese children, morbid obesity, eating behavior
HTR2C	11		BMI, obesity, antipsychotic-induced body-weight gain, weight change, BMI change
GNB3	13	2	BMI, obesity, fat mass, waist circumference, hip circumference, weight gain during pregnancy, lipolysis, weight loss with sibutramine, skinfolds, body weight at birth, change in fat mass, percent change in body weight, subcutaneous adrenoreceptor-mediated lipolysis, percent body fat
LEP	10	1	BMI, body weight, leptin, leptin secretion, obesity, abdominal subcutaneous fat change
LEPR	16	1	BMI, BMI > 25, fat mass, fat-free mass, body fat, lean mass, overweight/obesity, leptin, sagittal abdominal diameter, extreme obesity, energy expenditure, adipocyte size, subcutaneous abdominal, % body fat, abdominal total fat, abdominal subcutaneous fat, waist circumference
NR3C1	10		BMI, waist-to-hip ratio, waist circumference, abdominal visceral fat in lean subjects, leptin, overweight with type 2 diabetes, skinfolds, body-weight gain, lean mass
PPARG	30	14	BMI, obesity, fat mass, waist-to-hip ratios, waist circumference, leptin, change in BMI in obese and lean men, morbid obesity, weight increase and decrease (3 and 10 years), body weight, height, leptin, lipid oxidation and balance 24-hr, ponderal index at birth, body-weight gain, severe early onset obesity, lean body mass
UCP1	10	1	BMI, obesity, waist-to-hip ratio, % body fat, body weight, high-fat meal-induced thermogenesis, resting metabolic rate, fat increase (in high weight gainers)
UCP2	11	2	BMI, obesity, fat mass, 24-hr energy expenditure, 24-hr spontaneous physical activity, spontaneous sleeping physical activity, 24-hr respiratory quotient, 24-hr nonprotein fat oxidation, obesity, resting energy expenditure, glucose oxidation rate at rest, lipid oxidization rate at rest, body-weight increase, fat-mass increase, metabolic rate, percent body fat, body weight, percent overweight, skinfolds
UCP3	12	2	BMI, fat mass, waist-to-hip ratio, respiratory quotient, lean body mass, nonprotein fat oxidation, lean mass, percent body mass, resting energy expenditure, percent body fat, leptin, BMI in morbidly obese subjects, resting metabolic rate, body weight, current and maximum BMI

Abbrreviation: BMI, body mass index. *Source*: From Ref. 1.

Allelic test of association for case-control data				Genotypic test of association for case-control data				

Allele	A	a	Total	Genotype	AA	Aa	aa	Total
Case	N_{1A}	N_{1a}	$2* N_{cave}$	Case	N_{11}	N_{12}	N_{13}	N case
Control	N_{2A}	N_{2a}	$2* N_{control}$	Control	N_{21}	N_{22}	N_{23}	N control
Total	N allele A	N allele a	$2* (N_{cave} + N_{control})$	Total	N_{AA}	N_{Aa}	N_{aa}	N case + N control)

N_{ij} represents the count of alleles of type j found in sample i.

N_{ij} represents the count of individuals having genotype j found in sample i.

FIGURE 1   Difference between allelic and genotypic test.

the phenotype nor be linked to a gene that influences the phenotype. We define such an association as a spurious association.

Although the case-control study is a widely applied strategy for conducting genetic association studies, it is well known that it is susceptible to producing spurious associations due to population substructure. Examples of this confounding effect can be found in Knowler et al. (5) and Campbell et al. (6). In Knowler et al. (5), a negative relationship between type 2 diabetes and a Gm haplotype was found for the Pima and Papago Native American tribes. However, subsequent examination of the study discovered that the sample had recent European admixture and that the controls had higher European ancestry than the cases. Once the sample was stratified according to admixture, the authors concluded that it was most likely the presence European alleles and decrease of Indian alleles, and not the Gm haplotype, which decreased the individuals' susceptibility to type 2 diabetes. To address the issue of confounding due to population substructure, new statistical methods including family-based methods for association testing and estimation of genetic risks have been developed (7).

Family-Based Associations and TDT: Transmission Disequilibrium Test

Family-based tests of association in the presence of linkage (FTALs) (8,9), such as the transmission disequilibrium test (TDT), are one form of a method for dealing with confounding from admixture or population stratification. FTALs are effective at detecting linkage with association in case-control association studies. The TDT, as described by Spielman et al. (8) for binary traits, is a powerful method for detecting linkage between a marker locus and a trait locus in the presence of allelic association. The TDT uses information on the parent-to-offspring transmission status of the associated allele at a marker locus to assess linkage or association in the presence of the other. The key feature of the TDT is that alleles associated with disease have a higher probability of being found to have been transmitted to affected offspring. The TDT was mostly used for dichotomous traits, but Allison (9) extended it to quantitative traits. It is known as a family-based test because heterozygous parents and their affected offspring are required. The TDT approach has since been expanded to include genotypic tests (10,11,12).

A challenge in conducting family-based association tests is the difficulty and expense of recruiting parents and their affected offspring. Furthermore, the test is severely limited when parental data are unavailable. Additionally, if confounding from population stratification is suspected, the TDT will require many more subjects to achieve the level of power of a nonfamily-based association study (13,14). Other forms of family-based tests use siblings or other relatives (15–17).

Genomic Control

Genomic control provides a way to test for population stratification and adjust association tests accordingly. Genomic control was first coined by Devlin and Roeder (18), who noticed that the impact of population stratification on association studies can be quantified by a parameter they denoted λ (a variance inflation factor relative to trend test), which is larger when the degree of population stratification is larger. Under the null hypothesis of no association, but in the presence of population stratification, the Armitage trend test between case and control status and genotype is inflated by a multiplicative factor λ. Devlin and Roeder's genomic control method (18) corrects for spurious associations by applying Armitage's trend test to evaluate the association between genotype and case/control status for each of K randomly selected markers. The resulting vector of K Armitage test statistics is used to compute a correction factor ($\hat{\lambda}$) that is subsequently used to adjust the test statistic for each of the candidate loci. If there is no population stratification, the test statistics examining the association between the unlinked randomly selected genetic markers and the disease of interest will follow a chi-square distribution with one degree of freedom. However, if population stratification is present, then the distribution of test statistics will be inflated by λ as noted above. The solution is to remove the effect of the inflation factor by simply dividing the inflated association test by $\hat{\lambda}$ which is estimated from the randomly selected marker data. However, there is much variability in the estimation of $\hat{\lambda}$ (19). Bacanu et al. (19) provide an adjustment for $\hat{\lambda}$ values below 1. But it should be noted that this adjustment tends to make the adjusted association test more conservative.

Structured Association Tests

Structured association testing (SAT), on the other hand, actually incorporates population structure or stratification information into the association test (20–25). Although there are several forms of SAT, they all typically have two steps. Rather than just estimating a quantified inflation factor $\hat{\lambda}$ based on population structure or stratification, the SAT framework first estimates each individual's admixture proportion (the proportion of an individual's alleles that originated from a specific ancestral population). Once the admixture proportion is estimated for each individual, these estimates are incorporated into the model for the association test. Within the SAT framework, Pritchard and Rosenberg (26) developed a χ^2 test to detect population stratification. The test consists of randomly typing m unlinked markers from a sample of cases and controls. Under the null hypothesis, allele frequencies of each maker will be the same for cases and controls. If the null is rejected, then there is evidence of population stratification. Nevertheless, SAT models heavily rely on the precision of the inferred individual estimates (25,27–34). If the estimates are inaccurate, then the SAT tests may be invalid.

Conditional Conditioning

Under the SAT framework, it may seem reasonable to control for population substructure only after statistical evidence of population substructure is observed (25,35). However, if the goal is to control the overall Type I error rate at a prespecified rate, then this strategy is not valid. Although a covariate may not be statistically significant, the covariate can still be a confounder and not including in the model can lead to confounding (36). Hence, regardless of the significance of individual structure estimates, it should still be included in the SAT model in order to have valid tests of linkage in the presence of association.

MULTISTAGE ASSOCIATION STUDIES

GWA studies can be a powerful alternative to linkage analysis in localizing genetic variants with small contribution to the etiology of a disease. These large-scale studies face two related problems: (a) they require a sizable genotyping effort, which will increase the cost of the study; (b) all markers are to be tested for association with the phenotype of interest, which raises issues related to multiple testing. Several attempts have been made in recent years in order to address these problems. In this section, we discuss several multistage approaches and other methods to control the overall type I error in GWA studies.

The overall cost of a multistage study depends upon the total number of markers genotyped and the total number of individuals sampled. Strategies to maximize power while minimizing costs can be classified in two categories: group sequential methods and stepwise focusing methods.

Sequential and Group Sequential Methods

The sequential test procedures developed initially by Wald (37) were designed to reduce the sampling cost of different type of experiments. Compared to fixed sampling methods, they offer investigators greater control over both the type I error and power. Use of sequential procedures in genetic association studies was discussed by Sobell et al. (38) as a means of type I error control in multiple hypotheses testing settings. They proposed first genotyping all markers only on a subset of the total sample of individuals. Using this group of individuals, Sobell et al. (38) proposed dividing the markers to be tested into three groups on the basis of the P-values corresponding to the tests of association with the phenotype. The first group contains marker that are apparently unrelated to the pheno-type under consideration (i.e. have a P-value greater than some relatively large threshold, τ_L). Markers that are significantly associated with the phenotype (i.e. have a P-value less than some relatively small threshold, τ_S) are placed in the second category. The third group contains all the "ambiguous markers" for which a clear cut decision about the association between the marker and the phenotype could not be made (i.e. $\tau_L > P > \tau_S$). For these markers, more tests are required. More individuals are then genotyped and used as a second independent sample to further test the "ambiguous markers" for association. A third sample of genotyped individuals may be necessary in order to tests markers that remained ambiguous at the end of the second stage of testing.

Group sequential methods constitute an improvement over sequential designs since they do not require the evaluation of the test statistic for each unit of information collected. A group sequential association test works by dividing the overall sample into different subsets of individuals. A test for association between marker and phenotype is then conducted on the first group. The study stops if the test rejects the null hypothesis or shows signs of futility; otherwise the study continues to another stage. Within the second stage, all observations from the first and second stage are used to evaluate the hypothesis. The process continues through several stages until the null hypothesis of no association is either rejected, or it becomes obvious that this hypothesis will never be rejected or finally, when the entire sample is depleted. The key difference between the method of Sobell et al. (38) and group sequential methods is that group sequential methods accumulate information across the different stages of studies while Sobell et al. (38) consider each stage an independent sample and utilize only those observations within that stage to make inference. The gain in efficiency provided by the group sequential designs relative to the Sobell et al. approach (38) has been documented (39–42).

Stepwise Focusing Methods

There are two possible formulations of the stepwise approach to GWA studies. They correspond to the case where the investigator seeks to maximize the power of an association study under a budget constraint that limits the number of markers to be genotyped in the study (37,43). In some other cases, however, it is more important to design studies that achieve a desired power level. The focus in these situations is less about minimizing the genotyping effort than it is about controlling the size of sample to be selected.

The optimum allocation in these situations consists in spending most of the available resource on markers that are more susceptible to be associated with the phenotype under study. For studies that intend to identify only one true gene among a set of unlinked markers, Satagopan et al. (43) recommend using about 75% of the budget at the first stage to select the top 10% of markers more likely to be associated with the phenotype of interest. This ratio varies slightly however when the study is conducted using linked markers. For mildly correlated markers, use of about 25% of markers at the first stage and 75% of the available resource at the second stage is suggested to follow up the top 10% of markers. This rule-of-thumb also yields near optimal power when the objective is to identify a small number of genes from a very large pool of markers. It has been shown (43–45) that in this case, two-stage associations study can reduce the cost of a one-stage study by as much as 50%.

The two-stage design can also be optimal when the objective is to identify not just a subset of markers but specific haplotype groups associated with a specific phenotype (46). Other multistage approaches focus more on controlling the overall type I error rate. Measures like the false discovery rate (FDR) or the false-positive report probability (FPRP) are used to control the number of markers selected for further analysis at end of each stage. It has been shown that a *k*-stage selection procedure that uses high FDR at the first *k-1* stages and a stringent FDR at the last stage may result in a 50% to 70% reduction in genotyping cost (47). The FPRP produces weaker control than the family wise error rate (FWER) used in methods described in (43–45). In general, it can be shown that the designs that control for the FPRP are in general more powerful than those that use FWER to determine the number of markers that make it from one stage to another (48).

This improvement comes with the added cost that the number of false positives may be higher than what is observed with the methods that use FWER.

There have been very few studies that compared the efficiency of the group sequential methods to that of the stepwise focusing methods. However, the sequential methods offer the possibility to stop the study early when there is clear evidence to suggest which decision is more likely given the fraction of the data observed. Further research into this area is warranted.

OBESITY AND EPISTASIS

Epistasis or interaction among genes at different loci is a basic concept in genetics which can be traced back to Bateson (49) and Fisher (50). A common approach for exploring epistasis is to first search for loci which have moderate to large effects and then examine possible interactions among all such loci. However, interactions with small effect loci would be missed in this approach, and such interactions among loci of small effect could be the rule rather than exception for complex traits such as obesity (51). On the other hand, testing all possible interactions in GWA scans with thousands of SNP markers will lead to large number of tests, a situation referred to as the "curse of dimensionality" (52). Numerous methods have been proposed to resolve the issue of dimensionality and reduce the computational burden. Two methods have emerged, namely; multifactor dimensional reduction by Ritchie et al. (53) and recursive partitioning method by Culverhouse et al. (54). These methods are promising although, to our knowledge, they have not been applied to obesity data. Some authors have recommended using data-mining and neural networks (55,56) to overcome dimensionality problems. These methods to detect epistasis do not require a pre-specified statistical hypothesis, and in this respect are better suited to search for trends or patterns in high dimensional data sets. However, data-mining methods are prone to chance patterns in the data and may thereby result in false positives. Furthermore, models of neural networks are difficult to interpret and the results are not intuitive (57). Although the methodological issues in association and disequilibrium mapping of epistatic genes influencing obesity remain largely unresolved, there are substantial efforts directed in this direction.

ATTRIBUTABLE RISK: CALCULATION AND INTERPRETATION

Attributable risk (AR) can be defined as the excess risk of disease or condition for an individual with a risk factor relative to an individual without that risk factor, that is, the risk difference between individuals exposed to a risk factor and individuals not exposed to a risk factor. The rationale behind attributable risk calculations is to provide an alternative to simple relative risk measures in order to describe the rates in absolute terms instead of relative (58). In the context of this chapter, the risk factor can be a genetic factor (possibly an allele, a genotype, a haplotype, etc.) and the "disease" can be obesity or an obesity-related condition (e.g. diabetes). To illustrate the calculation, define the following four parameters:

- π_{11}, the probability of exposure and disease
- π_{12}, the probability of exposure and no disease
- π_{21}, the probability of no exposure and disease
- π_{22}, the probability of no exposure and no disease

The conditional probability of disease given exposure is $\varphi_1 = \pi_{11}/(\pi_{11} + \pi_{12})$ and the conditional probability of disease given no exposure is $\varphi_2 = \pi_{21}/(\pi_{21} + \pi_{22})$. MacMahon and Pugh (59) define AR $= \varphi_1 - \varphi_2$ which yields an expected $n(\varphi_1 - \varphi_2)$ excess cases among n exposures. The proportion of disease attributable to n exposures is calculated $\gamma = n(\varphi_1 - \varphi_2/n(\varphi_1) = (\varphi_1 - \varphi_2)/\varphi_1$ which can be also expressed as $\gamma = (\psi - 1)/\psi$ where $\psi = \varphi_1/\varphi_2$ is the relative risk of the exposed exhibiting disease compared to the nonexposed. The proportion of all cases attributable to the risk factor is typically of greatest public health interest (60). To achieve the estimate of the proportion of all cases attributable to the risk factor, define $\theta = \pi_{11} + \pi_{12}$ to be the prevalence of risk exposure. Levine (61) defined the proportion of all cases attributable to the risk factor as $\lambda = \theta(\psi - 1)/(\theta(\psi - 1) + 1)$. This statistic is also referred to as the population attributable fraction.

As with all investigations of risk factors, the design of the study must be considered. The risk ratio is directly estimable using prospective designs, however in a retrospective trails, where individuals are selected based upon disease states, odds ratios would be substituted for relative risks (58). Within genetic studies of complex phenotypes such as obesity, it is anticipated the attributable risks due to specific alleles or genotypes will be small given the multifactor nature of the trait. Other formulas and approaches are required to calculate population attributable fractions after adjusting for other risk factors. Regarding these approaches, the reader is referred to Benichou (62) and Walter (63). Finally, all the attributable risk estimates are simply descriptive estimates and we recommend reporting the 95% confidence intervals of these estimates (64). Table 2 presents estimated attributable risks from selected publications investigating the genetics of obesity and its related phenotypes (Table 2).

LACK OF REPLICATION

Lack of replication and contradictory results are two of the major concerns with association studies (65,66). Several of the genes identified in Rankinen et al. (1) which indicated association between obesity or obesity-related phenotypes were not consistently replicated in follow-up studies. Several reasons have been proposed to account for the lack of reproducibility. These include population heterogeneity (genetic stratification and environmental diversity), publication bias, epistasis, imprecise phenotypic measures, lack of type I error control and lack of statistical power to detect small effects (65).

Often, the argument is presented that failure to replicate may be due to the fact that the initial finding is in fact either a type I error (false positive result) or a spurious association attributed to population stratification. Inadequate adjustment for multiple hypothesis tests increases the probability of at least one type I error which may lead to numerous false positive results being published. Some debate exists as to whether population stratification is a likely cause of nonreplication. Some investigators have pointed out that although population stratification is the most common explanation given for spurious associations, there are few actual examples to support this assumption indicating the problem may be over emphasized (7). Other reasons for nonreplication may be over interpretation of marginal findings and under emphasis of publication bias for positive results, which is difficult to quantify.

TABLE 2 Selected Published Studies That Have Reported Attributable Risk Due to Genes/
Polymorphisms in Obesity Research

Reference	Gene and poly-morphism studied	Number of subjects	Phenotype	Estimated attributable risk
Bulotta et al. (67)	UCP2 866G/A polymorphism	746 Type II diabetics and 327 healthy controls	Type II diabetes	12%
Wernstedt et al. (68)	*IL6 174* G/C polymorphism	485 hypertensive individuals	Overweight	12%, 95% CI (2%, 21%)
Esterbauer et al. (69)	*UCP2* 866G/A	340 obese and 256 never obese individuals	Obesity	15%
Clement et al. (70)	*UCP2* 3826 G/A	238 obese and 91 nonobese individuals	Obesity	25%
Clement et al. (70)	*ADRB3* TPR64Arg	238 obese and 91 nonobese individuals	Obesity	9%

Abbrreviation: BMI, body mass index. *Source*: From Ref. 1.

Two other issues likely affecting the observed nonreplication of association studies is possibly low statistical power within some of the follow-up studies as well as population heterogeneity. If replication of a genetic finding is attempted in a readily available sample from a study of a different phenotype or marker, the replication study may have insufficient power due to numerous reasons including the variance of the phenotype or the magnitude of the effect size associated with the marker. If gene by environment interactions are occurring, then the fact that separate populations are investigated in nonidentical environments would explain variability in results.

Finally, consideration must be given to what defines "consistent" replication. Should replication be defined as observing statistically significant results in the same direction or observing biologically relevant results in the same direction across numerous studies? Addressing these issues, as well as adopting standard ascertainment criteria for obesity phenotypes may increase the replication of association studies (3).

META-ANALYSIS

Obesity is a somewhat unique trait in that its most commonly used anthropometric indicators (e.g. body mass index (BMI) in humans) and their "rodentometric" counterparts are easily and commonly measured by most biomedical researchers even if these researchers are not primarily obesity researchers. Perhaps for that reason, there have been many studies of obesity genetics. As these studies accumulate, the opportunity to try and seek greater power, precision, and clarity via meta-analysis comes to the fore. Here, we use the term "meta-analysis" broadly to refer to any activity that utilizes the data (whether raw data or published summary statistics) from two or more studies in a formal and quantitative manner to estimate quantities and/or test hypotheses.

Meta-analysis can be used to seek clarity when there are many studies that upon narrative review seem to give an equivocal answer about a particular question (e.g. whether a particular gene is associated with a particular phenotype). More and more, investigators are taking this approach with the report of a single study of the association of a polymorphism with a phenotype as a way of putting their latest result in the context of the existing research [e.g. Table 3, (71)]. Meta-analysis can also be used to refine estimates of an effect or

(Text continues on page 242.)

TABLE 3 Published Studies That Have Meta-Analyzed Genetic Findings in Obesity Research

Reference	Gene and polymorphism studied	Linkage or association	Number of studies	Number of subjects	Main finding	Comment
Sookoian et al. 2005 (89)	Tumor necrosis factor (*TNFA*) G-308A	Association	8 obesity, 16 BMI, 13 waist-to-hip ratio, 4 leptin	Obesity 2289; whites 41–60 y.o.; BMI 4647 Caucasian, Brazilian and Chinese	Association with obesity only significant in whites ages, 41–60; D = 1.32, 95% CI 1.09–1.63; *P* = 0.005 BMI significantly associated with D = 0.074, 95%CI 0.005–0.142; *P* = 0.034 no association with leptin or waist-to-hip ratio	
Swarbrick et al. 2005 (71)	Glutamate decorboxylase 2 (*GAD2*): -243 A > G, +61450 C > A, and +83897 T>A	Association	3	1252 cases; 1800, controls French, U.S. and Canadian	No association of -243G with Class III obesity (OR 1.11, 95% CI 0.90–1.36; *P* = 0.28)	
Paracchini et al. 2005 (90)	Leptin (*LEP*)A19G, leptin receptor (*LEPR* Q223R), Peroxisome proliferators-activated receptor gamma (*PPARG* P12A and C161T)	Association	1- *LEP* A19G 10- *LEPR* Q223R 7- *LEPR* K109R 7- *LEPR* K656N 6- *PPARG* P12A	Case/control *LEP* A19G- 141/65 *LEPR* Q223R-1430/1542 *LEPR* K109R-876/820 *LEPR* K656N-1147/917 *PPARG* P12A- 1622/2400	No association was seen with BMI (*LEPR* Q223R and *LEPR* K656N) or obesity (*LEP* A19G, *LEPR* K109R or *PPARG* P12A) in the mixed populations studied	
Johnson et al. 2005 (91)	NA	Linkage (genome wide)	13	2814 individuals (505 families)	Linkage of quantitative phenotype BMI to 8p (*P* < 0.0005)	

(Continued)

TABLE 3 Published Studies That Have Meta-Analyzed Genetic Findings in Obesity Research (*Continued*)

Reference	Gene and polymorphism studied	Linkage or association	Number of studies	Number of subjects	Main finding	Comment
Geller et al. 2004 (92)	Melanocortin 4 receptor (*MC4R*) V103I	Association	14	7713 individuals, mainly European origin	Negative association of *MC4R* V103I allele with obesity (OR 0.69; 95% CI 0.5–0.9, P = 0.03)	
Masud et al. 2003 (93)	Peroxisome proliferators activated receptor gamma (*PPARG*) Pro12Ala	Association	30	19136	Obese individuals only Ala12 carriers BMI 0.11d units (95% CI 0.05–0.18) higher than non-carriers (n = 2060/6305, P = 0.0006)	Pro12Ala may be genetic modifier of obesity
Heo et al. 2002 Heo et al. 2001 (94,95)	Leptin receptor (*LEPR*) K109R, Q223R and K656N	Association	9	3263 African American, Caucasian, Danish, Finish, French and Nigerian	No association with BMI or waist circumference at the 0.05 level in the overall population	
Wu et al. 2002 (96)	NA	Linkage (genome wide)	6849	6849 Caucasian, African American, Mexican American, and Asian	Linkage with BMI: 3q22.1 (LOD 3.45 in GENOA African American cohort) LOD > 2 3p24.1, 7p15.2, 7q22.3, 12q24.3, 16q12.2, and 17p11.2 in all populations using allele-sharing IBD (pi) for Caucasian, African Americans, and Mexican Americans, strong linkage at 3q27 (LOD 3.40, P = 0.03) linkage previously reported elsewhere	

Reference	Gene/region	Method		Sample	Result	Notes
Kurokawa et al. 2001 (97)	Beta3- adrenergic receptor gene (ADRB3) Trp64Arg	Association	22	2316 case 4266 controls Japanese	Mean difference in BMI cases and controls 0.26 kg/m(2), 95% CI 0.18–0.42, $P < 0.01$	No evidence for effect heterogeneity ($\chi^2 = 38.68$, df35, $P = 0.31$)
Allison et al. 1998 (98)	Beta3- adrenergic receptor gene (ADRB3) Trp64Arg	Association	27	7399	No significant association of AERB3 Trp64Arg with BMI weighted mean BMI difference Trp/Trp and Trp/Arg was 0.19 (s.e. = 0.11 $P = 0.07$)	
Fujisawa et al. 1998 (99)	Beta3-androgenic receptor (ADRB3) Trp64Arg	Association	31	2447 Trp64Arg 6789 Trp46Trp	Weighted mean difference in BMI between cases and controls was 0.30 (95% CI 0.13–0.47) indicating that Trp64Arg carriers exhibited higher BMI (on average 0.30 kg/m² higher)	
Allison and Heo 1998 (100)	LEP gene region	Linkage	5	1387	Evidence for linkage somewhere in OB gene region is extremely strong ($P = 1.5 \times 10^{-5}$)	
Keightley and Knott 1999 (101)	NA	Linkage	3	1803 F2 mice	No evidence of correlation between the position of previously mapped QTLs in any pair of experiments	

Abbreviations: CI, confidence interval; IBD, identical by descent; NA, Not applicable; OR, odds ratio; QTL, quantitative trait loci.

association. For example, three different meta-analyses have examined the association between the TRP64ARG polymorphism of the *ADRB3* (Table 3). Although they have differed with respect to their conclusions about statistical significance depending on the amount of data available and the population studied, the consistency of the point estimates of the association magnitude is remarkable. All three place the estimated mean BMI difference between carriers and non-carriers of this polymorphism between 0.19 and 0.30 BMI units which, for an average height US adult (~1.73 m) corresponds to a weight difference of between 0.57 and 0.89 kg.

Meta-analytic techniques for studying associations between specific polymorphisms and phenotypes are well-established and simple extensions of existing meta-analytic methodology. In contrast, methods for integrating linkage studies exist (72–87), but are in their infancy and require much further development. Finally methods for integrating quantitative trait loci (QTL) linkage studies across different experimental crosses (e.g. 81) let alone different species (88) are even less well developed and this is a critical topic for further methodologic research.

CONCLUSION

This chapter presented a brief overview of the ongoing research and the current approaches, techniques, and challenges in genetic research of obesity and obesity-related phenotypes. Research regarding these methodologic challenges is required for the continued advance of obesity-related genetics research.

REFERENCES

1. Rankinen T, Zuberi A, Chagnon YC, et al. The human obesity gene map: the 2005 update. Obesity (Silver Spring) 2006; 14(4):529–644.
2. Marti A, Moreno-Aliaga MJ, Hebebrand J, et al. Genes, lifestyles and obesity. Int J Obesity 2004; 28:S29–36.
3. Bell CG, Walley AJ, Froguel P. The genetics of human obesity. Nat Rev Genet 2005; 6:221–234.
4. Sasieni PD. From genotypes to genes: doubling the sample size. Biometrics 1997; 53:1253–61.
5. Knowler WC, Williams RC, Pettitt DJ, et al. Gm3-5,13,14 and Type-2 Diabetes-Mellitus—An association in American-Indians with genetic admixture. Am J Hum Genet 1988; 43:520–6.
6. Campbell C, Ogburn EL, Lunetta KL, et al. Demonstrating stratification in a European American population. Nat Genet 2005; 37:868–72.
7. Cardon LR, Bell IJ. Association studies design for complex diseases. Nat Genet 2002; 2:91.
8. Spielman RS., McGinnis RE, Ewens WJ. Transmission test for linkage disequilibrium: the insulin gene region and insulin-dependent diabetes mellitus (IDDM). Am J Hum Genet 1993; 52:506–16.
9. Allison DB. Transmission-disequilibrium tests for quantitative traits. Am J Hum Genet 1997; 60:676–90.
10. Schaid DJ, Sommer SS. Genotype relative risks: methods for design and analysis of candidate-gene association studies. Am J Hum Genet 1993; 53:1114–26.
11. Fallin D, Beaty T, Liang KY, et al. Power comparisons for genotypic vs. allelic TDT methods with >2 alleles. Genet Epidemiol 2002; 23:458–61.
12. Schaid DJ. Power comparisons for genotypic vs. allelic TDT methods with >2 alleles—Reply to Fallin et al. Genet Epidemiol 2002; 23:462–4.

13. Witte JS, Gauderman WJ, Thomas DC. Asymptotic bias and efficiency in case-control studies of candidate genes and gene-environment interactions: basic family designs. Am J Epidemiol 1999; 149:693–705.
14. McGinnis R, Shifman S, Darvasi A. Power and efficiency of the TDT and case-control design for association scans. Behav Genet 2002; 32:135–44.
15. Boehnke M, Langefeld CD. Genetic association mapping based on discordant sib pairs: the discordant-alleles test. Am J Hum Genet 1998; 62:950–61.
16. Lazzeroni LC, Lange K. A conditional inference framework for extending the transmission/disequilibrium test. Hum Hered 1998; 48:67–81.
17. Spielman RS, Ewens WJ. A sibship test for linkage in the presence of association: the sib transmission/disequilibrium test. Am J Hum Genet 1998; 62:450–8.
18. Devlin B, Roeder K. Genomic control for association studies. Biometrics 1999; 55(4):997–1004.
19. Bacanu SA, Devlin B, Roeder K. The power of genomic control. A J Hum Genet 2000; 66:1933–44.
20. Pritchard JK, Donnelly P. Case-control studies of association in structured or admixed populations. Theor Popul Biol 2001; 60:227–37.
21. Satten GA, Flanders WD, Yang Q. Accounting for unmeasured population substructure in case-control studies of genetic association using a novel latent-class model. Am J Hum Genet 2001; 68:466–77.
22. Chen HS, Zhu X, Zhao H et al. Qualitative semi-parametric test for genetic associations in case-control designs under structured populations. Ann Hum Genet 2003; 67:250–64.
23. Purcell S. Sample selection and complex effects in quantitative trait loci analysis. Dissertation, University of London, 2003.
24. Zhang SL, Zhu XF, Zhao HY. On a semiparametric test to detect associations between quantitative traits and candidate genes using unrelated individuals. Genet Epidemiol 2003; 24:44–56.
25. Hoggart CJ, Parra EJ, Shriver MD, et al. Control of confounding of genetic associations in stratified populations. Am J Hum Genet 2003; 72:1492–504.
26. Pritchard JK, Rosenberg NA. Use of unlinked genetic markers to detect population stratification in association studies. Am J Hum Genet 1999; 65:220–8.
27. Falush D, Stephens M, Pritchard JK. Inference of population structure using multilocus genotype data: linked loci and correlated allele frequencies. Genetics 2003; 164:1567–87.
28. Hoggart CJ, Shriver MD, Kittles RA, et al. Design and analysis of admixture mapping studies. Am J Hum Genet 2004; 74:965–78.
29. Montana G, Pritchard JK. Statistical tests for admixture mapping with case-control and cases-only data. Am J Hum Genet 2004; 75:771–89.
30. Patterson N, Hattangadi N, Lane B, et al. Methods for high-density admixture mapping of disease genes. Am J Hum Genet 2004; 74:979–1000.
31. Purcell S, Sham P. Properties of structured association approaches to detecting population stratification. Hum Hered 2004; 58:93–107.
32. Tang H, Peng J, Wang P, et al. Estimation of individual admixture: analytical and study design considerations. Genet Epidemiol 2005; 28:289–301.
33. Zhang C, Chen K, Seldin MF, et al. A hidden Markov modeling approach for admixture mapping based on case-control data. Genet Epidemiol 2004; 27:225–39.
34. Zhu XF, Cooper RS, Elston RC. Linkage analysis of a complex disease through use of admixed populations. Am J Hum Genet 2004; 74:1136–53.
35. Pritchard JK, Stephens M, Rosenberg NA, et al. Association mapping in structured populations. Am J Hum Genet 2000; 67:170–81.
36. Mickey RM, Greenland S. The impact of confounder selection criteria on effect estimation. Am J Epidemiol 1989; 129:125–37.
37. Wald A. Sequential Analysis. New York: John Wiley and Sons, 1947.
38. Sobell JL, Heston LL, Sommer SS. Novel association approach for determining the genetic predisposition to schizophrenia: case-control resource and testing of a candidate gene. Am J Med Genet 1993; 48:28–35.

39. Pampallona S, Tsiatis AA. Group sequential designs for one-sided and two-sided hypothesis testing with provision for early stopping in favor of the null hypothesis. J Stat Plan Inference 1994; 42:19–35.

40. O'Brien PC, Fleming TR. A multiple testing procedure for clinical trails. Biometrics 1979; 35:549–56.

41. Jennison C, Turnbull BW. Group Sequential Methods with Applications to Clinical Trials. Boca Raton: CRC Press, 2006.

42. Pocock SJ. Group sequential methods in the design and analysis of clinical trials. Biometrics 1977; 64(2):191–9.

43. Satagopan JM, Verbel DA, Venkatraman ES, Offit KE, Begg CB. Two-stage designs for gene-disease association studies. Biometrics 2002; 58:163–70.

44. Satagopan JM, Elston RC. Optimal two-stage genotyping in population-based association studies. Genet Epidemiol 2003; 25:49–157.

45. Elston RC, Guo XQ, Williams LV. Two-stage global search designs for linkage analysis using pairs of affected relatives. Genet Epidemiol 1996; 13:535–58.

46. Thomas D, Xie RR, Gebregziabher M. Two-stage sampling designs for gene association studies. Genet Epidemiol 2004; 27:401–14.

47. van den Oord EJCG, Sullivan PF. A framework for controlling false discovery rates and minimizing the amount of genotyping in the search for disease mutations. Hum Hered 2003; 56:188–99.

48. Kraft P. Efficient two-stage genome-wide association designs based on false positive report probabilities. Pacific Symposium on Biocomputing 11:523–34.

49. Bateson W. Facts limiting the theory of heredity. Science 1907; 26:649.

50. Fisher RA. The correlation between relatives on the supposition of Mendelian inheritance. Trans R Soc Edinb 1918; 52:399.

51. Frankel WN, Schork NJ. Who's afraid of epistasis? Nat Genet 1996; 14:371–3.

52. R. Bellman. Adaptive Control Processes: A Guided Tour. Princeton, NJ: Princeton University Press, 1961.

53. Ritchie MD, Hahn LW, Roodi N, et al. Multifactor-dimensionality reduction reveals high-order interactions among estrogen-metabolism genes in sporadic breast cancer. Am J Hum Genet 2001; 69:138.

54. Culverhouse R, Klein T, Shannon W. Detecting epistatic interactions contributing to quantitative traits. Genet Epidemiol 2004; 27:141.

55. Hoh J, Ott J. Mathematical multi-locus approaches to localizing complex human trait genes: statistical analysis methods for gene mapping originated. Nat Genet Rev 2003; 4:701.

56. Moore JH, Ritchie MD. The challenges of whole-genome approaches to common diseases. JAMA 2004; 291:1642.

57. Wu CH, McLarty JW. Neural Networks and Genome Informatics. New York, NY: Elsevier Science.

58. Walter SD. The estimation and interpretation of attributable risk in health research. Biometrics 1976; 32(4):829–49.

59. MacMahon B, Pugh TF. Epidemiology: Principle and Methods. Boston: Little Brown and Co., 1970.

60. Walter SD. The distribution of Levin's measure of attributable risk. Biometrika 1975; 62:371–5.

61. Levin ML. The occurrence of lung cancer in man. Acta Unio International Vontra Cancrum 1953; 19:531–41.

62. Benichou J. A review of adjusted estimators of attributable risk. Stat Methods Med Res 2001; 10:195–216.

63. Walter SD. Effect of interaction, confounding, and observational error on attributable risk estimation. Am J Epidemiol 1983; 117:598–604.

64. Benichou J, Gail MH. Variance calculations and confidence intervals for estimates of attributable risk based on logistic models. Biometrics 1990; 46:991–1003.

65. Redden DT, Allison DB. Non-replication in genetic association studies of obesity and diabetes research. J Nutr 2003; 133(11):3323–6.

66. Lyon H, Hirschorn J. Genetics of common forms of obesity: a brief overview. Am J Clin Nutr 2005; 82:215S–7S.

67. Bulotta A, Ludovico O, Coca A, et al. The common -866G/A polymorphism in the promoter region of the UCP-2 gene is associated with reduced risk of type 2 diabetes in Caucasians from Italy. J Clin Endocrinol Metab 2005; 90(2):1176–80.

68. Wernstedt I, Eriksson AL, Berndtsson A, et al. A common polymorphism in the interleukin-6 gene promoter is associated with overweight. Int J Obes Relat Metab Disord 2004; 28(10):272–9.

69. Esterbauer H, Schneitler C, Oberkofler H, et al. A common polymorphism in the promoter of UCP2 is associated with decreased risk of obesity in middle-aged humans. Nat Genet 2001; 28(2):78–83.

70. Clement K, Ruiz J, Cassard-Doulcier AM, Bouillaud F, et al. Additive effect of A–>G (-3826) variant of the uncoupling protein gene and the Trp64Arg mutation of the beta 3-adrenergic receptor gene on weight gain in morbid obesity. Int J Obes Relat Metab Disord 1996; 20(12):1062–6.

71. Swarbrick MM, Waldenmaier B, Pennacchio LA, et al. Lack of support for the association between GAD2 polymorphisms and severe human obesity. Plos Biol 2005; 3:1662–71.

72. Dempfle A, Loesgen S. Meta-analysis of linkage studies for complex diseases: an overview of methods and a simulation study. Ann Hum Genet 2004; 68:69–83.

73. Etzel CJ, Guerra R. Meta-analysis of genetic-linkage analysis of quantitative-trait loci. Am J Hum Genet 2002; 71:56–65.

74. Goffinet B, Gerber S. Quantitative trait loci: a meta-analysis. Genetics 2000; 155: 463–73.

75. Gu C, Province M, Todorov A, et al. Meta-analysis methodology for combining non-parametric sibpair linkage results: genetic homogeneity and identical markers. Genet Epidemiol 1998; 15:609–26.

76. Gu C, Province M, Rao DC. Meta-analysis of genetic linkage to quantitative trait loci with study-specific covariates: a mixed-effects model. Genet Epidemiol 1999; 17: S599–604.

77. Gu C, Province MA, Rao DC. Meta-analysis for model-free methods. Genetic Dissection of Complex Traits 2001; 42:255–72.

78. Guerra R, Etzel CJ, Goldstein DR, et al. Meta-analysis by combining p-values, Simulated linkage studies. Genet Epidemiol 1999; 17:S605–9.

79. Koziol JA, Feng AC. A note on the genome scan meta-analysis statistic. Ann Hum Genet 2004; 68:376–380.

80. Koziol JA, Feng AC. A note on generalized genome scan meta-analysis statistics. BMC Bioinformatics 2006; 6:32.

81. Li ZH, Rao DC. Random effects model for meta-analysis of multiple quantitative sibpair linkage studies. Genet Epidemiol 1996; 13:377–83.

82. Pardi F, Levinson DF, Lewis CM. Genome scan meta-analysis (GSMA), software implementation of the genome search meta-analysis method. Bioinformatics 2005; 21:4430–1.

83. Wise LH, Lanchbury JS, Lewis CN. Meta-analysis of genome searches. Ann Hum Genet 1999; 63:263–72.

84. Wise LH, Lewis CM. A method for meta-analysis of genome searches: application to simulated data. Genet Epidemiol 1999; 17:S767–71.

85. Zintzaras E, Ioannidis JPA. Heterogeneity testing in meta-analysis of genome searches. Genet Epidemiol 2005; 28:123–37.

86. Zintzaras E, Ioannidis JPA. HEGESMA, genome search meta-analysis and heterogeneity testing. Bioinformatics 2005; 21:3672–3.

87. Cooper M, Goldstein T, Maher B, et al. Identifying genomic regions for fine-mapping using genome scan meta-analysis (GSMA) to identify the minimum regions of maximum significance (MRMS) across populations. BMC Genetics 2005; 6:S42.

88. Serrano-Fernandez P, Ibrahim SM, Koczan D, et al. In silico fine-mapping, narrowing disease-associated loci by intergenomics. Bioinformatics 2005; 21:1737–8.

89. Sookoian SC, Gonzalez C, Pirola CJ. Meta-analysis on the G-308A tumor necrosis factor alpha gene variant and phenotypes associated with the metabolic syndrome. Obes Res 2005; 13:2122–31.

90. Paracchini V, Pedotti P, Taioli E. Genetics of leptin and obesity: a HuGE review. Am J Epidemiol 2005; 162:101–14.

91. Johnson L, Luke A, Deng HW, et al. Meta-analysis of five genome-wide linkage studies for body mass index reveals significant evidence for linkage to chromosome 8p. Int J Obes 2005; 29:413–9.

92. Geller F, Reichwald K, Dempfle A, et al. Melanocortin-4 receptor gene variant I103 is negatively associated with obesity. Am J Hum Genet 2004; 74:572–81.

93. Masud S, Ye S. Effect of the peroxisome proliferator activated receptor-{gamma} gene Pro12Ala variant on body mass index, a meta-analysis. J Med Genet 2003; 40:773–80.

94. Heo M, Leibel RL, Fontaine KR, et al. A meta-analytic investigation of linkage and association of common leptin receptor (*LEPR*) polymorphisms with body mass index and waist circumference. Int J Obes 2002; 26:640–6.

95. Heo M, Leibel RL, Boyer BB, et al. Pooling analysis of genetic data: the association of leptin receptor (*LEPR*) polymorphisms with variables related to human adiposity. Genetics 2001; 159:1163–78.

96. Wu XD, Cooper RS, Borecki I, et al. A combined analysis of genomewide linkage scans for body mass index, from the National Heart, Lung, and Blood Institute Family Blood Pressure Program. Am J Hum Genet 2002; 70:1247–56.

97. Kurokawa N, Nakai K, Kameo S, et al. Association of BMI with the beta 3-adrenergic receptor gene polymorphism in Japanese: meta-analysis. Obes Res 2001; 9:741–5.

98. Allison DB, Heo M, Faith MS, et al. Meta-analysis of the association of the Trp64Arg polymorphism in the beta(3) adrenergic receptor with body mass index. Int J Obes 1998; 22:559–66.

99. Fujisawa T, Ikegami H, Kawaguchi Y, et al. Meta-analysis of the association of Trp(64)Arg polymorphism of beta(3)-adrenergic receptor gene with body mass index. J Clin Endocrinol Metabol 1998; 83:2441–4.

100. Allison DB, Heo M. Meta-analysis of linkage data under worst-case conditions: a demonstration using the human OB region. Genetics 1998; 148:859–65.

101. Keightley PD, Knott SA. Testing the correspondence between map positions of quantitative trait loci. Genet Res 1999; 74:323–8.

6.2 Genome-Wide Approaches

Jorg Hager and Elke Roschman
IntegraGen SA, Evry, France

David Mutch
INSERM, U872, Nutriomique, Centre de Recherche des Cordeliers, Université Pierre et Marie Curie-Paris6, Paris, France

Karine Clément
INSERM, U872, Nutriomique, Centre de Recherche des Cordeliers, Université Pierre et Marie Curie-Paris6, UMRS 872, Université Paris Descartes, Assistance Publique Hôpitaux de Paris, AP-HP, and Department of Endocrinology and Nutrition, Pitié-Salpêtrière Hospital, Paris, France

GENOME-WIDE SCANS FOR HUMAN OBESITY

The identification of genes for complex human disease, such as obesity, has proved to be a challenge with so far limited success. Genetic studies using microsatellite markers have successfully identified genes for monogenic diseases, especially obesity syndrome like Bardet-Biedl diseases as described in Section 5, but have been notably poor in identifying genes for common obesity forms or obesity related complex traits. The genome-wide resolution that can be reasonably achieved using microsatellites is relatively low ranging between 10 centiMorgans and 5 centiMorgans. Higher resolutions can be achieved using high density single-nucleotide-polymorphism (SNP) chips for linkage mapping (1,2). To widely explore the genome of obese subjects, large DNA banks have been constituted in different populations through out the world: individuals and families with extreme obesity occurring during adulthood or childhood (European and American studies), cohorts issued from the general population (Quebec family study), and in particular groups (Pima Indians, Mexican Americans, African Americans and Amish) (3). Recently a population from the Pacific Island of Kosrae was also explored (4). The genome-wide scan task is performed without pre-conceptions about the functions of the genes and aims to identify known or unknown genes pre-disposing to obesity. Then molecular tools enable the newly identified genes to be positioned and eventually cloned. It is sometimes arduous to find the exact causative gene when genomic linked regions encompass thousand of bases and sometimes hundred of genes. The results of these genetic studies are reported each year in the international journal "Obesity Research" (4). The global picture of chromosomal regions linked to obesity illustrates the complexity of this multifactorial disease. At least, sixty-one genome-wide scans have been conducted and more than 250 regions, located on nearly all the chromosomes as shown on Figure 1, have been linked to different obesity related phenotypes such as fat mass, the distribution of adipose tissue, the occurrence of a metabolic syndrome, resting energy expenditure, energy and macronutrient intake, weight variation, the levels of circulating leptin, and insulin among other phenotypes (all references in (4). Some loci may be more specific for morbid obesity or childhood obesity (5,6) as detailed in Chapter 6.3. Interactions between chromosomal regions such as on chromosome 10 and 20 and

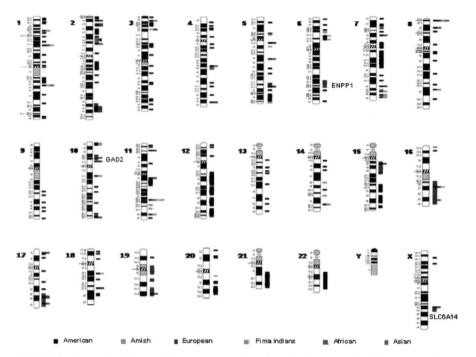

FIGURE 1 (*See color insert.*) Chromosomal regions linked with obesity in different populations. This figure illustrates the panel of chromosomal regions linked with obesity in different family studies. Linkage studies have been performed in different populations from Europe (blue blocks), North America (black blocks), Asia (pink blocks) as well as from Amish (green), Pima Indians (yellow blocks), and African Americans (red blocks). This map is built from information provided by the 2005 human obesity gene map (3).

between chromosome 13 and 2 (i.e. epistasis) were also shown. These regions may interact to influence extreme obesity (7,8). Candidate genes were also found in these regions linked with obesity phenotypes.

CANDIDATES DERIVED FROM THE GENOME-WIDE LINKAGE STUDIES IN CAUCASIANS

In the chromosomal regions linked with obesity phenotypes, associations between obesity and SNPs spanning candidate genes were sometimes found. SNPs spanning genes encoding SLC6A14 (solute carrier family 6 [neurotransmitter transporter], member 14) on chromosome X (9), the glutamic acid decarboxylase enzyme (GAD65) or GAD2 on chromosome 10 (10) and the ecto-nucleotide pyrophosphatase/phosphodiesterase 1 gene (ENPP1/PC-1). *ENPP1* on chromosome 6 were notably described (6).

SLC6A14 gene codes for an amino acid transporter able to regulate the availability of tryptophane during the synthesis of serotonin and may affect the regulation of the appetite and mood. The genetic association with the *SLC6A14* gene was replicated in an independent French population (11).

ENPP1 gene on chromosome 6q16.3 was first considered as a candidate gene for type-2 diabetes (12) but is located at a locus linked with both childhood and adult obesity and diabetes (6). A meta-analysis revealed that a common mutation K121Q is associated with type 2 diabetes but not clearly linked with obesity (13). Association studies in French Caucasians revealed a three-allele risk haplotype for these metabolic diseases. The results are detailed in Chapter 6.3. The physiological role of *ENPP1* is a matter of debate since *ENPP1* may inhibit the insulin receptor by interacting with a specific region in the α-subunit. The expression levels of *ENPP1* gene are increased in muscle and adipose tissue of insulin-resistant subjects. The role of K21Q change in *ENPP1* gene, associated with type 2 diabetes, might be mediated by a functional change induced in insulin signaling transduction from the α- to the β-subunit of the insulin receptor. The *ENPP1* haplotype associates with increased serum levels of soluble *ENPP1* protein in French children. It has been proposed that *ENPP1* variants contribute to establishing an individual's susceptibility to insulin resistance and the development of both obesity and diabetes. This study has provided clues for underlying common molecular mechanism to both conditions (6).

GAD2, the third gene derived from genome-wide scan approach encodes the 65 kDa subunit of the GAD65 which catalyzes the formation of gamma-aminobutyric acid (GABA) which can then interact with neuropeptide Y in the hypothalamus to stimulate food intake. Three SNPs showed an association with morbid obesity. A protective effect was attributed to the wild-type allele. A functional study found that the allele most frequently found in obese subjects exhibits greater transcriptional activity than the wild allele. This could result in an increase in hypothalamic GABA and a subsequent increase of food intake (10).

REPLICATION ISSUES

One of the greatest obstacles hindering progress is the issue of replication as described in Chapter 6.1. The results regarding the three main candidates found by the genome-wide scan approach illustrate the difficulty of confirming positive or linkage genetic studies in human population. For GAD2 independent replication could not be achieved in a large German population (14) and in obese population from Utah (15). Similarly, two recent reports failed to confirm the association between *ENPP1* and obesity and diabetes in very large groups of European individuals (16,17). Regarding other candidates identified by positional cloning the screening in large cohorts collected in Europe and North America will also be mandatory, as will be the functional studies required to confirm that the discovered genetic variation has a potential physiopathological implication. In the GAD2 study for example, the functional consequence of the risk genetic variant could not be confirmed (14). The diversity of genetic and environmental factors in humans has proved problematic for data replication (18). Globally, the result can be conflicting findings that cast doubt on potentially interesting candidate genes. The reasons for the lack of replication in most association and linkage studies performed in different populations are numerous and fully described in Chapter 6.1.

In addition, marker based systems in genome-wide linkage studies suffer from limited power without the availability of complete pedigree information. Complex diseases don't follow a Mendelian inheritance pattern and so nonparametric linkage methods must be and have been applied (19,20). Most of these studies rely on the estimation of the sharing of genomic fragments that are identical by decent (IBD) between two related individuals. The estimated IBD status is then compared to the expected value under the assumption of no linkage with the disease. A significant deviation from the expected IBD is evidenced for a disease gene at the linked locus. Where only one affected relative pair is available from each family it may not be possible to determine IBD unambiguously. In cases where no extended pedigree genotype information is available e.g. for late onset diseases, this can result in a significant decrease in the power to detect linkage (21). This has been reported for both microsatellite and SNP based methods (2,21,22). The major factor leading to this decrease in power is ambiguity in correct IBD prediction in a single relative pair with limited allele segregation data (23).

NEW METHOD CHARACTERIZING REGIONS IDENTICAL BY DESCENT

Direct identical by descent (IBD) mapping using an enzymatic process to enrich IBD regions should theoretically overcome these limitations, as the method does not rely on parental genetic information to determine IBD. The fact that non-IBD fragments will show sequence differences between two individuals is used to physically remove the non-IBD DNA. Concepts for physical enrichment of IBD DNA between related individuals were introduced by Ford and colleagues (24,25). Nelson et al. in 1993 proposed a technological solution termed Genomic Mismatch Scanning (GMS) (26). The principle relies on the fact that genomic fragments from non-IBD regions will be polymorphic in respect to the sequences of the homologous region between two individuals. When DNA from both individuals is mixed to form hybrid DNA, these sites will have base pair mismatches. These mismatches can be detected by specific DNA repair enzymes, which introduce nicks into the mismatched DNA making it susceptible to digestion by an exonuclease. Thereby, the non-IBD DNA can be removed physically from the solution. GMS held the promise to overcome the two major problems of marker based linkage mapping namely lack of resolution and ambiguity of IBD determination. With the development of high resolution SNP arrays for genotyping the method never achieved widespread application and there are probably multiple reasons for this. However, there are situations, especially in late onset diseases where the power of SNP based studies remains low and where a direct IBD typing method could be applied advantageously. However, the protocol described for the GMS method suffers from the complexity of its many steps and the absence of sufficient control within the process. A major challenge for the process is the efficient removal of DNA (self-self DNA and mismatched hybrid DNA) by the different enzymatic steps. For any relative pair whose ancestral chromosomes are unrelated, at least 75% of the DNA is targeted for removal, namely 50% self-self DNA plus 25% mismatched hybrids of paternal with maternal strands. Of the remaining 25% hybrid DNA of strands from the same parent the mismatched fraction depends on the relationship between the two individuals. Thus for sib-pairs an average of 87.5% of the total DNA must be eliminated. Careful titration of the enzymatic activities is therefore of prime importance. Obviously, the more process steps are required the higher will be the danger of any key step to fail. In addition one would ideally want to be able to evaluate the efficiency of the enzymatic steps within the process itself. Genome HIP is an improved method for direct IBD mapping. The method is both simpler in its application and more transparent in scoring the efficacy and success of each process step. The introduction of exogenous DNAs as internal controls of the process allows the tracking of each enzymatic step on the background of the genomic DNA.

This results in a significantly reduced risk to waste resources and time when a step has not worked as expected. The replacement of organic DNA extraction and ethanol precipitation by simple filtration allows easy handling of samples in standard microtiter plate format. The process can be applied with high robustness on many samples in parallel a pre-requisite for large-scale linkage studies in complex diseases. In addition, it facilitates adopting of the method to robotic liquid handling platforms. The current density of the genome-wide array used for GenomeHIP is 0.6 Megabases, enabling genome-wide scans at a 10 to 20-times higher resolution than the average microsatellite scan. SNP chips for linkage reach higher resolutions but the precision of the method cannot be judged only by array density. SNP chips need high density to overcome the relatively low information content for a single SNP. GenomeHIP is thus a new protocol for direct genome-wide IBD mapping that simplifies the process steps and improves the applicability of the procedure compared to earlier similar methods. The method allows the routine handling of large number of samples in parallel in a controlled process. The method provides a genome-wide resolution of 600 Kilobases using BAC chips. Results in CEPH sib-pairs show that the process is both robust and precise in its determination of IBD in this challenging application. This method should be especially advantageous over marker-based methods in situations where parental genotype data is not available. Future studies are on going in obese population using this new methodology.

GENOME-WIDE ASSOCIATION

Microarray-based SNP genotyping methods has increased the throughput as well as reduced the cost of SNP large scale genotyping. The International HapMap Consortium (27) published the first detailed haplotype map of the human genome, providing the possibility of exploring the SNP variations in human genes and thus to identify the genotypes that contribute to the predisposition to obesity and related phenotypes. Several groups are now conducting genome-wide association studies in case and controls and efficient platforms now provide the possibility of rapidly screening the human genome in large populations. Many companies provide tools and platforms for rapid screening. For example *Affymetrix* Company designed thousand of validated SNPs selected from both public SNP databases and a proprietary SNP database. This data is freely available, without any licensing, terms or conditions. *Affymetrix* is now using this SNP data base to develop a product that enables the genotyping of more than 100,000 SNPs in a single experiment. Another example is *Illumina* Company which also provides a high throughput SNP genotyping platform for custom and fixed content needs. These platforms are now used by leading genomics centers around the world. Although, the technology is rapidly improving, it still remains to chose for the best sample size and study design (e.g. case-control *vs.* family studies), the appropriate statistical methods for a given study design, and the control of multiple testing bias. Statistical approaches such as linkage of disequilibrium threshold values and permutation analyses have proven useful, but an ingenious approach recently described by Herbert and colleagues (28) will undoubtedly provide a template for future association studies. Using a multi-stage design, in which the number of SNPs considered is reduced at each step without sacrificing genome-wide significance, the authors selected the top 10 SNPs for further analysis and only one, a SNP variant near the *INSIG2* gene, was associated with obesity (see Chapter 6.3 for details). While more common statistical tests, such as the Bonferroni and Hochberg corrections, did not identify this variant, the multi-stage approach employed by the authors proved accurate as this variant was replicated in five independent populations. However, more studies necessary to determine the pertinence of this specific marker.

CONCLUSION

By looking at the complex picture of obesity-related susceptibility genes, one might stress that these genetic studies have mainly produced a large repertoire of predisposing alleles which importance is variable. In contrast to genes playing a major role in the development of monogenic obesity, variations in the genes associated with common obesity are not necessarily sufficient to express the obese phenotype. Association of a gene with a complex trait only proposes a factor of risk rather than the causative gene. As such, the researchers must err on the side of caution when positioning genes/SNPs in relation to disease. No single SNP will cause a complex disease; however, a combination of variants exposed to the so called "obesogenic" environmental stimuli will increase the relative risk that an individual develops the disease. Apart from the issues related to statistics, one can note that these studies have culminated in a list of common variants that may modify the risk of obesity or the associated downstream diseases with only a small degree of certainty. Even if confirmed in independent studies, these susceptibility alleles must be considered in the overall picture, where many contributing environment linked-factors may have an equal or even greater effect on the obese phenotype. In addition, combining these SNPs and defining the associated risks will be a real challenge.

More generally, when looking at the future promise of personalized medicine and nutrition, one must consider both sides of the coin. One side is purely beneficial, in which the health and well-being of an individual is improved based on their genetic blueprint. The other side concerns the ethics of possessing such knowledge, where information regarding an individual's genetic makeup may be used inappropriately (e.g. discrimination). Thus, while new technologies (such as genome HIP strategy) and international consortiums will enable the research community to unravel the genetics of complex traits and realize the ambitious goal of personalization more quickly, the future ethical handling of this information will prove to be a far greater challenge with the potential for drastic implications (29).

REFERENCES

1. Middleton FA, Pato MT, Gentile KL, et al. Genomewide linkage analysis of bipolar disorder by use of a high-density single-nucleotide-polymorphism (SNP) genotyping assay: a comparison with microsatellite marker assays and finding of significant linkage to chromosome 6q22. Am J Hum Genet 2004; 74(5):886–97.
2. Matsuzaki H, Loi H, Dong S, et al. Parallel genotyping of over 10,000 SNPs using a one-primer assay on a high-density oligonucleotide array. Genome Res 2004; 14(3):414–25.
3. Rankinen T, Zuberi A, Chagnon YC, et al. The human obesity gene map: the 2005 update. Obesity (Silver Spring) 2006; 14(4):529–644.
4. Shmulewitz D, Heath SC, Blundell ML, et al. Linkage analysis of quantitative traits for obesity, diabetes, hypertension, and dyslipidemia on the island of Kosrae, Federated States of Micronesia. Proc Natl Acad Sci U S A 2006; 103(10):3502–9.

5. Saar K, Geller F, Ruschendorf F, et al. Genome scan for childhood and adolescent obesity in German families. Pediatrics 2003; 111(2):321–7.

6. Meyre D, Bouatia-Naji N, Tounian A, et al. Variants of ENPP1 are associated with childhood and adult obesity and increase the risk of glucose intolerance and type 2 diabetes. Nat Genet 2005; 37(8):863–7.

7. Dong C, Li WD, Li D, Price RA. Interaction between obesity-susceptibility loci in chromosome regions 2p25-p24 and 13q13-q21. Eur J Hum Genet 2005; 13(1):102–8.

8. Dong C, Wang S, Li WD, et al. Interacting genetic loci on chromosomes 20 and 10 influence extreme human obesity. Am J Hum Genet 2003; 72(1):115–24.

9. Suviolahti E, Oksanen LJ, Ohman M, et al. The SLC6A14 gene shows evidence of association with obesity. J Clin Invest 2003; 112(11):1762–72.

10. Boutin P, Dina C, Vasseur F, et al. GAD2 on Chromosome 10p12 Is a Candidate Gene for Human Obesity. PLoS Biol 2003; 1(3):E68.

11. Durand E, Boutin P, Meyre D, et al. Polymorphisms in the amino acid transporter solute carrier family 6 (neurotransmitter transporter) member 14 gene contribute to polygenic obesity in French Caucasians. Diabetes 2004; 53(9):2483–6.

12. Abate N, Chandalia M, Satija P, et al. ENPP1/PC-1 K121Q polymorphism and genetic susceptibility to type 2 diabetes. Diabetes 2005; 54(4):1207–13.

13. Grarup N, Urhammer SA, Ek J, et al. Studies of the relationship between the ENPP1 K121Q polymorphism and type 2 diabetes, insulin resistance and obesity in 7,333 Danish white subjects. Diabetologia 2006; 49(9):2097–104.

14. Swarbrick MM, Waldenmaier B, Pennacchio LA, et al. Lack of Support for the Association between GAD2 Polymorphisms and Severe Human Obesity. PLoS Biol 2005; 3(9):e315.

15. Hunt SC, Xin Y, Wu LL, Hopkins PN, Adams TD. Lack of association of glutamate decarboxylase 2 gene polymorphisms with severe obesity in Utah. Obesity (Silver Spring) 2006; 14(4):650–5.

16. Weedon MN, Shields B, Hitman G, et al. No evidence of association of ENPP1 variants with type 2 diabetes or obesity in a study of 8,089 U.K. Caucasians. Diabetes 2006; 55(11):3175–9.

17. Lyon HN, Florez JC, Bersaglieri T, et al. Common variants in the ENPP1 gene are not reproducibly associated with diabetes or obesity. Diabetes 2006; 55(11):3180–4.

18. Laird NM, Lange C. Family-based designs in the age of large-scale gene-association studies. Nat Rev Genet 2006; 7(5):385–94.

19. Blackwelder WC, Elston RC. A comparison of sib-pair linkage tests for disease susceptibility loci. Genet Epidemiol 1985; 2(1):85–97.

20. Haseman JK, Elston RC. The investigation of linkage between a quantitative trait and a marker locus. Behav Genet 1972; 2(1):3–19.

21. Evans DM, Cardon LR. Guidelines for genotyping in genomewide linkage studies: single-nucleotide-polymorphism maps versus microsatellite maps. Am J Hum Genet 2004; 75(4):687–92.

22. Hoh J, Ott J. Scan statistics to scan markers for susceptibility genes. Proc Natl Acad Sci U S A 2000; 97(17):9615–7.

23. Kruglyak L, Daly MJ, Reeve-Daly MP, Lander ES. Parametric and nonparametric linkage analysis: a unified multipoint approach. Am J Hum Genet 1996; 58(6):1347–63.

24. Sanda AI, Ford JP. Genomic analysis I: inheritance units and genetic selection in the rapid discovery of locus linked DNA markers. Nucleic Acids Res 1986; 14(18):7265–83.

25. Casna NJ, Novack DF, Hsu MT, Ford JP. Genomic analysis II: isolation of high molecular weight heteroduplex DNA following differential methylase protection and Formamide-PERT hybridization. Nucleic Acids Res 1986; 14(18):7285–303.

26. Nelson SF, McCusker JH, Sander MA, et al. Genomic mismatch scanning: a new approach to genetic linkage mapping. Nat Genet 1993; 4(1):11–8.

27. www.hapmap.org.

28. Herbert A, Gerry NP, McQueen MB, et al. A common genetic variant is associated with adult and childhood obesity. Science 2006; 312(5771):279–83.

29. Mutch DM, Clement K. Unravelling the genetics of human obesity. PLoS Genet 2006; 2(12):e188.

Association and Linkage Studies in Caucasians

Anke Hinney and Johannes Hebebrand

Department of Child and Adolescent Psychiatry, University of Duisburg-Essen, Essen, Germany

Polygenic effects are relevant in human body weight regulation. However, most of the currently described confirmed genetic influences on obesity are conferred by a single gene either with a recessive (e.g. leptin deficiency), dominant or codominant (e.g. reduction in melanocortin-4 receptor tone) mode of inheritance. Genetic mechanisms of body weight regulation are complex; hence there is presumably a hundreds of genes involved in common obesity. Polygenic effects will each be rather small, but frequently affect a substantial proportion of obese individuals and, to a somewhat lesser extent, normal weight and even lean individuals. Association between genetic variants and common human disorders such as obesity could have implications for their prediction, prevention, and treatment.

ASSOCIATION AND LINKAGE STUDIES IN CHILDHOOD OBESITY

Genes with small but replicable effects (polygenes) on body weight have unambiguously been identified so far (1–3). Traditionally, two major routes for the detection/analysis of a candidate gene (polygene or major gene) have been followed, which can apply at the same time.

Genome wide linkage scans depict chromosomal regions harbouring candidate genes; fine mapping leads to a narrowed region for candidate gene analyses. Although this approach had been pursued for obesity and related phenotypes since 1997 (4), it took until 2003 to identify two candidate genes possibly underlying the linkage peaks on chromosomes 10 and X, respectively (5,6). In 2005, the first candidate gene for early onset obesity was identified via a genome scan (*ENPP1*; see below) (7). In general, linkage studies have been successful to detect major genes; however they have limited power to detect genes of modest effect (oligogenes, polygenes). A genome-wide association approach has a far greater power to detect these minor gene effects (8). Some genes will be considered because they are involved in relevant central or peripheral pathways as shown in animal models or via other evidence. Numerous association studies involving cases and controls (or family trios comprising an affected child and both parents) have been pursued; for single genes meta-analyses have been carried out (see Chapter 6.1). This approach should not solely be viewed as an alternative to the identification of genes contributing to linkage signals. Instead such studies can be complementary because linkage studies cannot readily lead to the detection of minor gene effects or infrequent major gene/allele effects. However, recent advances in chip technology make high-density, single nucleotide polymorphism (SNP)–based genome-wide approaches feasible; hence, nowadays high-density genome-wide association studies are becoming available.

Several genome wide linkage scans have been performed for adult obesity. Because single quantitative phenotypically-based genetic studies suggest a higher heritability of body weight in adolescence (9) and because genes that influence body weight in adulthood might not be the same as those that are relevant in childhood and adolescence (10), whole genome scans were also performed in young obese individuals. However, the number of linkage studies in early onset obesity is rather small.

The first of these scans was reported in 2003 (11). It was based on 89 families with two or more obese children. A total of 369 individuals were initially geno-typed for 437 micro-satellite markers. A second sample of 76 families was genotyped using micro-satellite markers that localize to regions for which max-imum likelihood binomial logarithm of the odd (MLB LOD) scores on use of the concordant sibling pair approach exceeded 0.7 in the initial sample. These regions with MLB LOD scores >0.7 were on chromosomes 1, 2, 4, 8, 9, 10, 11, 14, and 19 in the initial sample; MLB LOD scores on chromosomes 8 and 19 exceeded 1.5. In the second sample, MLB LOD scores of 0.68 and 0.71 were observed for chromosomes 10 and 11, respectively; none of the other regions detected in the first sample was linked to obesity in the second sample. Saar et al. (2003) noted that some of the nonsignificant linkage peaks overlap with regions detected in linkage studies encompassing adults. Interestingly, the linkage peak region on chromosome 10p11.23-12 harbours the *GAD2* gene in which SNPs were subsequently described to be associated with a pre-disposition to severe obesity (body mass index (BMI) > 40 kg/m^2). Boutin et al. (2003) specifically chose glutamic acid decarboxylase enzyme (*GAD2*) as a candidate gene because of (*i*) its location within the chromo-some 10p peak additionally identified in a number of linkage scans (12–15) and (*ii*) because of its potential functional involvement in weight regulation. *GAD2* encodes the 65-kD isoform of glutamate decarboxylase, which catalyzes the production of γ-aminobutyric acid, a major inhibitory neurotransmitter co-localized with neuropeptide Y in hypothalamic nuclei involved in the control of food intake. However, the confirmation of this result failed in well powered studies in four large Caucasian study groups, despite the fact that two [the aforementioned German and a British study group (15)] of these showed positive linkage signals in the chromosomal region harbouring *GAD2* (15,16). Hence, *GAD2* can currently not be regarded as a validated obesity polygene, oligogene or major gene.

The second linkage scan (17) based on individuals with early onset obesity was based on a longitudinal study using serial measurements of BMI from child-hood. 782 unselected white siblings from 342 families enrolled in the Bogalusa Heart Study were genotyped for a total of 357 autosomal micro-satellite markers. Siblings were followed up on average 20.2 years (ranging from 4.0 to 27.3 years) (17). A random effects model based on serial measurements of BMI from childhood to adulthood was used to develop a quadratic growth curve. The serial changes in BMI were measured in terms of long-term burden [area under the curve (AUC) divided by follow-up years] and long-term trend (incremental AUC, calculated as total AUC–baseline AUC). Linkage to the long-term measures of BMI was observed on six different chromosomes (1, 5, 7, 12, 13, and 18). For total AUC, linkage was detected on chromosomes 5, 7 and 12; for incremental AUC, chromosomes 1, 5, 7, 12, 13 and 18 were involved. Obesity-related candidate genes are located in these regions or near the markers showing positive linkage. The described evidence for linkage reported in this study indicated that these chromosomal regions might harbour genetic loci affecting the probability to develop obesity in childhood (17).

Meyre et al. (18) conducted a genome-wide search for childhood obesity-associated traits (BMI ≥ 95th percentile, ≥ 97th percentile, and ≥ 99th percentile as well as age of adiposity rebound, which represents a risk period for the development of obesity). 431 micro-satellite markers were genotyped in 506 subjects from 115 multiplex French Caucasian families, with at least one child with a BMI ≥95th percentile (97 pedigrees had at least two sibs with a BMI ≥95th percentile). Fine-mapping was performed at the seven most positive chromosomal regions. Nonparametric multipoint analyses revealed six regions of significant or suggestive linkage on chromosomes 2, 6, and 17 for a BMI above the 95th, 97th or 99th percentile. Regions on chromosomes 15, 16, and 19 were linked to the age of adiposity rebound. The strongest evidence of linkage was detected on chromosome 6q22.31 for a BMI above the 97th percentile (maximum likelihood score: 4.06) at marker D6S287. This logarithm of odds score met genome-wide significance tested through simulation. Eight independent genome scans in adults had previously reported quantitative trait loci on 6q linked to energy or glucose homeostasis-associated phenotypes. The identified locus on chromosome 6q16.3-q24.2 included 2.4 Mb that are common to eight genome scans for type 2 diabetes (T2D) or obesity.

Subsequent analysis of a candidate gene for insulin resistance, the (ectonucleotide pyrophosphatase/phosphodiesterase 1; also called PC-1) *ENPP1* gene, in more than 6,000 individuals showed association between a three-allele risk haplotype (K121Q, IVS20delT-11 and A>G+1044TGA; QdelTG) and childhood obesity (odds ratio; OR = 1.69, P = 0.0006), morbid or moderate obesity in adults (OR = 1.50, P = 0.006 or OR = 1.37, P = 0.02, respectively) and T2D (OR = 1.56, P = 0.00002). This *ENPP1* risk haplotype associated with obesity contributed to the observed chromosome 6q linkage with childhood obesity as suggested by the Genotype Identical By Descent Sharing Test. The haplotype conferred a higher risk of glucose intolerance and T2D to obese children and their parents and was associated with increased serum levels of soluble ENPP1 protein in children. Expression of a long *ENPP1* mRNA isoform, which includes the obesity-associated A>G+1044TGA SNP, was specific for pancreatic islet beta cells, adipocytes and liver. These findings suggested that several variants of *ENPP1* have a primary role in mediating insulin resistance and in the development of both obesity and T2D, suggesting that an underlying molecular mechanism is common to both conditions (7).

Very recently, association of the *ENPP1* K121Q polymorphism to obesity was shown in 670 Caucasian and 321 African-American adults comprising upper and lower extremes of the BMI distribution within the analysed study groups. Individuals homozygous for the K121 allele weighed approximately $1.3 \, \text{kg/m}^2$ more than individuals with all other genotypes. In both Caucasians and African-Americans, the K121 polymorphism in *ENPP1* was associated with increased BMI, but not with diabetes (19). However, the sample size was rather small for the described polygenic effect. Additionally, the analysis was only positive if the K121/K121 genotype was analysed in a recessive model; analysis of all genotypes rendered a negative result (P = 0.07). The data were not corrected for multiple testing. Finally, the two ethnic groups had been merged for the analysis although allele and genotype frequencies differed significantly between them. A meta-analysis pertaining to the haplotype described above or the K121Q SNP is lacking. Thus, the polygenic effect of SNPs/haplotypes in the *ENPP1* on obesity needs to be viewed with caution.

As genome wide linkage studies obviously have as yet not readily led to the elucidation of genetic mechanisms in body weight regulation, genome wide association approaches need to be pursued to detect oligo- to polygenic effects. Recently, these analyses have become feasible through the major improvements in the high throughput chip technologies that can process hundred-thousands of SNPs quickly and affordably.

IDENTIFICATION OF A CANDIDATE SNP VIA GENOME-WIDE ASSOCIATION

Recently, by use of a dense, whole-genome scan on 694 individuals from 288 families of the Framingham Heart Study a common single nucleotide polymorphism (SNP; rs7566605) in the vicinity of the insulin induced gene 2 (*INSIG2*) was found to be associated with obesity in both children and adults. The initial finding was confirmed in four of five separate samples comprised of individuals of Western European ancestry, African Americans and German children and adolescents, respectively. The CC genotype that pre-disposes to obesity was present in approximately 10% of individuals independent of their ethnicity (3).

The genome-wide association analysis in the Framingham families was performed employing a novel test strategy for quantitative traits in a family-based design (20,21). To circumvent the problem of multiple comparisons the analysis employed an initial screening and a subsequent test step (Pedigree-Based Association Test; PBAT) (21,22). The screening step used parental genotypes for selection of SNPs and genetic models that best predicted the phenotypes of the offspring. The second step used a family-based association test (FBAT) (23) to test the selected SNPs for association with BMI using measured genotypes of the offspring. FBAT is a more general version of the transmission disequilibrium test (TDT) (24) assessing transmission disequilibrium of an allele from the parents to the offspring in relation to the phenotype. It is crucial to bear in mind that the measured genotypes of the offspring are only used in the test step. As the screening step selected the alleles that are transmitted from the parent to the offspring merely on a stochastical basis, the test step is statistically independent from the screening step. Thus, the analyses in the screening step do not bias the significance level of the subsequently performed FBAT analyses in the actual test step (20). Hence, it is only necessary to adjust FBAT-results for the number of comparisons performed during the test step. Therefore, the SNP(s) that reached significance after adjustment for the number of tests performed in the test step is considered significant at a genome-wide level (20). In the Herbert et al. (3) study the 10 SNPs with the highest power estimates in the screening step were tested for association using FBAT (25,26). Only SNP rs7566605 10 kb upstream of the *INSIG2* gene turned out to be significant after this test procedure ($P = 0.0026$; after correction for testing 10 SNPs $P = 0.026$). The effect on body weight was conferred by a recessive effect of the minor (C) allele (3), as detected in the original screening step. The odds ratio of the effect was 1.3, so the risk for homozygotes of the C-allele to become obese was increased by about 30%. The average increase in BMI conferred by the risk genotype equalled to about 0.8–1 BMI units. However, apart from four independent confirmations the initial study (3) also reported a nonconfirmation in the "Nurses Health Study". The authors related the lack of association to the proportionately lower number of individuals with high BMI among the 2726 individuals of the "Nurses Health Study" as compared to the other study groups. One of the confirmation samples comprised Caucasian study groups from Poland and United States (1775 cases and 926 controls), which were combined for the analysis as there was no evidence of heterogeneity. Both single study groups would not have resulted in a confirmation. In three different family-based samples and three studies of unrelated individuals the rs7566605 CC genotype was associated with obesity. The best singular *P*-value was obtained in 368 Western European parent-child trios in which either a child or adolescent offspring was obese (mean BMI percentile 98.4 ± 1.93). The transmission disequilibrium test, which detects association in the presence of linkage (24), revealed an over-transmission of the C allele to the obese offspring ($P = 0.0017$), indicating that rs7566605 is associated with BMI from an early age. A meta-analysis that comprised all case-control samples showed that the CC genotype was, under a recessive model, significantly associated with obesity, with an OR of 1.22 (95% CI 1.05–1.42; $P = 0.008$) (3). Several attempts to replicate the *INSIG2* finding have been or are currently being undertaken. We are aware of both confirmations (27) as well as negative findings. Nevertheless, at this preliminary stage, we interpret the data as invoking *INSIG2* as a real obesity polygene.

ASSOCIATION STUDIES IN CANDIDATE GENES

To firmly establish a role of a variant in association studies large case numbers are required; whereby stratification according to weight class appears reasonable. Individuals could hence be categorized as underweight, normal weight, overweight, obese and extremely obese; allele frequencies would accordingly be expected to increase systematically. However, gene variations pre-disposing to leanness might not imply that other alleles increase in frequency in relationship to degree of adiposity. For every particular candidate gene it needs to be devised how to confirm that a specific allele indeed pre-disposes to obesity irrespective of the approach leading to the gene identification (28); stringent efforts to confirm an original finding are of crucial importance.

A vast amount of positive association studies has been published so far; just a minority of these been followed up systematically (29) and see Chapter 6.1. One needs to be aware of the fact that the majority of positive studies has not corrected for multiple tests; hence the reported "significant" finding should be viewed critically and not be taken for granted until confirmed in independent, sufficiently powered studies. It has, on the other hand, to be considered that negative findings also need to be published to avoid publication bias. Standards should be high for publication of such negative findings. The power of the study for a given (previously reported) effect should be stated, to allow a better interpretation of negative findings. The follow-up should be pursued in a systematic fashion to be sure if an identified gene/allele is involved in the phenotype or not.

Samples (and sampling strategies) rendering positive findings need to be delineated in detail so that the scientific community can get a balanced opinion. For this purpose, defined case-control and epidemiological/representative population samples could be referred to in addition to large trio samples to allow for TDT (24). Meta-analyses are exceedingly helpful as soon as a sufficient number of studies had been published. At some point a decision needs to be reached as to whether current evidence is sufficient to unequivocally conclude that a particular allele(s) is relevant for the phenotype. Whenever possible and feasible the decision should be based on the epidemiological level and on an appropriate meta-analysis of all available studies.

Clinical (e.g. assessment of the relevance of an obesity allele for co-morbid conditions), epidemiological and functional studies, as a general rule, only appear warranted, if an initial association finding can be confirmed. Otherwise, the risk of pursuing false positive findings appears too large. One candidate gene for which large scaled confirmatory studies were performed is illustrated in this paragraph. The transfer of results from animal models to humans has not only proven to be successful for rare syndromal monogenic forms of obesity (see Section 5). Mutations in the melanocortin-4 receptor gene (MC4R) that lead to a reduced receptor function are associated with obesity (see Chapter 5.6) (30–32), although their obesogenic effect was not confirmed in a population-based sample (33); a total of six carriers of *MC4R* mutations leading to a reduced function of the receptor were all within the normal weight range. Currently, more than 90 different infrequent nonsynonymous, nonsense and frameshift mutations in the *MC4R* have been described in extremely obese individuals (see e.g. 33). Most of these mutations lead to total or partial loss of function in in vitro assays. Combined frequencies for all functionally relevant mutations typically range from 2% to 3% in extremely obese individuals; approximately 0.5% of the normal weight population also harbors such mutations. The quantitative effect of functionally relevant human *MC4R* mutations on body weight was recently determined in a family setting based on obese index cases harboring a mutation. Carriers of these mutations had a significantly higher current BMI than their wild type relatives equivalent to 4.5 and 9.5 kg/m^2 in males and females, respectively. Obviously, additional genetic and/or environmental factors are also operative in these families, which accordingly also contribute to the obesity of the index cases (34).

Apart from this major gene effect, it was shown that a variant (V103I, rs2229616) in the *MC4R* is negatively associated with obesity (1,2). This rather small polygenic effect can only be detected and confirmed in large study groups, particularly if the respective allele is infrequent (allele frequency $\leq$ 5%) as is the case with the V103I polymorphism, which occurs in 2–9% of different populations (2). The *MC4R* V103I polymorphism underscores that it will be especially difficult to pinpoint the effect of gene variants that exert only a minor influence on body weight. V103I had been detected by several groups (e.g. 30,35,36). Because both association and functional studies had initially been negative, this polymorphism had originally been considered as irrelevant for body weight regulation. However, a family-based association test (TDT) () in 520 trios ascertained via an obese child or adolescent revealed a reduced transmission of the I103-allele (10 transmissions, 25 nontransmissions; *P*-value: 0.02). This finding led to a meta-analysis. Most groups had reported a (slightly) higher frequency of the I103-allele in controls than in obese cases. A meta-analysis considering newly generated data (including 2,334 subjects of the epidemiological KORA-S4 sample, which is representative of the Augsburg region in Germany) and all previously published reports (7,713 individuals in total; 3,631 obese and 4,082 controls) provided clear evidence for a negative association of the I103-allele with obesity (odds ratio: 0.69; 95%-confidence interval: 0.59–0.99). Sex- and age-adjusted regression analysis resulted in an effect estimate of −0.48 kg/m^2 for I103 carrier status ($P = 0.22$), which is approximately equivalent to a reduction of 1.6 kg in a 1.8-m-tall individual (1).

BMI is a complex trait influenced by many genes and environmental factors; in light of previous negative functional findings the two receptor variants were again compared in *in vitro* assays (1). However, no differences were found although minor functional differences cannot be excluded via such assays. Additionally, the 5′ and 3′ regions of the *MC4R* were re-sequenced and four other SNPs were detected, three of which were in total linkage disequilibrium with the original polymorphism. None of these readily explained the negative association with obesity (1). However, the negative association with obesity could subsequently be reconfirmed in a large epidemiologic study group (7937 individuals, an extension of the original KORA S2000 cohort) (2). Recently, a second meta-analysis comprising a total of approximately 30,000 individuals also confirmed the initial finding (37).

Since this V103I polymorphism shows normal endogenous agonist binding properties and normal cell surface receptor expression levels, it had been difficult to link the I103 allele with a potential molecular effect. Recently, the 103I *MC4R* revealed a modest (2-fold) but statistically significant decrease in antagonist hAGRP(87-132) potency, which is consistent with the protective effect conferred by this variant (38). The effect of β-MSH, a potent agonist at the *MC4R* (39), seemed, on the other hand, to be increased for the 103I-allele (38). Hence, both, the lower antagonist and the increased agonist potencies are compatible with an elevated *MC4R* function, which could explain the weight reducing effect of the variant.

CONCLUSION

Only one of the genome scans described for children and adolescents so far led to the identification of a candidate gene for early onset obesity (*ENPP1* gene) (7,18). There is no complete confirmation of these results in an independent population yet; hence the positive data have to be treated rather cautiously as an independent confirmation represents a pre-requisite for validation of a candidate gene with a general implication for the analysed phenotype. However, a novel genome wide scan employing a high density SNP set that was performed in adults led to the identification of a SNP in the vicinity of the *INSIG2* gene. This gene seemingly is also implicated in early onset obesity. As the frequency of homozygotes for the relevant C-allele is high (about 10%) and the conferred risk relatively small (OR = 1.33), *INSIG2* can currently be regarded as a polygene for obesity.

The 103I allele of the *MC4R* is to our knowledge the first confirmed polygene conferring a protection from obesity that has been detected in extremely obese children and adolescents. The polygenic effect is obviously also exerted in adults as most of the studies included in the meta-analyses comprised adult obese cases. Whereas the effect size of this allele on mean BMI has been shown to be $-0.5 \, \text{kg/m}^2$, its effect size in children and adolescents has not been assessed.

REFERENCES

1. Geller F, Reichwald K, Dempfle A, et al. Melanocortin-4 receptor gene variant I103 is negatively associated with obesity. Am J Hum Genet 2004; 74(3):572–81 (Epub 2004, Feb 17).
2. Heid IM, Vollmert C, Hinney A, et al. KORA Group. Association of the 103I MC4R allele with decreased body mass in 7937 participants of two population based surveys. J Med Genet 2005; 42(4):e21.
3. Herbert A, Gerry NP, McQueen MB, et al. A common genetic variant is associated with adult and childhood obesity. Science 2006; 312(5771):279–83.
4. Comuzzie AG, Hixson JE, Almasy L, et al. A major quantitative trait locus determining serum leptin levels and fat mass is located on human chromosome 2. Nat Genet 1997; 15(3):273–6.
5. Boutin P, Dina C, Vasseur F, et al. GAD2 on chromosome 10p12 is a candidate gene for human obesity. PLoS Biol 2003; 1(3):E68. (Epub 2003, Nov 3).

6. Suviolahti E, Oksanen LJ, Ohman M, et al. The SLC6A14 gene shows evidence of association with obesity. J Clin Invest 2003; 112(11):1762–72.
7. Meyre D, Bouatia-Naji N, Tounian A, et al. Variants of ENPP1 are associated with childhood and adult obesity and increase the risk of glucose intolerance and type 2 diabetes. Nat Genet 2005; 37(8):863–7.
8. Risch N, Merikangas K. The future of genetic studies of complex human diseases. Science 1996; 273(5281):1516–7.
9. Pietilainen KH, Kaprio J, Rissanen A, et al. Distribution and heritability of BMI in Finnish adolescents aged 16 yr and 17 yr: a study of 4884 twins and 2509 singletons. Int J Obes Relat Metab Disord 1999; 23(2):107–15.
10. Fabsitz RR, Carmelli D, Hewitt JK. Evidence for independent genetic influences on obesity in middle age. Int J Obes Relat Metab Disord 1992; 16(9):657–66.
11. Saar K, Geller F, Ruschendorf F, et al. Genome scan for childhood and adolescent obesity in German families. Pediatrics 2003; 111(2):321–7.
12. Hager J, Dina C, Francke S, et al. A genome-wide scan for human obesity genes reveals a major susceptibility locus on chromosome 10. Nat Genet 1998; 20(3):304–8.
13. Lee JH, Reed DR, Li WD, et al. Genome scan for human obesity and linkage to markers in 20q13. Am J Hum Genet 1999; 64(1):196–209. (Erratum in Am J Hum Genet 2000; 66(4):1472.
14. Dong C, Wang S, Li WD, et al. Interacting genetic loci on chromosomes 20 and 10 influence extreme human obesity. Am J Hum Genet 2003; 72(1):115–24 (Epub 2002, Dec 11).
15. Groves CJ, Zeggini E, Walker M, et al. Significant linkage of BMI to chromosome 10p in the U.K. Population and Evaluation of GAD2 as a Positional Candidate. Diabetes 2006; 55(6):1884–9.
16. Swarbrick MM, Waldenmaier B, Pennacchio LA, et al. Lack of support for the association between GAD2 polymorphisms and severe human obesity. PLoS Biol 2005; 3(9):e315 (Epub 2005, Aug 30).
17. Chen W, Li S, Cook NR, et al. An autosomal genome scan for loci influencing longitudinal burden of body mass index from childhood to young adulthood in white sibships: the Bogalusa heart study. Int J Obes Relat Metab Disord 2004; 28(4):462–9.
18. Meyre D, Lecoeur C, Delplanque J, et al. A genome-wide scan for childhood obesity-associated traits in French families shows significant linkage on chromosome 6q22. 31-q23.2. Diabetes 2004; 53(3):803–11.
19. Matsuoka N, Patki A, Tiwari HK, et al. Association of K121Q polymorphism in ENPP1 (PC-1) with BMI in Caucasian and African-American adults. Int J Obes (Lond) 2006; 30(2):233–7.
20. Van Steen K, McQueen MB, Herbert A, et al. Genomic screening and replication using the same data set in family-based association testing. Nat Genet 2005; 37(7):683–91 (Epub 2005, Jun 5).
21. Lange C, DeMeo D, Silverman EK, et al. PBAT: tools for family-based association studies. Am J Hum Genet 2004; 74(2):367–9.
22. Lange C, Lyon H, DeMeo D, et al. A new powerful non-parametric two-stage approach for testing multiple phenotypes in family-based association studies. Hum Hered 2003; 56(1–3):10–7.
23. Laird NM, Horvath S, Xu X. Implementing a unified approach to family-based tests of association. Genet Epidemiol 2000; 19(Suppl. 1):S36–42.
24. Spielman RS, McGinnis RE, Ewens WJ. Transmission test for linkage disequilibrium: the insulin gene region and insulin-dependent diabetes mellitus (IDDM). Am J Hum Genet 1993; 52(3):506–16.
25. Horvath S, Xu X, Laird NM. The family based association test method: strategies for studying general genotype–phenotype associations. Eur J Hum Genet 2001; 9(4):301–6.
26. Lange C, DeMeo DL, Laird NM. Power and design considerations for a general class of family-based association tests: quantitative traits. Am J Hum Genet 2002; 71(6): 1330–41. (Epub 2002, Nov 21).

27. Lyon HN, Emilsson V, Hinney A, et al. The association of a SNP upstream of INSIG2 with body mass index is reproduced in several but not all cohorts. PLoS Genet 2007; 3(4):e61 (Epub 2007 Mar 7).
28. Campbell H, Rudan I. Interpretation of genetic association studies in complex disease. Pharmacogenomics J 2002; 2(6):349–60 (Review).
29. Rankinen T, Zuberi A, Chagnon YC, et al. The human obesity gene map: the 2005 update. Obesity (Silver Spring) 2006; 14(4):529–644.
30. Hinney A, Hohmann S, Geller F, et al. Melanocortin-4 receptor gene: case-control study and transmission disequilibrium test confirm that functionally relevant mutations are compatible with a major gene effect for extreme obesity. J Clin Endocrinol Metab 2003; 88(9):4258–67.
31. Farooqi IS, O''Rahilly S. Monogenic obesity in humans. Annu Rev Med 2005; 56:443–58 (Review).
32. Lubrano-Berthelier C, Dubern B, Lacorte JM, et al. Melanocortin 4 receptor mutations in a large cohort of severely obese adults: prevalence, functional classification, genotype-phenotype relationship, and lack of association with binge eating. J Clin Endocrinol Metab 2006; 91(5):1811–8 (Epub 2006, Feb 28).
33. Hinney A, Bettecken T, Tarnow P, et al. Prevalence, spectrum, and functional characterization of melanocortin-4 receptor gene mutations in a representative population-based sample and obese adults from Germany. J Clin Endocrinol Metab 2006; 91(5):1761–9 (Epub 2006, Feb 21).
34. Dempfle A, Hinney A, Heinzel-Gutenbrunner M, et al. Large quantitative effect of melanocortin-4 receptor gene mutations on body mass index. J Med Genet 2004; 41(10):795–800.
35. Gotoda T, Scott J, Aitman TJ. Molecular screening of the human melanocortin-4 receptor gene: identification of a missense variant showing no association with obesity, plasma glucose, or insulin. Diabetologia 1997; 40(8):976–9.
36. Hinney A, Schmidt A, Nottebom K, et al. Several mutations in the melanocortin-4 receptor gene including a nonsense and a frameshift mutation associated with dominantly inherited obesity in humans. J Clin Endocrinol Metab 1999; 84(4):1483–6.
37. Young EH, Wareham NJ, Farooqi S, et al. The V103I polymorphism of the MC4R gene and obesity: population based studies and meta-analysis of 29563 individuals. Int J Obes (Lond) 2007; Mar 13 (Epub ahead of Print).
38. Xiang Z, Litherland SA, Sorensen NB, et al. Pharmacological Characterization of 40 Human Melanocortin-4 Receptor Polymorphisms with the Endogenous Proopiomelanocortin-Derived Agonists and the Agouti-Related Protein (AGRP) Antagonist. Biochemistry 2006; 45(23):7277–88.
39. Biebermann H, Castaneda TR, van Landeghem F, et al. A role for beta-melanocyte-stimulating hormone in human body-weight regulation. Cell Metab 2006; 3(2):141–6.

7.1 Genetics of Eating Behavior

Antonio Tataranni
Sanofi-Aventis, Bridgewater, New Jersey, U.S.A.

Monica Bertolini
Cattedra e Servizio di Endocrinologia e malattie del metabolismo, University degli Studi di Modena e Reggio Emilia, Modena, Italy

Obesity that results from chronic positive energy balance (1) has serious health consequences (2), and despite recent advances in the understanding of the molecular biology controlling energy homeostasis (3) and large efforts to uncover the genetic underpinnings of obesity in human populations (4), the exact cause of weight gain in the majority of people remains unknown. This is not entirely surprising because it is inherently difficult to study the etiology of obesity in humans. The methodologies available to measure various components of daily energy metabolism are either barely precise (energy expenditure) or profoundly inaccurate (energy intake) and thus unable to detect the small differences in energy balance that, when chronically sustained, are likely to be responsible for the development of obesity in the majority of people. For the past 30 years, regulation of energy expenditure has been a dominant theme in human obesity research. The majority of studies have been conducted under the controlled, artificial conditions of a metabolic study unit and often in the resting state. Some studies have indicated that low resting energy expenditure (5) and low whole-body lipid oxidation rates (6,7) are inherited phenotypes, which can predispose some individuals to development of obesity. However, these findings are not universal, and an unequivocal molecular explanation for their regulation is still missing (8). It is only recently, with the advent of the doubly labeled water technique (9), that a limited number of studies have started to provide information on energy expenditure in individuals who are unencumbered by the confines of the laboratory setting. However, to date these areas of research have not produced convincing evidence that abnormal regulation of energy expenditure is either a common or a major risk factor for weight gain in humans. The study of molecular mechanisms and resulting behaviors that underlie energy intake in humans has been even less conclusive. In the vast majority of studies, eating behavior, food intake, and macronutrient preferences are measured by instruments (Visual Analog Scales, food frequency questionnaires, diaries, recalls, diet histories, weighed records) sharing the same weakness; they depend on subjects honestly telling researchers their interoceptive sensations and what they consumed (Table 1). The inability of accurately measuring what people eat and, why, represents the most fundamental flaw in obesity research (10). Faced with these difficulties, many researchers in this field continue to shy away from measurements of eating behavior and food intake as the proximal, genetically dissectible phenotypes and rely instead on measurements of body weight and body composition to identify the molecular cause(s) of the disease.

TABLE 1 Methodologies to Measure Food Intake in Humans

Methodology	Phenotype measured	Technical and experimental complexity	Precision	Cost	Other considerations
Questionnaires	Total energy intake, macronutrient preferences, taste preferences, subjective feelings of hunger and satiation, restraint, dishinibition, etc.	Low	Low	Low	Very widely used, some self administered, subject to reporting biases
Vending machines	Total energy intake, macronutrients	Medium	High	High	Requires support of fully staffed metabolic kitchen
Doubly labelled water	Total energy intake	High	Medium	High	Requires mass spectrometry, relies on precise measurements of body weight to estimate total energy intake from total energy expenditure
Neuroimaging	Neuroanatomical correlates of hunger, taste and satiation	Very high	Unknown	Very high	Requires fMRI and/or PET, methodology development in its infancy

Indeed, studies in twins (11), adoptees (12), and family members (13) indicate that obesity is heritable and that a large portion (up to 70%) of the between-person variance in adiposity is genetically determined (See Section 2). It is likely that several genes control both energy intake and expenditure. Because familial traits such as energy expenditure and nutrient partitioning explain only a minor portion of the genetic variability of weight gain, it is then assumed that the main cause of obesity in humans is an inherited tendency to overeat. If the innate risk for weight gain is mainly the consequence of eating in excess of daily energy expenditure (14), then the brain, which controls eating behavior, must play a major role in the etiology of the disease.

This conclusion is not only based on deductive reasoning. The discovery of complex neuropeptidergic pathways that control energy balance has irrefutably demonstrated that body fat content is, at least in part, under nonconscious homeostatic control in the hypothalamus (15). However, animals and humans seldom eat in response to acute changes in energy balance. Eating is not a simple, stereotypical behavior. It requires a set of tasks to be carried out by the central and peripheral nervous systems to coordinate the initiation of a meal episode, procurement of food, consumption of the procured food, and termination of the meal (16). Most of these tasks are behaviors learned after weaning. Accordingly, there is now universal recognition that the hypothalamus is not likely to be the only or even the major compartment of the brain involved in the control of eating behavior. Thus obesity, once the prototypical metabolic disorder, is increasingly recognized as a neurological disease due to inherited and localized neurochemical defects (17). By subscribing to the notion that the brain plays a critical role in the control of energy homeostasis and, ultimately, the genesis of obesity, one must acknowledge that the greatest challenge following the identification of the genetic makeup of obese individuals will be to understand how these molecular defects work together to alter the neurophysiology of those regions of the brain that control eating behavior and, ultimately, energy balance.

EATING BEHAVIOR IN RARE FORMS OF OBESITY

Molecular mechanisms that control energy balance and lead to a thrifty metabolism (18–20) are being discovered at an unprecedented rate in animal models of obesity. The same cannot be said for humans. However, as with other complex phenotypes, there are rare examples of mono- and oligogenic causes for obesity that serve as models for understanding the complex hormonal and neural networks that regulate eating behavior in humans (Tables 2 and 3). As described in Section 3 in details the genetic mutation causing massive obesity in *ob/ob* mice was described and the mutated gene was found to encode a previously unknown adipocyte-derived hormone, named leptin from the Greek word leptos (lean), which described its catabolic effects (21). In mice lacking circulating leptin, hormone replacement therapy rapidly corrected the severe, early onset obesity and many associated metabolic and hormonal abnormalities including hyperphagia, defective thermogenesis, infertility, and type 2 diabetes (22). In accord with Dr. Coleman's parabiosis experiments in the 1970s (23), the genetic mutation causing massive obesity in the *db/db* mouse was shown to be a molecular defect of the leptin receptor gene (24,14). Animals homozygous for this mutation exhibited a phenotype virtually identical to *ob/ob* mice, but had elevated plasma leptin concentrations (25). These landmark discoveries and the need to understand

TABLE 2 Monogenic Forms of Human Obesity

Gene	Chromosomal location	Number of cases	Abnormal eating behavior	Abnormal energy expenditure	Phenotype
MC4R	18q22	3–5% of morbid obesity	⇑	⇔	Hyperphagia, moderate to severe obesity
LEP	7q31.3	6	⇑	⇔	Hyperphagia, severe early onset obesity, hypogonadism
LEPR	1p31	3	⇑	⇔	Hyperphagia, severe early onset obesity, hypogonadism
POMC	2p23.3	2	⇑	?	Severe obesity, ACTH deficiency, red hair
PCSK1	5q15-q21	1	?	?	Childhood onset obesity, IGT, hypogonadism, hypocortisolism
SIM1	6q16.3-q21	1	?	?	Severe obesity

the central mechanisms mediating the effect of leptin on food intake and energy expenditure led to the ongoing effort to unravel the complex neurohormonal system that controls energy homeostasis. This regulatory system originates mostly in the hypothalamus, but involves many other sub-cortical and cortical regions of the brain. Studies in mice, genetically engineered to suppress or overexpress specific gene products, indicate that food intake and body weight regulation depend on the balance between anabolic-[Neuropeptide Y (NPY), Agouti-related

TABLE 3 Summary of Loci with Evidence of Linkage with Eating Behaviors

TFEQ	QFS		AFDS	
	Peak of linkage	Candidate gene or marker locus	Peak of linkage	Candidate gene or marker locus
Restraint	–		3p	D3S1304
			6p	D6S276
				GLP1
				TNF
Dysinhibition	19p13	D19S215	7	PAI
	15q24-q25	ARNT2	16	
		NMB		
Hunger	15q21	LHNLAIII	3	PPARG
	15q24-q25	ARNT2		
		NMB		
	17q23-q24	D17S1290		
		D17S1351		

Note: LHNLAIII is a genetic marker.
Abbreviations: AFOS, Amish Family Diabetes Study; ARNT2, Aryl-hydrocarbon receptor nuclear translocator 2; NMB, Neuromedin B; QFS, Quebec Family Study.

protein (AgRP), melanin-concentrating hormone (MCH), orexins (OX), and ghrelin (GHRL)) and catabolic (proopiomelanocortin (POMC/MSH), cocaine- and amphetamine-related transcript (CART)] neurotransmitters and their receptors (see Section 3). These central pathways are, in turn, modulated by peripheral hormones secreted by the stomach (e.g., ghrelin, cholecystokinin (CCK), intestine (e.g., peptide YY (PYY)), pancreas (e.g., insulin) and adipose tissue (e.g., leptin). Many of the same hormones and neurotransmitters have been shown to also affect energy expenditure and nutrient partitioning. A detailed description of the physiologic characteristics and functional properties of this complex regulatory system is detailed in many excellent reviews on this topic (26–30) and in chapter 9.5.

Since many of the hormones and neuropeptides mentioned above have profound effects on energy homeostasis and body weight regulation in animals, their discovery has renewed hope of a definitive understanding of the etiology of abnormal eating behaviour, human obesity and, possibly, their treatment. However, expectations of an easy explanation are hindered by the constitutive redundancy of the central system that controls energy homeostasis (29) and by the fact that we do not know if the contribution made by some molecules that affect energy metabolism in animals necessarily translates to similar effects in humans. These concerns are somewhat diminished by evidence that key molecules governing energy homeostasis are conserved across mammalian species (30).

The identification of severe hyperphagia in individuals with mutations of the leptin, leptin receptor, and MC4-receptor genes confirms that energy intake is likely to be regulated in a similar, albeit not identical, manner in humans and animals (Table 2) (31). Such mutations are extremely rare among humans, although molecular defects of the MC4-R have been shown to be present in 3% to 5% of morbidly obese individuals (see Chapter. 5.6). Interestingly, a recent meta-analysis of available data based on case-control studies revealed no association between obesity and genetic variability in the leptin/leptin receptor genes. The most likely explanation of these findings is that most of the investigated polymorphisms have little or no functional impact on the biologic properties of either leptin or its receptor (32).

A set of over 25 inherited diseases, sometimes grouped under the term of syndromic obesity (see Chapter. 5.1), in which obesity is occurring in the clinical context of a distinct set of associated clinical phenotypes, has also been identified (33). The genetic bases of some of these syndromes such as Prader-Willi syndrome, Bardet-Biedel syndrome, Alström syndrome, Cohen syndrome and Borjerson-Forssmann-Lehmann syndrome has been elucidated. However, while interesting theories have been advanced, to date, mutations in the genes causing syndromic obesity have not been shown to be present in, linked, or associated with nonsyndromic foms of obesity. Furthermore, how mutations in these genes may result in dysregulated eating behavior remains pure speculation (33).

POSITIONAL CLONING

Predictably, due to methodological difficulties of measuring what people eat and why, there have been few attempts to determine the contribution of genes to variance of food intake, macronutrient preferences, or more general eating behavior. Nonetheless, despite the putatively large influence of environmental factors, heritability estimates for eating behavior–related variables range from $h^2 = 0.08$ to $h^2 = 0.65$, indicating that up to two thirds of interindividual variance is attributable to genetic factors (34).

Therefore, it is not surprising that positional cloning strategies to find susceptibility alleles for abnormal eating behavior have been explored using whole genome-
wide linkage analysis that utilizes polymorphic genetic markers of many affected
sibling pairs (35). This analysis does not require a priori knowledge of the involvement
of particular genes in the condition to be studied, but is less powerful in finding
complex disease susceptibility alleles than in determining single genes responsible for
rare Mendelian disorders. The limited power of this approach typically leads to a
putative linkage results on broad genomic regions. It is generally accepted that finer
mapping of genotype markers on chromosomal regions with suggestive linkage is
required to narrow down the regions by association testing, which means that until the
regions are completely sequenced (in most cases the appropriate mapping density can
only be determined empirically) the success of this effort is still not guaranteed (35).

In the Quebec Family Study, 4 chromosomal regions were identified as
linked to abnormal eating behavior (Table 3) and the best positional candidate
gene, neuromedin β, was located near the peak of linkage on chromosome 15.
A mutation in this gene was found to be associated with disinhibition and susceptibility to hunger as well as changes of fatness over time (36). Neuromedin β is a
bombesin-like petide, a family of not very well characterized proteins with many
biological effects, including modulation of the serotoninegic system, secretion of
thyrotropin in the pituitary gland and the stimulation of PYY (36). Eating
behaviors were also examined in the Amish Family Diabetes Study. This genome-
wide multipoint linkage analysis also identified loci on four chromosomal regions
as possible regions containing genes controlling eating behaviors (Table 3). Functional candidate genes, located within the region of peak linkage to disinhibition
and restraint, encode leptin, peroxisome proliferator-activated receptor gamma
(PPARG), Glucagon-like peptide-1 (GLP1), tumor necrosis factor (TNF) and lymphotoxin (LTA) respectively. Leptin, TNF and lymphotoxin are adipocytokines.
PPARG is expressed in many tissues, but the highest concentrations are found in
adipose tissue and large intestine (31). Glucagon like peptide is a hormone derived
from tissue-specific post-translational processing of the proglucagon gene in the
intestinal L cells. The role of signals originating in peripheral tissues to control
complex cognitive functions such as disinhibition and restraint can only be
speculated at this time. However, it is worth noting that leptin receptors are
widely distributed throughout the brain and that the hypothalamus, the main site
of action of leptin and other peripheral signals involved in the regulation of eating
behavior, has direct and indirect neuronal connections with several other regions
of the brain involved in hedonic and cognitive control of food intake.

Over the past five years, a larger number of genetic linkage studies have
focused on obesity itself, rather than eating behavior. Genome-wide scans completed in several populations (4,38–43) have led to the identification of loci linked
to obesity on many chromosomes, including chromosome 2, 4, 5, 10, 11 and 20 (4).
These areas of the genome are currently under intense investigation and may lead
to the cloning of human obesity susceptibility genes, including those controlling
food intake. It seems, however, that because of the complex relationships in the
polygenic nature of diseases such abnormal eating behavior and obesity
(individuals who carry only one or some of these alleles may still not develop the
disease because they either lack another allele (gene-gene interaction) or are not
exposed to the precipitating environment (44) (gene-environment interaction)
multifaceted genetic strategies are required for the identification of their molecular
underpinnings. While the search for the genetic causes of abnormal eating

behavior and obesity often begins with positional cloning strategies, it is increasingly recognized that positional cloning strategies will not provide all the answers.

TRANSCRIPTOMICS PROFILING AND HUMAN OBESITY

Abnormal eating behavior and obesity may turn out to be a diverse set of discrete diseases (4). However, it is possible that, as a consequence of the multiple primary mutations causing each of these discrete diseases, alterations in the expression and or activity of downstream genes along a smaller number of biochemical pathways may commonly develop. Identification of these putative and potentially more common, secondary molecular defects may not be possible by genetic studies based exclusively on single nucleotide polymorphism discovery. A recent technological advancement that allows the assessment of multitude of genes simultaneously has emerged in the field of transcriptomics using microarray gene expression profiling.

The term gene expression profiling refers to the study of the expression level of thousands of genes simultaneously in a given cell/tissue, which has been made possible by a number of recent technological advances such as cDNA microarrays. The promise of this technology is that it should allow capturing the molecular complexity of physiological processes on a global scale (as opposed to the reductionistic, one-transcript-at-a-time approach) and consequently facilitate the understanding of how multiple molecular defects may lead to the same disease. Work has begun to identify genes which are locally expressed under normal conditions (providing, in part, a neurochemical map of the normal human brain) and efforts are already underway to investigate the interacting set of genes that may give rise to other neurological diseases such as schizophrenia, Alzheimer's disease, and autism. However, to the best of our knowledge, the potential use of this technology in understanding the molecular signature of abnormal eating behavior and obesity remains largely untested in the brain. In the only experiment conducted to date, the differential expression of approximately 600 genes was tested in the human hypothalamus of five obese and five lean donors (45). Nineteen transcripts were down regulated and seven transcripts were up regulated in obese versus lean donors. None of these transcripts has been previously identified as a candidate gene for human obesity in association or linkage studies (Fig. 1). While some of the differentially expressed genes, such as histidine decarboxylase (*HDC*) (46) and neuropeptide Y receptor Y2 (*NPY2R*) (47), are known to participate in the control of energy homeostasis in experimental animals, none of these transcripts has been previously identified as a candidate gene for human obesity in association or linkage studies. This may be partially due to the very small experimental sample size and/or limited number of transcripts arrayed on this particular microarray.

Gene expression profiling of the human brain has significant intrinsic limitations, which have been discussed elsewhere (see Chapter. 9.5). Selection of appropriate controls (cause of death, agonal period, postmortem interval, accuracy and consistency in dissecting the brain regions of interest), sensitivity of microarray techniques to detect significant changes in gene expression of rare transcripts, large technical variation, and region and time specificity of the expression of transcripts of interest are some of the overarching concerns complicating the use this methodology for the study of the human brain. Notwithstanding these limitations, we expect transcriptomic approaches to complement gene discovery efforts and increase the chance to identify the putative common neurochemical abnormalities that result from the primary genetic defects underlying the etiology of eating behavior and obesity.

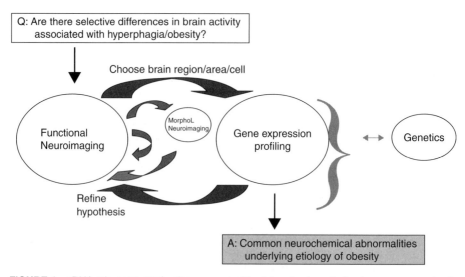

FIGURE 1 cDNA microarray technology was used to determine hypothalamic gene expression in five obese (2M/3F, age at death=51.8 ± 21.3 y, BMI=48.5 ± 12.5 kg/m^2, mean $\pm$ SD) and five lean (2M/3F, 50.8 ± 17.7 y, 23.0 ± 2.6 kg/m^2) humans. All donors were free of cancer, diabetes, or neurodegenerative diseases and not known to be on any chronic drug treatment at time of death. Five pair-matched (by sex and age at death) assays were conducted using a human neurobiology array (Clontech Laboratories, Palo Alto, CA) consisting of 588 genes. Prior to hybridization, the integrity of the RNA samples was verified using bioanalyzer. Each obese array was normalized to the paired lean array by a normalization coefficient [Σ (intensity-background)$_\text{all genes Lean}$/ Σ intensity-background)$_\text{all genes Obese}$]. Only genes with a background-adjusted signal intensity at least two-fold greater than background and not affected by signal bleed were called present. Based on paired t-tests of log-transformed adjusted intensities, we identified ($p < 0.05$) 19 genes that were downregulated and seven that were upregulated in obese versus lean donors.

CONCLUSION

To live up to the scientific challenge posed by the discovery of the etiology of human obesity, we will most likely have to face the complexity of the human brain and its role in the regulation of eating behavior and energy homeostasis. Lockhart & Barlow (48) recently wrote that "...it is because the brain is complex, brain functions are diverse and varied, and the number of genes involved in neural processes is likely to be large (and largely unknown at this point), that it is important to move beyond conventional approaches to strategies that look broadly..." at the pathophysiology of neurological diseases. Consequently, positional cloning or transcriptomic strategies are unlikely to provide all the answers. One of the greatest challenges following the identification of the genetic makeup of obese individuals will be to understand how mutations in known and unknown genes contribute to the brain alterations that cause people to eat in excess of their energy needs (46). Which research strategies will fulfill this unmet scientific need remains to be seen. However, it has been suggested that neuroimagenomics, an iterative experimental approach combining neuroimaging, gene expression profiling of the human brain, and genetics (Fig. 2) may provide an especially promising way to investigate the molecular biology of eating behavior and obesity and assist in the discovery of novel drugs to treat this extraordinary public health problem.

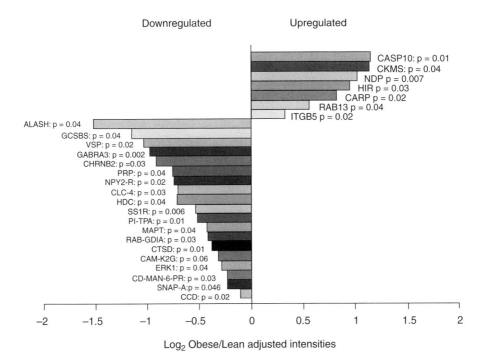

FIGURE 2 Neuroimagenomics consists of an iterative experimental approach combining neuro-imaging and gene-expression profiling of the human brain. We plan to use the results of ongoing neurofunctional studies to make informed choices on the regions where we should begin to investigate the gene-expression profile of the brains of obese and lean individuals; in turn, we fully expect the outcome of the latter to suggest how to formulate and/or refine our hypothesis for future neuroimaging studies. This may apply to redefining where to look (increasing the region specificity of the hypothesis) and how to look (choosing the radiolabeled probe(s) that best suit the hypothesis). We expect neuroimagenomics to complement gene discovery efforts and increase the chance to identify the putative common neurochemical abnormalities that result from the primary genetic defects underlying the etiology of obesity.

REFERENCES

1. Tataranni PA, Ravussin E. Energy Metabolism and Obesity. In: Wadden TA, Stunkard AJ, eds. Handbook of Obesity Treatment. New York: The Guilford Press, 2002,42–72.
2. WHO. Obesity: Preventing and managing the global epidemic. WHO, 1997.
3. Xu AW, Kaelin CB, Morton CJ, et al. Effects of hypothalamic neurodegeneration on energy balance. PLoS Biol. 2005; 3(12):e415.
4. Rankinen T, Zuberi A, Chagnon YC, et al. The human obesity gene map: the 2005 update. Obesity (Silver Spring). 2006; 14(4):529–644.
5. Ravussin E, Lillioja S, Knowler WC, et al. Reduced rate of energy expenditure as a risk factor for body-weight gain. N Engl J Med. 1988; 318:467–72.
6. Zurlo F, Lillioja S, Esposito-Del PA, et al. Low ratio of fat to carbohydrate oxidation as predictor of weight gain: study of 24-h RQ. Am J Physiol. 1990; 59:E650–7.
7. Seidell JC, Muller DC, Sorkin JD, et al. Fasting respiratory exchange ratio and resting metabolic rate as predictors of weight gain: the Baltimore Longitudinal Study on Aging. Int J Obes Relat Metab Disord 1992; 16:667–74.
8. Ravussin E, Bogardus C. Energy balance and weight regulation: genetics versus environment. Br J Nutr 2000; 83(Suppl 1):S17–20.

9. Schoeller DA, Taylor PB. Precision of the doubly labelled water method using the two-point calculation. Hum Nutr Clin Nutr 1987; 41:215–23.

10. Winkler JT. The fundamental flaw in obesity research. Obes Rev. 2005; 6(3):199–202.

11. Bouchard C, Perusse L. Heredity and body fat. Annu Rev Nutr 1988; 8:259–77.

12. Allison DB, Kaprio J, Korkeila M, et al. The heritability of body mass index among an international sample of monozygotic twins reared apart. Int J Obes Relat Metab Disord 1996; 20:501–6.

13. Sakul H, Pratley R, Cardon L, et al. Familiality of physical and metabolic characteristics that predict the development of non-insulin-dependent diabetes mellitus in Pima Indians. Am J Hum Genet 1997; 60:651–6.

14. Tataranni PA. Mechanisms of weight gain in humans. Eur Rev Med Pharmacol Sci 2000; 4:1–7.

15. Williams DL, Schwartz MW. The melanocortin system as a central integrator of direct and indirect controls of food intake. Am J Physiol Regul Integr Comp Physiol 2005; 289(1):R2–3.

16. Berthoud HR. An overview of neural pathways and networks involved in the control of food intake and selection. In: Berthoud HR, Seeley RJ, eds. Neural and Metabolic Control of Macronutrient Intake. Whashington, D.C.: CRC Press 2000:361-87.

17. Bray GA. Obesity is a chronic, relapsing neurochemical disease. Int J Obes Relat Metab Disord 2004; 28(1):34–8.

18. Neel JV. A "thrifty" genotype renedered detrimental by "progress". Am J Hum Genet 1962; 14:353–62.

19. Ravussin E, Bogardus C. Energy expenditure in the obese: is there a thrifty gene? Infusionstherapie 1990; 17:108–12.

20. Swinburn B, Egger G, Raza F. Dissecting obesogenic environments: the development and application of a framework for identifying and prioritizing environmental interventions for obesity. Prev Med 1999; 29:563–70.

21. Zhang Y, Proenca R, Maffei M, et al. Positional cloning of the mouse obese gene and its human homologue (published erratum appears in Nature 1995 Mar 30; 374(6521):479) (see comments). Nature 1994; 372:425–32.

22. Campfield LA, Smith FJ, Guisez Y, et al. Recombinant mouse ob protein: evidence for a peripheral signal linking adiposity and central neural networks. Science 1995; 269:546–9.

23. Coleman DL. Effects of parabiosis of obesity with diabetes and normal mice. Diabetologia 1973; 9:294–8.

24. Tartaglia LA, Dembski M, Weng X, et al. Identification and expression cloning of a leptin receptor, OB-R. Cell 1995; 83:1263–71.

25. Maffei M, Halaas J, Ravussin E, et al. Leptin levels in human and rodent: measurement of plasma leptin and ob RNA in obese and weight-reduced subjects. Nat Med 1995; 1:1155–61.

26. Cummings DE, Schwartz MW. Genetics and pathophysiology of human obesity. Annu Rev Med 2003; 54:453–71.

27. Barsh GS, Schwartz MW. Genetic approaches to studying energy balance: perception and integration. Nat Rev Genet 2002; 3:589–600.

28. Friedman JM. Obesity in the new millennium. Nature 2000; 404:632–4.

29. Saper CB, Chou TC, Elmquist JK. The need to feed: homeostatic and hedonic control of eating. Neuron 2002; 36:199–211.

30. Tschop M, Heiman ML. Rodent obesity models: an overview. Exp Clin Endocrinol Diabetes 2001; 109:307–19.

31. Barsh GS, Farooqi IS, O'Rahilly S. Genetics of body-weight regulation. Nature 2000; 404:644–51.

32. Paracchini V, Pedotti P, Taioli E. Genetics of leptin and obesity: a HuGE review. Am J Epidemiol. 2005; 15:162(2):101–14. Epub 2005 Jun 22.

33. Chung WK, Leibel RL. Molecular physiology of syndromic obesities in humans. Trends Endocrinol Metab 2005; 16(6):267–72.

34. Faith MS, Keller KL. Genetic architecture of ingestive behavior in humans. Nutrition 2004; 20(1):127–33.

35. Bogardus C, Baier L, Permana P, et al. Identification of susceptibility genes for complex metabolic diseases. Ann N Y Acad Sci 2002; 967:1–6.
36. Bouchard L, Drapeau V, Provencher V, et al. Neuromedin beta: a strong candidate gene linking eating behaviors and susceptibility to obesity. Am J Clin Nutr 2004; 80(6):1478–86.
37. Steinle NI, Hsueh W, Snitker S, et al. Eating behavior in the Old Order Amish: heritability analysis and a genome-wide linkage analysis. Am J Clinical Nutrition 2002; 75:1098–106.
38. Comuzzie AG, Hixson JE, Almasy L, et al. A major quantitative trait locus determining serum leptin levels and fat mass is located on human chromosome 2. Nat Genet 1997; 15:273–6.
39. Stone S, Abkevich V, Hunt SC, et al. A major predisposition locus for severe obesity, at 4p15-p14. Am J Hum Genet 2002; 70:1459–68.
40. Hanson RL, Ehm MG, Pettitt DJ, et al. An autosomal genomic scan for loci linked to type II diabetes mellitus and body-mass index in Pima Indians. Am J Hum Genet 1998; 63:130–8.
41. Norman RA, Tataranni PA, Pratley R, et al. Autosomal genomic scan for loci linked to obesity and energy metabolism in Pima Indians. Am J Hum Genet 1998; 62:659–68.
42. Lee JH, Reed DR, Li WD, et al. Genome scan for human obesity and linkage to markers in 20q13. Am J Hum Genet 1999; 64:196–209.
43. Hager J, Dina C, Francke S, et al. A genome-wide scan for human obesity genes reveals a major susceptibility locus on chromosome 10. Nat Genet 1998; 20:304–8.
44. Ravussin E, Valencia ME, Esparza J, et al. Effects of a traditional lifestyle on obesity in Pima Indians. Diabetes Care 1994; 17:1067-74.
45. Del Parigi A, Page GP, Beach TG, et al. Differential gene expression in the hypothalamus of obese and lean humans: a preliminary report. Diabetologia 2003, 46 (abstr).
46. Fulop AK, Foldes A, Buzas E, et al. Hyperleptinemia, visceral adiposity, and decreased glucose tolerance in mice with a targeted disruption of the histidine decarboxylase gene. Endocrinology 2003; 144:4306–14.
47. Sainsbury A, Schwarzer C, Couzens M, et al. Important role of hypothalamic Y2 receptors in body weight regulation revealed in conditional knockout mice. Proc Natl Acad Sci U.S.A 2002; 99:8938–43.
48. Lockhart DJ, Barlow C. Expressing what's on your mind: DNA arrays and the brain. Nat Rev Neurosci 2001; 2:63–8.

7.2 Genetics of Physical Activity

Tuomo Rankinen and Claude Bouchard

Human Genomics Laboratory, Pennington Biomedical Research Center, Baton Rouge, Louisiana, U.S.A.

The beneficial effects of regular physical activity on primary and secondary prevention of several common chronic diseases have been well established and reduction of sedentarism is one of the main goals of public health initiatives. The main challenge for implementation of these recommendations is the poor compliance to physical activity interventions. Since physical activity is a behavioral trait, research has mainly focused on finding psychological, social and environmental factors that contribute to levels of physical activity. Interest on the biological basis of physical activity has re-emerged recently (1,2) and advances in techniques of molecular genetic research have opened new avenues to test for the role of specific genes and mutations. The purpose of this review is to summarize the data from genetic epidemiology studies, and potential candidate genes for physical activity levels.

EVIDENCE FROM GENETIC EPIDEMIOLOGY STUDIES

Studies on the genetics of physical activity level are not extensive, but evidence from both twin and family studies suggests that genetic factors could be involved in the determination of physical activity level. Several twin studies have addressed the role of genetic factors in physical activity level and the findings from these studies are summarized in Table 1.

Twin Studies

In a large cohort of mono- and dizygotic (MZ and DZ, respectively) male twin pairs over 18 years of age from the Finnish Twin Registry (3), information on intensity and duration of activity, years of participation in a given activity, physical activity on the job, and subjective opinion of the subject's own activity level was obtained from a questionnaire. A physical activity score was generated from these variables using factor analysis, which was then used to compute correlations within MZ and DZ twin pairs. The results indicated an estimated heritability of 62% for age-adjusted physical activity level. Heller et al. reported a significantly higher concordance within 94 pairs of MZ twins than within 106 pairs of DZ twins for participation in vigorous exercise in the previous two weeks, and derived a heritability estimate of 39% for this phenotype (4). In a cohort of Finnish teenage twins, leisure-time physical activity level outside the school was assessed using a questionnaire with two questions: one concerning the frequency and the other the intensity of the activities (5). Based on these two questions the subjects were assigned to one of five classes of activity level. The results revealed greater intraclass correlations for MZ twins that for DZ twins for activity level (Table 1).

In the USA Vietnam Era Twin Registry cohort, levels of moderate and vigorous activities were assessed in 3344 male twin pairs aged 33 to 51 years (6).

TABLE 1 Summary of the Intraclass Correlations from Twin Studies for Physical Activity Level and Physical Activity-Related Phenotypes

Source	Physical activity trait	Age	Sex	Number of pairs		Correlation coefficients	
				MZ	DZ	MZ	DZ
Kaprio et al. (3)	Total physical activity	>18	Male	1537	3507	0.57	0.26
Koopmans et al. (7)	Sports participation	18–22	Male	249	241	0.89	0.60
			Female	329	303	0.85	0.72
Aarnio et al. (5)	Leisure-time physical activity outside the school	16	Male	147	191	0.72	0.45
		16	Female	231	179	0.64	0.41
Lauderdale et al. (6)	Intermittent moderate activities	33–51	Male	1006	530	0.38	0.12
	Jogging/running (>10 miles/wk)					0.53	0.07
	Strenuous racquet sports (>5 h/wk)					0.52	0.28
	Bicycling (>50 miles/wk)					0.58	0.14
	Swimming (>2 miles/wk)					0.39	0.35
Beunen and Thomis (8)	Sports participation	15	Male	17	19	0.66	0.62
			Female	17	19	0.98	0.71
Maia et al. (9)	Sports participation index	12–25	Male	85	68	0.82	0.46
			Female	118	85	0.90	0.53
	Leisure-time physical activity		Male	85	68	0.69	0.22
			Female	118	85	0.72	0.56
Stubbe et al. (12)	Sports participation	13–14	Male	115	87	0.88	0.82
		15–16	Male	136	112	0.80	0.68
		17–18	Male	100	96	0.88	0.65
		19–20	Male	92	82	0.86	0.35
		13–14	Female	161	109	0.87	0.84
		15–16	Female	185	115	0.83	0.81
		17–18	Female	148	113	0.80	0.68
		19–20	Female	158	97	0.83	0.53
Franks et al. (13)	Physical activity index	4–10	Mixed[a]	62	38	0.78	0.80
	Physical activity energy expenditure	4–10	Mixed[a]	62	38	0.87	0.76
Joosen et al. (14)	Physical activity (accelerometer)	18–39	Mixed	12	8	0.88	0.42
	Activity-induced energy expenditure	18–39	Mixed	12	8	0.82	0.64
McGue et al. (10)	Self-rated ability on athletic competition	27–80	Male	226	202	0.50[b]	0.26[b]
		27–86	Female	452	345		
McGuire et al. (11)	Perceived athletic self-competence	10–18	Male	45	49	0.58[b]	0.23[b]
		10–18	Female	47	48		

[a]55% and 50% males in MZ and DZ twins, respectively
[b]Coefficients adjusted for sex

Both moderate and vigorous activities showed significant familial clustering. The odds ratios for a twin to engage in physical activity when his co-twin also engaged in the same activity ranged from 1.25 (95%CI 1.21–.30) to 4.60 (2.89–7.30). For the heritability analyses, only twin pairs who were in contact with each other at least once per month as adults were selected. Twin correlations for all activities were greater in MZ pairs ($n=1006$) than in DZ pairs ($n=530$). However, the heritability estimates were greater for vigorous activities such as jogging/running (0.53), racquet sports (0.48) and bicycling (0.58) than for moderate activities (from 0.12 to 0.40).

Participation in sports activity may be influenced by genetic factors. In a study based on 1294 families including both parents and 1587 pairs of MZ and DZ twins, an estimated heritability of 45% for sports participation was reported (7). The remaining phenotypic variance was attributed to shared familial environment (44%) and environmental factors unique to each individual (11%). In the Leuven Longitudinal Twin Study, Beunen and Thomis reported that additive genetic factors explained 44% and 83% of the variation in a sports participation index in 15-year-old girls and boys, respectively (8). Similarly, Maia et al. detected greater heritabilities for a sports participation index and leisure-time physical activity in Portuguese boys (63–68%) than in girls (32–40%) (9). Moreover, it was suggested that psychological factors affecting sports participation may be characterized by a significant genetic component. In a cohort of 678 MZ and 547 DZ twin pairs, aged 27 to 86 years, an index of self-rated ability in athletic competition showed a genetic effect of 50.5% while the remaining 49.5% of the variance was due to nonshared environmental factors (10). A similar estimate of genetic effect was derived from data of 92 MZ twin pairs, 97 DZ twin pairs and 94 full sibling pairs, aged 10 to 18 years. The genetic effect for perceived athletic self-competence was 54% whereas nonshared environmental factors contributed an additional 42% of the variance (11).

Stubbe et al. investigated sport participation in a cohort of 2628 Dutch twin pairs aged 13 to 20 years (12). Sports participation was defined as engagement in leisure-time sports activities (competitive or non-competitive) with an intensity of 4 METs or more for at least 60 minutes per week. The cohort was divided in four 2-year age strata for statistical analyses. In younger twins (13–14 and 15–16 years), the tetrachoric twin correlations for sports participation were high (0.68–0.88) and did not differ between mono- and dizygotic twins. In older twins (17–18 and 19–20 years), however, the correlations were high (0.80–0.88) in monozygotic twins, but low to moderate (0.35–0.68) in dizygotic twins. Structural equation models confirmed that shared environmental factors explained the majority of the variance (c^2 from 0.78–0.84) in sports participation in younger twins, whereas the contribution of genetic factors started to emerge in older twins. The heritability estimates for sports participation were 36% and 85% in 17- to 18-year-old and 19- to 20-year-old twins, respectively (12).

The lack of genetic effect on sports participation in younger twins is in agreement with the observations by Franks and co-workers in 100 sex-concordant, 4- to 10-year-old twin pairs (13). Neither questionnaire-based physical activity level nor physical activity energy expenditure (assessed with doubly labelled water) showed significant genetic component. Shared and unique environmental factors explained 65% to 69% and 31% to 35% of the variance in these two physical activity traits, respectively (13). Joosen et al. investigated activity-induced energy expenditure (2-week doubly labelled water) and physical activity levels (triaxial accelerometer) in a small sample of 20 pairs of 18- to 39-year old twins (14). In agreement with the observations in older twins by Stubbe et al. intraclass correlations for both activity traits were higher in MZ than in DZ twins. Genetic factors explained 72% and 78% of the variance in activity-induced energy expenditure and physical activity level, respectively, while shared environment explained the remaining variance (14).

Family Studies
Physical activity levels and patterns in children and their parents tend to be similar. Only a few studies of familial aggregation of activity level and sports participation will be summarized here. In 100 children, aged 4 to 7 years, and 99 mothers and 92 fathers from the Framingham Children's Study (15), data on habitual physical activity were obtained with an accelerometer for about 10 hours per day for an average of 9 days in children and 8 days in fathers and mothers over the course of one year. Active fathers or active mothers were more likely to have active offspring than inactive fathers or mothers, with odds ratios of 3.5 and 2.0, respectively. When both parents were active, the children were 5.8 times more likely to be active as children of two inactive parents. These results are thus compatible with the notion that genetic or other factors transmitted across generations predispose a child to be active or inactive.

In the 1981 Canada Fitness Survey, a total of 18,073 individuals living in households across Canada completed a questionnaire on physical activity habits (16). Detailed information on the frequency, duration and intensity of activities performed on a daily, weekly, monthly and yearly basis was used to estimate average daily energy expenditure for each individual. Familial correlations were 0.28, 0.12 and 0.21 for spouses ($n = 1024$ pairs), parents and offspring ($n = 1622$ pairs), and sibling pairs ($n = 1036$), respectively. The lower correlations in parent-offspring and sibling pairs compared to spouses suggest only a small contribution of genetic factors in the familial aggregation of leisure-time energy expenditure.

In the Phase 1 of the Québec Family Study (QFS), path analysis procedures (17) were used to estimate the relative contribution of genetic and non-genetic factors to activity level. Two different indicators of physical activity, habitual physical activity and participation in moderate to vigorous physical activity, were obtained from a 3-day activity record completed by 1610 subjects from 375 families encompassing nine types of relatives by descent or adoption. Most of the variation in the two indicators of habitual physical activity level was accounted for by non-transmissible environmental factors, with values reaching 71% for habitual physical activity and 88% for exercise participation. The transmission effect across generations was also significant. The estimate for habitual physical activity was 29%, and it was entirely attributable to genetic factors. The corresponding estimate for participation in moderate to vigorous physical activity was 12%, and it was accounted for by cultural transmission with no genetic effect. Since habitual physical activity was computed as the sum of all activities, and participation in moderate to vigorous activity included only more vigorous activities, low intensity activities were probably those characterized by the significant genetic effect. The results were thus interpreted as an indication of inherited differences in the propensity to be spontaneously active or inactive (17). Simonen et al. investigated familial aggregation of physical activity level in nuclear families from the Phase 2 of the QFS (18). Maximal heritabilities derived from the maximum likelihood estimates of familial correlations reached 25%, 16% and 19% for the degree of inactivity, time spent in moderate to strenuous physical activities, and total level of physical activity, respectively (18).

EVIDENCE FROM MOLECULAR STUDIES

Data on molecular genetics of physical activity levels in humans are still scarce. However, animal studies provide several examples how naturally occurring mutations and artificially–induced changes in key genes may affect physical activity patterns. For example, mice lacking the dopamine transporter gene exhibit marked hyperactivity (19), whereas dopamine receptor D2 (Drd2) deficient mice are characterized by reduced physical activity levels (20). Likewise, disruption of the melanin-concentrating hormone pathway leads to hyperactivity. Mice lacking the pro-melanin-concentrating hormone (*PMCH*) gene or carrying an inactive form of the PMCH gene are lean and hyperactive, although their food intake is normal (21–23). In addition, melanin-concentrating hormone receptor knockout mice develop the same hyperactivity phenotype as the PMCH deficient animals (21,24,25).

An example of the potential involvement of a spontaneous gene mutation in physical activity regulation comes from the fruit fly (*Drosophila melanogaster*). These insects exhibit two distinct activity patterns related to food-search behavior; rovers move about twice the distance while feeding compared to sitters. This activity pattern is genetically determined and is regulated by the *dg2* gene, which encodes a cGMP-dependent protein kinase (PKG) (26). PKG activity is significantly higher in wild-type rovers than in wild type and mutant sitters and activation of the *dg2* gene reverts foraging behavior from a sitter to a rover. Furthermore, overexpression of the *dg2* gene in sitters changed their behavior to the rover phenotype (26).

Association Studies

Only a few association studies on DNA sequence variation in candidate genes and physical activity traits are available. The candidate genes with positive findings include *DRD2*, angiotensin-converting enzyme (*ACE*), leptin receptor (*LEPR*), melanocortin 4 receptor (*MC4R*), calcium-sensing receptor (*CASR*), and aromatase (*CYP19A1*). The first four genes were investigated with an a priori hypothesis on the association between physical activity and DNA sequence variation (27–30). In the other studies, the activity traits were treated as covariates in association analyses focusing on other target traits (bone mineral density) (31,32).

Simonen et al. investigated the associations between physical activity phenotypes and DNA sequence variation in the *DRD2* gene locus in the QFS and the HERITAGE Family Study subjects (29). In both cohorts, a C/T transition in codon 313 of the gene was associated with physical activity levels in White women. The T/T homozygote women of the QFS reported significantly less weekly activities during the previous year than the heterozygotes and the C/C homozygotes. Similarly, among the White women of the HERITAGE Family Study, the T/T homozygotes showed lower sports and work indices derived from the ARIC-Baecke questionnaire than the other genotypes. No associations were found in males or in Black women (29). Also in the QFS cohort, Loos et al. reported significant associations between a C/T polymorphism located 2745 base pairs upstream of the *MC4R* gene start codon and physical activity phenotypes (30). Homozygotes for the rare T-allele had significantly lower moderate-to-strenuous physical activity levels and higher inactivity score than the other genotypes (Fig. 1).

In Pima Indians, a glutamine (Gln) to arginine (Arg) substitution in codon 223 of the *LEPR* gene was associated with total physical activity, calculated by dividing 24-hour energy expenditure by sleeping energy expenditure measured in a respiratory chamber. The Arg233Arg homozygotes showed about 5% lower physical activity level than the Gln223Gln homozygotes (27). Winnicki et al. investigated the determinants of habitual physical activity level in a group of never-treated stage I hypertensives (28). Physical activity was assessed by a questionnaire and the subjects were classified as sedentary or exercisers (leisure or sports activities at least once a week during the previous two months). The *ACE* I/D genotype, age, sex, marital status, profession, and coffee and alcohol consumption were included as predictors of physical activity level in the regression model. The *ACE* genotype and marital status were the strongest contributors to physical activity status. The frequency of the D/D genotype was significantly higher in the sedentary group than among active subjects approximately 76% of the D/D homozygotes were sedentary, whereas the corresponding frequency in the I-allele homozygotes was 48% (28).

Lorentzon et al. investigated the associations between the *CASR* gene polymorphism and bone mineral density and its predictors, including habitual physical activity, in adolescent Swedish girls (31). The weekly amount of weight-bearing

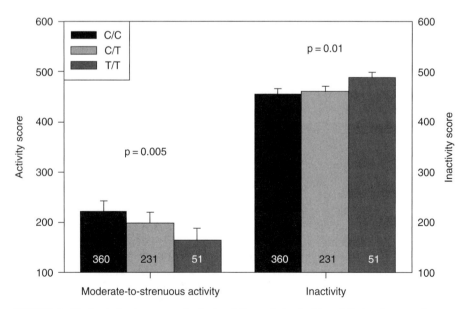

FIGURE 1 Moderate-to-strenuous physical activity and physical inactivity levels according to a melanocortin 4 receptor (*MC4R*) genotype in the Quebec Family Study cohort. The MC4R polymorphism is a C/T transition located 2745 base pairs upstream of the *MC4R* gene start codon. *Source*: From Ref. 30.

physical activity during the previous year was estimated using a standardized questionnaire, and a G/T transversion in codon 986 inducing an alanine to serine substitution was genotyped with a polymerase chain reaction – restriction fragment length polymorphism method. Carriers of the serine allele reported about 1.4 hours less physical activity per week than the homozygotes for the alanine allele (31). In post-menopausal Finnish women, a TTTA repeat in intron 4 of the *CYP19A1* gene was not associated with bone mineral density, fracture risk or circulating estradiol levels (32). Physical activity was the only predictor of bone health that was associated with the *CYP19A1* genotype. The proportion of physically active persons, defined as 3 or more hours of physical activity per week, was 36.6%, 25.7%, and 19.6% in women with short, midsize and long TTTA repeats, respectively (32).

Linkage Studies

The first genome-wide linkage scan for physical activity traits was carried out in the Québec Family Study cohort (33). The scan was based on 432 polymorphic markers genotyped in 767 subjects from 207 families. Physical activity measures were derived from a 3-day activity diary (total daily activity, inactivity, moderate to strenuous activity), and an 11-item questionnaire (weekly physical activity during the past year). The strongest evidence of linkage (P = 0.0012) was detected on chromosome 2p22-p16 with the physical inactivity phenotype. Suggestive linkages were also found on 13q22 with total daily activity and moderate to strenuous activity phenotypes, and on 7p11 with both inactivity and moderate to strenuous activity. In addition, weekly activity during the past year showed suggestive evidence of linkage on 11p15 and 15q13, inactivity on 20q12, and moderate to strenuous activity on 4q31 and 9q31 (33).

ARE THERE EPIGENETIC EFFECTS?

In recent years, a growing body of evidence has emphasized that DNA sequence variation was extremely important in accounting for individual differences in behavior, physiology and response to drugs or lifestyle interventions. However, another line of evidence has highlighted that DNA and histone chemical modifications (see Chapters 7.1 and 7.2) could also translate in phenotypic differences that often mimicked those associated with DNA sequence variants. These DNA and nucleoproteins alterations have been collectively referred to as "epigenetic events". These epigenetic events begin to occur early after fertilization, are thought to take place in utero and even throughout the lifespan, are typically stable and influence gene expression. Is there any evidence for a contribution of epigenetics to human variation in physical activity levels?

There is no direct evidence for a contribution of any DNA methylation event or histone biochemical alterations to physical activity level for the simple reason that the issue has not been considered yet. However, there are experimental data which are highly compatible with the hypothesis that epigenetics has the potential to influence the spontaneous level of physical activity. For instance, in one such experiment, Vickers et al. investigated whether maternal undernutrition throughout pregnancy resulted in differences in postnatal locomotor behavior (34). Female Wistar rats received only 30% of the ad libitum intake of the control females during pregnancy. The offspring of restricted mothers were significantly smaller at

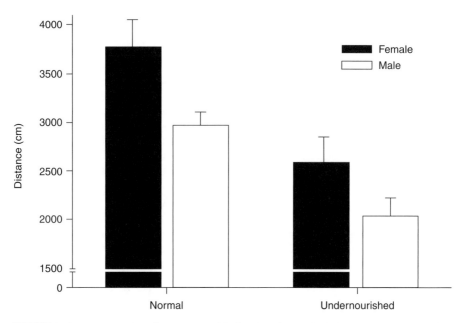

FIGURE 2 Locomotor activity in 14-month-old offspring of normally fed and undernourished (30% of normal intake) mothers. Effects of fetal maternal nutrition and gender are statistically significant ($P < 0.005$ for both). *Source*: From Ref. 34.

birth. At ages, 35 days, 145 days and 420 days, the voluntary locomotor activity of the offspring of the two groups were assessed. At all ages, the offspring of the undernourished mothers were significantly less active, and the findings are illustrated in Fig. 2 for the 420 days time point. These results suggested that the effects of undernutrition during pregnancy persisted during postnatal life. This effect persisted even when offspring were overnourished during postnatal life.

CONCLUSION

The lack of regular physical activity has been recognized as a major risk factor for several chronic diseases, including cardiovascular diseases (CVD), type 2 diabetes and obesity. Regular exercise training has been shown to have beneficial effects on several risk factors of CVD and diabetes. However, low adherence to exercise programs impedes the preventive and therapeutic potential of regular exercise as a preventive measure. Thus, it is important to understand the factors contributing to the likelihood that an individual will adopt a physically active lifestyle. Contribution of genetic factors to physical activity levels has been evaluated in twin and family studies. Maximal heritability estimates derived from studies using mono- and dizygotic twins have ranged from 20% to 80% for various physical activity traits. Family studies have also indicated that a child is more likely to be physically active if at least one of the parents is active, with heritability estimates being between 19% and 30%. In terms of molecular basis, the research on genetics of physical activity in humans is still in its infancy. However, data from the first human studies and several animal models suggest that several genes encoding neurotransmitters, their transporters and receptors contribute to variation in spontaneous physical activity patterns.

REFERENCES

1. Rowland TW. The biological basis of physical activity. Medicine and Science in Sports and Exercise 1998; 30:392–9.
2. Thorburn AW, Proietto J. Biological determinants of spontaneous physical activity. Obes Rev 2000; 1:87–94.
3. Kaprio J, Koskenvuo M, Sarna S. Cigarette smoking, use of alcohol, and leisure-time physical activity among same-sexed adult male twins. Prog Clin Biol Res 1981; 69:37–46.
4. Heller RF, O'Connell DL, Roberts DC, et al. Lifestyle factors in monozygotic and dizygotic twins. Genetic Epidemiology 1988; 5:311–21.
5. Aarnio M, Winter T, Kujala UM, et al. Familial aggregation of leisure-time physical activity – a three generation study. Int J Sports Med 1997; 18:549–56.
6. Lauderdale DS, Fabsitz R, Meyer JM, et al. Familial determinants of moderate and intense physical activity: a twin study. Medicine and Science in Sports and Exercise 1997; 29:1062–8.
7. Koopmans JR, Van Doornen LJP, Boomsma DI. Smoking and sports participation. In: Godlbourt U, De Faire U, Berg K, eds. Genetic factors in coronary heart disease. Lancaster: Kluwer Academic, 1994:217–35.
8. Beunen G, Thomis M. Genetic determinants of sports participation and daily physical activity. Int J Obes Relat Metab Disord 1999; 23:S55–63.
9. Maia JA, Thomis M, Beunen G. Genetic factors in physical activity levels. A twin study. Amer J Prev Med 2002; 23:87–91.
10. McGue M, Hirsch B, Lykken DT. Age and the self-perception of ability: a twin study analysis. Psychol Aging 1993; 8:72–80.
11. McGuire S, Neiderhiser JM, Reiss D, et al. Genetic and environmental influences on perceptions of self-worth and competence in adolescence: a study of twins, full siblings, and step- siblings. Child Dev 1994; 65:785–99.
12. Stubbe JH, Boomsma DI, De Geus EJ. Sports participation during adolescence: a shift from environmental to genetic factors. Med Sci Sports Exerc 2005; 37:563–70.
13. Franks PW, Ravussin E, Hanson RL, et al. Habitual physical activity in children: the role of genes and the environment. Am J Clin Nutr 2005; 82:901–8.
14. Joosen AM, Gielen M, Vlietinck R, et al. Genetic analysis of physical activity in twins. Am J Clin Nutr 2005; 82:1253–9.
15. Moore LL, Lombardi DA, White MJ, et al. Influence of parents' physical activity levels on activity levels of young children. J Pediatr 1991; 118:215–9.
16. Perusse L, Leblanc C, Bouchard C. Familial resemblance in lifestyle components: results from the Canada Fitness Survey. Can J Public Health 1988; 79:201–5.
17. Perusse L, Tremblay A, Leblanc C, et al. Genetic and environmental influences on level of habitual physical activity and exercise participation. Am J Epidemiol 1989; 129:1012–22.
18. Simonen RL, Perusse L, Rankinen T, et al. Familial aggregation of physical activity levels in the Quebec family study. Medicine and Science in Sports and Exercise 2002; 34:1137–42.
19. Gainetdinov RR, Wetsel WC, Jones SR, et al. Role of serotonin in the paradoxical calming effect of psychostimulants on hyperactivity. Science 1999; 283:397–401.
20. Kelly MA, Rubinstein M, Phillips TJ, et al. Locomotor activity in D2 dopamine receptor-deficient mice is determined by gene dosage, genetic background, and developmental adaptations. J Neurosci 1998; 18:3470–9.
21. Zhou D, Shen Z, Strack AM, et al. Enhanced running wheel activity of both Mch1r- and Pmch-deficient mice. Regul Pept 2005; 124:53–63.
22. Kokkotou E, Jeon JY, Wang X, et al. Mice with MCH ablation resist diet-induced obesity through strain-specific mechanisms. Am J Physiol Regul Integr Comp Physiol 2005; 289:R117–24.
23. Segal-Lieberman G, Bradley RL, Kokkotou E, et al. Melanin-concentrating hormone is a critical mediator of the leptin-deficient phenotype. Proc Natl Acad Sci USA 2003; 100:10085–90.

24. Astrand A, Bohlooly YM, Larsdotter S, et al. Mice lacking melanin-concentrating hormone receptor 1 demonstrate increased heart rate associated with altered autonomic activity. Am J Physiol Regul Integr Comp Physiol 2004; 287:R749–58.

25. Marsh DJ, Weingarth DT, Novi DE, et al. Melanin-concentrating hormone 1 receptor-deficient mice are lean, hyperactive, and hyperphagic and have altered metabolism. Proc Natl Acad Sci U SA 2002; 99:3240–5.

26. Osborne KA, Robichon A, Burgess E, et al. Natural behavior polymorphism due to a cGMP-dependent protein kinase of Drosophila. Science 1997; 277:834–6.

27. Stefan N, Vozarova B, Del Parigi A, et al. The Gln223Arg polymorphism of the leptin receptor in Pima Indians: influence on energy expenditure, physical activity and lipid metabolism. Int J Obes Relat Metab Disord 2002; 26:1629–32.

28. Winnicki M, Accurso V, Hoffmann M, et al. Physical activity and angiotensin-converting enzyme gene polymorphism in mild hypertensives. Am J Med Genet A 2004; 125:38–44.

29. Simonen RL, Rankinen T, Perusse L, et al. A dopamine D2 receptor gene polymorphism and physical activity in two family studies. Physiol Behav 2003; 78:751–7.

30. Loos RJ, Rankinen T, Tremblay A, et al. Melanocortin-4 receptor gene and physical activity in the Quebec Family Study. Int J Obes (Lond). 2005; 29:420–8.

31. Lorentzon M, Lorentzon R, Lerner UH, et al. Calcium sensing receptor gene polymorphism, circulating calcium concentrations and bone mineral density in healthy adolescent girls. European J Endocrinol 2001; 144:257–61.

32. Salmen T, Heikkinen AM, Mahonen A, et al. Relation of aromatase gene polymorphism and hormone replacement therapy to serum estradiol levels, bone mineral density, and fracture risk in early postmenopausal women. Ann Med 2003; 35:282–8.

33. Simonen RL, Rankinen T, Perusse L, et al. Genome-wide linkage scan for physical activity levels in the Quebec Family study. Med Sci Sports Exerc 2003; 35:1355–9.

34. Vickers MH, Breier BH, McCarthy D, et al. Sedentary behavior during postnatal life is determined by the prenatal environment and exacerbated by postnatal hypercaloric nutrition. Am J Physiol Regul Integr Comp Physiol 2003; 285:R271–3.

7.3 Interaction Between Genes and Lifestyle Factors

Ruth J.F. Loos, Karani S. Vimaleswaran, and Nicholas J. Wareham
Medical Research Council (MRC) Epidemiology Unit, Cambridge, U.K.

The current global obesity epidemic has developed only over the past three decades and cannot be explained by changes in our genome. It is more likely due to a changing environment that promotes excessive calorie intake and discourages physical activity, behaviors that are poorly compensated for, by our pre-agricultural hunter-gatherer genes. Our genome has evolved in times of food scarcity, when the risk of famine was ever present and large amounts of physical effort were required to obtain food. Genes that may have provided a survival advantage under these circumstances may, in the present-day sedentary, food-abundant society, predispose to obesity (1). It is likely that susceptibility to obesity is partly determined by genetic factors, but that an 'obesity-promoting' lifestyle is necessary for its phenotypic expression.

This chapter describes the evidence for gene-lifestyle interactions in the etiology of obesity. The terminology in this field is still contentious and the concept of 'gene-environment interaction' means different things to different people largely depending on the type of research they are involved with. To the epidemiologist and statistician, a gene-environment interaction is defined as the relationship between an environmental exposure (e.g., diet and physical activity) and a disease phenotype that differs in magnitude (Fig. 1A) or differ in direction (Fig. 1B) depending on the genotype carried at a specific locus. The biologist might interpret it as the direct biological effect of one factor on another within the same biological pathway. These definitions have different implications. Throughout this chapter, we will use the epidemiological definition of interaction.

In this overview, we first describe how epidemiological studies have provided evidence for gene-lifestyle interaction in the etiology of obesity. Subsequently, we review candidate gene studies that have examined how lifestyle factors, such as diet and physical activity, influence the association between gene variants and weight change and how genetic variation modifies an individual's responsiveness to diet and physical activity in relation to weight change.

EVIDENCE FROM EPIDEMIOLOGICAL STUDIES

There is a synergistic relationship between genes and environment in the etiology of obesity. The severity of obesity will be determined by lifestyle and environmental conditions on a background of the individual's genetic predisposition. Individuals with a high genetic predisposition for obesity who live in an obesogenic environment will gain the most weight. In an environment that does not favor obesity, these individuals would still be overweight. Individuals with a slight predisposition to obesity will be normal weight in a restrictive environment, whereas in an obesogenic environment many of them will become overweight or

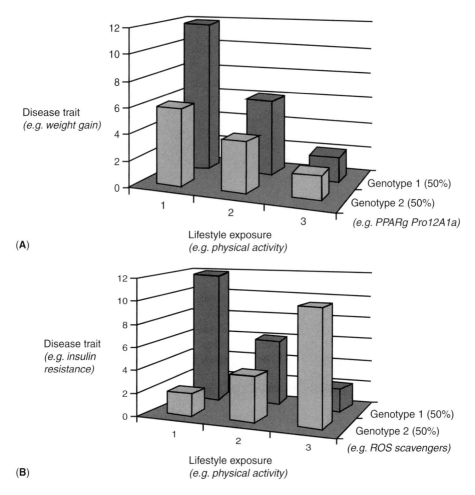

FIGURE 1 (**A**) A gene-lifestyle interaction occurs when the relationships between an environmental exposure and a phenotypic outcome differ in magnitude when stratified by genetic subgroup. (**B**) Where the direction of association between the lifestyle factor and disease trait differ when stratified by genotype, the main effects of the genetic or lifestyle factors may be indiscernible unless the effect of interaction is taken into account. *Abbreviations*: PPARG, peroxisome proliferation-activated receptor gamma; ROS, reactive oxygen species. *Source*: Adapted from Ref. 163.

obese. Some are genetically resistant to obesity and will remain normal weight in a wide range of obesogenic conditions.

Migration Studies
Suggestive evidence for gene-lifestyle interaction in the development of chronic disease such as obesity was first provided by migration studies in which genetically related populations living different lifestyles are compared.

An example of such a gene-lifestyle interaction comes from the Pima Indians, a population apparently predisposed to obesity and type 2 diabetes. Of the Pima Indians living in the 'restrictive' environment of the remote Mexican Sierra Madre Mountains only 13% (BMI: 24.9 (SD 4.0) kg/m^2 (mean (SD)) are obese compared to 69% of those living in the 'obesogenic' environment of Arizona (BMI: 33.4 (7.5) kg/m^2) ($p < 0.0001$) (3). Although Mexican and USA Pima Indians are genetically closely related, the environment they live in is very different. Mexican Pima Indians get 26% of their energy intake from dietary fat and spend 23.9 (13.3) h/wk on occupational activities, whereas USA Pima Indians' diet consists of 35% of dietary fats, while they spend only 12.6 (13.9) h/wk on occupational activities (4). These findings show that, despite a similar genetic predisposition to obesity, different lifestyles result in a clearly different prevalence of obesity.

Prospective studies have reported significant increases in BMI following migration to a new country. A study of 654 Tokelauans who migrated from a Pacific Atoll living a subsistence lifestyle to New Zealand living a Westernized lifestyle showed an increase in BMI from 24.1 to 28.7 kg/m^2 between 1968 and 1982, whereas BMI of non-migrants rose only from 24.8 to 26.1 kg/m^2 (5). Similar findings were reported in Japanese migrating to the USA or Hawaii (6).

Other studies compared first generation with second and third generation migrants, under the assumption that the first generation migrants will hold on longer to the traditional lifestyle, whereas the later generation migrants will adopt the lifestyle of the 'new' country more thoroughly. In a study with 2791 Mexican-American men and women from the third National Health and Nutrition Examination Survey (NHANES III), waist circumference and BMI of Mexico-born and US-born Mexicans were compared. The Mexico-born women and men had a smaller waist circumference (90.4 (13.1) cm and 94.0 (9.9) cm, respectively) and lower BMI (27.8 (5.5) kg/m^2 and 26.9 (4.0) kg/m^2, respectively) than the US-born English speaking Mexican Americans (93.6 (15.0) cm ($p = 0.02$) and 97.3 (13.0) ($p < 0.001$) cm for waist circumference and 29.1 (6.8) kg/m^2 and 28.2 (5.0) kg/m^2 for BMI, respectively) (7). Similar findings had been reported by the Hispanic Health and Nutrition Examination Survey (HHANES); i.e., Mexican-Americans of the second generation had a significantly higher BMI ($+1.15$ kg/m^2 ($p < 0.0001$) for men and $+1.76$ kg/m^2 ($p < 0.0001$) for women) compared to the first generation (8).

These migration studies have provided first suggestive evidence for gene-environment interaction in the development of obesity; i.e., despite a similar genetic background, lifestyle changes/differences resulted in increased obesity. However, these studies explain only one part of gene-environment interaction as they did not allow comparison with other populations that had a different genetic background but that underwent the same lifestyle changes. This should be kept in mind when interpreting the findings of migration studies in view of gene-lifestyle interaction.

Twin Studies

Several well-controlled twin studies have provided additional evidence concerning the role of genetic factors in the response to diet and exercise intervention.

In a 100-day overfeeding study (9), 12 male monozygotic pairs ate a 1000 kcal per day surplus (6 day/wk) over the energy cost for weight maintenance. Overfeeding induced significant increases in weight and fat mass. The mean weight gain for the 24 participants was 8.1 kg, but there were considerable differences in the adaptation to excess energy intake with a threefold difference between the lowest and highest gainers (range about 4–12 kg). However, this heterogeneity in the response was not randomly distributed across genotypes; there was at least three times more variance between pairs than within pairs in the gains of weight and fat mass (F ratios $= 3.4$ ($p < 0.02$) and 3.0 ($p < 0.05$), respectively). Significant genotype-overfeeding interactions were also observed for most of the other body composition and fat distribution phenotypes.

Along the same lines, 14 pairs of female MZ twins completed a 4-week, very low-calorie diet (1.6 MJ/d) (10). The twins lost on average 8.8 kg of weight and 6.5 kg of fat mass. The weight loss, however, varied from 5.9 to 12.4 kg for body weight and 3.5 to 12 kg for fat mass. Again, these changes were not randomly distributed. There was 12.8 times ($p < 0.001$) more variability in weight loss between pairs than within pairs, and the F ratio for fat mass change was even greater (17.0; $p < 0.001$).

Similar results were found in another weight loss study with twins in whom a negative energy balance was induced by exercise training (11). In this study, seven MZ twin pairs of young adult men completed a study protocol during which they exercised on cycle ergometers twice a day, 9 out of 10 days, over a period of 93 days while being kept on a constant daily energy intake. The mean total energy deficit caused by exercise above the estimated energy cost of weight maintenance reached about 58,000 Kcal (244 MJ). The men lost on average 5.0 kg in body weight, ranging from 1 kg to about 8 kg. Intra-pair resemblance was observed for changes in weight, fat mass, fat percentage and subcutaneous fat. Even though there were large individual differences in response to the negative energy balance, men with the same genotype responded more alike than men with different genotypes. The F ratio of the between-pair to the within-pair variance was 6.8 ($p = 0.01$) for weight loss and 14.1 ($p < 0.01$) for fat mass.

These findings indicate that, in response to overfeeding, a short-term, very low-calorie diet, or an exercise training intervention, some individuals will gain or lose weight more easily than others, but that individuals of the same genotype respond in a more similar way than unrelated individuals.

EVIDENCE FROM CANDIDATE GENE STUDIES

The evidence that both genetic and environmental factors are important in the atiology of obesity is strong (12,13), but biological basis for their interactions need to be determined. Various genes are now being studied for their potential interactions with diet and physical activity (14,15). There has been a growing recognition that diet and physical activity can have important effects on gene expression by interacting directly with transcription factors that control the expression of specific genes through regulatory elements in the promoter region or by altering the stability of mRNA (16–18). For example, glucose and fatty acids, mainly Polyunsaturated fatty acids (PUFAs), regulate fundamental adipose cell and liver functions through binding to nuclear receptors that act as nutrient sensors such as peroxisome proliferator-activated receptors (PPARs), sterol regulatory element binding transcription factors (SREBPs or SREBFs) and carbohydrate responsive element-binding protein (ChREBP), leading to changes in their transcriptional activity (18). Subsequently, these nuclear receptors bind in the promoter region of a large number of genes involved in metabolic pathways that are important in energy homeostasis. Physical activity and exercise increase the expression of many genes in the skeletal muscle through transcriptional activity and increased mRNA stability (16). The molecular mechanisms linking exercise to the transcriptional regulation of exercise-responsive genes remain to be fully elucidated. However, a number of initiating stimuli that activate specific signaling pathways, including calcium, energy charge (ATP/ADP), redox state (NAD/NADH), oxygen tension, mechanical stretch, neuroregulatory peptides, free radicals, growth factors and cytokines (Interleukine, IL6), known to be altered in the skeletal muscle in response to exercise and contractile activity, have been proposed as exercise-induced gene regulators (19–21). An acute bout of exercise is sufficient to increase the expression of genes, both during and in the period following exercise, whereas habitual endurance exercise training enhances the oxidative capacity and metabolic efficiency of the muscle (22) through cumulative effects of transient changes in gene expression that occur in response to each exercise bout (23). Increases in solute carrier family 2 (facilitated glucose transporter), member 4 (*SLC2A4* or *GLUT4*) (24,25), pyruvate dehydrogenase kinase 4 (*PDK4*) (26), NRF1 (27,28), peroxisome proliferator-activated receptor gamma (*PPARG*), coactivator 1 alpha (*PPARGC1A*) (27,29,30), lipoprotein lipase (*LPL*) (31,32), hexokinase 2 (*HK2*) (33) and Uncoupling protein (*UCP3*) mRNA (34,35) have been observed in response to various exercise protocols in both rats and humans.

In this chapter, we summarise the evidence for gene-diet and gene-physical activity interactions for sets of genes that in at least three studies have been associated with changes in body weight and body fatness in response to specific experimental conditions, such as weight loss interventions, short-term overfeeding interventions, or exercise training interventions. We also include observational studies that examine weight change over time. Although less controlled than interventions studies, these longitudinal studies reflect individual responsiveness to the obesogenic environment they share. Table 1– 4 summarize the findings on these and other candidate genes that have been reported for their association with weight change in interaction with the environment.

Peroxisome Proliferation-Activated Receptor Gamma

Peroxisome proliferation-activated receptors (PPARs) are members of the nuclear hormone receptor subfamily of ligand-regulated transcription factors (99). PPARs act by binding to the promoter region as a heterodimer with retinoid X receptor (RXR) and regulate the transcription of genes involved in lipid and glucose metabolism (100,101). There are currently three known isoforms; peroxisome proliferator-activated receptor alpha (PPARA); peroxisome proliferator-activated receptor delta (PPARD); and PPARG. They bind to similar peroxisome proliferator response elements (PPREs), but exhibit different transactivation functions that are mediated, in part, by tissue distribution, ligand specificity, and coactivator recruitment (100-102). The peroxisome proliferation-activated receptor gamma (PPARG) isoform, which represents a more restricted pattern of expression than PPARA and PPARD, is predominantly expressed in white adipose tissue and, at lower levels, in skeletal muscle (103,104). PPARG has a regulatory role in adipogenesis by modulating the expression of target genes involved in adipocyte differentiation (105,106). Both diet and exercise influence *PPARG* expression. Antagonism of PPARG using a synthetic ligand has been shown to suppress the increased adiposity observed in high-fat diet-induced obesity (107). Fatty acids, in particular PUFAs, are potent ligands for PPARG that through binding the receptor change PPARG conformation

(*Text continues on page 307*)

TABLE 1 Intervention Trials and Observational Studies Reporting Gene-Environment Interactions in Relation to Weight Change for ADRB-genes

Gene	Polymorphism	Population	Interaction with overfeeding (intervention) or weight gain over time (observational)	Interaction with weight loss (intervention) and specific nutrient intake (observational)	Interactions with exercise training (intervention) and physical activity level (observational)
ADRB1	Gly49Ser	761 healthy women (36)	Gly49-allele carriers gained more weight during a 15-year follow-up compared to Ser49Ser homozygotes ($p = 0.018$)		
ADRB2	Gln27Glu	836 men and women between 35 and 64 yrs (37)			In sedentary men, Gln27Gln homozygotes had a 3.45 increased risk of obesity compared to Glu27-allele carriers ($p = 0.002$). The risk was not increased in physically active men. (p for interaction = 0.009)
		24 normal weight young adult twins (134)	Gln27Gln homozygotes gained more weight ($p < 0.001$) and subcutaneous fat ($p < 0.005$) after 100 days overfeeding compared to Glu27-allele carriers		
		139 obese and 113 lean women (38)			In physically active women, the Glu27-allele carriers have a higher BMI compared to the Gln27Gln homozygotes ($p = 0.003$). No differences in BMI in sedentary women. (p for interaction = 0.005)
	Arg16Gly	1151 African American children and adolescents (40)	Over 24-yr follow-up, Gly16Gly men had a more pronounced increase in BMI and subscapular skinfold ($p < 0.05$) than Arg16-allele carriers		
		286 young adults who gained 12.8 kg vs. 296	In men, weight gainers were more often Gly16Gly or Arg16Arg		

	who were weight stable over the previous 6.8 yrs (41)	homozygous than Arg16Gly heterozygous ($p = 0.04$). In women, Gly16gly homozygotes were more often weight stable ($p = 0.05$).
	482 Caucasian men and women of the HERITAGE Family Study (42)	In women, Gly16-allele carriers lost less weight ($p = 0.04$) and body fat ($p = 0.0003$) after a 20-wk endurance-training program than Arg16Arg homozygotes.
	160 young nonobese men (43)	Weight gainers, defined as gaining >10% increase in BMI over 5 yrs, were more often Gly16-allele carriers than Arg16Arg homozygotes ($p < 0.05$).
ADRB3 Trp64Arg	185 morbidly obese patients (44)	Trp64Trp homozygotes gained less weight over a period of 25 yrs that Arg64-allele carriers ($p = 0.007$)
	Non-diabetic obese Japanese women (45)	Arg64-allele carriers lost less weight after a 12-wk weight loss program (diet + exercise) than Trp64Trp homozygotes ($p < 0.05$)
	292 morbidly obese men and women (46)	In women, Arg64-allele carriers have gained more weight over a 20-yr follow-up than Trp64Trp homozygotes ($p = 0.017$).
	186 normal weight Japanese men (47)	Trp64Trp homozygotes gained more weight over a period of 25 years ($p = 0.013$) than Arg64-allele carriers.
	61 diabetic obese Japanese women (48)	Arg64-allele carriers lost less weight after a 12-wk weight loss program (diet + exercise) than Trp64Trp homozygotes ($p < 0.05$)

(Continued)

TABLE 1 Intervention Trials and Observational Studies Reporting Gene-Environment Interactions in Relation to Weight Change for ADRB-genes *(Continued)*

Gene	Polymorphism	Population	Interaction with overfeeding (intervention) or weight gain over time (observational)	Interaction with weight loss (intervention) and specific nutrient intake (observational)	Interactions with exercise training (intervention) and physical activity level (observational)
		457 men of an unselected sample of Southern Italy (49)	Arg64-allele carriers have a higher probability of developing overweight over a 20-yr follow-up than Trp64Trp homozygotes ($p = 0.02$).		
		313 obese and lean Spanish men and women between 20–60 yrs (50)			In sedentary individuals, Arg64-carriers had an increased obesity risk compared to Trp64Trp64 homozygotes ($p = 0.05$). The obesity risk in physically active people was not different between genotypes. (*p* for interaction = 0.06)
		76 perimenopausal Japanese women (51)		Arg64-allele carriers lost less weight after a 12-wk weight loss program (diet + exercise) than Trp64Trp homozygotes ($p = 0.035$)	
		46 Japanese children of short stature (52)	The Arg64-allele carriers gained more weight during a 5-year follow-up period (from age 1–6 years) than Trp64Trp homozygotes ($p < 0.05$).		
		295 healthy Japanese men (53)	The prevalence of overweight is 3.37 95%CI[1.12–10.16] higher in the Arg64-allele carriers than in Trp64Trp homozygotes, but only in men with the highest energy intake.		

TABLE 2 Intervention Trials and Observational Studies Reporting Gene-Environment Interactions for PPARG2 in Relation to Weight Change

Gene	Variant	Population	Interaction with overfeeding (intervention) or weight gain over time (observational)	Interaction with weight loss (intervention) and specific nutrient intake (observational)	Interactions with exercise training (intervention) and physical activity level (observational)
PPARG2	Pro12Ala	752 obese and 869 nonobese men (54)	In the obese group: Ala12Ala homozygotes gained more weight over 24 yrs ($p = 0.004$) In the lean group: Ala12Ala homozygotes gained less weight over 24 yrs ($p = 0.002$)		
		119 nondiabetic men and women (55)	Ala12-allele carriers gained more weight over a 10-yr period ($p = 0.009$)		
		70 postmenopausal overweight women (56)	Ala12-allele carriers gained more weight over a 12-mo follow-up after a weight loss intervention ($p < 0.01$)		
		592 nondiabetic men and women (57)		BMI is negatively related to the ratio of poly-unsaturated fats to saturated fats, but only in the Ala12-allele carriers (p for interaction $= 0.004$)	
		490 overweight individuals with impaired glucose tolerance (58)		Ala12Ala homozygotes lost more weight compared to Pro12-allele carriers after a 3-yr intensive diet and exercise intervention ($p = 0.043$)	

(Continued)

TABLE 2 Intervention Trials and Observational Studies Reporting Gene-Environment Interactions for PPARG2 in Relation to Weight Change (*Continued*)

Gene	Variant	Population	Interaction with overfeeding (intervention) or weight gain over time (observational)	Interaction with weight loss (intervention) and specific nutrient intake (observational)	Interactions with exercise training (intervention) and physical activity level (observational)
		2141 women of the Nurses' Health Study (59)		BMI is negatively related to the ratio of polyunsaturate fats to saturated fats and positively to the total dietary fat intake, but only in the Pro12Pro homozygotes ($p < 0.0001$), (p for interaction = 0.003) BMI is positively related to the total dietary fat intake, but only in the Pro12Pro homozygotes ($p = 0.0001$) (p for interaction < 0.005)	
		720 men and women of the QFS (63)			
		311 Finnish men and women followed up from birth and at age 7, 20, and 41 yrs (61)	Ala12-allele carriers gained less weight between age 7–20 yrs ($p = 0.043$). Ala12-allele carriers gained more weight between age 20–41 yrs ($p = 0.001$)		
		29 healthy young adults with a family history of type 2 diabetes (62)			Ala12-allele carriers lost more weight after a 10-wk training program ($p < 0.05$)

Abbreviations: ADRB, adrenergic receptor beta; QFS, Quebec Family study.

TABLE 3 Intervention Trials and Observational Studies Reporting Gene-Environment Interactions for UCP Genes in Relation to Weight Change

Gene	Variant	Population	Interaction with overfeeding (intervention) or weight gain over time (observational)	Interaction with weight loss (intervention) and specific nutrient intake (observational)	Interactions with exercise training (intervention) and physical activity level (observational)
UCP1	Bcl A > G(3826)	57 unrelated individuals from the Quebec Family Study (63)	G-allele was more frequent in high gainers for percentage body fat during a 12-yr follow-up period ($p = 0.02$)		
		238 morbidly obese men and women (64)	G-allele carriers gained more body weight during adult life ($p = 0.02$)		
		163 patients with BMI > 27 kg/m² (65)		The G-allele was associated with less weight loss in response to a 10-week low calorie diet (25% reduction) ($p < 0.05$)	
		113 obese Japanese women (66)		G/G homozygotes lost less weight after a 12-week weight loss program ($p < 0.05$)	
		24 normal weight young adult twins (67)		G-allele carriers lost less body weight during 4 mos after an overfeeding intervention ($p = 0.007$)	
		99 premenopausal Japanese women (68)	G-allele carriers gained more body weight during 4-yr follow-up ($p < 0.05$)		
UCP2	A55V	24 normal weight young adult twins (67)		A55V heterozygotes lost less subcutaneous fat during 4 months after a 100-day overfeeding intervention ($p = 0.024$)	

(Continued)

TABLE 3 Intervention Trials and Observational Studies Reporting Gene-Environment Interactions for UCP Genes in Relation to Weight Change (*Continued*)

Gene	Variant	Population	Interaction with overfeeding (intervention) or weight gain over time (observational)	Interaction with weight loss (intervention) and specific nutrient intake (observational)	Interactions with exercise training (intervention) and physical activity level (observational)
	I/D	41 patients with chronic renal failure (69)	D/D homozygotes gained more weight during peritoneal dialysis treatment ($p < 0.01$)		
		24 normal weight young adult twins (67)	D/D homozygotes gained more weight during 5 years following an overfeeding intervention ($p = 0.008$)		
UCP3	−55C>T	338 morbidly obese (70)			A higher physical activity level was associated a lower BMI, but only in C/C homozygotes ($p = 0.015$)
		157 obese and 150 normal weight (BMI < 25 kg/m^2) men and women (71)			T-allele carriers have a lower risk of obesity, but only among those with a higher recreational physical activity level ($p = 0.05$)

Y210Y(C>T)	24 normal weight young adult twins (67)	C/C homozygotes lost less body weight during 4 months after an overfeeding intervention ($p = 0.008$)
(GA)IVS6	503 Caucasian men and women of the HERITAGE Family Study (72)	240/240 homozygotes decreased BMI and sum of skinfold more than 240/242 and 242/242 individuals after a 20-wk endurance-training program ($p = 0.01$)
Haplotype of 6 SNPs	214 overweight Korean women (73)	The common haplotype [CGTACC] is associated with a more pronounced reduction in body weight ($p = 0.006$ and 0.001), waist-hip ratio ($p = 0.039$ and 0.014) and BMI ($p = 0.006$ and 0.002) in the codominant and recessive models, after the completeion of the 1-month weight control program [a very low-energy diet- 2900 kJ/d]

TABLE 4 Intervention Trials and Observational Studies Reporting Gene-Environment Interactions in Relation to Weight Change

Gene	Variant	Population	Interaction with overfeeding (intervention) or weight gain over time (observational)	Interaction with weight loss (intervention) and specific nutrient intake (observational)	Interactions with exercise training (intervention) and physical activity level (observational)
ACE	I/D	80 young male army recruits (74)			I/I homozygotes gained more fat mass ($p = 0.04$) and fat free mass ($p = 0.01$) after a 10-wk intensive training program compared to D-allele carriers.
		314 men (49)	D/D homozygotes gained more weight during a 20-yr follow up than I-allele carriers ($p = 0.033$).		
ADIPO Q	−11391 G > A	648 obese men and women (75)		After 10-wk intervention of hypoenergetic -600 kcal/d diets with a targeted fat energy of 20–25% or 40–45%, interaction of the genotype with the diet was observed. Codominant: weight loss: −1.6 kg (CI: -2.9; -0.2), $p= 0.027$ Dominant: weight loss: −1.6 kg (CI: -2.9; -0.2), $p= 0.023$	
ADRA2 B	^{12}Glu^9	126 nondiabetic men and women (76)	Glu^9/Glu^9 homozygotes gained more weight during a 5-yr follow-up than Glu^{12}-allele carriers ($p = 0.04$).		

Gene	Polymorphism	Sample		
AGT	−6 A > G	135 essential hypertensive patients (< 50 yrs) (77)	A-allele carriers gained more weight during a 3-yr follow-up than G/G homozygotes ($p<0.001$).	
APO A5	−1131T > C	606 hyperlipaemic and overweight men (78)		C-allele carriers lost more weight in response to a 12-week low-fat diet than T/T homozygotes ($p = 0.002$)
ATP1A2	BglII (8.0 kb > 3.3 kb)	24 normal weight young adult twins (79)	8.0/8.0kb homozygotes gained more fat mass during 100 days of overfeeding than 3.3 k-allele carriers ($p < 0.05$).	
CYPT19	IVS4 (TTTA)n	173 postmenopausal overweight and obese women (80)		Homozygotes for the 11-repeat alleles had a greater decrease in body fat% after a 1-yr intervention of moderate-intensity exercise ($p = 0.01$).
COMT	$Val^{108/158}Met$	173 postmenopausal overweight and obese women (80)		Met/Met homozygotes had a smaller decrease in body fat% than Val/Val homozygotes after a 1-year intervention of moderate-intensity exercise ($p < 0.05$).
DF	HincII (6.5 kb > 3.5 kb)	24 normal weight young adult twins (81)	3.5/3.5kb homozygotes gained more weight during 100 days of overfeeding than 6.5 kb-allele carriers ($p < 0.05$).	

(Continued)

TABLE 4 Intervention Trials and Observational Studies Reporting Gene-Environment Interactions in Relation to Weight Change (*Continued*)

Gene	Variant	Population	Interaction with overfeeding (intervention) or weight gain over time (observational)	Interaction with weight loss (intervention) and specific nutrient intake (observational)	Interactions with exercise training (intervention) and physical activity level (observational)
ENPP1	1044 A > G	648 obese men and women (75)		After a 10-wk intervention of hypoenergetic (−600 kcal/d) diets with a targeted fat energy of 20–25% or 40–45%, interaction of the genotype with the diet was observed. Recessive: weight loss: 2.1 kg (CI: −4.1; 0.0), $p = 0.045$	
GNB3	C825T	47 white and 255 black men and women of the HERITAGE Family Study (82)		In blacks, T/T homozygotes lost more fat mass ($p = 0.012$) and body fat% (0.006) after a 20-wk aerobic endurance training program than C-allele carriers.	
		111 individuals treated with either placebo or sibutramine (83)		After a 54-wk structured weight loss program, T-allele carriers of the placebo group lost more weight than C/C homozygotes ($p = 0.031$), and T/T homozygotes of the sibutramine group lost more weight than the C-allele carriers ($p = 0.01$).	
GRL (*NR3C1*)	BclI (2.3 kb > 4.5 kb) 24 normal weight young adult twins (84)		2.3/2.3 kb homozygotes gained more weight ($p = 0.002$) and abdominal visceral fat ($p = 0.04$) in		

Gene	Polymorphism	Population	Findings
		173 pre-adolescents and adolescents (85)	response to 100-day overfeeding than 4.5 kb-allele carriers. 4.5/2.3 kb heterozygotes increased sum of skinfolds more during a 12-y follow-up than 4.5/4.5 kb and 2.3/2.3 kb homozygotes ($p < 0.01$).
HT2CR	Cys23Ser	148 healthy teenage girls, of whom 75 displayed weight loss and 91 had a stable, normal weight (86)	The Ser23 allele was more frequent in the group that displayed weight loss ($p = 0.0001$)
KCNJ11	Glu23Lys	648 obese men and women (75)	After 10-wk intervention of hypoenergetic (-600 kcal/d) diets with a targeted fat energy of 20–25% or 40–45%, interaction of the genotype with the diet was observed. Codominant: weight loss: 0.8 kg (CI: -0.1; 1.6), $p= 0.032$
IL6	-174G > C	41 men and women (87)	G/G homozygotes decreased body weight significantly more than C-allele carriers after a 24-wk aerobic exercise training program ($p<0.05$)
IL15RA	PstI C > A	153 young (18–31 yrs) men and women (88)	A-allele carriers gained more lean mass after 10 wks of resistance exercise training than C/C homozygotes ($p<0.05$)

(Continued)

TABLE 4 Intervention Trials and Observational Studies Reporting Gene-Environment Interactions in Relation to Weight Change (*Continued*)

Gene	Variant	Population	Interaction with overfeeding (intervention) or weight gain over time (observational)	Interaction with weight loss (intervention) and specific nutrient intake (observational)	Interactions with exercise training (intervention) and physical activity level (observational)
INS	VNTR	256 nonobese adolescent girls (89)	III/III homozygotes gained more weight between age 12 and 16 yrs than I-allele carriers		
LEP	D7S2519, D7S649	252 morbidly obese patients (90)		D7S2519 and D7S649 showed significant association with weight loss during a 16-wk, very low calorie diet intervention ($p = 0.007$)	
LEPR	Ser(T)343Ser(C)	98 overweight patients (91)		C-allele carriers lost more weight in response to a low-calorie diet than T/T homozygotes ($p = 0.006$).	
	Pro(G)1019Pro(A)	335 healthy white Australian women (92)	A/A homozygotes gained more weight during a 2-yr follow-up than the G-allele carriers ($p = 0.02$).		
	Lys656 Asn	67 obese (18 men and 49 women) (93)		Lys656Lys homozygotes have a more pronounced decrease in weight, BMI, fat mass, and waist circumference ($p < 0.05$) after 3 wks of hypocaloric diet (1520 kcal, 52% carbohydrates, 25% lipids, and 23% proteins) and an exercise program (60 min of aerobic exercise training > 3/wk) than Asn656-allele carriers.	

LPL	PvuII C > T	24 normal weight young adult twins (94)	C/C homozygotes gained more weight after 100 days overfeeding than T-allele carriers ($p = 0.015$).	
	BamHI 33kb > 19kb	24 normal weight young adult twins (94)	19 kb-allele carriers gained more weight after 100 days overfeeding than 33/33 kb homozygotes ($p = 0.039$)	
	S447X	741 black and white men and women of the HERITAGE Family Study (95)		In women, both black and white, X447-allele carriers lost more weight and body fat after a 20-wk endurance-training program than S4474S homozygotes ($p < 0.05$). No associations were found in men.
MC4R	Val103Ile	1013 elderly men and women (96)	103Ile-allele carriers gained more weight during a 3.5-yr follow-up period than Val103Val homozygotes ($p = 0.038$).	
PLIN	11482G > A	48 obese men and women (97)		G/G homozygotes lost more weight after a 1-yr low-energy diet compared to A-allele carriers ($p = 0.02$) (p for interaction = 0.015).
	11482G → A and 14995A → T	1909 men and 2198 Asian women (aged 18–69 years)		
PON1	R192Q	71 nondiabetic healthy men (98)		Q192Q homozygotes decreased BMI more than R192-allele carriers after

(Continued)

TABLE 4 Intervention Trials and Observational Studies Reporting Gene-Environment Interactions in Relation to Weight Change (*Continued*)

Gene	Variant	Population	Interaction with overfeeding (intervention) or weight gain over time (observational)	Interaction with weight loss (intervention) and specific nutrient intake (observational)	Interactions with exercise training (intervention) and physical activity level (observational)
				a 12-wk calorie restriction intervention ($p < 0.05$). R192-allele carriers decreased waist-to-hip ratio more than Q192Q homozygotes after a 12-wk calorie restriction intervention ($p < 0.05$).	
SLC6A1 4	+22510 C > G	481 obese women (75)		After 10-wk intervention of hypoenergetic (−600 kcal/d) diets with a targeted fat energy of 20–25% or 40–45%, interaction of the genotype with the diet was observed. Dominant: weight loss: 1.8 kg (CI: −0.3; 3.3), $p = 0.019$	
TNF	−308 G > A	648 obese men and women (75)		After 10-wk intervention of hypoenergetic (−600 kcal/d) diets with a targeted fat energy of 20%–25% or 40–45%, interaction of the genotype with the diet was observed. Codominant: weight loss: 1.0 kg (CI: −0.0; 2.0), $p = 0.047$ Dominant: weight loss: 1.4 kg (CI: −0.3; 2.5), $p = 0.015$	

such that it binds with high affinity to coactivators and influences cellular transcription activity? (105,108,109). Although the mechanisms through which exercise mediates PPARG activity have not been fully elucidated, some studies have shown evidence for an exercise-PPARG interaction. A 16-wk exercise training program in spontaneous hypertensive rats significantly upregulated *PPARG* expression in skeletal muscle (110). Similarly, rats with a low intrinsic exercise capacity expressed lower amounts of key proteins, including PPARG, that are required for mitochondrial function in skeletal muscle as compared to rats with a high intrinsic exercise capacity (111). However, in human skeletal muscle, 9 days of aerobic exercise training (60 min cycling per day) resulted in a significantly ($p = 0.04$) reduced expression of *PPARG* (112). Multiple *PPARG* mRNA isoforms have been identified which are formed by alternative promoters and differential splicing (113). In vivo disruption of the PPARG2 isoform has metabolic consequences, with reduced adipose tissue mass observed in some, but not all, studies (114–116). *PPARG2* mRNA expression is elevated in adipocytes of morbidly obese individuals (104) and several studies have shown association between *PPARG2* gene variants and obesity-related phenotypes (12). The Pro12Ala variant is the most commonly studied *PPARG2* gene variant, located in an alternatively spliced exon B of the PPARG2 isoform. The Pro12Ala substitution decreases the affinity of the PPARG2 protein for its response elements in target genes and decreases its transcriptional activity by 50% (117,118). Although a meta-analysis has shown that the Pro12-allele is associated with a modest (1.25 fold) but significant ($p = 0.002$) increase in diabetes risk (119), the role of the Pro12Ala variant in the development of obesity remains controversial. Several studies have attempted to elucidate the association between the Pro12Ala variant and obesity on its own or in interaction with lifestyle factors (12). Here, we describe studies that, with an epidemiological approach, have examined the interaction between the Pro12Ala *PPARG2* variant and lifestyle factors in the development of obesity (Table 1).

In a Danish study, the Pro12Ala polymorphism was examined in relation to weight gain over a 24y follow-up period in 1621 draftees; 752 were obese and 869 non-obese (54). In the group of obese individuals, the Ala12Ala homozygotes had a significantly ($p = 0.004$) faster increase in BMI ($0.27 \, \text{kg/m}^2$ per y) compared to the Pro12-allele carriers ($0.1 \, \text{kg/m}^2$ per y). However, the opposite was seen in the lean group, with the Ala12Ala homozygotes showing a slower increase ($p = 0.002$) in BMI ($0.11 \, \text{kg/m}^2$ per y) compared to the Pro12-allele carriers ($0.17 \, \text{kg/m}^2$ per y). In agreement with the results for the obese individuals in the Danish study, a Finnish follow-up study reported a positive association between the Ala12-allele and weight gain over 10-y period in 119 non-diabetic middle-aged men and women (mean BMI: $27.1 \, \text{kg/m}^2$) (55). The Ala12-allele carriers gained significantly ($p = 0.009$) more weight over a 10-y period; Ala12Ala homozygotes increased body weight by 11.2%, the Pro12Ala heterozygotes by 4.9% and Pro12Pro homozygotes by only 1.8% (55). Two studies reported on weight loss during a weight loss intervention (56,58); 70 postmenopausal overweight women completed 6 months of a hypocaloric diet and were followed for 12 months after the intervention (56). Weight loss did not differ by genotype, however weight regain during follow-up was greater ($p < 0.01$) in the Ala12-allele carriers (5.4 kg) compared to the Pro12Pro homozygotes (2.8 kg), which is consistent with the long-term follow-up studies in overweight and obese individuals (54,55). In the Finnish Diabetes Prevention study, 490 overweight individuals with impaired glucose tolerance were randomly allocated to a control group or an intensive diet and exercise intervention group (58).

In the intervention group, Ala12Ala homozygotes −8.3%) lost significantly (*p* = 0.043) more weight during the 3-year intervention than the Pro12Ala heterozygotes (−4%) and the Pro12Pro homozygotes (−3.4%) (58). In an exercise training intervention study, the Ala12-allele was associated with a greater weight loss, but only in 29 healthy offspring with family history of type 2 diabetes, not in the control group (62). After 10 weeks of training Ala12- allele carriers lost 1.8 kg, whereas the Pro12Pro homozygotes lost −0.3 kg (*p* < 0.05).

In an observational study of 592 nondiabetic men and women, the Pro12Ala PPAR-γ variant affected the association between BMI and the poly unsaturated to saturated fat ratio (P:S) ratio (57). In Ala12-allele carriers, the P:S ratio increases was negatively associated with BMI. However, no association was observed in the Pro12Pro homozygotes (*p* for gene-diet interaction = 0.004). However, opposite results were reported by two other gene-diet interaction studies. In 2141 women of the Nurses' health Study, the P:S ratio was negatively associated with BMI in the Pro12Pro homozygotes (*p* < 0.0001), but no association was found in the Ala12-allele carriers (*p* for gene-diet interaction = 0.003) (59). Similarly, a positive association was found between total dietary fat intake and BMI in the Pro12Pro homozygotes (*p* = 0.0001), but not in the Ala12-allele carriers of the Québec Family Study (n = 720) (*p* for gene-diet interaction = 0.005) (60).

These studies show that the Pro12Ala *PPARG2* polymorphism may affect weight change in response to diet or exercise. However, in some studies the Ala12-allele is associated with an increased risk; i.e. more weight gain or less weight loss (55,56,118), whereas others report that the Ala12-allele is associated with a reduced risk; i.e., less weight gain or more weight loss (58,62,120). The reasons for these opposite results are not clear but may be related to the difference in age of the populations studied. In a Finnish study, weight and height of 311 men and women was measured at birth and again at age 7, 20 and 41 years (61). Ala12-allele carriers gained significantly (*p* = 0.043) less weight during childhood and adolescence (7–12 y) compared to Pro12Pro homozygotes. However, the opposite was seen between the ages of 20 and 41 during which time the Ala12-carriers gained more weight than the Pro12Pro homozygotes (*p* = 0.001). In a similar way to the epidemiological data, the biology of PPARG has proven to be paradoxical as PPARG is involved in increasing lipid uptake and decreasing insulin sensitivity at the same (121). These opposing functions may underlie the opposite epidemiological findings.

Hence, PPARG represents a potential direct link between adiposity, response to food, control of appetite and energy balance and is also one of the most critical genetic factors predisposing to positive energy balance and, ultimately, obesity.

Uncoupling Proteins

Uncoupling proteins (UCPs) may play a role in the regulation of energy metabolism by uncoupling respiration from phosphorylation, leading to the generation of heat instead of ATP, and thus increasing energy expenditure. UCP1 was the first characterized mitochondrial transmembrane carrier protein, and was shown to be responsible for the high thermogenic capacity of brown adipose tissue. However, the lack of substantial brown adipose tissue in adult humans suggests that UCP1 has a limited role in thermogenesis in man. UCP2 and UCP3 proteins have high amino acid similarities with UCP1. UCP2 is widely expressed, whereas UCP3 is predominantly expressed in skeletal muscle. Although the primary physiological functions of UCP2 and UCP3 are still a matter of debate, animal and human studies have suggested that both UCPs have uncoupling properties that may affect energy metabolism (122). Therefore, UCPs have been extensively studied for association with obesity-related phenotypes (12). Both diet and exercise influence the expression of *UCP* genes. For example, rats fed a high fat diet showed an increased *UCP1*, *UCP2* and *UCP3* mRNA expression in the brown adipose tissue (123), white adipose tissue (124,125) and skeletal muscle (124) respectively. However, similar responses in *UCP2* and *UCP3* mRNA expression in skeletal muscle were also seen following fasting, i.e., total food restriction for 1 or 2 days (126–130). Moderate food restriction downregulated *UCP3*, but not *UCP2* expression (126,131–133). The mechanism responsible for the upregulation of *UCP* gene expression after fasting or a high fat diet may be the increased fatty acids plasma levels that accompany both high fat diets and total fasting. Elevated circulating levels of free fatty acids are associated with higher expression of *UCP3* mRNA in muscle (133,134), suggesting that the expression of *UCP3* in muscle is increased under conditions of higher fatty acid use as fuel (135,136). It was shown that UCPs possibly play a role in promoting a greater proportion of fat oxidation during short term exposure to high protein diets or an increase in protein-carbohydrate ratio in high fat diets in rats (137). Physical inactivity has been associated with significantly increased levels of *UCP2* and *UCP3* mRNA in skeletal muscle (138), whereas endurance training downregulates UCP2 and UCP3 mRNA expression and protein content (138–140). Swim training-induced transcriptional activation of hepatic *UCP2* has been shown to prevent body weight gain and adiposity in genetically obese db/db mice (141). *UCP3* mRNA expression and protein levels were found to be significantly lower in endurance-trained athletes than in untrained individuals and the level of *UCP3* mRNA was negatively correlated with aerobic capacity (142–144). However, several studies in rodents and humans have shown that *UCP3* mRNA expression is upregulated after an acute bout of exercise (26,34,35,145), which might be due to elevated plasma FFA levels during exercise (146,147). Taken together, these results show that endurance training downregulates UCP in humans, which coincides with an improved mechanical energy efficiency, whereas acute exercise up regulates *UCP3* mRNA expression, which may play a role in the elevated post-exercise energy expenditure. Given the role of UCPs in energy metabolism and the regulation of *UCP* mRNA expression through diet and physical activity, interactions between *UCP* gene variants and lifestyle factors on obesity have been extensively studied (Table 2).

Several studies have found that the *Bcl*I polymorphism of the *UCP1* gene, which is a result of an A/G transition in the 5′ untranslated region (−3826 bp) of the gene, modifies weight change in response to alterations in the energy balance (63–68). In a 12-year follow-up of 57 unrelated individuals of the Québec Family Study, the −3826A>G polymorphism was found to be significantly associated with increase in percentage body fat (63). The G-allele frequency was higher ($p = 0.02$) in the high weight gainers (62.1%) compared to the low weight gainers (32.1%). Concordant findings were reported by a small Japanese study that showed that in premenopausal women ($n = 20$) G-allele carriers gained significantly ($p < 0.05$) more weight compared to the A/A homozygotes during a 4-year follow-up (68). These findings are consistent with a French study that examined 238 morbidly obese men and women (64). The G-allele carriers gained significantly more weight during adult life compared to A/A homozygotes (OR: 1.4, $p = 0.02$). Weight gain was even more pronounced when UCP1 −3826G-allele carriers were also carriers of the Arg64 beta-adrenergic receptor (ADRB) allele (OR: 4.95, $p = 0.05$). The synergistic effect between the –3826A>G UCP1 variant and the Trp64Arg adrenergic, beta-3-, receptor (*ADRB3*) variant was also observed in a Finish 10 year follow-up study (148). Carriers of both the G-allele for the *UCP1* variant and the Arg64-allele for the *ADRB3* variants gained 6.5% in weight, whereas the weight of the homozygotes for both variants remained unchanged (–0.2%) ($p = 0.036$). These three studies consistently show that carriers of the G-allele of the –3826A>G *UCP1* are more prone to gain weight over time.

In the twin overfeeding study, the association of the –3826A>G polymorphism with weight gain during 100 days of overfeeding was examined, as well as with the weight changes four months and five years after the overfeeding intervention (67). No associations were found with body weight gain during overfeeding. However, during the four months after the overfeeding period, body weight decreased significantly ($p = 0.007$) less in the G-allele carriers than in the A/A homozygotes. The association of the –3826A>G polymorphism with weight loss was also studied in 163 patients with BMI greater than 27 (65). The G/G homozygotes lost less weight (–4.6 kg) on a 10-week low calorie diet (25% energy restriction) compared to the heterozygotes (–5.7 kg), who in turn lost less than the A/A homozygotes (–7.1 kg) ($p < 0.05$). These findings are partially in agreement with a Japanese study that examined the synergic effect of the –3826A>G UCP1 and Trp64Arg *ADRB3* polymorphism (66). The study included 113 obese women who were treated with a combined low-calorie diet and exercise program for 12 weeks. The G/G homozygotes lost significantly ($p < 0.05$) less weight (–4.3 kg) compared to the A/G (–7.7 kg) and A/A (–7.4 kg) genotypes. The weight loss was even less in G/G homozygotes who were also *ADRB3* Arg64 allele carriers (–3.3 kg). These findings are in agreement with a Finnish 12 week weight loss intervention, followed by a 40 week maintenance follow-up. Carriers of both the G-allele of the *UCP1* variant and the Arg64-allele of the *ADRB3* variant showed a smaller weight reduction compared to those homozygous for both variants (–10.5 kg vs. –14.0 kg, $p = 0.05$). During the 40 week maintenance period, carriers of both *UCP1* and *ADRB3* alleles gained 5.8 kg, whereas the weight of women homozygous for both variants remained unchanged (–0.5 kg, $p = 0.04$). Taken together, these observational and intervention studies consistently suggest that the G-allele of the *UCP1* –3826A>G polymorphism is associated with 'obesity proneness' and with less success in weight loss programs. In addition, the effect of the *UCP1* G-allele on weight change seems to be more pronounced in the presence of the *ADRB3* Arg64-allele. Interestingly, this *UCP1-ADRB3* synergistic effect has also been associated with a lower autonomic nervous system activity (149) and lower basal metabolic rate (150) and chronic stimulation of the ADRB3 can induce the expression of *UCP* genes in white adipose tissue and skeletal muscle (151–153).

In the twin overfeeding study, the effect of two *UCP2* gene polymorphisms, A55V and I/D, were examined (67). Both variants have been associated with sleeping metabolic rate and 24-h energy expenditure in Pima Indians, with the A55A and D/D homozygotes have the lowest energy expenditure (154,155). The UCP2 A55V polymorphism is located in exon 4 and results in a conservative amino acid substitution at codon 55. Little is known about the tertiary structure of the UCP2 protein, but based on what is known of the UCP1 protein topology, it is predicted that the UCP2 A55V polymorphism would probably not result in any major change in the tertiary structure of the protein (156). The *UCP2* 45 bp

I/D polymorphism is located in the 3′-untranslated region of exon 8 of the *UCP2* gene. It has been hypothesized that this polymorphism is involved in the mRNA processing or in the stability of the transcript (157). None of the two polymorphisms showed significant association with weight gain during the overfeeding period in the twin study (67). However, during the 4 months after the over-feeding intervention, the A55V heterozygotes lost significantly ($p<0.03$) less subcutaneous fat (–32%) than the A55A homozygotes (–55%). During the 5-year period after the overfeeding intervention, the twins gained on average 3.6 kg, but the D/D homozygotes gained significantly ($p=0.008$) more weight than the I-allele carriers. Similar results were reported for patients who were treated with peritoneal dialysis (69). A side effect of this treatment is weight gain and fat accumulation. In a study with 41 patients with chronic renal failure, it was found that the D/D homozygotes increased body weight (+ 3.0 kg) and body fat mass (+3.8 kg) significantly more than the I/D heterozygotes (−1.0 kg ($p<0.01$) and +0.8 kg ($p<0.05$), respectively) (69). In contrast, lack of interaction between physical activity and I/D variant on subsequent weight changes during a 10-year follow-up was reported in a Danish study (158).

The twin overfeeding study also examined the effect of the *Rsa*I poly-morphisms of the *UCP3* gene, which is a C>T transition resulting in a silent Y210Y variant in exon 5 (67). This polymorphism was not associated with weight gain during the 100d overfeeding intervention, however, four months after the intervention, body weight had decreased less ($p=0.008$) in the C/C homozygotes compared to the C/T heterozygotes. A dinucleotide GA microsatellite located in intron 6, (GA)IVS6, was found to be associated with change in BMI and sum of skinfolds in 503 white men and women of the HERITAGE Family Study (72). After a 20 wk endurance training program, BMI in individuals that were homo-zygous for the (GA) IVS6 240-allele decreased (–0.44 kg/m^2), whereas BMI increase in those with genotypes 242/242 or 240/242 (+0.30 kg/m^2) ($p=0.01$). In the same population, a genomewide linkage scan showed suggestive evidence for linkage at the *UCP2-UCP3* locus and change in body fat percentage after 20 weeks of endurance training (159). It is not known whether this polymorphism in intron 6 influences *UCP3* mRNA, protein content or uncoupling activity. Another *UCP3* variant, the –55C>T variant that is located in the promoter region and associated with *UCP3* expression (160), was examined for gene-physical activity interaction in 338 morbidly obese women (70). High physical activity levels were associated with a lower BMI, but only in women that were C/C homozygotes ($p=0.015$), not in T-allele carriers (70). In another study, six SNPs [–55C>T, Int2-143G>C, Tyr99Tyr, Int3-47G>A, Int4-498C>T and Tyr210Tyr] were examined in association with obesity phenotypes and the outcomes of very low energy diet in 214 Korean women, who had completed 1-month weight control program involving an intake of 2900 kJ/d. A significant association of the common *UCP3* haplotype [CGTACC] with very low-energy diet-induced changes in body weight ($p=0.006$ and 0.001), waist-hip ratio ($p=0.039$ and 0.014) and BMI ($p=0.006$ and 0.002) in the codominant and recessive models was observed (73). A gene-physical activity interaction was also reported in a case-control study with 157 obese and 150 normal weight men and women (71). The association between the –55C>T *UCP3* variant and the risk of obesity was only manifest among those with higher recreational physical activity (OR: 0.46, $p=0.05$) and not among those with lower physical activity levels (OR: 0.84, $p=0.84$).

Adrenergic Receptors

The adrenergic receptors belong to a large family of G protein-coupled receptors that regulate a wide variety of physiological responses. They can be divided in two main types, the alpha- and beta-adrenergic receptors. The alpha-adrenergic receptors can be found in adipose tissue where they inhibit lipolysis. However, they are mainly located in blood vessels and play an important role in cardiovascular regulation. The beta-adrenergic system plays a key role in regulating energy balance as ADRBs mediate the catecholamine-induced lipolysis and thermogenesis in adipose tissue. Several studies have shown that in obese individuals the relative increase in fat oxidation after β-adrenergic stimulation is blunted (161–164). Of the three ADRBs, the *ADRB2* and *ADRB3* subtypes are highly plausible candidate genes for obesity. ADRB2 is the dominant lipolytic adrenergic receptor subtype and plays an important role in the regulation of energy homeostasis by controlling glycogen breakdown and lipid mobilization (165–167). *ADRB3* is primarily expressed in white adipose tissue, where it stimulates lipolysis, but it is also expressed in skeletal muscle at lower levels (165,168,169). Gene variants in the *ADRB* genes have been extensively studied for their association with obesity (12). Although there is little evidence that nutrients and diet affect the *ADRB* gene expression or protein activity, animal studies have shown that *ADRB* genes mediate the susceptibility for obesity when on a high-fat diet. Mice that lack one or all three *ADRB* genes had a reduced metabolic rate and were slightly obese when on a chow diet (170,171). However, on a high fat diet, these *ADRB*-less mice developed massive obesity that was entirely due to a failure of the diet-induced thermogenesis (170). Furthermore, exercise-induced weight change might be mediated through the adrenergic system. Exercise results in elevated plasma concentrations of catcholamines that stimulate lipolysis and energy expenditure through the ADRBs (172). Adults who exercise on a regular basis have increased thermogenic responsiveness to β-adrenergic stimulation compared to sedentary individuals (173). Taken together, these data make the *ADRB* genes good candidates for gene-lifestyle interaction studies in relation to diet and exercise induced weight change (Table 3).

Polymorphisms in the *ADRB2* have been associated with many obesity related phenotypes (12). One of the frequently studied *ADRB2* polymorphisms is the Gln27Glu missense mutation, which affects the extracellular N-terminus of the receptor (174). Although the mutated receptors display normal agonist binding and functional coupling to G-proteins, the mutation markedly alters the degree of agonist-promoted downregulation of the receptor expression (174,175). Ukkola et al. (38) studied the effect of the Gln27Glu polymorphism on weight gain in the twin overfeeding study. Overfeeding induced a greater gain in body weight ($p < 0.001$) and in total subcutaneous fat ($p < 0.005$), as assessed from the sum of eight skinfolds, in Gln27Gln homozygotes compared to Glu27-allele carriers. The *ADRB2* Gln27Glu polymorphism accounted for about 7% of the variance in body weight and subcutaneous fat gains. A significant interaction (p for interaction $= 0.009$) between the *ADRB2* Gln27Glu polymorphism and daily physical activity in relation to obesity risk was observed in men of a French population (37). Gln27Gln homozygotes had a 3.45 times higher risk of obesity compared to Glu27-allele carriers ($p = 0.002$), but only in sedentary men. In men who were physically active, the risk of obesity was not significantly increased for the Gln27Gln homozygotes. An interaction (p for interaction $= 0.005$) between the Glu27Gln *ADRB2* variant and physical activity was also found a Spanish women (176). However, the findings were different from the French study. In sedentary women, BMI of Gln27Gln and Glu27-allele carriers was not significantly different, whereas in physically active women, the Glu27-allele carriers had a higher BMI compared to the Gln27Gln homozygotes ($p = 0.003$); suggesting that the Glu27-allele carriers do not benefit equally from physical activity compared to non-carriers. Other studies did not find significant interactions with this *ADRB2* variant and lifestyle in relation to obesity risk (41–43).

Another *ADRB2* variant, Arg16Gly, was studied in 1151 African-American and Caucasian children and adolescents, who were followed every three years for 24 years (40). The Arg16Gly *ADRB2* polymorphism has been associated with a decrease in β2-receptor density and efficiency (175,177). This *ADRB2* variant seemed to moderate weight gain only in men; by age 32, BMI and subscapular skinfold had increased more ($p < 0.05$) in the Gly16Gly men (+8% and +50% more, respectively) compared to the Arg16Arg men (40). The results of a Dutch study that compared 286 men and women who had gained an average of 12.8 kg during a 6.8-year follow-up of with those who had remained weight stable over the same period were harder to interpret (41). In men, weight gainers were more often Gly16Gly or Arg16Arg homozygous than Arg16Gly heterozygous compared to weight stable men ($p = 0.04$). In women, however, Gly16gly homozygotes were more often weight stable ($p = 0.05$). In a similar study with 160 young non-obese men, weight gainers, defined as having gained ≥10% BMI over 5 y follow-up, were compared to those that remained stable. The Gly16-allele was more frequent in weight gainers as compared to weight stable men who were more often Arg16Arg homozygotes ($p < 0.05$) (43). In the HERITAGE Family Study, white and black individuals followed a 20-week endurance training program. A significant association between the Arg16Gly variant and loss in weight and body fat was observed, but only in white women (42). Women who were Gly16-allele carriers lost less weight (Arg16Gly: +0.03 kg/m^2 and Gly16Gly: –0.04kg/m^2) and body fat % (–0.50 % and –0.63%) compared to Arg16Arg homozygotes (BMI: –0.34 kg/m^2 ($p = 0.04$) and body fat %: –1.9% ($p = 0.0003$)). No associations were observed in blacks or in white men. Overall, these findings suggest that the Gly16-allele is associated with an increased risk of weight gain and with resistance to weight loss through endurance training. However, the effect seemed to be sex-specific and no consistency is observed between studies for the type of genetic model (recessive or dominance).

The polymorphism at codon 64 (Trp64Arg) of the *ADRB3* gene, located in the first intracellular loop of the receptor, has been extensively studied for its association with obesity-related phenotypes on its own or in synergy with variants in other genes (12). The Arg64-allele is associated with a marked decrease in beta 3-adrenoreceptor function (178,179) and was found to be related to a reduced metabolic rate (150,180,181). In 185 morbidly obese patients, body weight at age 20-year was not different between the Trp64Trp homozygotes and the Trp64Arg heterozygotes (44). However, over a follow-up period of about 25 years, the heterozygous patients (+ 67 kg) gained significantly ($p = 0.007$) more weight compared to the homozygous patients (+51 kg). Similar results were reported in another group of French morbidly obese women, but not in men (46). Women who carried the Arg64-allele gained more weight than Trp64Trp homozygotes (+ 62.2 kg vs. + 47 kg, $p = 0.017$) over a 20-year follow-up period. This is in agreement with the findings in an unselected sample of 457 men from Southern Italy for whom 20-year follow-up data were available (49). The incidence of overweight was significantly ($p = 0.02$) higher in the Arg64-allele carriers (44.7%)

compared to Trp64Trp homozygotes (27.0%). In Japanese children who were followed-up for five years between one and six years of age, Arg64-allele carriers gained more weight (from –5.3% of ideal body weight at one year to 17.7% at six years ($p < 0.05$)) compared to Trp64Trp homozygotes (from –5.0% to 1.3%) (152). A gene-energy intake interaction was observed in 295 healthy Japanese men (53). The risk of being overweight was higher (OR: 3.37, 95%CI [1.12–10.2]) in the Arg64-allele carriers compared to the Trp64Trp homozygotes, but only in those with the highest energy intake (4th quartile). Opposite findings were reported in another Japanese study in which annual body weight data were available for 128 normal weight men between 25 and 50 years of age (47). Body weight gain over a 25-year follow-up was greater ($p = 0.013$) in the Trp64Trp homozygotes (+6.2 kg) than in the Arg64 allele carriers (+3.8 kg). These studies suggest that the *ADRB3* Trp64Arg mutation affects weight gain over time, with most studies suggesting that the Arg64-allele carriers have an increased risk to gain weight over time. The opposite outcome in the Japanese study may be due to ethnic differences, differences in environmental exposures or the fact that the individuals were within the range of normal weight.

The ADRB3 Trp64Arg mutation has also been reported to affect the outcome of weight loss interventions. In two different studies, non-diabetic (45) and diabetic (48) obese Japanese women underwent a 12-week weight reduction program (exercise and diet). After the weight loss intervention, both studies reported that the Arg64-allele carriers tended to lose less weight than the Trp64Trp homozygotes. Furthermore, both studies reported that the Arg64-allele carriers had a lower resting metabolic rate compared to the Trp64Trp homozygotes. Similar results were found in a group of non-diabetic obese and non-obese perimenopausal Japanese women (51). The Arg64-allele carriers (–0.01 (1.17) kg) did not lose weight during a 12-week weight loss intervention program, whereas Trp64Trp homozygotes (–0.74 (0.15) kg, $p = 0.035$) did. A cross-sectional study with 313 Spanish men and women found that the effect of the Trp64Arg polymorphism on obesity risk was modified by physical activity level (p for interaction = 0.06) (50). In sedentary individuals, Arg64-allele carriers had a higher obesity risk compared to Trp64Trp homozygotes (OR: 2.98, 95% CI: 1.00–8.56, $p = 0.05$), whereas no difference between the two genotypes groups were observed when the individuals were physically active.

Taken together, these studies suggest that carriers of the Arg64-allele tend to be 'resistant to weight loss' and, in some cases, 'prone to weight gain', which might in part be due to a lower resting metabolic rate.

So far, most studies have examined only one or two candidate genes at a time. Only one study (Nugenob study: *www.nugenob.org*) considered 26 genes, including *PPARG2*, *UCP2* and *UCP3*, in relation to weight loss after a 10-week intervention. In this study 648 obese adult individuals were given a hypo-energetic diet; 336 were randomly assigned to a low fat diet (20–25% of total energy from fat, 15% from protein and 60–65% from carbohydrate), and 312 to high fat diet (40–45% of total energy from fat, 15% from protein, and 40–45% from carbohydrate). The weight loss after the 10-week intervention was studied in relation to genotypes of 42 SNPs in 26 obesity-related candidate genes. Overall, heterozygotes showed weight loss differences that ranged from −0.6 to 0.8 kg, and homozygotes, from –0.7 to 3.1 kg, compared with the noncarriers of each of the SNPs, and after adjusting for gender, age, baseline weight and centre. Genotype-dependent additional weight loss on low fat diet ranged from 1.9 to

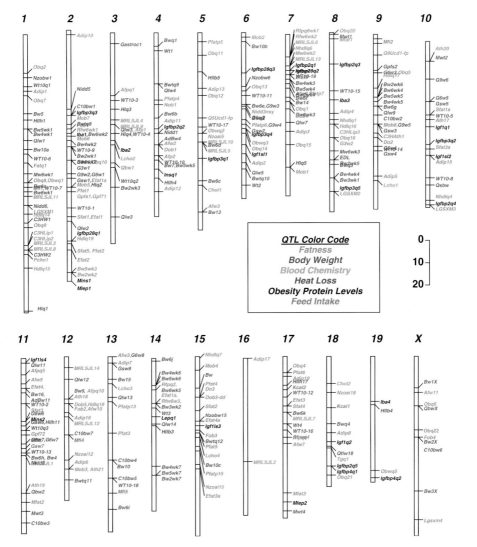

FIGURE 3.4.1 Consensus predisposition (QTL) map for obesity-related traits in the mouse (through June 2006), representing most of the loci from the experiments detailed. *Abbreviation*: QTL, quantitative trait loci.

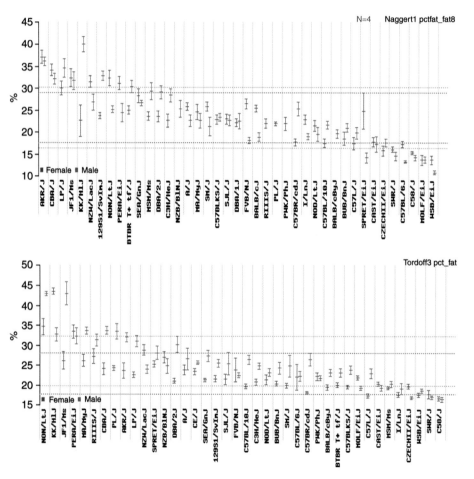

FIGURE 3.4.2 Percent body fat after high fat (*top*) (6) and normal fat (*bottom*) (3) diets from the 40 inbred lines of the Mouse Phenome Project.

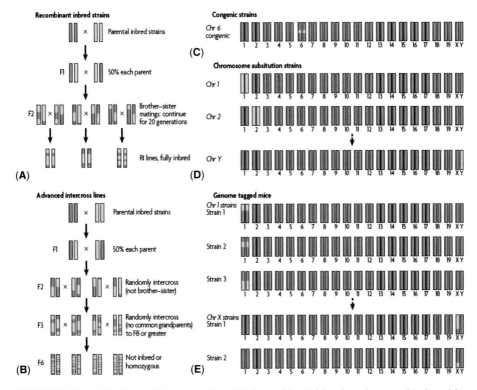

FIGURE 3.4.3 Derivatives of inbred strains. (**A**) Recombinant inbred strains are developed by crossing two different inbred parental strains to produce F1 offspring (obligate heterozygotes at all loci). From there, a series of brother-sister matings are established, and their offspring are repeatedly intercrossed for at least 20 generations. This produces fully inbred strains, each of which is homozygous at all loci for a unique combination of the original parental genomes. (**B**) In advanced intercross lines (AILs), the goal is to increase recombination frequency, so matings between siblings and cousins are avoided. By providing large numbers of animals that carry many additional genetic breakpoints, AILs were particularly useful in narrowing quantitative trait loci (QTL) confidence intervals. (**C**) Congenic strains are produced with the goal of transferring a single locus, such as a mutant gene, from one genetic background to another. In this example, a chromosome 6 (chr 6) locus is illustrated. The mouse carrying the locus to be transferred is mated, or "outcrossed," to the strain of choice to produce obligate heterozygotes. The heterozygotes are then intercrossed, and the process of outcrossing and intercrossing, with selection for the locus of interest at all outcross generations, is repeated. (**D**) In chromosome-substitution strains (CSS, formerly called consomic strains), one chromosome in its entirety is transferred from one strain background to another. (**E**) Genome tagged mice (GTM) are similar in concept to a congenic strain, but the idea is to not only transfer a single locus to another genetic background, but to transfer large, overlapping regions of each chromosome from one strain to another, and to build up a collection of such strains that covers the whole genome. *Source*: From Ref. 2.

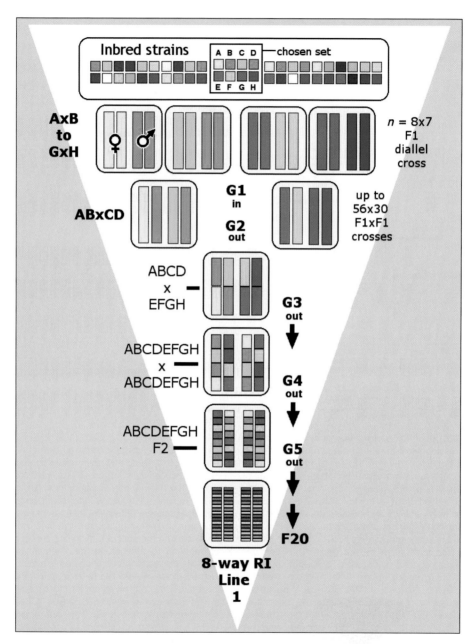

FIGURE 3.4.4 Outline of the production of a set of recombinant inbred strains originating from a cross of eight inbred lines (The Collaborative Cross). Production of approximately 1000 such recombinant inbred strains will enable very high-resolution mapping of QTL, effective dissection of epistatic interactions, powerful analysis of gene × environment interactions, and application of systems biology to the dissection of complex traits. *Abbreviation*: QTL, quantitative trait loci.

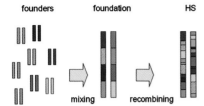

founders   foundation   HS

mixing   recombining

FIGURE 3.4.6 Construction of the heterogeneous stock (HS) mice, showing one chromosome pair from each of the eight founder inbred strains and how they eventually recombine into one chromosome pair from an HS mouse that is a mosaic of the progenitors. *Source*: Courtesy of William Valdar and Richard Mott.

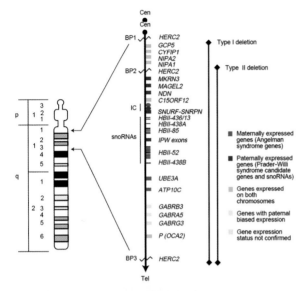

FIGURE 5.2.1 Physical map of Prader-Willi syndrome genes. *Source*: Adapted from Ref. 59.

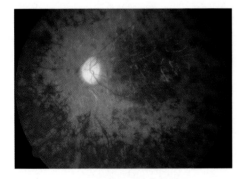

FIGURE 5.3.3 Fundus picture of a Bardet-Biedl syndrome patient showing retinitis pigmentosa (pigment migrations cover degenerated retina).

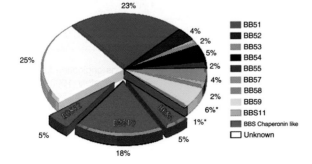

FIGURE 5.3.4 Schematic colored representation of the identified Bardet-Biedl syndrome (BBS) genes and their percentage of mutation detected in the BBS patient population.

MC4R variant reported in human obesity

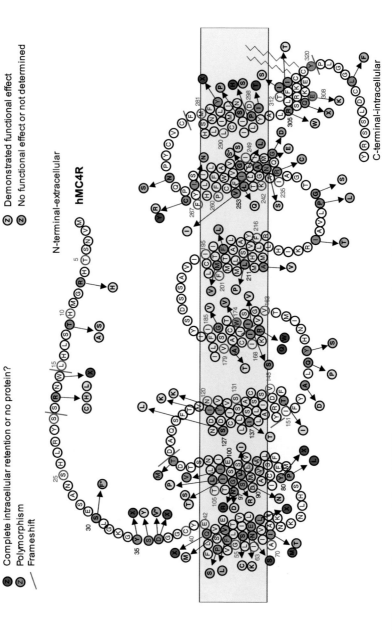

FIGURE 5.6.1 Schematic representation of MC4R and the sequence variants detected in human obesity. The positions of the sequence variants are indicated on the secondary structure of MC4R. Amino acids are indicated as circles in single-letter code. Amino acids affected by a mutation are indicated in purple circles. S30F*/G252S* and Y35STOP**/D37V** are double mutants. Note that the mutations are not clustered in a specific functional domain of the protein.

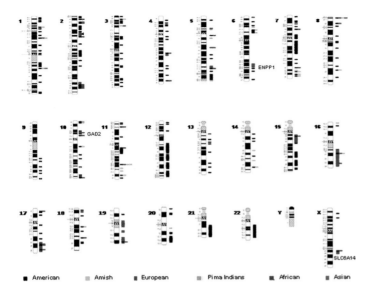

FIGURE 6.2.1 Chromosomal regions linked with obesity in different populations. This figure illustrates the panel of chromosomal regions linked with obesity in different family study. Linkage studies have been performed in different populations from Europe (blue blocks), North America (black blocks), Asia (pink blocks) as well as from Amish (green), Pima Indians (yellow blocks), and African Americans (red blocks). This map is built from information provided by the 2005 human obesity gene map (3).

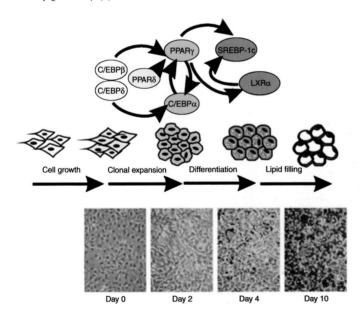

FIGURE 9.3.1 The differentiation of preadipocytes into mature adipocytes is a highly regulated, multistep process that requires a coordinated program of transcriptional events leading to changes in gene expression. When confluent 3T3-L1 preadipocytes are treated with differentiation inducers, CEBPD and CEBPB are rapidly induced; the cells synchronously reenter the cell cycle and undergo approximately two rounds of cell division, a process termed "mitotic clonal expansion". (*For full caption, see page 431.*)

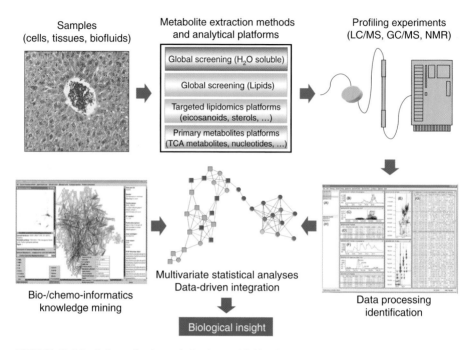

Samples
(cells, tissues, biofluids)

Metabolite extraction methods
and analytical platforms

Global screening (H₂O soluble)

Global screening (Lipids)

Targeted lipidomics platforms
(eicosanoids, sterols, ...)

Primary metabolites platforms
(TCA metabolites, nucleotides, ...)

Profiling experiments
(LC/MS, GC/MS, NMR)

Bio-/chemo-informatics
knowledge mining

Multivariate statistical analyses
Data-driven integration

Biological insight

Data processing
identification

FIGURE 10.2.6   Schematic of metabolomics and lipidomics.

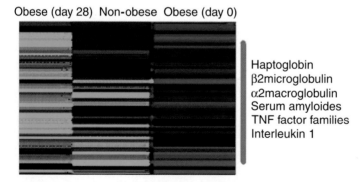

Obese (day 28) Non-obese Obese (day 0)

Haptoglobin
β2microglobulin
α2macroglobulin
Serum amyloides
TNF factor families
Interleukin 1

FIGURE 10.3.1   Cluster of inflammatory-related gene expression in adipose tissue of non-obese subjects and obese patients before and after VLCD. Each row represents one gene and each column represents one clinical situation or nutritional condition. The intensity of colors of each gene represents the mean in $\log_2$ of gene expression ratios of 7 non-obese subjects and 10 obese subjects before and after VLCD. Green, red, and black colors represent, respectively, the genes down-regulated, upregulated, and equal to median. Examples of inflammatory genes are given beside the cluster. *Abbreviation*: VLCD, very low-calorie diet.

−1.6 kg in heterozygotes, and from 3.8 kg to −2.1 kg in homozygotes relative to the noncarriers. None of the associations was statistically significant with respect to the multiple testing. The SNPs in these candidate genes play only a minor role in modulating weight changes induced by a moderate hypo-energetic low-fat or high-fat diet (75).

FUTURE DIRECTIONS

The responsiveness to alteration in energy balance induced by diet or physical activity can vary considerably between individuals. Although little is known about the causes of the heterogeneity in responsiveness, the available evidence suggests that genetic factors may play an important role. Diet, physical activity and genetic factors are intimately related in the etiology of obesity and, although the impact of the genotype is generally modest, it can be considerably amplified in an obesity-promoting environment. Unravelling these interactions will undoubtedly shed light on the etiology of obesity and may have wide implications for the public health initiatives focused on promoting weight loss and preventing weight gain. As gene-by-environment research proceeds, generalized nutrition and exercise recommendations will give way to interventions that are targeted to specific molecular mechanisms that underlie energy homeostasis. The expected advances from gene-lifestyle interaction research will enable individuals to make personalized dietary and other lifestyle choices. Dieticians and exercise experts will advise individuals with a particular genotype on how to maximize their genetic potential and minimize their risk of obesity. Although personalized diets and exercise/physical activity recommendations would be an interesting application of this gene-lifestyle interaction knowledge, we believe, however, that the implementation of such an approach lies far ahead of us.

Current research towards gene-lifestyle interactions is plagued with problems similar to those encountered in other epidemiological studies (182,183), and additional ones that are specific to gene-environment interaction studies. These problems include small, underpowered sample sizes, irreproducible results, poor reporting on significance of interaction, and selective reporting of 'positive' results. In addition, the fields of nutrition and physical activity epidemiology are both seriously affected by exposure measurement error.

The choice of an appropriate study design is a first step towards overcoming some of these problems. The classical epidemiological methods for detecting gene-environment interactions include either cross-sectional case-control studies or case-control studies nested within a cohort. The cross-sectional case-control is relatively simple and would be fine for purely genetic studies. However, the examination of environmental influences is likely to be affected by recall bias. The normal response to this situation is to design prospective case-control or nested case-control studies in which diet and physical activity are assessed before the occurrence of disease. One of the disadvantages of the case-control design is that it reduces 'obesity' to a binary trait, which is rather artificial, as obesity is only the extreme of a continuum. Obesity is a heterogeneous disorder that results from an increase energy intake or reduced energy expenditure or a combination of these processes. Studying the impact of genetic and environmental influences on continuously distributed obesity-related or intermediate phenotypes, such as BMI, body fat percentage, energy expenditure, fat oxidation and plasma hormone levels may provide a clearer and more refined insight into the causal pathways under-lying weight gain and obesity than studies of the obesity state itself, which is simply the final common shared phenotype.

Observational designs have been commonly used to study gene-environment interactions for weight change. A limitation of this design is that the environmental exposure (diet and physical activity) is generally not precisely measured and affected by recall bias, which reduces the power of the study. This can be overcome by large well-controlled lifestyle intervention studies in which the cohort is randomized to a control group or to one or more intervention groups that are subsequently followed up for several weeks. The key attributes to these studies is to maximize the difference between control and intervention group and to strictly control the intervention. The response to the lifestyle intervention is then compared across the genotypes of the gene variant of interest. Generally, sample sizes of lifestyle intervention studies will be smaller than of observational studies, but the increased measurement precision and control of the exposure should compensate for the smaller sample size. Lifestyle intervention designs can be particularly useful for replicating gene-environment interaction results of gene variants that are rare. Recruitment will be based on genotype such that the study group is enriched with individuals that carry the rare variant which will allow more powerful analyses.

In gene-environment interaction studies power is even more of an issue than in studies that examine main genetic effects only. The problems of power can be dealt with by increasing the size of studies, limiting the number of hypotheses tested and by improving the precision of exposure measurement formulas and tables have been published for estimating power and sample size for case-control studies, where both the outcome and environmental risk factors are reduced to a categorical state (184,185), as well as for quantitative analyses, where outcome and environmental exposure are continuous traits (186). These formulas and tables indicate that samples sizes need to be relatively large to detect moderate interaction effects. With a case-control design, for example, a sample size of at least 7500 is required to achieve 80% power for detecting a moderate interaction effect ($\theta = OR_{E|G=1}/OR_{E|G=0} = 1.5$) with a common gene variant (allele-frequency = 0.25) and significance at 5%. Thousand individuals would be required to detect a stronger interaction effect ($\theta = 3$), but such strong interactions are rare (185). In a study with a quantitative trait and a continuous environmental exposure, a sample of 5000 would be powered ($\beta = 80\%$ at $\alpha = 0.05$) to detect an interaction effect of 1.2 ($slope_{rare\ allele}/slope_{common\ allele}$) when the allele frequency is 0.30 and domi-nant, whereas larger interaction effects (e.g., 1.5) can be detected with 500 individuals (186). The power and sample size depend on the study design, the allele frequency, the strength of the association between outcome and exposure and the magnitude of the interaction (185,186). In addition, the measurement error in the assessment of the outcome and exposure has been shown to be critical for the power to detect interactions on continuous traits (187). Smaller studies with repeated and more precise measurement of exposure and outcome will be as powerful as studies even 20 times bigger, which necessarily employ less precise measures because of their size (187). Of the 65 studies that are summarized in Tables 1–4, only three (5 %) contained more than 1000 individuals, 12 (18%) had more than 500 individuals, whereas 20 (31%) studies contained fewer than 100 individuals. The results of studies published so far should be interpreted with caution, not just because of the problems of false discovery but also because many of these studies fail to report the statistical significance of the gene-lifestyle interaction term and did not correct for multiple testing.

The epidemiological evidence of gene-environment interaction requires replication. However, for 30 (75%) of the 40 gene variants for which interactions with lifestyle factors have been reported (Tables 1–4) no replication data were available yet. For only five (13%) of the gene variants were there more than two reported interactions. Even when replication data is available, studies are difficult to compare because study designs, methods, populations and analyses differ substantially which hampers future meta-analyses.

The search for gene-environment interaction is likely to result in fewer false positive findings if it is based on an understanding of biology rather than a random search for statistical interaction. However, for several genes for which statistical gene-environment interactions have been reported (Tables 1–4), the evidence for a biological effect of diet and/or physical activity on gene expression, protein levels, function or activity is weak or not existing. The causal inference from an observation based on an interaction on a quantitative trait is raised by (1) its biological plausibility, (2) the known links between the continuous trait and disease risk, and (3) by the observation in meta-analyses of case-control studies of an association with obesity. This combination of different types of evidence is perhaps a model for future studies of gene-environment interaction.

CONCLUSION

So far, genetic association studies, including gene-environment interaction studies, have focussed on one or two polymorphisms per gene at a time. Some of these polymorphisms were identified through gene sequencing and were studied because they result in an amino acid change or are located in the promoter region and, therefore, potentially affect the mRNA stability, processing or transcription and/or protein translation. However, most studies examined polymorphisms that have no functional significance. The polymorphisms were 'inherited' from previous studies that had historically identified these gene variants through labor intensive, time consuming and expensive methods. Recent advances in high-throughput genotyping technologies, coupled with the development of massive databases such as the International HapMap Project (http://www.hapmap.org/) that catalogues millions of SNPs, have set the stage for an in depth characterization of the genetic variation and haplotype structure of candidate genes. Genetic association studies are already applying a more comprehensive approach that makes optimal use of the newly available resources.

Although the evidence base is growing, consistent data are lacking which hampers the ability to make recommendations. Therefore, large well-designed studies with accurately measured diet and physical activity that integrate existing knowledge of molecular biology will be needed to build the foundation upon which gene-directed nutrition and exercise therapy will be based. This can be addressed with population studies of appropriate experimental design, intervention trials of adequate size and quality and trials in individuals selected for specific gene variants.

REFERENCES

1. Eaton SB, Konner M, Shotak M. Stone agers in the fast lane: chronic degenerative diseases in evolutionary perspective. Am J Med 1988; 84:739–49.

2. Franks PW, Loos RJF. PGC-1alpha gene and physical activity in type 2 diabetes mellitus. Exercise Sport Science Rev 2006; 34:171–5.
3. Ravussin E, Valencia ME, Esparza J, et al. Effects of a traditional lifestyle on obesity in Pima Indians. Diab Care 1994; 17:1067–74.
4. Esparza J, Fox C, Harper IT, et al. Daily energy expenditure in Mexican and USA Pima indians: low physical activity as a possible cause of obesity. Int J Obes Relat Metab Disord 2000; 24:55–9.
5. Salmond CE, Prior IA, Wessen AF. Blood pressure patterns and migration: a 14-year cohort study of adult Tokelauans. Am J Epidemiol 1989; 13:37–52.
6. Curb JD, Marcus EB. Body fat and obesity in Japanese Americans. Am J Clin Nutr 1991; 53:S1552–5.
7. Sundquist J, Winkleby M. Country of birth, acculturation status and abdominal obesity in a national sample of Mexican-American women and men. Int J Epidemiol 2000; 29:470–7.
8. Khan LK, Sobal J, Martorell R. Acculturation, socioeconomic status, and obesity in Mexican Americans, Cuban Americans, and Puerto Ricans. Int J Obes Relat Metab Disord 1997; 21:91–6.
9. Bouchard C, Tremblay A, Despres JP, et al. The response to long-term overfeeding in identical twins. N Engl J Med 1990; 322:1477–82.
10. Hainer V, Stunkard AJ, Kunesova M, et al. Intrapair resemblance in very low calorie diet-induced weight loss in female obese identical twins. Int J Obes Relat Metab Disord 2000; 24:1051–7.
11. Bouchard C, Tremblay A, Despres JP, et al. The response to exercise with constant energy intake in identical twins. Obes Res 1994; 2:400–10.
12. Rankinen T, Zuberi A, Chagnon YC, et al. The human obesity gene map: the 2005 update. Obesity (Silver Spring). 2006; 4(4):529–644.
13. Swinburn BA, Caterson ID, Seidell JC, et al. Diet, nutrition and the prevention of excess weight gain and obesity. Public Health Nutrit 2004; 7(1A):123–46.
14. Wolfharth B, Bray MS, Hagberg JM, et al. The human gene map for performance and health-related fitness phenotypes: the 2004 update. Med Sci Sports Exercise 2005; 37:881–903.
15. Loos RJF, Rankinen T. Gene-diet interactions on body weight changes. J Am Diebet Assoc 2005; 105:29–34.
16. De Caterina R, Madonna R. Role of nutrients and physical activity in gene expression. World Rev Nutr Diet 2005; 94:107–19.
17. Corthesy-Theulaz I, Van Dunnen JT, Ferre P, et al. Nutrigenomics: he impact of biomics technology on nutrition research. Ann Nutr Metab 2005; 49:355–65.
18. Muller M, Kersten S. Nutrigenomics: goals and strategies. Nat Rev Genet 2003; 4:315–22.
19. Scarpulla RC. Nuclear activators and coactivators in mammalian mitochondrial biogenesis. Biochimica et Biophysica Acta (BBA)—ene Structure Express 2002; 1576:1–14.
20. Winder WW. Energy-sensing and signaling by AMP-activated protein kinase in skeletal muscle. J Appl Physiol 2001; 91:1017–28.
21. Olson EN, Williams RS. Calcineurin signaling and muscle remodeling. Cell 2000; 101:689–92.
22. Saltin B, Gollnick PD. Skeletal muscle adaptability: significance for metabolism and performance. In: Anonymous Handbook of physiology: Skeletal muscle. American Physiology Society, Bethesda, MD, 1983; 555–632.
23. Hood DA. Plasticity in skeletal, cardiac, and smooth muscle: invited review: contractile activity-induced mitochondrial biogenesis in skeletal muscle. J Appl Physiol 2001; 90:1137–57.
24. Kraniou Y, Cameron-Smith D, Misso M, et al. Effects of exercise on GLUT-4 and glycogenin gene expression in human skeletal muscle. J Appl Physiol 2000; 88:794–6.
25. Kraniou GN, Cameron-Smith D, Hargreaves M. Effect of short-term training on GLUT-4 mRNA and protein expression in human skeletal muscle. Exp Physiol 2004; 89:559–63.

26. Pilegaard H, Ordway GA, Saltin B, et al. Transcriptional regulation of gene expression in human skeletal muscle during recovery from exercise. Am J Physiol 2000; 279: E806–14.

27. Baar K, Wende A, Jones TE, et al. Adaptations of skeletal muscle to exercise: rapid increase in the transcriptional coactivator PGC-1. The FASEB J 2002; 16:1879–86.

28. Murakami T, Shimomura Y, Yoshimura A, et al. Induction of nuclear respiratory factor-1 expression by an acute bout of exercise in rat muscle. Biochim Biophys Acta 1998; 1381(1):113–22.

29. Pilegaard H, Saltin B, Neufer PD. Exercise induces transient transcriptional activation of the PGC-1alpha gene in human skeletal muscle. J Physiol (Lond) 2003; 546:851–8.

30. Goto M, Terada S, Kato M, et al. cDNA Cloning and mRNA analysis of PGC-1 in epitrochlearis muscle in swimming-exercised rats. Biochem Biophys Res Commun 2000; 274:350–4.

31. Hamilton MT, Etienne J, McClure WC, et al. Role of local contractile activity and muscle fiber type on LPL regulation during exercise. Am J Physiol 1998; 275: E1016–22.

32. Seip RL, Mair K, Cole TG, et al. Induction of human skeletal muscle lipoprotein lipase gene expression by short-term exercise is transient. Am J Physiol 1997; 272: E255–61.

33. O'Doherty RM, Bracy DP, Osawa H, et al. Rat skeletal muscle hexokinase II mRNA and activity are increased by a single bout of acute exercise. Am J Physiol 1994; 266:E171–8.

34. Cortright RN, Zheng D, Jones JP, et al. Regulation of skeletal muscle UCP-2 and UCP-3 gene expression by exercise and denervation. Am J Physiol 1999; 276:E217–21.

35. Tsuboyama-Kasaoka N, Tsunoda N, Maruyama K, et al. Up-regulation of uncoupling protein 3 (UCP3) mRNA by exercise training and down–regulation of UCP3 by denervation in skeletal muscles. Biochem Biophys Res Commun 1998; 247: 498–503.

36. Linne Y, Dahlman I, Hoffstedt J. [beta]1-Adrenoceptor gene polymorphism predicts long-term changes in body weight. Int J Obesity 2005; 29:458–62.

37. Meirhaeghe A, Helbecque N, Cottel D, et al. Beta2-adrenoceptor gene polymorphism, body weight, and physical activity. Lancet 1999; 353:896.

38. Ukkola O, Tremblay A, Bouchard C. Beta-2 adrenergic receptor variants are associated with subcutaneous fat accumulation in response to long-term overfeeding. Int J Obes Relat Metab Disord 2001; 25:1604–8.

39. Corbalan MS, Marti A, Forga L, et al. The risk of obesity and the Trp64Arg polymorphism of the beta(3)-adrenergic receptor: effect modification by age. Ann Nutr Metab 2002; 46:152–8.

40. Ellsworth DL, Coady SA, Chen W, et al. Influence of the 2-adrenergic receptor Arg16Gly polymorphism on longitudinal changes in obesity from childhood through young adulthood in a biracial cohort: the Bogalusa Heart Study. Int J Obes Relat Metab Disord 2002; 26:928–37.

41. Van Rossum CTM, Hoebee B, Seidell JC, et al. Genetic factors as predictors of weight gain in young adult Dutch men and women. Int J Obes Relat Metab Disord 2002; 26:517–28.

42. Garenc C, Perusse L, Chagnon YC, et al. Effects of {beta}2-adrenergic receptor gene variants on adiposity: the HERITAGE family study. Obes Res 2003; 11:612–8.

43. Masuo K, Katsuya T, Fu Y, et al. {beta}2- and {beta}3-adrenergic receptor polymorphisms are related to the onset of weight gain and blood pressure elevation over 5 years. Circulation 2005; 111:3429–34.

44. Clement K, Vaisse C, Manning BS, et al. Genetic variation in the 3-adrenergic receptor and an increased capacity to gain weight in patients with morbid obesity. N Engl J Med 1995; 333:352–4.

45. Yoshida T, Sakane N, Umekawa T, et al. Mutation of beta 3-adrenergic-receptor gene and response to treatment of obesity. Lancet 1995; 346:1433–44.

46. Clement K, Manning BS, Basdevant A, et al. Gender effect of the Trp64Arg mutation in the beta 3 adrenergic receptor gene on weight gain in morbid obesity. Diabete Metab 1997; 23:424–7.

47. Nagase T, Aoki A, Yamamoto M, et al. Lack of association between the Trp64Arg mutation in the {beta}3-adrenergic receptor gene and obesity in Japanese men: a longitudinal analysis. J Clin Endocrinol Metab 1997; 82:1284–7.

48. Sakane N, Yoshida T, Umekawa T, et al. Effects of Trp64Arg mutation in the beta 3-adrenergic receptor gene on weight loss, body fat distribution, glycemic control, and insulin resistance in obese type 2 diabetic patients. Diabet Care 1997; 20: 1887–90.

49. Strazzullo P, Iacone R, Siani A, et al. Relationship of the Trp64Arg polymorphism of the beta3-adrenoceptor gene to central adiposity and high blood pressure: interaction with age. Cross-sectional and longitudinal findings of the Olivetti Prospective Heart Study. J Hypertens 2001; 19:399–406.

50. Marti A, Corbalan MS, Martinez-Gonzales MA, et al. TRP64ARG polymorphism of the beta 3-adrenergic receptor gene and obesity risk: effect modification by a sedentary lifestyle. Diabet Obes Metab 2002; 4:428–30.

51. Shiwaku A, Nogi A, Anuurad E, et al. Difficulty in losing weight by behavioral intervention for women with Trp64Arg polymorphism of the beta3-adrenergic receptor gene. Int J Obes Relat Metab Disord 2003; 27:1028–36.

52. Matsuoka H, Iwama S, Miura GI, et al. Impact of polymorphisms of beta2- and beta3-adrenergic receptor genes on longitudinal changes in obesity in early childhood. Acta Paediatr 2004; 93:430.

53. Miyaki K, Sutani S, Kikuchi H, et al. Increased risk of obesity resulting from the interaction between high energy intake and the Trp64Arg polymorphism of the beta3-adrenergic receptor gene in healthy Japanese men. J Epidemiol 2005; 15:203–10.

54. Ek J, Urhammer SA, Soø TI, et al. Homozygosity of the Pro12Ala variant of the peroxisome proliferation-activated receptor-gamma2 (PPAR-gamma2): divergent modulating effects on body mass index in obese and lean Caucasian men. Diabetologia 1999; 42:892–5.

55. Lindi V, Sivenius K, Niskanen LK, et al. Effect of the Pro12Ala polymorphism of the PPAR-gamma2 gene on long-term weight change in Finnish non-diabetic subjects. Diabetologia 2001; 44:925–6.

56. Nicklas BJ, Van Rossum EFC, Berman DM, et al. Genetic variation in the peroxisome proliferator-activated receptor-{gamma}2 gene (Pro12Ala) affects metabolic responses to weight loss and subsequent weight regain. Diabetes 2001; 50:2172–6.

57. Luan J, Browne PO, Harding AH, et al. Evidence for gene-nutrient interaction at the PPAR{gamma} locus. Diabetes 2001; 50:686–9.

58. Lindi VI, Uusitupa MIJ, Lindstrom J, et al. Association of the Pro12Ala polymorphism in the PPAR-{gamma}2 gene with 3-year incidence of type 2 diabetes and body weight change in the Finnish diabetes prevention study. Diabetes 2002; 51:2581–6.

59. Memisoglu A, Hu FB, Hankinson SE, et al. Interaction between a peroxisome proliferator-activated receptor {gamma} gene polymorphism and dietary fat intake in relation to body mass. Hum Mol Genet 2003; 12:2923–9.

60. Robitaille J, Despres JP, Perusse L, et al. The PPAR-gamma P12A polymorphism modulates the relationship between dietary fat intake and components of the metabolic syndrome: results from the Quebec Family Study. Clin Genet 2003; 63: 109–16.

61. Pihlajamaki J, Vanhala M, Vanhala P, et al. The Pro12Ala Polymorphism of the PPAR{gamma}2 Gene Regulates Weight from Birth to Adulthood. Obes Res 2004; 12:187–90.

62. Ostergard T, Ek J, Hamid Y, et al. Influence of the PPAR-gamma2 Pro12Ala and ACE I/D polymorphisms on insulin sensitivity and training effects in healthy offspring of type 2 diabetic subjects. Horm Metab Res 2005; 37:99–105.

63. Oppert JM, Vohl MC, Chagnon M, et al. DNA polymorphism in the uncoupling protein (UCP) gene and human body fat. Int J Obes Relat Metab Disord 1994; 18: 526–31.

64. Clement K, Ruiz J, Cassard-Doulcier AM, et al. Additive effect of A–>G (-3826) variant of the uncoupling protein gene and the Trp64Arg mutation of the beta 3-

adrenergic receptor gene on weight gain in morbid obesity. Int J Obes Relat Metab Disord 1996; 20:1062–6.

65. Fumeron F, Durack-Brown I, Betoulle D, et al. Polymorphisms of uncoupling protein (UCP) and beta 3 adrenoreceptor genes in obese people submitted to a low calorie diet. Int J Obes Relat Metab Disord 1996; 20:1051–4.

66. Kogure A, Yoshida T, Sakane N, et al. Synergic effect of polymorphisms in uncoupling protein 1 and b_3-adrenergic receptor genes on weight loss in obese Japanese. Diabetologia 1998; 41:1399.

67. Ukkola O, Tremblay A, Sun G, et al. Genetic variation at the uncoupling protein 1, 2 and 3 loci and the response to long-term overfeeding. Eur J Clin Nutr 2001; 55: 1008–15.

68. Matsushita H, Kurabayashi T, Tomita M, et al. Effects of uncoupling protein 1 and beta3-adrenergic receptor gene polymorphisms on body size and serum lipid concentrations in Japanese women. Maturitas 2003; 45:39–45.

69. Nordfors L, Heimburger O, Lonnqvist F, et al. Fat tissue accumulation during peritoneal dialysis is associated with a polymorphism in uncoupling protein 2. Kidney Int 2000; 57:1713–9.

70. Otabe S, Clement K, Dina C, et al. A genetic variation in the 5′ flanking region of the UCP3 gene is associated with body mass index in humans in interaction with physical activity. Diabetologia 2000; 43:245–9.

71. Alonso A, Marti A, Corbalan MS, et al. Association of UCP3 gene −55C>T polymorphism and obesity in a Spanish population. Ann Nutr Metab 2005; 49:183–8.

72. Lanouette CM, Chagnon YC, Rice T, et al. Uncoupling protein 3 gene is associated with body composition changes with training in HERITAGE study. J Appl Physiol 2002; 92:1111–8.

73. Cha MH, Shin HD, Kim KS, et al. The effects of uncoupling protein 3 haplotypes on obesity phenotypes and very low-energy diet-induced changes among overweight Korean female subjects. Metabolism 2006; 55:578–86.

74. Montgomery HE, Clarkson P, Barnard M, et al. Angiotensin-converting-enzyme gene insertion/deletion polymorphism and response to physical training. Lancet 1999; 353:541–5.

75. Sørensen TIA, Boutin P, Taylor MA, et al. Genetic Polymorphisms and Weight Loss in Obesity: A Randomised Trial of Hypo-Energetic High- versus Low-Fat Diets. Plos Clin Trials 2006; 1(2):e12.

76. Sivenius K, Lindi VI, Niskanen Lk, et al. Effect of a three-amino acid deletion in the alpha2B-adrenergic receptor gene on long-term body weight change in Finnish non-diabetic and type 2 diabetic subjects. Int J Obes Relat Metab Disord 2001; 25: 1609–14.

77. Chaves FJ, Giner V, Corella D, et al. Body weight changes and the A-6G polymorphism of the angiotensinogen gene. Int J Obes Relat Metab Disord 2002; 26: 1173–8.

78. Aberle J, Evans D, Beil FU, et al. A polymorphism in the apolipoprotein A5 gene is associated with weight loss after short-term diet. Clinical Genetics 2005; 68:152–4.

79. Ukkola O, Joanisse DR, Tremblay A, et al. Na+-K+−ATPase alpha 2-gene and skeletal muscle characteristics in response to long-term overfeeding. J Appl Physiol 2003; 94:1870–4.

80. Tworoger SS, Chubak J, Aiello EJ, et al. The Effect of CYP19 and COMT Polymorphisms on Exercise-Induced Fat Loss in Postmenopausal Women. Obes Res 2004; 12:972–81.

81. Ukkola O, Chagnon YC, Tremblay A, et al. Genetic variation at the adipsin locus and response to long-term overfeeding. Eur J Clin Nutr 2003; 57:1073–8.

82. Rankinen T, Rice T, Leon AS, et al. G protein (beta)3 polymorphism and hemodynamic and body composition phenotypes in the HERITAGE Family Study. Physiol Genomics 2002; 8:151–7.

83. Hauner H, Meier M, Jockel KH, et al. Prediction of successful weight reduction under sibutramine therapy through genotyping of the G-protein beta3 subunit gene (GNB3) C825T polymorphism. Pharmacogenetics 2003; 13(8):4539.

84. Ukkola O, Rosmond R, Tremblay A, et al. Glucocorticoid receptor Bcl I variant is associated with an increased atherogenic profile in response to long-term overfeeding. Atherosclerosis 2001; 157:221–4.

85. Tremblay A, Bouchard L, Bouchard C, et al. Long-term adiposity changes are related to a glucocorticoid receptor polymorphism in young females. J Clin Endocrinol Metab 2003; 88:3141–5.

86. Westberg L, Bah J, Rastam M, et al. Association between a polymorphism of the 5-HT2C receptor and weight loss in teenage girls. Neuropsychopharmacology 2002; 26:789–93.

87. McKenzie JA, Weiss EP, Ghiu IA, et al. Influence of the interleukin-6 -174 G/C gene polymorphism on exercise training-induced changes in glucose tolerance indexes. J Appl Physiol 2004; 97:1338–42.

88. Riechman SE, Balasekaran G, Roth SM, et al. Association of interleukin-15 protein and interleukin-15 receptor genetic variation with resistance exercise training responses. J Appl Physiol 2004; 97:2214–9.

89. Thorsby BM, Berg JP, Birkeland KI. Insulin gene variable number of tandem repeats is associated with increased fat mass during adolescence in non-obese girls. Scan J Clin Lab Invest 2005; 65(2):163–8.

90. Oksanen L, Ohman M, Heiman ML, et al. Markers for the gene ob and serum leptin levels in human morbid obesity. Human Genet 1997; 99:559–64.

91. Mammes O, Aubert R, Betoulle D, et al. LEPR gene polymorphisms: associations with overweight, fat mass and response to diet in women. European J Clin Invest 2001; 31:398–404.

92. de Silva AM, Walder KR, Boyko EJ, et al. Genetic variation and obesity in Australian women: a prospective study. Obes Res 2001; 9:733–40.

93. de Luis Roman D, de la Fuente RA, Sagrado MG, et al. Leptin Receptor Lys656Asn Polymorphism Is Associated with Decreased Leptin Response and Weight Loss Secondary to a Lifestyle Modification in Obese Patients. Arch Med Res 2006; 37:854–9.

94. Ukkola O, Tremblay A, Bouchard C. Lipoprotein lipase polymorphisms and responses to long-term overfeeding. J Int Med 2002; 251:429–36.

95. Garenc C, Perusse L, Bergeron J, et al. Evidence of LPL gene-exercise interaction for body fat and LPL activity: the HERITAGE Family Study. J Appl Physiol 2001; 91:1334–40.

96. Rutanen J, Pihlajamaki J, Karhapaa P, et al. The Val103Ile Polymorphism of Melano-cortin-4 Receptor Regulates Energy Expenditure and Weight Gain. Obes Res 2004; 12:1060–6.

97. Corella D, Qi L, Sorli JV, et al. Obese Subjects Carrying the 11482G>A Polymorphism at the Perilipin Locus Are Resistant to Weight Loss after Dietary Energy Restriction. J Clin Endocrinol Metab 2005; 90:5121–6.

98. Obata T, Ito T, Yonemura A, et al. R192Q paraoxonase gene variant is associated with a change in HDL-cholesterol level during dietary caloric restriction in nondiabetic healthy males. J Atheroscler Thromb 2003; 10:57–62.

99. Spiegelman BM. PPAR-gamma: adipogenic regulator and thiazolidinedione receptor. Diabetes 1998; 47:507–14.

100. Kersten S, Desvergne B, Wahli W. Roles of PPARs in health and disease. Nature 2000; 405:421–4.

101. Lazar MA. Progress in cardiovascular biology: PPAR for the course. Nature Medicine 2001; 7:23–4.

102. Rosen ED, Walkey CJ, Puigserver P, et al. Transcriptional regulation of adipogenesis. Genes Dev 2000; 14:1293–307.

103. Fajas L, Auboeuf D, Raspe E, et al. The Organization, Promoter Analysis, and Expression of the Human PPARgamma Gene. J Biol Chem 1997; 272:18779–89.

104. Vidal-Puig AJ, Considine RV, Jimenez-Linan M, et al. Peroxisome Proliferator-activated Receptor Gene Expression in Human Tissues. Effects of Obesity, Weight Loss, and Regulation by Insulin and Glucocorticoids. J Clin Invest 1997; 99:2416–22.

105. Tontonoz P, Hu E, Spiegelman BM. Stimulation of adipogenesis in fibroblasts by PPAR[gamma]2, a lipid-activated transcription factor. Cell 1994; 79:1147–56.

106. Wu Z, Xie Y, Bucher NL, et al. Conditional ectopic expression of C/EBP beta in NIH-3T3 cells induces PPAR gamma and stimulates adipogenesis. Genes Dev 1995; 9:2350–63.
107. Nakano R, Kurosaki E, Yoshida S, et al. Antagonism of peroxisome proliferator-activated receptor [gamma] prevents high-fat diet-induced obesity in vivo. Biocheml Pharmacol 2006; 72:42–52.
108. Xu HE, Lambert MH, Montana VG, et al. Molecular Recognition of Fatty Acids by Peroxisome Proliferator-Activated Receptors. Molecular Cell 1999; 3:397–403.
109. Desvergne B, Wahli W. Peroxisome Proliferator-Activated Receptors: Nuclear Control of Metabolism. Endocr Rev 1999; 20:649–88.
110. Kawamura T, Yoshida K, Sugawara A, et al. Regulation of skeletal muscle peroxisome proliferator-activated receptor gamma expression by exercise and angiotensin-converting enzyme inhibition in fructose-fed hypertensive rats. Hypertension Res 2004; 27(1):61–70.
111. Wisloff U, Najjar SM, Ellingsen O, et al. Cardiovascular risk factors emerge after artificial selection for low aerobic capacity. Science 2005; 307:418–20.
112. Tunstall RJ, Mehan KA, Wadley GD, et al. Exercise training increases lipid metabolism gene expression in human skeletal muscle. Am J Physiol 2002; 283:E66–72.
113. Auwerx J. PPARgamma, the ultimate thrifty gene. Diabetologia 1999; 42:1033–49.
114. Koutnikova H, Cock TA, Watanabe M, et al. Compensation by the muscle limits the metabolic consequences of lipodystrophy in PPAR{gamma} hypomorphic mice. PNAS 2003; 100:14457–62.
115. Medina-Gomez G, Virtue S, Lelliott C, et al. The link between nutritional status and insulin sensitivity is dependent on the adipocyte-specific peroxisome proliferator-activated receptor-{gamma}2 isoform. Diabetes 2005; 54:1706–16.
116. Zhang J, Fu M, Cui T, et al. Selective disruption of PPAR{gamma}2 impairs the development of adipose tissue and insulin sensitivity. PNAS 2004; 101:10703–8.
117. Deeb SS, Fajas L, Nemoto M, et al. A Pro12Ala substitution in PPARgamma2 associated with decreased receptor activity, lower body mass index and improved insulin sensitivity. Nature Genet 1998; 20:284–7.
118. Masugi J, Tamori Y, Mori H, et al. Inhibitory effect of a proline–to-alanine substitution at codon 12 of peroxisome proliferator-activated receptor-gamma 2 on thiazolidine-dione-induced adipogenesis. Biochem Biophys Res Commun 2000; 268:178–82.
119. Altshuler D, Hirschhorn JN, Klannemark M, et al. The common PPAR(gamma) Pro12Ala polymorphism is associated with decreased risk of type 2 diabetes. Nature Genet 2000; 26:76–80.
120. Ek J, Andersen G, Urhammer SA, et al. Studies of the Pro12Ala polymorphism of the peroxisome proliferator-activated receptor-gamma2 (PPAR-gamma2) gene in relation to insulin sensitivity among glucose tolerant caucasians. Diabetologia 2001; 44: 1170–6.
121. Lehrke M, Lazar MA. The Many Faces of PPAR [gamma]. Cell 2005; 123:993–9.
122. Schrauwen P, Hesselink M. UCP2 and UCP3 in muscle controlling body metabolism. J Exp Biol 2005; 205:2275–85.
123. Giraudo SQ, Kotz CM, Grace MK, et al. Rat hypothalamic NPY mRNA and brown fat uncoupling protein mRNA after high-carbohydrate or high-fat diets. Am J Physiol Regul Integr Comp Physiol 1994; 266:R1578–83.
124. Matsuda J, Hosoda K, Itoh H, et al. Cloning of rat uncoupling protein-3 and uncoupling protein-2 cDNAs: their gene expression in rats fed high-fat diet. FEBS Lett 1997; 418:200–4.
125. Fleury C, Neverova M, Collins S, et al. Uncoupling protein-2: a novel gene linked to obesity and hyperinsulinemia. Nature Genet 1997; 15:269–72.
126. Boss O, Samec S, Kuhne F, et al. Uncoupling Protein-3 Expression in Rodent Skeletal Muscle Is Modulated by Food Intake But Not by Changes in Environmental Temperature. J Biol Chem 1998; 273:5–8.
127. Millet L, Vidal H, Andreelli F, et al. Increased uncoupling protein-2 and -3 mRNA expression during fasting in obese and lean humans. J Clin Invest 1997; 100: 2665–70.

128. Boss O, Samec S, Dulloo A, et al. Tissue-dependent upregulation of rat uncoupling protein-2 expression in response to fasting or cold. FEBS Lett 1997; 412:111–4.

129. Sivitz WI, Fink BD, Donohoue PA. Fasting and Leptin Modulate Adipose and Muscle Uncoupling Protein: Divergent Effects Between Messenger Ribonucleic Acid and Protein Expression. Endocrinology 1999; 140:1511–19.

130. Hildebrandt AL, Neufer PD. Exercise attenuates the fasting-induced transcriptional activation of metabolic genes in skeletal muscle. Am J Physiol 2000; 278:E1078–86.

131. Vidal-Puig A, Rosenbaum M, Considine RC, et al. Effects of obesity and stable weight reduction on UCP2 and UCP3 gene expression in humans. Obes Res 1999; 7:133–140.

132. Cusin I, Zakrzewska KE, Boss O, et al. Chronic central leptin infusion enhances insulin-stimulated glucose metabolism and favors the expression of uncoupling proteins. Diabetes 1998; 47:1014–19.

133. Brun S, Carmona MC, Mampel T, et al. Uncoupling protein-3 gene expression in skeletal muscle during development is regulated by nutritional factors that alter circulating non-esterified fatty acids. FEBS Lett 1999; 453:205–9.

134. Boss O, Bobionni-Harsch E, Assimacopoulos-Jeannet F, et al. Uncoupling protein-3 expression in skeletal muscle and free fatty acids in obesity. Lancet 1998; 351(9120):1933.

135. Samec S, Seydoux J, Dulloo AG. Role of UCP homologues in skeletal muscles and brown adipose tissue: mediators of thermogenesis or regulators of lipids as fuel substrate? FASEB J 1998; 12:715–24.

136. Samec S, Seydoux J, Dulloo AG. Interorgan signaling between adipose tissue metabolism and skeletal muscle uncoupling protein homologs: is there a role for circulating free fatty acids? Diabetes 1998; 47:1693–8.

137. Petzke KJ, Riese C, Klaus S. Short-term, increasing dietary protein and fat moderately affect energy expenditure, substrate oxidation and uncoupling protein gene expression in rats. J Nutrit Biochem 2007; 18(6):400–7.

138. Hjeltnes N, Fernström M, Zierath JR, et al. Regulation of UCP2 and UCP3 by muscle disuse and physical activity in tetraplegic subjects. Diabetologia 1999; 42:826–30.

139. Schrauwen P, Hesselink M. An alternative function for human uncoupling protein 3: protection of mitochondria against accumulation of nonesterified fatty acids inside the mitochondrial matrix. FASEB J 2001; 15:2497–502.

140. Schrauwen P, Van Aggel-Leijssen DPC, Hul G, et al. The effect of a 3-month low-intensity endurance training program on fat oxidation and acetyl-CoA carboxylase-2 expression. Diabetes 2002; 51:2220–6.

141. Oh KS, Kim M, Lee J, et al. Liver PPAR[alpha] and UCP2 are involved in the regulation of obesity and lipid metabolism by swim training in genetically obese db/db mice. Biochem Biophys Res Commun 2006; 345:1232–9.

142. Schrauwen P, Troost FJ, Xia J, et al. Skeletal muscle UCP2 and UCP3 expression in trained and untrained male subjects. Int J Obes Relat Metab Disord 1999; 23:966–72.

143. Russell AP, Wadley GD, Snow R, et al. Slow component of [V]O(2) kinetics: the effect of training status, fibre type, UCP3 mRNA and citrate synthase activity. Int J Obes Relat Metabol Disord 2002; 26(2):157–64.

144. Russell AP, Wadley GD, Hesselink M, et al. UCP3 protein expression is lower in type I, IIa and IIx muscle fiber types of endurance-trained compared to untrained subjects. Pflügers Archive—Eur J Physiol 2003; 445(5):563–9.

145. Zhou M, Lin BZ, Coughlin S, et al. UCP-3 expression in skeletal muscle: effects of exercise, hypoxia, and AMP-activated protein kinase. Am J Physiol 2000; 279:E622–9.

146. Schrauwen P, Hesselink MKC, Vaartjes I, et al. Effect of acute exercise on uncoupling protein 3 is a fat metabolism-mediated effect. Am J Physiol 2002; 282:E11–17.

147. Pilegaard H, Keller C, Steensberg A, et al. Influence of pre-exercise muscle glycogen content on exercise-induced transcriptional regulation of metabolic genes. J Physiol (Lond) 2002; 541:261–71.

148. Sivenius K, Valve R, Lindi V, et al. Synergistic effect of polymorphisms in uncoupling protein 1 and beta3-adrenergic receptor genes on long-term body weight change in Finnish type 2 diabetic and non-diabetic control subjects. Int J Obes Relat Metab Disord 2000; 24:514–9.

149. Shihara N, Yaduda K, Moritani T, et al. Synergistic effect of polymorphisms of uncoupling protein 1 and beta3-adrenergic receptor genes on autonomic nervous system activity. Int J Obes Relat Metab Disord 2001; 25:761–6

150. Valve R, Heikkinen S, Rissanen A, et al. Synergistic effect of polymotphisms in uncoupling protein 1 and b_3-adrenergic receptor genes on basal metabolic rate in obese Finns. Diabetologia 1998; 41:357–61.

151. Nagase I, Yoshida T, Kumamoto K, et al. Expression of Uncoupling Protein in Skeletal Muscle and White Fat of Obese Mice Treated with Thermogenic beta 3-Adrenergic Agonist. J Clin Invest 1996; 97:2898–904.

152. Yoshida T, Umekawa T, Kumamoto K, et al. beta 3-Adrenergic agonist induces a functionally active uncoupling protein in fat and slow-twitch muscle fibers. Am J Physiol 1998; 274:E469–75.

153. Nakamura H, Nagase I, Asano A, et al. Beta 3-adrenergic agonist up-regulates uncoupling proteins 2 and 3 in skeletal muscle of the mouse. J Vet Med Sci 2001; 63(3):309–14.

154. Walder K, Norman RA, Schrauwen P, et al. Association between uncoupling protein polymorphisms (UCP2-UCP3) and energy metabolism/obesity in Pima indians. Hum Mol Genet 1998; 7:1431–5.

155. Kovacs P, Ma L, Hanson RL, et al. Genetic variation in *UCP2* (uncoupling protein-2) is associated with energy metabolism in Pima Indians. Diabetologia 2005; 48(11):2242–50.

156. Urhammer SA, Dalgaard LT, Sørensen TIA, et al. Mutational analysis of the coding region of the uncoupling protein 2 gene in obese NIDDM patients: impact of a common amino acid polymorphism on juvenile and maturity onset forms of obesity and insuline resistance. Diabetologia 1997; 40:1227–30.

157. Barbe P, Millet L, Larrouy D, et al. Uncoupling protein-2 messanger ribonucleic acid expression during very-low-calorie diet in obese premenopausal women. J Clin Endocrinol Metab 1998; 83:2450–3.

158. Berentzen T, Dalgaard LT, Petersen L, et al. Interactions between physical activity and variants of the genes encoding uncoupling proteins -2 and -3 in relation to body weight changes during a 10-y follow-up. Int J Obes Relat Metab Disord 2004; 29:93–9.

159. Chagnon YC, Rice T, Perusse L, et al. Genomic scan for genes affecting body composition before and after training in Caucasians from HERITAGE. J Appl Physiol 2001; 90:1777–87.

160. Schrauwen P, Xia J, Walder K, et al. A novel polymorphism in the proximal UCP3 promoter region: effect on skeletal muscle UCP3 mRNA and obesity in male non-diabetic Pima Indians. Int J Obes Relat Metab Disord 1999; 23:1242–5.

161. Blaak EE, Van Baak MA, Kemerinck GJ, et al. Beta-adrenergic stimulation of energy expenditure and forearm skeletal muscle metabolism in lean and obese men. Am J Physiol 1994; 267:E306–15.

162. Blaak EE, Van Baak MA, Saris WHM. (Beta)-adrenergically stimulated fat oxidation is diminished in middle-aged compared to young subjects. J Clin Endocrinol Metab 1999; 84(10):3764–9.

163. Schiffelers SLH, Van Harmelen VJA, de Grauw HAJ, et al. Dobutamine as selective beta 1-adrenoceptor agonist in in vivo studies on human thermogenesis and lipid utilization. J Appl Physiol 1999; 87:977–81.

164. Webber J, Taylor J, Greathead H, et al. A comparison of the thermogenic, metabolic and haemodynamic responses to infused adrenaline in lean and obese subjects. Int J Obes Relat Metab Disord 1994; 18:717–24.

165. Enocksson S, Shimizu M, Lonnqvist F, et al. Demonstration of an in vivo functional beta 3-adrenoceptor in man. J Clin Invest 1995; 95(5):2239–45.

166. Lafontan M. Differential recruitment and differential regulation by physiological amines of fat cell beta-1, beta-2 and beta-3 adrenergic receptors expressed in native fat cells and in transfected cell lines. Cell Signal 1994; 6:363–92.

167. Barbe P, Millet L, Galitzky J, et al. In situ assessment of the role of the beta 1-, beta 2- and beta 3-adrenoceptors in the control of lipolysis and nutritive blood flow in human subcutaneous adipose tissue. Brit J Pharmacol 1996; 117(5):907–13.

168. Tavernier G, Barbe P, Galitzky J, et al. Expression of beta3-adrenoceptors with low lipolytic action in human subcutaneous white adipocytes. J Lipid Res 1996; 37:87–97.

169. Chamberlain PD, Jennings KH, Paul F, et al. The tissue distribution of the human beta3-adrenoceptor studied using a monoclonal antibody: direct evidence of the beta3-adrenoceptor in human adipose tissue, atrium and skeletal muscle. International J Obes Relat Metabol Disord 1999; 23(10):1057–65.
170. Bachman ES, Dhillon H, Zhang CY, et al. Beta AR Signaling Required for diet-induced thermogenesis and obesity resistance. Science 2002; 297:843–5.
171. Susulic VS, Frederich RC, Lawitts J, et al. Targeted disruption of the beta(3)-adrenergic receptor gene. J Biol Chem 1995; 270:29483–92.
172. Kjaer M, Secher NH, Galbo H. Physical stress and catecholamine release. Baillieres Clin Endocrinol Metabol 1987; 1(2):279–98.
173. Bell C, Stob NR, Seals DR. Thermogenic Responsiveness to (beta)-adrenergic stimulation is augmented in exercising vs. sedentary adults: role of oxidative stress. J Physiol (Lond) 2005.
174. Green SA, Turki J, Innis M, et al. Amino-terminal polymorphisms of the human beta 2-adrenergic receptor impart distinct agonist-promoted regulatory properties. Biochemistry 1994; 33:9414–9.
175. Liggett SB. Polymorphisms of the beta 2-Adrenergic Receptor and Asthma. Am J Respir Crit Care Med 1997; 156:156S–62S.
176. Corbalan MS, Marti A, Forga L, et al. The 27Glu polymorphism of the beta2-adrenergic receptor gene interacts with physical activity influencing obesity risk among female subjects. Clin Genet 2002; 61:305–7.
177. McGraw DW, Forbes SL, Kramer LA, et al. Polymorphisms of the 5' Leader istron of the human beta 2-adrenergic receptor regulate receptor expression. J Clin Invest 1998; 102:1927–32.
178. Hoffstedt J, Poirier O, Thorne A, et al. Polymorphism of the human beta3-adrenoceptor gene forms a well-conserved haplotype that is associated with moderate obesity and altered receptor function. Diabetes 1999; 48:203–5.
179. Pietri-Rouxel F, St John Manning B, Gros J, et al. The biochemical effect of the naturally occurring Trp64–>Arg mutation on human beta3-adrenoceptor activity. Eur J Biochem 1997; 247(3):1174–9.
180. Sipilainen R, Uusitupa M, Heikkinen S, et al. Polymorphism of the beta3-adrenergic receptor gene affects basal metabolic rate in obese Finns. Diabetes 1997; 46:77–80.
181. Walston J, Andersen RE, Seibert M, et al. Arg64 {beta}3-adrenoceptor variant and the components of energy expenditure. Obes Res 2003; 11:509–11.
182. Von Elm E, Egger M. The scandal of poor epidemiological research. BMJ 2004; 329:868–9.
183. Ioannidis JPA, Gwinn M, Little J, et al. A road map for efficient and reliable human genome epidemiology. Nature Genet 2006; 38:3–5.
184. Hwang SJ, Beaty TH, Liang KY, et al. Minimum sample size estimation to detect gene-environment interaction in case-control designs. Am J Epidemiol 1994; 140(11):1029–37.
185. Foppa I, Spiegelman D. Power and sample size calculations for case–control studies of gene–environment interactions with a polytomous exposure variable. Am J Epidemiol 1997; 146(7):596–604.
186. Luan JA, Wong MY, Day NE, et al. Sample size determination for studies of gene-environment interaction. Int J Epidemiol 2001; 30:1035–40.
187. Wong MY, Day NE, Luan JA, et al. The detection of gene-environment interaction for continuous traits: should we deal with measurement error by bigger studies or better measurement? Int J Epidemiol 2003; 32:51–7.

Roland Rosmond
Partille, Sweden

During the past decade, mutations affecting liability to obesity have been discovered at a phenomenal rate, and despite very few consistently replicated findings, a number of intriguing results have emerged in the literature (1). The obesity gene map shows putative loci on all chromosomes except Y. More than 600 genes, markers, and chromosomal regions have been associated or linked with human obesity phenotypes (1). However, researchers are still looking for the gene variants that cause most cases of obesity. Genome-wide scans in different ethnic populations have localized major obesity loci on chromosomes 2, 5, 10, 11 and 20 (2). This indicates that the common forms of obesity arises in individuals who carry a cluster of genes each of which creates only a minor tendency towards energy accretion, but whose combined effects can lead to a pronounced weight gain.

This chapter reviews evidence concerning the role of genetic variants in circulating hormone concentrations and human obesity. Because of space limitation, much material cannot be incorporated in this overview. The discussion of the more common alterations in endocrine function that are characteristic of human obesity is focused primarily on those occurring as a result of mutations in single genes.

OBESITY: A HETEROGENEOUS PHENOTYPE

Obesity with an increased number of adipocytes (i.e., hypercellular obesity) typically begins in early or middle childhood, and usually accompanies a body mass index (BMI) above $40 \, kg/m^2$. In contrast, obesity with enlarged adipocytes (i.e., hypertrophic obesity) tends to correlate with truncal fat distribution, which in turn is an important predictor of the health hazards of obesity. Certainly, differences in clinical symptomatology favor a separation of obesity into two broad categories: *visceral* and *nonvisceral* obesity. Since there may be some degree of overlap between these conditions, it could be argued that the etiology of these disorders may be shared. However, from an analytic as well as from an investigational point of view, we will presume that etiologies differ. Given the differences in number and size of fat cells (3), this seems a reasonable assumption.

GENETIC VARIANTS AND MAJOR ENDOCRINE DETERMINANTS OF OBESITY
Insulin

From a whole body perspective, insulin has a fat-sparing effect. Not only does it drive most cells to preferentially oxidize carbohydrates instead of fatty acids for energy, insulin indirectly stimulates accumulation of fat in adipose tissue. The human insulin gene (*INS*) is located at 11p15.5 (4). Over ten years ago, Weaver et al. performed the first study indicating a potential association between *INS* gene mutation, insulin and central, visceral obesity (5). A polymorphisms in the

5′-flanking region of the *INS* gene was studied in 56 severely obese (mean BMI 40 kg/m^2), unrelated British young non-diabetic women for associations of restriction fragment length polymorphism (RFLP) of *INS* with anthropometric measurements and indices of insulin secretion and resistance. An association of the class 3 allele of the hypervariable region in the 5′-flanking region of the *INS* gene was found with upper segment obesity. Furthermore, the class 3 allele was also associated with fasting hyperinsulinemia and stimulated insulin secretion. To determine which genetic factors predispose obese patients to beta-cell dysfunction, Le Stunff et al. studied single-nucleotide polymorphisms (SNPs) in the region of the *INS* gene among 615 obese children (6). They found that young obese patients homozygous for class I variable number of tandem repeat alleles secrete more insulin than those with other genotypes.

Variants in the insulin receptor gene (*INSR*) have long been considered possible candidates for the underlying cause of hyperinsulinemia/insulin resistance and obesity. With in situ hybridization and Southern blot analysis of somatic cell hybrid DNA, Yang-Feng et al. (7) assigned the *INSR* gene to 19p13.3-p13.2. Insulin binding stimulates autophosphorylation of the intracellular region of the receptor β-subunit (8). In obese subjects, there is a decrease in the number of insulin receptors on the cell membranes of insulin-sensitive target cell, such as adipocytes (9). This downregulation of the number of insulin receptors is thought to occur as a result of the increased circulating insulin levels (9).

In addition to insulin-related genes, a number of other genes appear to be involved in the association between insulin secretion and obesity. Below are just a few examples to highlight the diversity of genes affecting both insulin and obesity.

In 1995, a series of papers published in the *New England Journal of Medicine* indicated a potential relevance of a missense mutation in the adrenergic, beta-3-, receptor (*ADRB3*) to human obesity (10–12). A cytosine-to-thymidine substitution was identified resulting in the replacement of tryptophan by arginine (Trp64Arg) in the first intracellular loop of the receptor. Those with the mutation had a higher waist-to-hip ratio (WHR) and a greater increase in the serum insulin response after the oral administration of glucose (11).

In a recent association study using a 9-bp insertional polymorphism, AGC AGC GGC, between nucleotides 6979 and 6998 of the proopiomelanocortin (*POMC*) gene, was performed in 380 (185 girls) Italian obese children and adolescents (13). Interestingly, the results showed that this polymorphism, in the obese patients, was associated with differences in fasting insulin levels; this finding persisted after correction for age, sex, and pubertal stage. Heterozygotes had 24% higher mean insulin levels than those homozygous for the wild allele and showed a stronger correlation between insulin and BMI (13).

Peroxisome proliferator-activated receptors are members of the nuclear hormone receptor subfamily of ligand-dependent transcription factors (14). The isoform peroxisome proliferator-activated receptor gamma 2 (PPARG2) is mainly expressed in adipose tissue (15), where it modulates the expression of target genes involved in adipocyte differentiation (14). To date, at least two naturally occurring mutations in this gene have been identified, which impair the function of PPARG2 (16,17). The C → G mutation in exon B of the *PPARG2* gene leads to the substitution of alanine for proline at codon 12 (Pro12Ala) (18). The *PPARG2* Ala allele has reduced ability to activate transcription of PPARG2 target genes (18). Some, but not all studies, have indicated a role for this variant in the pathogenesis of obesity and obesity-associated insulin resistance (17,19–21).

Catecholamines

The principal catecholamines are epinephrine (adrenaline), norepinephrine (noradrenaline) and dopamine. In addition to their effects as neurotransmitters, norepinephrine and epinephrine can influence the rate of metabolism. This influence works both by modulating endocrine function such as insulin secretion and by increasing the rate of glycogenolysis and fatty acid mobilization. The catecholamines bind to two different classes of receptors termed the adrenergic, alpha and beta, receptors. Recently, a meta-analysis of 40 published papers with a total of 12,805 subjects was performed with the objective to elucidate the potential impact of a Trp64Arg polymorphism of the *ADRB3* gene on insulin resistance (22). Significant associations emerged in subjects with obesity as well as in subjects with diabetes (22). Since adrenergic, beta-3-, receptor plays a significant role in the control of lipolysis and thermogenesis in brown adipose tissue through autonomic nervous system activity, the association of the Trp64Arg polymorphism with autonomic nervous system activity have previously been examined (23). The autonomic nervous system activity was examined during supine rest and standing by electrocardiogram R-R interval power spectral analysis. With a postural change to standing, the parasympathetic and sympathetic nervous system activity indexes of heterozygotes showed a higher response than those of normal subjects (23).

The polymorphisms in codon 16 (Arg16Gly) and codon 27 (Gln27Glu) of adrenergic, beta-2-, receptor (*ADRB2*) is associated with central fat mass and BMI (24,25). In a small group of obese women with the Glu27Glu genotype, epinephrine and norepinephrine were quantified by high-performance liquid chromatography (26). The respiratory quotient was higher in the Glu27Glu obese women along the study, and fat oxidation was significantly lower. However, epinephrine and norepinephrine levels did not differ between women with the Glu27Glu genotype compared with those with Gln27Gln genotype (26).

In 2003, Sivenius et al investigated the impact of a three-amino acid deletion (12Glu9) polymorphism in the adrenergic, alpha-2B-, receptor (*ADRA2B*) on autonomic nervous function (27). The short form (Glu(9)/Glu(9)) of the polymorphism has previously been associated with a reduced basal metabolic rate in obese subjects. Data of a 10-year follow-up study with 126 nondiabetic control subjects and 84 type 2 diabetic patients were used to determine the effects of the 12Glu9 polymorphism on autonomic nervous function. The nondiabetic men with the Glu(9)/Glu(9) genotype, especially those with abdominal obesity, had significantly lower total and low-frequency power values in the power spectral analysis when compared with other men (27). These results suggest that the 12Glu9 polymorphism of the *ADRA2B* gene modulates autonomic nervous function in nondiabetic men with central obesity.

Glucocorticoids

Progressive weight gain is the most universal symptom in subjects with elevated circulating glucocorticoid (cortisol) levels. Obesity is truncal, and the subjects have thin extremities due to muscle wasting. Glucose intolerance with hyperglycemia and eventually diabetes mellitus is common. The human glucocorticoid receptor gene (*NR3C1*) is located on chromosome 5q31 (28). Mutations in the *GRL* were first reported in 1991. To date, a number of mutations within the human *GRL* gene have been described. Subjects with a polymorphism at nucleotide position 1220; resulting in an asparagine-to-serine change at codon 363 in the *GRL*, have a higher sensitivity to exogenously administered glucocorticoids, with respect to both cortisol suppression and insulin response (29). Comparison between N363S carriers and controls show that the N363S carriers have a higher BMI than controls (29). In the Quebec Family Study, a biallelic (4.5- and 2.3-kb alleles) *Bcl*I RFLP was found to be associated with a higher abdominal visceral fat area in both men and women, independently of total body fat mass (30). In a general population of nonCushingoid middle-aged men, the 4.5-kb fragment was associated with elevated BMI, WHR, and abdominal sagittal diameter (31). Moreover, salivary cortisol levels were elevated in the men with the 4.5-kb allele (31). The molecular identity of the *Bcl*I polymorphism has recently been determined as a G-to-C transition in the second intron, 646 base pair from the exon 2/intron 2 junction (32).

Over 90% of circulating cortisol is bound, predominantly to the alpha-2-globulin cortisol-binding globulin. Alterations in cortisol-binding globulin concentrations change total circulating cortisol concentrations accordingly but free cortisol concentrations are normal. In a recent study in 44 obese pre-menopausal women, a microsatellite located within the cortisol-binding globulin showed a strong correlation between salivary cortisol after 0.25-mg dexamethasone suppression test and WHR (33).

Since the melanocortin-4 receptor (MC4-R) regulates food intake and possibly energy expenditure, a $G \rightarrow A$ substitution at codon 103 (Val-103Ile) of the MC4R gene was examined for the influence on abdominal obesity and salivary cortisol in 284 unrelated men born in 1944 (34). The frequency of allele G was 0.97 and 0.03 for allele A. The heterozygotes had lower WHR and trends for lower BMI and abdominal sagittal diameter compared to G/G homozygotes. The heterozygotes had also, in comparison to G/G subjects, significantly higher mean cortisol concentrations in the morning (21.4 vs. 14.6 nmol/l), and after a standardized lunch (15.3 vs. 8.0 nmol/l) (34).

The hypothalamus-pituitary-adrenal axis that regulates cortisol production and secretion has extensive and complex central neural connections, and receives afferent regulatory signals from different parts of the brain. For instance, the hypothalamic neurons are excitatory influenced on by serotoninergic (5-HT) central pathways (35). Inhibitory effects are exerted by gamma-aminobutyric acid (GABA) (36). Catecholamines can exert both inhibitory and excitatory effects (37). Lately, an *Msp*I RFLP in the promoter region of the 5-hydroxytryptamine (serotonin) receptor 2A (*5-HT2A*) gene (–1438G/A) has been described (38). The human $5\text{-}HT_{2A}$ gene is located on 13q14–q21 (39), and consists of 3 exons separated by 2 introns and spans over 20 kb (40). The potential impact of the $5\text{-}HT_{2A}$ –1438G/A promoter polymorphism on obesity and salivary cortisol was examined in a group of unrelated Swedish men (41). Homozygotes for the –1438G allele had, in comparison with –1438A/A subjects, higher BMI, WHR, and abdominal sagittal diameter. Moreover, cortisol escape from 0.25-mg dexamethasone suppression was found in subjects with the –1438A/G genotype. From these results, it is suggested that an abnormal production rate of the $5\text{-}HT_{2A}$ gene product might lead to the development of abdominal obesity. The pathophysiology could involve stress factors that destabilize the serotonin-hypothalamic-pituitary-adrenal system in those with genetic vulnerability in the serotonin receptor gene (41).

Clinical evidence suggests that alprazolam, a benzodiazepine that activates GABAergic receptors, inhibits the activity of the hypothalamic-pituitary-adrenal axis (42,43). In obese subjects, pretreatment with alprazolam blunts the hypothalamic-pituitary-adrenal axis response to pharmacological challenge tests (44). Recently, a novel SNP in the 3' non-coding region of the gamma-aminobutyric acid (GABA) A receptor, alpha 6 (*GABRA6*) gene has been described (45). DNA sequencing has shown that it is a T to C substitution resulting in the loss of an *Alw*NI restriction site at nucleotide 1519 (45). The *GABRA6* gene is located on chromosome 5q31.1-q35 (46). With this background, the potential impact of the 1519T>C polymorphism in the *GABRA6* gene on obesity and obesity-related phenotypes as well as salivary cortisol were examined in a group of unrelated Swedish men born in 1944 (47). Carriers for the T allele had borderline significantly higher WHR and abdominal sagittal diameter compared to homozygotes for the C allele. The homozygotes for the T allele had, in comparison to heterozygotes, significantly higher mean cortisol levels before and after a standardized lunch. In addition, T/T subjects had significantly higher diurnal cortisol secretion compared to T/C subjects. These findings suggest a role of the 1519T>C polymorphism in the *GABRA6* gene in the predisposition to hypercortisolism and abdominal obesity. As with $5\text{-}HT_{2A}$ −1438G/A promoter polymorphism, the pathophysiology may involve various environmental factors, particularly stress, that destabilizes the GABA-hypothalamic-pituitary-adrenal systems in those with genetic vulnerability (47).

Leptin

Leptin is a 16-kD adipocyte hormone that functions as the afferent signal in a negative feedback loop regulating body weight. Defects in leptin production cause severe hereditary obesity in rodents and humans. Leptin acts through the leptin receptor (LEPR), a single-transmembrane-domain receptor of the cytokine receptor family, which is found in many tissues in several alternatively spliced forms. The leptin (*LEP*) gene is the human homolog of the gene (ob) mutant in the mouse "obese" phenotype, and is located on chromosome 7q31.3. In a group of 419 obese subjects (BMI >40 kg/m^2), a DNA variant in exon 1 of the *LEP* gene (A→G substitution, base +19) showed a prevalence of 62% (48). Furthermore, obese individuals homozygous for the G-allele showed significantly lower leptin concentrations compared to obese patients either heterozygous or homozygous for the A-allele after correction for BMI (48). In two independent Caucasian cohorts of obese girls, a frequent promoter variant of the *LEP* gene was found to be associated with changes in the relationship between serum leptin and body fatness (49). Girls of comparable adiposity had different circulating leptin levels, depending on their genotype at this locus. Girls with the −/− *LEP* -2549 genotype had 25% lower mean leptin levels than the girls with other genotypes, as reflected by differences in the regression slopes of leptin-to-fat mass (49).

The human *LEPR* gene contains a number of SNPs, including Gln223Arg, which changes an amino acid on the extracellular region common to all isoforms of the receptor (50). In a community-based cohort of Caucasian postmenopausal women from the Sheffield area, genotypes at that locus are associated with differences in BMI, fat mass and serum leptin levels (50). Measurement of serum leptin-binding activity indicates that this may reflect changed receptor function associated with genotype. These observations indicate that functional variations in the *LEPR* gene are important factors in the regulation of adiposity and BMI. In another cohort study of two hundred eighty-four 51-year-old men anthropometric and endocrine variables were examined in relation to *LEPR* polymorphisms by RFLP analysis (51). Three polymorphisms were examined: Lys109Arg in exon 4, Gln223Arg in exon 6, and Lys656Asn in exon 14. Measurements of body fat mass correlated with leptin concentration in Lys109 homozygotes and in Lys109 heterozygotes but not in Arg109 homozygotes (51).

A major quantitative trait locus determining leptin levels has been linked to the *POMC* region on chromosome 2. Most studies, based on fewer than 350 lean or obese subjects, have shown no association between *POMC* SNP 8246 C/T and serum leptin, but significant associations have been reported with *RsaI* 8246 C/T SNP haplotypes. Recently, the association of four *POMC* SNPs with body composition and serum leptin was investigated in 2758 normal Caucasian female subjects from the St Thomas' UK Adult Twin Registry (52): *RsaI* and 51 G/C in the 5 UTR and 8246 C/T and 7965 C/T in the 3'UTR. Under the recessive model, the 8246 T allele was significantly associated with higher mean BMI and total fat. Significant associations were maintained in sib-TDT with waist circumference, total fat and emerged with serum leptin (52). The potential impact of a cryptic trinucleotide repeat polymorphism in exon 3 of *POMC* on serum leptin levels and obesity was examined in 284 unrelated Swedish men born in 1944 (53). The amplification of the microsatellite locus yielded a 155-bp fragment and a fragment with one additional copy of the 9-bp repeat unit GGCAGCAGC (164 bp). Tests for differences in phenotype showed that subjects with the longer PCR repeat product had significantly higher serum leptin concentrations compared with subjects with the shorter PCR product (53). Obesity and its related metabolic perturbations were the same across the *POMC* genotypes. The observed association might reflect variations in melanocortin expression and/or activity, because exon 3 contains, among others, the coding sequences for melanocortins (53).

CONCLUSION

Obesity is a fundamental disorder of energy balance. While genetic factors influence obesity through endocrine mechanisms, several endocrine changes observed in obese subjects are likely consequences of obesity. Interesting findings have been reported with several candidate genes suggesting that they may play a role in susceptibility to illness or modification of the course of illness, at least in a subset of individuals with endocrine-related obesity. However, identification of an effect of a genetic variant will be the first, simple step on a more challenging path towards elucidation of the biological pathways involved, and crucially, the gene-gene and gene-environment interactions. If a genotype-phenotype relationship is to be found, then as much of the background noise from non-genetic factors as can be eliminated should be, and future studies must fulfill more stringent criteria that those adopted in the majority of reports published.

REFERENCES

1. Rankinen T, Zuberi A, Chagnon YC et al. The human obesity gene map: the 2005 update. Obesity (Silver Spring). 2006; 14:529–644.
2. Mutch DM, Clement K. Unravelling the genetics of human obesity. PLoS Genet 2006; 2:e188.
3. Bray GA. Contemporary Diagnosis and Management of Obesity. Newtown: Handbooks in Health Care Co. 1998.
4. Harper ME, Ullrich A, Saunders GF. Localization of the human insulin gene to the distal end of the short arm of chromosome 11. Proc Natl Acad Sci USA 1981; 78:4458–60.

5. Weaver JU, Kopelman PG, Hitman GA. Central obesity and hyperinsulinaemia in women are associated with polymorphism in the 5' flanking region of the human insulin gene. Eur J Clin Invest 1992; 22:265–70.
6. Le Stunff C, Fallin D, Schork NJ et al. The insulin gene VNTR is associated with fasting insulin levels and development of juvenile obesity. Nat Genet 2000; 26:444–6.
7. Yang-Feng TL, Francke U, Ullrich A. Gene for human insulin receptor: localization to site on chromosome 19 involved in pre-B-cell leukemia. Science 1985; 228:728–31.
8. Kasuga M, Karlsson FA, Kahn CR. Insulin stimulates the phosphorylation of the 95,000-dalton subunit of its own receptor. Science 1982; 215:185–7.
9. Kolterman OG, Insel J, Saekow M et al. Mechanisms of insulin resistance in human obesity: evidence for receptor and postreceptor defects. J Clin Invest 1980; 65:1272–84.
10. Walston J, Silver K, Bogardus C et al. Time of onset of non-insulin-dependent diabetes mellitus and genetic variation in the β3-adrenergic-receptor gene. N Engl J Med 1995; 333:343–7.
11. Widén E, Lehto M, Kanninen T et al. Association of a polymorphism in the β3-adrenergic-receptor gene with features of the insulin resistance syndrome in Finns. N Engl J Med 1995; 333:348–51.
12. Clement K, Vaisse C, Manning BS et al. Genetic variation in the β3-adrenergic receptor and an increased capacity to gain weight in patients with morbid obesity. N Engl J Med 1995; 333:352–4.
13. Santoro N, del Giudice EM, Cirillo G et al. An insertional polymorphism of the proopiomelanocortin gene is associated with fasting insulin levels in childhood obesity. J Clin Endocrinol Metab 2004; 89:4846–9.
14. Spiegelman BM. PPAR-γ: adipogenic regulator and thiazolidinedione receptor. Diabetes 1998: 47:507–14.
15. Elbrecht A, Chen Y, Cullinan CA et al. Molecular cloning, expression and characterization of human peroxisome proliferator activated receptors γ1 and γ2. Biochem Biophys Res Commun 1996; 224:431–7.
16. Ristow M, Muller-Wieland D, Pfeiffer A et al. Obesity associated with a mutation in a genetic regulator of adipocyte differentiation. N Engl J Med 1998; 339:953–9.
17. Deeb SS, Fajas L, Nemoto M et al. A Pro12Ala substitution in PPARγ2 associated with decreased receptor activity, lower body mass index and improved insulin sensitivity. Nat Genet 1998; 20:284–7.
18. Yen CJ, Beamer BA, Negri C et al. Molecular scanning of the human peroxisome proliferator activated receptor γ (hPPARγ) gene in diabetic Caucasians: identification of a Pro12Ala PPARγ2 missense mutation. Biochem Biophys Res Commun 1997; 241:270–4.
19. Altshuler D, Hirschhorn JN, Klannemark M et al. The common PPARγPro12Ala polymorphism is associated with decreased risk of type 2 diabetes. Nat Genet 2000; 26:76–80.
20. Clement K, Hercberg S, Passinge B et al. The Pro115Gln and Pro12Ala PPARγ gene mutations in obesity and type 2 diabetes. Int J Obes Relat Metab Disord 2000; 24:391–3.
21. Rosmond R, Chagnon M, Bouchard C. The Pro12Ala PPARγ2 gene missense mutation is associated with obesity and insulin resistance in Swedish middle-aged men. Diabetes Metab Res Rev 2003; 19:159–63.
22. Zhan S, Ho SC. Meta-Analysis of the Association of the Trp64Arg polymorphism in the β3 adrenergic receptor with insulin resistance. Obes Res 2005; 13:1709–19.
23. Shihara N, Yasuda K, Moritani T et al. The association between Trp64Arg polymorphism of the β3-adrenergic receptor and autonomic nervous system activity. J Clin Endocrinol Metab 1999; 84:1623–7.
24. Large V, Hellström L, Reynisdottir S et al. Human β-2 adrenoceptor gene polymorphisms are highly frequent in obesity and associate with altered adipocyte β-2 adrenoceptor function. J Clin Invest 1997; 100:3005–13.
25. Rosmond R, Ukkola O, Chagnon M et al. Polymorphisms of the β2-adrenergic receptor gene (ADRB2) in relation to cardiovascular risk factors in men. J Intern Med 2000; 248:239–44.
26. Macho-Azcarate T, Marti A, Gonzalez A et al. Gln27Glu polymorphism in the β2 adrenergic receptor gene and lipid metabolism during exercise in obese women. Int J Obes Relat Metab Disord 2002; 26:1434–41.

27. Sivenius K, Niskanen L, Laakso M et al. A deletion in the α2B-adrenergic receptor gene and autonomic nervous function in central obesity. Obes Res 2003; 11:962–70.
28. Rosmond R. The glucocorticoid receptor gene and its association to metabolic syndrome. Obes Res 2002; 10:1078–86.
29. Huizenga NA, Koper JW, De Lange P et al. A polymorphism in the glucocorticoid receptor gene may be associated with and increased sensitivity to glucocorticoids in vivo. J Clin Endocrinol Metab 1998; 83:144–51.
30. Buemann B, Vohl MC, Chagnon M et al. Abdominal visceral fat is associated with a *Bcl*I restriction fragment length polymorphism at the glucocorticoid receptor gene locus. Obes Res 1997; 5:186–92.
31. Rosmond R, Chagnon YC, Holm G et al. A glucocorticoid receptor gene marker is associated with abdominal obesity, leptin, and dysregulation of the hypothalamic-pituitary-adrenal axis. Obes Res 2000; 8:211–8.
32. Fleury I, Beaulieu P, Primeau M et al. Characterization of the *Bcl*I polymorphism in the glucocorticoid receptor gene. Clin Chem 2003; 49:1528–31.
33. Barat P, Duclos M, Gatta B et al. Corticosteroid binding globulin gene polymorphism influences cortisol driven fat distribution in obese women. Obes Res 2005; 13:1485–90.
34. Rosmond R, Chagnon M, Bouchard C et al. A missense mutation in the human melanocortin-4 receptor gene in relation to abdominal obesity and salivary cortisol. Diabetologia 2001; 44:1335–8.
35. Dinan TG. Serotonin and the regulation of hypothalamic-pituitary-adrenal axis function. d Life Sci 1996; 58:1683–94.
36. Calogero AE, Gallucci WT, Chrousos GP et al. Interaction between GABAergic neurotransmission and rat hypothalamic corticotropin-releasing hormone secretion in vitro. Brain Res 1988; 463:28–36.
37. Al-Damluji S. Adrenergic control of the secretion of anterior pituitary hormones. Baillieres Clin Endocrinol Metab 1993; 7:355-92.
38. Collier DA, Arranz MJ, Li T et al. Association between 5-HT2A gene promoter polymorphism and anorexia nervosa. Lancet 1997; 350:412.
39. Sparkes RS, Lan N, Klisak I et al. Assignment of a serotonin 5HT-2 receptor gene (HTR2) to human chromosome 13q14-q21 and mouse chromosome 14. Genomics 1991; 9:461–5.
40. Chen K, Yang W, Grimsby J et al. The human 5-HT2 receptor is encoded by a multiple intron-exon gene. Brain Res Mol Brain Res 1992; 14:20–6.
41. Rosmond R, Bouchard C, Björntorp P. 5-HT(2A) receptor gene promoter polymorphism in relation to abdominal obesity and cortisol. Obes Res 2002; 10:585–9.
42. Curtis GC, Abelson JL, Gold PW. Adrenocorticotropic hormone and cortisol responses to corticotropin-releasing hormone: changes in panic disorder and effects of alprazolam treatment. Biol Psychiatry 1997; 41:76–85.
43. Arvat E, Maccagno B, Ramunni J et al. The inhibitory effect of alprazolam, a benzodiazepine, overrides the stimulatory effect of metyrapone-induced lack of negative cortisol feedback on corticotroph secretion in humans. J Clin Endocrinol Metab 1999; 84:2611–5.
44. Grottoli S, Arvat E, Gauna C et al. Alprazolam, a benzodiazepine, blunts but does not abolish the ACTH and cortisol response to hexarelin, a GHRP, in obese patients. Int J Obes Relat Metab Disord 2000; 24 S136–7.
45. Loh EW, Ball D. Role of the GABA(A)β2, GABA(A)α6, GABA(A)α1 and GABA(A)γ2 receptor subunit genes cluster in drug responses and the development of alcohol dependence. Neurochem Int 2000; 37:413–23.
46. Hicks AA, Bailey ME, Riley BP et al. Further evidence for clustering of human GABAA receptor subunit genes: localization of the alpha 6-subunit gene (GABRA6) to distal chromosome 5q by linkage analysis. Genomics 1994; 20:285–8.
47. Rosmond R, Bouchard C, Björntorp P. Allelic variants in the GABA(A)α6 receptor subunit gene (GABRA6) is associated with abdominal obesity and cortisol secretion. Int J Obes Relat Metab Disord 2002; 26:938–41.
48. Hager J, Clement K, Francke S et al. A polymorphism in the 5′ untranslated region of the human ob gene is associated with low leptin levels. Int J Obes Relat Metab Disord 1998; 22:200–5.

49. Le Stunff C, Le Bihan C, Schork NJ et al. A common promoter variant of the leptin gene is associated with changes in the relationship between serum leptin and fat mass in obese girls. Diabetes 2000; 49:2196–200.
50. Quinton ND, Lee AJ, Ross RJ et al. A single nucleotide polymorphism (SNP) in the leptin receptor is associated with BMI, fat mass and leptin levels in postmenopausal Caucasian women. Hum Genet 2001; 108:233–6.
51. Rosmond R, Chagnon YC, Holm G et al. Hypertension in obesity and the leptin receptor gene locus. J Clin Endocrinol Metab 2000; 85:3126–31.
52. Chen Y, Snieder H, Wang X et al. Proopiomelanocortin gene variants are associated with serum leptin and body fat in a normal female population. Eur J Hum Genet 2005; 13:772–80.
53. Rosmond R, Ukkola O, Bouchard C et al. Polymorphisms in exon 3 of the proopiomelanocortin gene in relation to serum leptin, salivary cortisol, and obesity in Swedish men. Metabolism 2002; 51:642–4.

7.5 Genetics and Drugs

Yvon C. Chagnon
Psychiatric Genetic Unit, Laval University Research Center Robert-Giffard, Beauport, Quebec, Canada

Paola Artioli
Department of Psychiatry, San Raffaele Institute, Milan, Italy

Alessandro Serretti
Institute of Psychiatry, University of Bologna, Bologna, Italy

Drug-induced weight gain is a serious side effect of many commonly used drugs leading both to non-compliance with treatment and to the development of comorbid conditions related to obesity. Drug-induced weight gain has been observed following insulin therapy in patients with type 1 or type 2 diabetes, in psychiatric therapy using antipsychotics, antidepressants, or mood stabilizers, in neurologic treatments with antiepileptic drugs, and in hypertension or steroid hormone therapies (1). Weight gain observed could be less then 1 kg for some antidepressants to up to 50 kg for some antipsychotic or antiepileptic-treated patients (1). Modest weight loss of 5% to 10% of initial body weight is clinically significant (2), and even modest weight gain is an undesirable side-effect of drugs.

Predictive markers of the adverse effects of drugs may provide more tailored, effective, and safer courses of treatment (3). It is thought that individual susceptibility to drug therapeutic and adverse effects could stem from different genetic backgrounds (4). This means that each individual could be evaluated for his potential response to medications, and for his susceptibility to develop different adverse effects according to his own genetic variations (5,6), the so-called individualized medicine. Associated variations in genes could fuel future research by better understanding the genetic mechanisms of drug response in patients. The identification of gene variants involved in the variable susceptibility to develop drug-induced obesity is in its infancy. We have reviewed the effects on weight of the few of the genes studied in relation to antipsychotics and the antidepressants (PA, AS).

CANDIDATES GENE STUDIES
Antipsychotics
Adverse metabolic effects of antipsychotics on weight are not observed in all patients or to the same extent, and vary according to the antipsychotic used (7). We have estimated that 15% of the patients using antipsychotics developed obesity, and observed that the susceptibility to become obese under antipsychotics varied among families (8). Few genes have yet to be studied in relation to body weight gain under antipsychotics, only four genes showing confirmation results (Table 1). Variations in genes from the neurotransmitter systems, from enzymes metabolizing these drugs, and from body weight regulation pathways were shown to be associated with weight changes (26).

TABLE 1 Candidate Genes Showing Significant Effect at $p \leq 0.05$ for the Antipsychotic Side Effect on Weight

Gene	Variant	Antipsychotics	Effect	Reference
CCK 3p22-p21	rs747455 C > T	Clozapine	CC greater weight change	(9)
LEP 7q31.3	−2548A > G	Chlorpromazine Risperidone	GG/AG smaller BMI change than AA	(10)
		Olanzapine Risperidone	AA/AG smaller BMI change than GG	(11)
		Clozapine	GG/AG smaller weight change than AA	(9)
ADRA2A 10q24-q26	−1291C > G	Clozapine	GG greater weight change than CC	(12)
BDNF 11p13	Val66Met	Clozapine	ValVal greater weight change	(9)
		Risperidone	MetMet smaller weight gain than ValVal	(13)
GNB3 12p13	825C > T	Clozapine	TT greater weight change than CT/CC	(14)
	−4521G > A	Olanzapine	GG greater BMI than AA	(15)
PMCH 12q24	+3127G > A		GG greater BMI than GA	
CYP2D6 22q13.1	*1/*1, *1/*3, *4	Olanzapine	*1/*3, *4 greater % change in BMI	(16)
	188C > T	Risperidone	CC smaller weight gain than CT/TT	(13)
HTR6 1p36-p35	267 T > C	Risperidone	TC/CC greater weight gain than TT	(13)
		Clozapine	No effect	(17)
HTR2A 13q14-q21	102T > C	Risperidone	CC smaller weight gain than TT	(13)
		Clozapine	No effect	(18)
		Clozapine	No effect	(17)
	His452Tyr	Clozapine	No effect	(18)
HTR2C Xq24	−759C > T	Chlorpromazine Risperidone	T/TC smaller BMI change than C/CC C greater frequency in patients with 7% BMI change	(19)
		Olanzapine Risperidone	T/TC smaller BMI change than C/CC C greater frequency in patients with 7% BMI change	(11)
		Clozapine	T/TC smaller BMI change than C/CC C greater frequency in patients with 7% BMI change	(20)
		Clozapine	T smaller BMI change than C in males	(21)
		Clozapine	T *greater* BMI change than C in males	(22)
		Olanzapine	C greater frequency in patients with 10% BMI change	(23)
		Risperidone	T smaller BMI change than C	(13)
		Clozapine	No effect	(24)
		Clozapine	No effect	(25)

Abbreviations: ADRA2A, adrenergic receptor alpha 2a; BDNF, brain-derived neurotrophic factor; CCK, cholecystokinin; CYP2D6, cytochrome P450, subfamily IID (debrisoquine, sparteine, -metabolizing), polypeptide 6; GNB3, guanine nucleotide binding protein (G protein), beta polypeptide 3; HTR6, HTR2A, HTR2C: 5-hydroxytryptamine (serotonin) receptor 6, 2A, 2C; LEP, leptin; PMCH, promelanin concentrating hormone.

Neurotransmitter Receptor Genes

In Chinese schizophrenic patients, those carrying the −759T allele of the functional −759C > T variant (27) in the 5-hydroxytryptamine (serotonin) receptor 2C (*HTR2C*) located on the chromosome Xq24, showed a weight gain three times lower than those not carrying the T variant allele (19). This result was confirmed in males only (21), but not in a third sample of antipsychotic-resistant patients (24). This suggested that resistance to the therapeutic effect of a previous anti-psychotic medication could be related to negative association results with weight change (28). However, this association was confirmed recently in other ethnic groups, whether resistant or not to antipsychotics (11,20). In contrast, Basile et al. (22) reported that carriers of the −759T alleles showed a "higher" gain in weight than non-carriers in a mixed population of antipsychotic-resistant Caucasians and African Americans. The second *HTR2C* variant Cys23Ser possibly functional (29) or nonfunctional (30), showed no association with body weight gain in antipsychotic-naïve or resistant clozapine-treated schizophrenic of Caucasian or African-American origins (17,18,31). The brain-derived neurotrophic factor (*BDNF*) located at 11p13 is involved in many brain processes and the Val allele of the Val66Met variant was shown to be associated with a greater weight gain under clozapine (9) or risperidone (13).

Drug Metabolizing Genes

A significant effect of the cytochrome P450, family 2, subfamily D, polypeptide 6 (*CYP2D6*) genotypes on the percent change of body mass index (BMI) have been reported in Caucasian males taking olanzapine and carrying the poor *4 and intermediate *1/*3 metabolizer genotypes (32,16). Similarly, CC homozygotes of the 188C > T variant showed smaller weight gain under risperidone (13). However, clearance of olanzapine is not reduced in subjects who are deficient in CYP2D6, and the significance of this association remains unclear. No association was observed with a di-nucleotide repeat polymorphism of the cytochrome P450 1A2 (18), which is one of the main metabolizing enzyme of clozapine with CYP2D6 and cytochrome P450, family 3, subfamily A, polypeptide 4 (CYP3A4).

Body-Weight Control Genes

In Chinese antipsychotic-naïve schizophrenic patients, homozygote for the A allele of the −2548A > G polymorphism of the leptin gene (*LEP*) showed higher changes in body weight than patients carrying A/G and G/G genotypes (10). This result was confirmed in a first sample of antipsychotic-resistant Caucasians (9), while a "higher" BMI change was observed in homozygotes for the G allele in antipsychotic-naïve Caucasian (11). Chinese schizophrenic patients treated with clozapine showed a three times higher weight gain while carrying the GG genotype of the adrenergic, alpha–2A-, receptor (*ADRA2A*) in contrast to CC genotype of the −1291C > G variant (12). Similarly, a two to three times higher weight gain was observed in those carrying the TT genotype of the guanine binding protein 3 825C > T variant in contrast to carriers of the CT or CC genotypes (14). Negative results were reported previously for these two genes (18,33). Finally, homozygotes −4521GG of the pro-melanin-concentrating hormone (PMCH) showed five more units of BMI than AA homozygotes ($p < 0.05$) in schizophrenic males younger than 50 years of age taking olanzapine (15). It was also reported recently that the first receptor of PMCH showed affinity for the antipsychotic haloperidol (34).

Eleven genes showed no relation to antipsychotic-induced weight changes. Genes were the tumor necrosis factor alpha (TNF) and the cytochrome P450, family 1, subfamily A, polypeptide 2 (CYPA12) (18), the 5-hydroxytryptamine (serotonin) receptor 1A (HTR1A), the histamine receptor H1 and H2 receptors (HRH1, HRH2), and the adrenergic, beta-3-, receptor (ADRB3) and the adrenergic, alpha1A, receptor (ADRA1A) (17,18,33,35), the serotonin transporter (17), the dopamine receptor 3 and 4 (DRD2, DRD3) (13,36), and the synaptosomal-associated protein 25 kDa (SNAP23) (37).

Antidepressants

The effects on weight gain exerted by tricyclic antidepressant are well established (38,39). For selective serotonin reuptake inhibitors (SSRIs), no weight gain (40) or long-term weight gains between 17.9% and 33% (41,42) were reported. Liability (43) and the probability and extent of weight gain (38) appear to differ substantially between MAO-I and individual tricyclic antidepressants. Weight gain was more pronounced during acute treatment with amitriptyline than with imipramine or desipramine. Weight gain correlated positively with dosage and duration of treatment, and the resulting body weight was higher than prior to the current depressive episode.

Body weight effects associated with SSRI treatment of depression are far less well understood. In a double-blind multicenter study comparing treatment of depression with the SSRIs, fluoxetine and paroxetine, weight loss was observed more often in the fluoxetine (12%) than in the paroxetine group (3%) (44). In a double-blind placebo-controlled study covering 26 to 32 weeks, a significant mean increase in body weight of 3.6% compared to baseline was found with paroxetine, while patients on sertraline (+1%) or fluoxetine (−0.2%) showed no significant weight change (45). There are also studies reporting weight gain during treatment with fluoxetine (40), citalopram, and sertraline (46). In a meta-analysis of the placebo-controlled studies performed during the licensing process, mirtazapine showed the highest liability to cause weight gain with 10% to 11% *versus* 1% to 2% of patients developing increased appetite and weight gain. Mirtazapine also induced body weight increase of 2.4 kg within 4 weeks in 11 patients, while nine patients on venlafaxine lost 0.4 kg during the same period (47). The weight gain associated with mirtazapine might be confined to the first weeks of treatment with body weight reaching a plateau after 2 months despite ongoing treatment (45,46). Other newer antidepressants are currently not thought to affect body weight (45,46), which is somewhat surprising for venlafaxine given its structural similarity to sibutramine that effectively reduces body weight. Other data indicate a weight loss by 0.4 kg within the first 4 weeks of treatment of major depression with venlafaxine (47).

The different liabilities of tricyclic antidepressants to induce weight gain were explained by their different patterns of stimulation or functional antagonism of dopamine, norepinephrine, serotonin, and histamine receptors. In general, alpha-adrenergic neurotransmission is thought to stimulate appetite, while beta-adrenergic, histaminergic, dopaminergic, and serotoninergic signal transduction confers satiety (38). This concept explains why tricyclic antidepressants with a strong antihistaminergic effect, e.g., amitriptyline or doxepin, induce marked weight gain. Of the numerous 5-hydroxytryptamine (serotonin) receptor subtypes currently identified, 5-hydroxytryptamine receptors (HTR) 1B and 2C receptors are believed to mediate the 5-HT induced satiety. De Vry and Schreiber (48) stated that the relative contribution of the multiple HTR1 and HTR2 receptors underlying the hypophagic effect remains unclear and is difficult to dissociate from typical side effects such as nausea and anxiogenesis. Clinically significant weight loss over a year or more can be produced by both d-fenfluramine and sibutramine treatment, but apparently not by the SSRIs fluoxetine (49). The weight loss observed during the first few weeks of treatment is compatible with their serotoninergic effect, but the weight gain occurring during long-term treatment with SSRIs cannot be explained by this concept.

Two studies addressed the effect on leptin secretion of antidepressant drugs (50,51). During 6 weeks of treatment with tricyclic drugs or paroxetine, plasma leptin levels did not change (52) while body weight increased by 3.5 and 1.0 kg, respectively, in treated patients in contrast to untreated patients. In another study, only a very small increase in plasma leptin compared to baseline in 11 patients gaining 2.4 kg of body weight during 4 weeks of mirtazapine treatment for major depression was found (47). A number of recent studies have addressed the relationship between the effects of psychotropic drugs on weight and on the TNF system. Surprisingly, all drugs investigated so far, which induce clear-cut weight gain (clozapine, olanzapine, amitriptyline, and mirtazapine), also clearly activated the TNF system. This activation resulted in increased plasma levels of sTNF-R p75 (tumor necrosis factor receptor superfamily, member 1B) for all these drugs, and of sTNF-R p55 (tumor necrosis factor receptor superfamily, member 1A) and TNF alpha levels for some of them. Activation of the TNF system seems to be specific for psychotropic drugs that induce weight gain, since drugs which did not affect or even decreased weight (haloperidol, paroxetine, and venlafaxine) did not influence the TNF system at all (47,52).

Although the efficacy of antidepressant drugs has been studied relatively extensively with molecular genetic approaches, adverse events induced by antidepressant drugs, including weight gain, hypotension, sedation, anticholinergic effects, sleep disturbance, and antidepressant-induced mania have received little attention. Several genes warrant investigation: these include the 5-hydroxytryptamine (serotonin) receptor 2C, proopiomelanocortin, leptin, ghrelin, tumor necrosis factor alpha, adiponectin, dopamine D2 receptor, histamine receptor H1, and alpha1, beta2 and beta3 adrenergic receptor genes. Actually, no gene has been specifically investigated for its effect on antidepressant induced weight gain, but we may hypothesize that partially similar mechanism compared to antipsychotics may be involved, but this is only speculatory.

Other Drugs
Mood Stabilizers
Treatment with lithium has long been recognized to be associated with metabolic adverse effects notably weight gain (53). The incidence of weight gain has been reported to be as high as 62% of starting weight (54), with 64% of patients gaining more than 10 kg (55). No evidence for an association has been observed between two polymorphisms (+35A>G in intron 3 and +7T>G in intron 10) in the subunit of the guanine nucleotide binding protein (G protein), alpha activating activity polypeptide, olfactory type (*GNAL*) gene and weight gain in response to lithium treatment (56).

Antiepileptic Drugs

Treatment of epilepsy or bipolar disorder with valproic acid induces weight gain and increases serum levels for the leptin, but lowers its secretion (57). Valproic acid induces reduction in the levels of mRNA encoding estrogen receptor-alpha that may account for the weight gain that occur in a proportion of women treated with Valproic acid for epilepsy or for bipolar mood disorder (58). Genetic factors may have an influence on the weight change induced by Valproic acid since all five pairs of monozygotic twins concordant for epilepsy and treated with Valproic acid showed similar weight courses (59). Lamotrigine is an antiepileptic drug that is weight-neutral, while topiramate and zonisamide may induce weight loss. It has been shown that the antipsychotic olanzapine-induced weight gain can be lowered using topiramate (60,61) or nizatidine (62). Topiramate is an anticonvulsant known to block AMPA/kainate-gated ions and sodium channels and positively modulate GABA receptors (63). Topiramate has also been used successfully to treat obesity but with severe side effects (64). Nizatidine is an antagonist of histamine receptor 2, and may reduce, but not stop, the antipsychotic quetiapine-induced weight gain (65).

Insulin Sensitizer

Thiazolidinediones, also called glitazones, are insulin sensitizers that act as agonists of the peroxisome proliferator-activated receptors-gamma (PPAR) and can be used for treating patients with type 2 diabetes mellitus. The combination of glitazones with insulin may favor weight gain due to enhanced adipogenesis. Patients with the *PPARG* Pro12Ala genotype show a better response to rosiglitazone treatment than those with the Pro12Pro genotype do, with no difference in weight or BMI (66).

GENOME-WIDE SCAN STUDIES

These results highlighted that associations of genes with weight gain could be observed in different ethnic groups, in specific gender, under different categories of antipsychotics, and in patient naïve or previously resistant to an antipsychotic. Candidate gene analysis is central to pharmacogenetic studies but integrated genome approaches are needed to quickly identify all of the genes involved, and to define individual susceptibility. Genome-wide linkage and association studies, and whole genome expression analysis, or both combined should highlight candidate genes and pathways involved in drug-induced weight gain. Kirkwood et al. (67) studied olanzapine-treated 20% extreme weight gainers ($N = 255$) and 20% least weight gainers ($N = 258$) in a genome-wide association study where 30,000 SNPs were genotyped from the ~1.6 million SNPs tested. Three hundred and eleven SNPs were identified as associated ($p < 0.001$) to weight gain under olanzapine, top hit being the gene polycystic kidney and hepatic diseases 1, and the gene peptidylglycine alpha-amidating monooxygenase. Whole-genome expression profiling was used to analyze primary neuronal cell culture stimulated at pharmaceutically relevant doses with one of eight antipsychotics, 20 antidepressants, or eight opioid drugs, and gene expression data could predict to which classes the different drugs belonged (68). These results demonstrated a genomic signature for the different drugs, and therefore genes possibly related to the specific effects of these drugs. In conclusion, the analysis of the genetics of adverse effects of drugs, particularly weight gain, is in its infancy and will need, as the analysis of the genetics of other complex traits, concerted research efforts. Drug-induced weight gain in human is also a powerful tool to identify genes related to obesity because of its inducible and reversible properties.

CONCLUSION

Most of the drugs induced unwanted side effects including weight gain that in some cases could be detrimental to the compliance and health of the patients. Drug-induced weight gain has been observed in psychiatric therapy using antipsychotics, antidepressants, or mood stabilizers, in neurologic treatments with antiepileptic drugs, following insulin therapy in patients with type 1 or type 2 diabetes and in hypertension or steroid hormone therapies. The identification of gene variants involved in the variable susceptibility to develop drug-induced weight gain and obesity is in its infancy. We have reviewed the few of the genes studied in relation to antipsychotics, antidepressants, and to other drugs. Some ten genes, including the serotonin receptor 2C, the cytochrome P-450 2D6, the brain-derived neurotrophic factor and the leptin genes, give positive associations with weight or body mass index gain under antipsychotics and 11 give no clear association. No gene has been studied yet for antidepressant effect on weight. The mood stabilizer lithium and the insulin sensitiser thiazolidinediones showed no association each with a different candidate gene. Genes involved in the adverse effects of drugs on weight may provide candidate genes and pathways for obesity per se.

REFERENCES

1. Ness-Abramof R, Apovian CM. Drug-induced weight gain. Drugs Today (Barc) 2005; 41(8):547–55.
2. Anonymous. Clinical guidelines on the identification, evaluation, and treatment of overweight and obesity in adults. Obesity Res 1998; 6:S51–S209.
3. Lazarou J, Pomeranz BH, Corey PN. Incidence of adverse drug reactions in hospitalized patients: a meta-analysis of prospective studies. Jama 1998; 279(15):1200–5.
4. Evans WE, Johnson JA. Pharmacogenomics: the inherited basis for interindividual differences in drug response. Annu Rev Genomics Hum Genet 2001; 2:9–39.
5. Evans WE, Relling MV. Moving towards individualized medicine with pharmacogenomics. Nature 2004; 429(6990):464–8.
6. Bentley DR. Genomes for medicine. Nature 2004; 429(6990):440–5.
7. Allison DB, Mentore JL, Heo M, et al. Antipsychotic-induced weight gain: a comprehensive research synthesis. Am J Psychiatry 1999; 156(11):1686–96.
8. Chagnon YC, Merette C, Bouchard RH, et al. A genome wide linkage study of obesity as secondary effect of antipsychotics in multigenerational families of eastern Quebec affected by psychoses. Mol Psychiatry 2004; 9(12):1067–74.
9. Muller DJ, Sicard T, De Luca V, et al. Antipsychotic treatment-emerging weight gain: adding light on some important candidate genes. Pharmacogenetics in Psychiatry Annual Meeting, 2005; Abstract.
10. Zhang ZJ, Yao ZJ, Mou XD, et al. Association of −2548G/A functional polymorphism in the promoter region of leptin gene with antipsychotic agent-induced weight gain. Zhonghua Yi Xue Za Zhi 2003; 83(24):2119–23.
11. Templeman LA, Reynolds GP, Arranz B, et al. Polymorphisms of the 5-HT2C receptor and leptin genes are associated with antipsychotic drug-induced weight gain in Caucasian subjects with a first-episode psychosis. Pharmacogenet Genom 2005; 15(4):195–200.

12. Wang YC, Bai YM, Chen JY, et al. Polymorphism of the adrenergic receptor alpha 2a −1291C>G genetic variation and clozapine-induced weight gain. J Neural Transm 2005; 112(11):1463–8.

13. Lane HY, Liu YC, Huang CL, et al. Risperidone-related weight gain: genetic and nongenetic predictors. J Clin Psychopharmacol 2006; 26(2):128–34.

14. Wang YC, Bai YM, Chen JY, et al. C825T polymorphism in the human G protein beta3 subunit gene is associated with long-term clozapine treatment-induced body weight change in the Chinese population. Pharmacogenet Genom 2005; 15(10):743–8.

15. Chagnon YC, Bureau A, Gendron D, et al. Possible association of the pro-melanin concentrating gene and the body mass index as a side-effect of the antipsychotic olanzapine. Am J Med Genet 2007; Published Online May 31.

16. Ellingrod VL, Miller D, Schultz SK, et al. CYP2D6 polymorphisms and atypical antipsychotic weight gain. Psychiatr Genet 2002; 12(1):55–8.

17. Hong CJ, Lin CH, Yu YW, et al. Genetic variants of the serotonin system and weight change during clozapine treatment. Pharmacogenetics 2001; 11(3):265–8.

18. Basile VS, Masellis M, McIntyre RS, et al. Genetic dissection of atypical antipsychotic-induced weight gain: novel preliminary data on the pharmacogenetic puzzle. J Clin Psychiatry 2001; 62(Suppl 23):45–66.

19. Reynolds GP, Zhang ZJ, Zhang XB. Association of antipsychotic drug-induced weight gain with a 5-HT2C receptor gene polymorphism. Lancet 2002; 359(9323):2086–7.

20. Miller D, Ellingrod VL, Holman TL, et al. Clozapine-induced weight gain associated with the 5HT2C receptor −759C/T polymorphism. Am J Med Genet B Neuropsychiatr Genet 2005; 133(1):97–100.

21. Reynolds GP, Zhang Z, Zhang X. Polymorphism of the promoter region of the serotonin 5-HT(2C) receptor gene and clozapine-induced weight gain. Am J Psychiatry 2003; 160(4):677–9.

22. Basile VS, Masellis M, De Luca V, et al. 759C/T genetic variation of 5HT(2C) receptor and clozapine-induced weight gain. Lancet 2002; 360(9347):1790–1.

23. Ellingrod VL, Perry PJ, Ringold JC, et al. Weight gain associated with the −759C/T polymorphism of the 5HT2C receptor and olanzapine. Am J Med Genet B Neuropsychiatr Genet 2005; 134B(1):76–8.

24. Tsai SJ, Hong CJ, Yu YW, et al. −759C/T genetic variation of 5HT(2C) receptor and clozapine-induced weight gain. Lancet 2002; 360(9347):1790.

25. Theisen FM, Hinney A, Bromel T, et al. Lack of association between the −759C/T polymorphism of the 5-HT2C receptor gene and clozapine-induced weight gain among German schizophrenic individuals. Psychiatr Genet 2004; 14(3):139–42.

26. Chagnon YC. Susceptibility genes for the side effect of antipsychotics on body weight and obesity. In LLerena A, Licinio J. eds. Pharmacogenet Pharmacogenom in Curr Drug Targets 2006; 7:1681–95.

27. Buckland PR, Hoogendoorn B, Guy CA et al. Low gene expression conferred by association of an allele of the 5-HT2C receptor gene with antipsychotic-induced weight gain. Am J Psychiatry 2005; 162(3):613–5.

28. Malhotra AK. The relevance of pharmacogenetics to schizophrenia. Curr Opin Psychiatry 2003; 16:171–4.

29. Okada M, Northup JK, Ozaki N, et al. Modification of human 5-HT(2C) receptor function by Cys23Ser, an abundant, naturally occurring amino-acid substitution. Mol Psychiatry 2004; 9(1):55–64.

30. Fentress HM, Grinde E, Mazurkiewicz JE, et al. Pharmacological properties of the Cys23Ser single nucleotide polymorphism in human 5-HT(2C) receptor isoforms. Pharmacogenom J 2005; 5(4):244–54.

31. Rietschel M, Naber D, Fimmers R, et al. Efficacy and side-effects of clozapine not associated with variation in the 5-HT2C receptor. Neuroreport 1997; 8(8):1999–2003.

32. Brockmoller J, Kirchheiner J, Schmider J, et al. The impact of the CYP2D6 polymorphism on haloperidol pharmacokinetics and on the outcome of haloperidol treatment. Clin Pharmacol Ther 2002; 72(4):438–52.

33. Tsai SJ, Yu YW, Lin CH, et al. Association study of adrenergic beta3 receptor (Trp64Arg) and G-protein beta3 subunit gene (C825T) polymorphisms and weight change during clozapine treatment. Neuropsychobiology 2004; 50(1):37–40.

34. Theisen FM, Haberhausen M, Firnges MA, et al. No evidence for binding of clozapine, olanzapine and/or haloperidol to selected receptors involved in body weight regulation. Pharmacogenom J 2006, online publication, 19 September 2006; doi:10.1038/sj.tpj.6500418.

35. Hong CJ, Lin CH, Yu YW, et al. Genetic variant of the histamine-1 receptor (glu349asp) and body weight change during clozapine treatment. Psychiatr Genet 2002; 12(3):169–71.

36. Rietschel M, Naber D, Oberlander H, et al. Efficacy and side-effects of clozapine: testing for association with allelic variation in the dopamine D4 receptor gene. Neuropsychopharmacology 1996; 15(5):491–6.

37. Muller DJ, Klempan TA, De Luca V, et al. The SNAP-25 gene may be associated with clinical response and weight gain in antipsychotic treatment of schizophrenia. Neurosci Lett 2005; 379(2):81–9.

38. Garland EJ, Remick RA, Zis AP. Weight gain with antidepressants and lithium. J Clin Psychopharmacol 1988; 8(5):323–30.

39. Fernstrom MH, Kupfer DJ. Antidepressant-induced weight gain: a comparison study of four medications. Psychiatry Res 1988; 26(3):265–71.

40. Michelson D, Amsterdam JD, Quitkin FM, et al. Changes in weight during a 1-year trial of fluoxetine. Am J Psychiatry 1999; 156(8):1170–6.

41. Sachs GS, Guille C. Weight gain associated with use of psychotropic medications. J Clin Psychiatry 1999; 60(Suppl 21):16–9.

42. Sussman N. Review of atypical antipsychotics and weight gain. J Clin Psychiatry 2001; 62(Suppl 23):5–12.

43. Fernstrom MH. Drugs that cause weight gain. Obes Res 1995; 3(Suppl 4):435S–9S.

44. Chouinard G, Saxena B, Belanger MC, et al. A Canadian multicenter, double-blind study of paroxetine and fluoxetine in major depressive disorder. J Affect Disord 1999; 54(1–2):39–48.

45. Fava M, Judge R, Hoog SL, et al. Fluoxetine versus sertraline and paroxetine in major depressive disorder: changes in weight with long-term treatment. J Clin Psychiatry 2000; 61(11):863–7.

46. Fava M. Weight gain and antidepressants. J Clin Psychiatry 2000; 61(Suppl 11):37–41.

47. Kraus T, Haack M, Schuld A, et al. Body weight, the tumor necrosis factor system, and leptin production during treatment with mirtazapine or venlafaxine. Pharmacopsychiatry 2002; 35(6):220–5.

48. De Vry J, Eckel G, Kuhl E, et al. Effects of serotonin 5-HT(1) and 5-HT(2) receptor agonists in a conditioned taste aversion paradigm in the rat. Pharmacol Biochem Behav 2000; 66(4):797–802.

49. Halford JC, Harrold JA, Lawton CL, et al. Serotonin (5-HT) drugs: effects on appetite expression and use for the treatment of obesity. Curr Drug Targets 2005; 6(2):201–13.

50. Himmerich H, Koethe D, Schuld A, et al. Plasma levels of leptin and endogenous immune modulators during treatment with carbamazepine or lithium. Psychopharmacology (Berl) 2005; 179(2):447–51.

51. Himmerich H, Schuld A, Haack M, et al. Early prediction of changes in weight during six weeks of treatment with antidepressants. J Psychiatr Res 2004; 38(5):485–9.

52. Hinze-Selch D, Schuld A, Kraus T, et al. Effects of antidepressants on weight and on the plasma levels of leptin, TNF-alpha and soluble TNF receptors: a longitudinal study in patients treated with amitriptyline or paroxetine. Neuropsychopharmacology 2000; 23(1):13–9.

53. Livingstone C, Rampes H. Lithium: a review of its metabolic adverse effects. J Psychopharmacol 2006; 20(3):347-55.

54. Peselow ED, Dunner DL, Fieve RR, et al. Lithium carbonate and weight gain. J Affect Disord 1980; 2(4):303–10.

55. Vendsborg PB, Bech P, Rafaelsen OJ. Lithium treatment and weight gain. Acta Psychiatr Scand 1976; 53(2):139–47.

56. Zill P, Malitas PN, Bondy B, et al. Analysis of polymorphisms in the alpha-subunit of the olfactory G-protein Golf in lithium-treated bipolar patients. Psychiatr Genet 2003: 13(2):65–9.

57. Lagace DC, McLeod RS, Nachtigal MW. Valproic acid inhibits leptin secretion and reduces leptin messenger ribonucleic acid levels in adipocytes. Endocrinology 2004; 145(12):5493–503.

58. Reid G, Metivier R, Lin CY, et al. Multiple mechanisms induce transcriptional silencing of a subset of genes, including oestrogen receptor alpha, in response to deacetylase inhibition by valproic acid and trichostatin A. Oncogene 2005; 24(31):4894–907.

59. Klein KM, Hamer HM, Reis J, et al. Weight change in monozygotic twins treated with valproate. Obes Res 2005; 13(8):1330–4.

60. Levy E, Margolese HC, Chouinard G. Topiramate produced weight loss following olanzapine-induced weight gain in schizophrenia. J Clin Psychiatry 2002; 63(11):1045.

61. Nickel MK, Nickel C, Muehlbacher M, et al. Influence of topiramate on olanzapine-related adiposity in women: a random, double-blind, placebo-controlled study. J Clin Psychopharmacol 2005; 25(3):211–7.

62. Atmaca M, Kuloglu M, Tezcan E, et al. Nizatidine treatment and its relationship with leptin levels in patients with olanzapine-induced weight gain. Hum Psychopharmacol 2003; 18(6):457–61.

63. White HS, Brown SD, Woodhead JH, et al. Topiramate enhances GABA-mediated chloride flux and GABA-evoked chloride currents in murine brain neurons and increases seizure threshold. Epilepsy Res 1997; 28(3):167–79.

64. Anghelescu I, Klawe C, Szegedi A. Add-on combination and maintenance treatment: case series of five obese patients with different eating behavior. J Clin Psychopharmacol 2002; 22(5):521–4.

65. Atmaca M, Kuloglu M, Tezcan E, et al. Nizatidine for the treatment of patients with quetiapine-induced weight gain. Hum Psychopharmacol 2004; 19(1):37–40.

66. Kang ES, Park SY, Kim HJ, et al. Effects of Pro12Ala polymorphism of peroxisome proliferator-activated receptor gamma2 gene on rosiglitazone response in type 2 diabetes. Clin Pharmacol Ther 2005; 78(2):202–8.

67. Kirkwood SC, Fu D-J, Mukhopadhyay N, et al. Genome-wide association study for olanzapine treatment-emergent weight gain. Pharmacogenetics in Psychiatry Annual Meeting, 2005; Abstract.

68. Gunther EC, Stone DJ, Gerwien RW, et al. Prediction of clinical drug efficacy by classification of drug-induced genomic expression profiles in vitro. Proc Natl Acad Sci USA 2003; 100(16):9608–13.

8.1   Molecular Basis of Epigenetic Memory

C. Gallou-Kabani, A. Vigé, M.S. Gross, and C. Junien
*INSERM, AP-HP, Université Paris Descartes and Faculté de Médecine, INSERM
Unit 781, Clinique Maurice Lamy, Hôpital Necker-Enfants Malades, Paris, France*

The term "epigenetics"—from "epi" the Greek for "above"—was first coined in the 1940s by Conrad Waddington, who defined epigenetics as "the causal interactions between genes and their products which bring phenotype into being" (1). The term "epigenetics" is now used to refer to stably maintained mitotically (and potentially meiotically) heritable patterns of gene expression occurring without changes in DNA sequence.

MOLECULAR BASIS OF EPIGENETIC MEMORY
The Epigenetic Codes and Machinery

The epigenetic code comprises several levels of interconnected and interdependent codes: the DNA methylation code, the histone code (histone methylation, acetylation and phosphorylation), and the coregulator code that "orchestrates" the activity of the genome, together with RNA interference. The epigenetic codes define a process involving the recruitment of a myriad of chromatin-remodeling complexes, insulator proteins, histone exchange chaperones, enzymes, coregulators, and effectors, directing appropriate chromatin remodeling (2).

Many covalent epigenetic modifications are involved in keeping genes stably repressed or active. DNA methylation remains the best studied epigenetic modification. In mammalian genomes, this covalent modification often occurs at cytosine residues followed by a guanine residue—CpG dinucleotides. In most cases, the acquisition and maintenance of "CpG methylation" leads to the silencing of gene expression. Gene expression is also controlled by the organization of histones in the nucleosomes around which the DNA is wrapped. These post-translational modifications of histone proteins modulate chromatin structure (2). The core histones (H2A, H2B, H3, and H4) are subject to dozens of different modifications, the "histone code," including acetylation, methylation, and phosphorylation. In general, active genes are heavily acetylated and methylated on histone H3 lysine 4, resulting in the recruitment of nucleosome remodeling enzymes and histone acetylases, thereby regulating transcription. Conversely, deacetylation and lys 27 methylation negatively regulate transcription by promoting a compact chromatin structure. Chromatin modification requires a complex machinery, including chromatin remodeling complexes, coactivators, and corepressors and several entities with DNA/protein binding properties and enzymatic activities, such as heterochromatin protein 1 (HP1), histone deacetylase (HDAC), histone acetyl transferase (HAT), DNA methyl transferase (DNMT), histone methyl transferase (HMT), and methyl binding domain (MBD) proteins with demethylase activity. Specific epigenetic patterns condition the accessibility of chromatin to transcription factors, facilitating the recognition by these factors of genes to be expressed (to various extents) and of genes to be silenced transiently or permanently, in a stage- and/or tissue-specific manner.

Our understanding of the regulation of gene expression is likely to change with the recent discovery of microRNAs. MicroRNAs are short non-coding RNAs that regulate gene expression by binding to target mRNAs, leading to reduced protein synthesis and sometimes decreased steady-state levels. MicroRNAs or siRNAs regulate gene expression, directing silencing machinery to promoters, heterochromatin formation, and genome stability; they often arise from the demethylation of tandem repeats, which are common in pericentromeric sequences (3). There are several hundreds of microRNAs, some of which are regulators of important biological processes, including cellular differentiation, proliferation, and developmental timing. Several studies also suggest that micro-RNAs are also regulators of a broad range of metabolic pathways. Yet, almost nothing is known of their function in mammalian systems in vivo. It has been proposed that microRNAs may contribute to common metabolic diseases and that targeting microRNAs may represent novel therapeutic tools (4). Genetic studies will shed light on whether variations in miRNA genes or their respective targets can predispose to common metabolic diseases (5).

Plausible Target-Candidate Sequences for Adaptation?

What type of sequence could be the epigenetic support of such changes transmitted without erasure to subsequent generations? What type of epigenetic mark on DNA (methylation), histones, or other components of chromatin or on RNA or proteins could resist erasure and be passed on to subsequent generations? Genomically imprinted genes or transposable elements adjacent to or within genes are good candidates for epigenetic marks. With the exception of a brief period of global demethylation in the early stages of mammalian embryonic development, transposons are normally silenced by promoter CpG methylation (6).

When investigating the potential role of epigenetic alterations in biological functions, it is important to be able to determine which sequence and what type of alteration (DNA methylation and/or histone alterations), which tissue, and which developmental stage are concerned: candidate gene or genes and/or genome-wide? Where are the CpGs susceptible to methylation located within the gene: in the regulatory, promoter sequences, or within the gene, in coding or noncoding sequences? Are these changes correlated with gene expression? Alternatively DNA methylation may not be the mark. The recent study of the epigenetic regulation of Maspin expression in the human placenta shows that selective histone modifications, not DNA methylation, are associated with differential placental gene expression in human gestation (7). Specific subsets of genes are particularly sensitive to early nutritional effects on epigenetic regulation: genomically imprinted genes and genes adjacent to or containing transposable elements. Alternatively chromatin may not be the only support. The existence of yet another type of non-Mendelian epigenetic mechanism—inherited RNA transcripts mediating transgenerational changes in gene expression has been discovered in the mouse (8).

Promoter CpG Islands, Transcription Factor Binding Sites, or Other Sites?

About 4% to 8% of the C residues in the human genome are methylated, and 5-mC accounts for about 1% of all the residues comprising the genome (9). There are 100 million potential CpG dinucleotide methylation targets in the mammalian diploid genome. The CpG dinucleotide occurs about once every 80 dinucleotides, throughout 98% of the genome. However, certain sequences, known as CpG islands, contain a higher frequency of this dinucleotide. There are approximately 29,000 CpG islands in the human genome, and 50% to 60% of all genes contain a CpG island (9). CpG sequences dispersed throughout the genome are often heavily methylated, but those located in CpG islands display a lower level of methylation. Genes with CpG islands may remain unmethylated, regardless of transcription state. Genes without CpG islands may display various methylation patterns, not necessarily reflecting transcriptional activity. The hypermethylation of CpG islands in the promoters of tumor suppressor genes has been extensively documented in cancer (10,11).

The methylation of CpG dinucleotides within gene promoters is emerging as a major epigenetic mechanism controlling transcription. Epigenetic alterations, such as DNA methylation, may occur at sites within promoter sequences involved in the differential regulation of DNA-protein interactions required for definition of the three-dimensional chromatin structure necessary for gene transcription (12). One of the mechanisms by which methylation represses gene expression involves the inhibition of transcription factor binding to methylated binding sites or the promotion of repressor binding. The methylation of specific CpG sites might lead to the binding of repressors to functionally defined *cis*-acting elements, thereby compromising promoter function (13). Variations in maternal behavior are associated with differences in estrogen receptor (ER)-alpha (*ESRRA*) expression in the medial preoptic area and are transmitted across generations. The regions identified as differentially regulated included a signal transducer and activator of transcription (STAT5) binding site, and chromatin immunoprecipitation assays showed lower levels of Stat5b binding to the ESRRA 1B promoter in the adult offspring of mothers with low-licking/grooming than in the adult offspring of high-licking/grooming mothers (14–16).

Moreover, changes in the methylation status of a particular CpG, such as those in the promoter of the glucocorticoid receptor (GR), the estrogen receptor alpha (ESRRA), and P53 genes may play a major role in the adaptation of mammals to their environment and can be reversed by trichostatin A (TSA), a HDAC inhibitor; or methionine, a methyl donor (14–17).

Transposable Elements Adjacent to or Located Within Genes

One of the key functions of epigenetic modifications in the eukaryotic cell genome is to abolish the transcriptional activity of retroelements. Retrotransposons are thought to be maintained in a predominantly methylated state to prevent retrotransposition events that might lead to deleterious mutations and cancer. The aberrant methylation of transposable elements next to genes can affect the level of transcription of those genes, as shown for the intracisternal A particle (IAP) sequence next to the Agouti and Axin loci in rodents. However, some transposons, such as IAP retrotransposon escape this epigenetic silencing and may interfere with the expression of neighboring genes in several ways (18,19). Specific transposable elements induce epigenetic instability, allowing early diet to influence epigenotype. Both transposons and imprinted genes are therefore good candidate supports (20). The proximity of such elements may render many human genes epigenetically labile, as demonstrated for two mutant mice—Agouti viable yellow A^{vy} and Axin Fused Axin^{Fu} mice—harboring an insertion of an IAP retrotransposon and more recently a third one, the $Cabp^{IAP}$ locus (21).

The A^{vy} allele was generated by insertion of the IAP retrotransposon into the 5′-end of the A allele (19,20). The A^{vy} metastable allele is the best studied example of this phenomenon in mice (see Chapter 3.1). In A^{vy}/a mice, transcription originating from an IAP retrotransposon inserted upstream from the agouti gene (A) leads to the ectopic production of agouti protein, resulting in yellow fur, obesity, diabetes and an increase in susceptibility to tumors. Expression at this locus is controlled by the long terminal repeat of the retrotransposon. The intensity of expression is variable in isogenic mice, resulting in mice with a range of coat colors, from yellow to agouti or rather "pseudoagouti." These pseudoagouti mice have a methylated long terminal repeat. CpG methylation of the long terminal repeat of the transposable IAP sequence in the Agouti region varies considerably in A^{vy} mice, and is inversely correlated with ectopic *agouti* expression. The gene is expressed to various extents in isogenic mice, resulting in a range of coat colors, from yellow to agouti. Agouti mice have a methylated long terminal repeat. The agouti locus displays epigenetic inheritance if inherited from the mother but not if inherited from the father; the distribution of phenotypes in the offspring depends on the phenotype of the dam: A^{vy} dams with the agouti phenotype are more likely to have agouti offspring, whereas yellow dams produce a higher proportion of yellow offspring than agouti mothers (22).

Another mutation—the "fused" mutation in the house mouse (Sheldon Reed), $Axin^{Fu}$—also displays variable levels of expression: the tail may be kinked, bifurcated, or normal. Like Agouti A^{vy}, $Axin^{Fu}$ is caused by IAP insertion. The phenotype is correlated with the methylation state of the long terminal repeat (19). $Axin^{Fu}$ displays inter-individual variation for both DNA methylation and phenotype. Unlike the A^{vy} allele, for which the epigenetic transmission of methylation at the IAP sequence is limited to the female germline, the $Axin^{Fu}$ locus displays epigenetic inheritance following both maternal and paternal transmission, but depends on the genetic background of the strain (19).

How many such metastable epialleles exist? There are thousands of IAP retrotransposons in mice, but many may not be transcriptionally active. Other examples have been reported in other animals and plants (23). The transposable elements present in humans include endogenous retroviral sequences (ERVs), Alu sequences, and diverse long interspersed element-1 (LINE-1 or L1) LINE sequences, that are usually hypermethylated (24). The sequencing of the human genome has shown that transposable elements (SINEs, LINEs, etc.) account for about 35% to 40% of the genome and are found in about 4% of human genes (25). It would be interesting to determine whether these genes are involved in the regulation of energy homeostasis. However, no transposable elements able to resist demethylation during preimplantation like murine IAP sequences have yet been identified in humans (18).

Studies in patients with schizophrenia and other complex diseases have shown that some genomic retroelements (Alu elements) are transcribed in the affected tissues. Kan et al. identified retroelements in the hypomethylated fraction of brain genomic DNA from patients, and showed that a substantial portion of these elements were located close to or within potentially interesting target genes for future genetic transcription and epigenetic studies (24). Some human endogenous retroviruses displaying aberrant transcriptional activity due to epigenetic reorganization are potential candidates (26). A systematic analysis of recent L1-mediated retrotranspositional events causing human genetic disease was carried out to provide a more complete picture of the impact of L1-mediated retrotransposition on the architecture of the human genome. 48 L1 retrotransposition-linked mutations were identified, including L1-mediated retrotransposons and insertions reported to contain a poly(A) tail. This analysis also suggested that about 10% of L1-mediated retrotranspositional events are associated with significant genomic deletions in humans (27). Thus in humans, specific retroelements may represent potential targets for environmentally triggered epigenetic alterations important for developmental programming, lifelong deteriorations, and transgenerational transmission.

Genomically Imprinted Genes

Imprinted genes appear to be plausible candidates for adaptation. For most human genes, the two alleles contribute equally to production of the gene product. Imprinted genes are monoallelically expressed (from either the paternal or the maternal allele) and are therefore functionally haploid. Most imprinted genes are grouped in clusters, which may comprise reciprocally imprinted genes—some maternally and some paternally expressed—at about 15 different sites on the chromosomes of the human genome. More than 80 genes have been shown to be imprinted in humans and mice, and it is postulated that 100–500 imprinted genes may exist in the entire human genome. These imprinted domains are regulated coordinately, via long-range mechanisms such as antisense RNA interference and methylation-sensitive boundary elements. The complexity of imprinted domain regulation may render these domains particularly susceptible to environmental dysregulation via nutrition (28–30). There is compelling evidence that DNA methylation at imprinted genes varies with aging (both hyper- and hypomethylation are observed), between tissues, individuals, and disease conditions in humans and various animals, and during the course of pathological processes leading to cancer or atherosclerosis (28,31–33). Imprinted genes are dosage-sensitive, and encode proteins involved in common pathways. Changes in the relative expression levels of these genes may therefore have a major effect on phenotype. Loss-of-imprinting may be more likely for genes indirectly regulated by epigenetic marks, remote from imprinting control elements, displaying naturally leaky expression of the silenced allele, or for which multiple elements act in combination to ensure silencing (34). Individuals with colorectal neoplasia were found to have a 5.1-fold increased risk of insulin-like growth factor 2 (IGF2) loss-of-imprinting in peripheral blood leucocytes than people without colorectal neoplasia (details are provided in Chapter 8.2). Thus loss-of-imprinting of IGF2 represents a potential heritable biomarker for the early detection of colorectal neoplasia predisposition (35,36). Although not formally demonstrated, abundant evidence from genomic (or parental) imprinting studies suggests that monoallelically expressed imprinted genes are among the most promising targets for programming, evolutionary modifications, and transgenerational effects in response to rapid changes in the nutritional environment, such as those associated with the worldwide epidemic of metabolic syndrome, obesity, and type-2 diabetes:

(1) Intrauterine growth: Genomic imprinting and placentation emerged at about the same time in mammalian evolution (37). Most imprinted genes are strongly expressed in the placenta and recent studies in the mouse suggest that placenta-specific imprinting involves repressive histone modifications and non-coding RNAs (38,39).

(2) Imprinted genes in the placenta control the supply of nutrients, whereas, in fetal compartments, they control nutrient demand by regulating the growth rate of the fetal tissues (40,41). Consistent with conflict theory, the results of knockout

experiments have shown that paternally expressed genes (insulin-like growth factor 2, *Igf2*, mesoderm-specific transcript homolog (mouse) *Mest* or paternally expressed gene 1, *Peg1*, paternally expressed gene 3, *Peg3*, delta-like 1 homolog (Drosophila) (*Dlk*), solute carrier family 38, member 4, *Slc38a4*) aim to maximize resource acquisition by the current offspring, whereas maternally expressed genes (insulin-like growth factor 2 receptor, *Igf2r*; H19, imprinted maternally expressed untranslated mRNA *H19*; growth factor receptor-bound protein 10, *Grb10*, *Ipl*, *Mash*) aim to conserve resources.

(3) Postnatal growth: Imprinted genes may also affect postnatal metabolic adaptation to feeding, through the allocation of acquired resources to growth and, during lactation, through milk release, suckling, fat reserves and homeostatic mechanisms, such as glucose and temperature regulation, growth, feeding behavior and emotional cues, with opposing parental influences on growth and metabolism (43,44).

(4) Imprinted genes have direct and/or indirect effects on adult metabolism. Imprinted genes probably act at multiple levels in pathways regulating energy homeostasis. For the *Gnas/Gnasxl* (GNAS complex locus) gene pair, antagonistic effects are consistent with the conflict hypothesis, according to which maternal and paternal genes have opposing interests in the offspring (45). The *Mest* (mesoderm-specific transcript)/*Peg1* (paternally expressed gene 1) expression ratio is much higher in the white adipose tissue of mice with diet-induced and genetic obesity/diabetes than in that of other mice (46).

(5) Behavior and brain: Imprinted genes play an important role in the development of regions of the brain, such as the hypothalamus, contributing to energy homeostasis regulation, and in social, cognitive, and maternal behavior (37,47–49).

(6) Adaptation/evolution: the epigenetic lability (metastable alleles) of imprinted genes in response to nutrients (19,20,50,51) or behavioral reactivity to new environments (49,52–54) and aging (55) seems to be important. Imprinted genes are probable targets of nutritional or environmental programming: variations in the expression of the normally active allele may serve as a highly sensitive substrate for nutritional or environmental programming.

(7) Culture conditions and the manipulation of early embryos, assisted-reproduction technologies, and nuclear transfer experiments may disrupt genomic imprinting (56–58).

(8) Diabetes and obesity/lean-ness often accompany syndromes (see Chapters 5.1, 5.2, 5.3) or genetic manipulations (transgenic and knockout mouse models) associated with changes in imprinting (uniparental disomy, loss-of-imprinting) (59,60).

(9) Unusual erasure of epigenetic marks: as epigenetic marks of imprinted genes, unlike those of non-imprinted genes, are not erased after fertilization, the acquired changes may lead to stable transgenerational effects. Parental imprinting marks originate in sperm and oocytes and are generally protected from this genome-wide reprogramming. Early primordial germ cells possess imprinting marks similar to those of somatic cells. However, rapid DNA demethylation after mid-gestation erases these parental imprints, in preparation for sex-specific de novo methylation during gametogenesis. In the case of imprinted genes, promoter-restricted H3 Lys 4 di-methylation is an epigenetic mark for monoallelic expression. Methylation of histone tails has been implicated in long-term epigenetic memory. This pattern of promoter-restricted H3 Lys 4 di-methylation, already present in totipotent cells, is causally related to the long-term programming of allelic expression and provides an epigenetic mark for monoallelically expressed genes (61).

Changes in circumstances over several generations may result in the re-recruitment of alleles to the active genome, accounting for the reversibility of adaptive changes. Genomic imprinting may act as a buffering system or "rheostat," supporting adaptation to environmental conditions by silencing or increasing the expression of monoallelically expressed genes (62). The nonerasure of these epimutations in the germline would lead to stable transgenerational effects (47,62–66).

EPIGENETIC REPROGRAMMING

Epigenetic reprogramming of the genome is an essential process that occurs during both primordial germ cell development and early embryogenesis. It allows epigenetic marks to be cleared and reset between generations to ensure the totipotency of the zygote.

After fertilization, the paternal and maternal genomes in the zygote undergo rapid demethylation at coding sequences (genes) and at repetitive sequences (transposable elements). In theory, epigenetic marks are largely erased and reset in a lineage-specific fashion. However, this demethylation may not be complete. After implantation, active de novo methylation takes place, to various extents, depending on the part of the embryo concerned. The bulk of the genome becomes hypermethylated in the embryonic ectoderm and mesoderm, whereas the genome of extra-embryonic cells, such as the primary endoderm and trophoblast, remains hypomethylated. A sequence of de novo methylation dictates the structure and function of each somatic tissue, through a finely tuned pattern involving the switching on and off of gene expression (18,67–75).

However, epigenetic marks characteristic of imprinted genes, whatever these marks are since methylation may not be the only relevant epigenetic mark—at the DMRs and probably elsewhere—are passed on to the somatic tissues of the next generation, ensuring that mom's alleles and dad's alleles are recognized as such throughout life. In contrast, in germ cells these marks are reversible but at a later stage. In germ cells, parental methylation imprints in imprinted genes escape this process of demethylation and de novo methylation. The imprints of these genes are not eliminated until just before the primordial germ cells reach the gonadal ridge and are appropriately reinstalled during male and female gametogenesis, this process being completed during the slow growth period before puberty (68,76–78).

The incomplete erasure of methylation in genes associated with a measurable phenotype results in unusual patterns of inheritance from one generation to the next, referred to as transgenerational epigenetic inheritance. Such responses add an entirely new dimension to the study of gene-environment interactions and it is tempting to assume that the same mechanisms are also involved in humans. Since 1999, evidence has accumulated suggesting that epigenetic chromatin remodeling is one of the mechanisms underlying both developmental programming and non-Mendelian transgenerational inheritance in plants and mammals. Thus demethylation is not complete, with global DNA methylation being reduced to about 10% its initial level (68,79). Is this methylation evenly distributed? Do some sequences and/or individuals resist methylation erasure more strongly than others? Is the extent of demethylation constant or variable and does it depend on environment? Are some tissues or differentiation states more susceptible than others to demethylation? Depending on the distribution of methylation between coding and noncoding sequences, up to 90% of methylated genes may be demethylated, with 10% of genes retaining their methylation. The fate of histone modifications during these demethylation phases remains unclear. With the exception of a brief period of global demethylation—active for the paternal haploid genome and passive for the maternal genome—in the early mammalian embryo, transposons are normally silenced by promoter CpG methylation. Epigenetic marks in the paternal genome are actively cleared within hours of fertilization, whereas those in the maternal genome are cleared over a period of days. Transposon-like IAP sequences may escape this epigenetic silencing (18). Thus, information can be passed from parent to offspring in a form other than DNA sequence.

Marks may be cleared and re-established in the germline or early in development. An analysis of DNA methylation at the A^{vy} and $Axin^{Fu}$ loci in mature gametes, zygotes, and blastocysts revealed that the paternally and maternally inherited alleles are treated differently. The paternally inherited allele is demethylated rapidly, whereas the maternal allele is demethylated more slowly, in a manner similar to that for nonimprinted single-copy genes. There is no obvious clearing of the DNA methylation marks at A^{vy} during oogenesis, no active demethylation at this locus following maternal inheritance and no methylation of this locus in blastocysts. Thus, no DNA methylation of this allele is observed in the blastocyst, suggesting that C methylation is not the mark transmitted across generations. Thus, this maternal epigenetic effect is not the result of maternal environment. Instead, these data show that this effect results from the incomplete erasure of an epigenetic modification when a silenced A^{vy} allele is passed through the female germline, resulting in inheritance of the epigenetic modification (19,22,66,80–86).

Covalent histone modifications are also involved in early embryonic reprogramming events. During oocyte maturation and pre-implantation, mouse development histone modifications could be classified into two strikingly distinct categories. The first contains stable "epigenetic" marks such as histone H3 lysine 9 methylation [Me(Lys9)H3], histone H3 lysine 4 methylation [Me(Lys4)H3], and histone H4/H2A serine 1 phosphorylation [Ph(Ser1)H4/H2A]. The second group contains dynamic and reversible marks and includes hyperacetylated histone H4, histone H3 arginine 17 methylation [Me(Arg17)H3] and histone H4 arginine 3 methylation [Me(Arg3)H4]). Removal of these marks in eggs and early embryos occurs during metaphase suggesting that the enzymes responsible for the loss of these modifications are probably cytoplasmic in nature (87).

Maintenance of pluripotency is achieved by a novel chromatin-based mechanism, a bivalent chromatin structure that marks key developmental genes in embryonic stem cells. Bernstein et al. identified a specific modification pattern, termed "bivalent domains" consisting of large regions of H3 lysine 27 methylation harboring smaller regions of H3 lysine 4 methylation in mouse embryonic stem (ES) cells. Bivalent domains tend to coincide with transcription factor genes expressed at low levels. Thus, bivalent domains silence developmental genes in ES cells while keeping them poised for activation. A striking correspondence was found between genome sequence and histone methylation in ES cells, which become notably weaker in differentiated cells (88).

EPIGENETIC CHANGES WITHIN THE LIFETIME

In addition to epigenetic programming during crucial periods of development, stochastically and/or genetically and/or environmentally triggered epigenetic changes within the lifetime can generate epimutations. These epimutations can result from replication-dependent and replication-independent events and will accumulate overtime, increasing the "epigenetic burden" even more.

Replication-Dependent Events

Maintenance of the epigenome is crucial for normal gene expression and preservation of cell identity. The epigenome is the set of heritable properties encoded by elements other than DNA-based sequences. At each cycle, during S phase, this is achieved by duplication of chromatin structure in tight coordination with DNA replication. Such a coordinate process requires histone synthesis and their deposition onto DNA by chromatin assembly factors to be efficiently coupled to DNA synthesis (89). Rather than enzymes that act in isolation to copy methylation patterns after replication, the types of interactions discovered thus far indicate that DNA methyl transferase (DMNT) may be components of larger complexes actively involved in transcriptional control and chromatin structure modulation, i.e., participate in tumorigenesis by methylation-independent as well as methylation-dependent pathways. DNA methylation controls all genetic processes in the cell (replication, transcription, DNA repair, recombination, gene transposition) and it is a mechanism of cell differentiation, gene discrimination, and silencing. DNMT1 plays a central role in cell cycle regulation. Deregulation of DNMT1 leads to triggering of a newly described epigenetic checkpoint, the DNA replication stress checkpoint (90). Thus the DNA methylation machinery represents an attractive therapeutic target (91). The maintenance DNA methyltransferase, Dnmt1, which is involved in propagating the methylation mark at a CpG dinucleotide over successive rounds of replication, with a low rate of de novo methylation, has an estimated error rate of up to 5% (92,93). Epigenetic modifications to DNA generate reversible and clonally heritable alterations in transcription state. Errors in the elaborate epigenetic silencing apparatus of higher eukaryotes can lead to "epimutation" and the abnormal silencing of a gene.

There is compelling evidence to suggest that DNA methylation varies between tissues, individuals, and disease conditions in humans and various animals. Intra- and interindividual epigenetic variations have been detected in human germ cells. The male germline displays locus, cell-, and age-dependent differences in DNA methylation, and these significant differences in DNA methylation have been reported between unrelated individuals, with these differences far greater than those achieved by DNA sequence variation. Variation is greatest for promoter CpG islands and pericentromeric satellites in single-copy DNA fragments and repetitive elements, respectively (33).

An epigenetic drift is observed during aging, with global hypomethylation and the hyper- or hypomethylation of CpG dinucleotides in the promoters of several genes, leading to major changes in the level of expression of these genes (2–7%). Thus, epigenetic alterations do occur but are reversed more frequently than genetic changes; they often produce mosaic patterns of gene expression or silencing and can be inherited through the germline (34,71) and result in promoting the occurrence of age-related diseases. The intrinsic plasticity of the epigenetic state has been demonstrated through studies of aging, carcinogenesis, and atherogenesis in mice and human twins and suggests that the labile nature of the epigenetic state may facilitate the manipulation of the adult phenotype during development (33,94–111). A recent study analyzed DNA methylation and histone acetylation in 80 pairs of human MZ twins between 3 and 74 years of age, using a combination of global and locus-specific methods. One-third of these MZ twins had significantly dissimilar epigenetic profiles that increased with age. The most disparate profiles were those of older twins and of twins with a history of nonshared environments (112).

Replication-Independent events

Replication-independent events underlie transcription of genes. The maintenance of the structural organization of DNA into chromatin—of key importance to regulate genome function and stability—is crucial to preserve cellular identity. Besides S phase related histones, minor forms of histones have been found expressed also outside of S phase. These histone variants, called replacement histones, have been identified for all histones except H4. They are structurally similar to replication-associated histones but functionally distinct due to limited differences in their amino-acid sequences. Replacement histones are generally constitutively synthesized at low amount throughout interphase in cycling cells but also in nonproliferative cells during differentiation or quiescence (113). The H3 variants H3.1 and H3.3 are coupled to DNA synthesis, or can be deposited at any stage of the cell cycle independently of DNA synthesis, respectively. The deposition mechanism of such histone variants onto DNA involves dedicated histone chaperones, histone interacting factors that stimulate histone transfer reactions without being part of the final product. The Chromatin Assembly Factor-1 (CAF-1) and histone regulator A (HIRA) are both involved in the initial step of nucleosome formation i.e., deposition of H3 and H4 histones onto DNA but they promote distinct nucleosome assembly pathways, DNA-synthesis dependent (CAF-1) or independent (HIRA). In mammalian cells, certain active gene promoters are enriched with H3.3. A transcription-coupled deposition for H3.3 is thus an attractive hypothesis.

Lysine methylation is absent prior to histone incorporation into chromatin except at H3K9. H3.1 contains more K9me1 than H3.3. In addition, H3.3 presents other modifications, including K9/K14 diacetylated and K9me2. These initial modifications seem to impact final posttranscriptional modifications within chromatin (114). However, the underlying molecular mechanism and the associated chaperones and/or remodeling factors still need to be characterized. Thus, the existence of distinct pathways involved in the deposition of each variant may have interesting therapeutic implications as it should be possible to target specific candidate proteins.

Valproic acid has been used for decades in the treatment of epilepsy, and is also effective as a mood stabilizer and in migraine therapy. It has been shown that valproic acid is also a histone deacetylase inhibitor. Valproate induces replication-independent active DNA demethylation owing to the participation of MBD2/dMTase (MBD2 is a transcriptional repressor belonging to the MeCP1 histone deacetylase complex). Valproic acid enhances intracellular demethylase activity through its effects on histone acetylation. Chromatin acetylation and DNA methylation are found in a dynamic inter-relation and the consequences of HDAC inhibitors are not limited to changes in histone acetylation but they also bring about a change in the state of modification of DNA. This raises the possibility that DNA methylation is reversible, independent of DNA replication by commonly prescribed drugs (115,116). Future work should help to unveil the position of the epigenetic events within the rhythmic cascade in order to gain more insights into their contribution to the circadian regulation of gene expression.

It is currently thought that most epigenetic changes are coupled to DNA replication. However, emerging evidence that DNA methylation and chromatin modification can occur in a replication-independent manner has challenged this notion. This epigenetic plasticity may facilitate changes in gene expression in response to the oscillatory, circadian, and seasonal rhythms responsible for the rhythmic modulation of the expression of a substantial proportion of the genes during the course of the day and to environmental events throughout the entire life of the cell (117). Chromatin dynamics cycles with a 24 h periodicity are characteristic of some circadian patterns of gene activity. It has been estimated that, depending on the tissue, approximately 10% of our genes display rhythmic modulation with the rhythmic expression of HAT in liver, adipose tissue, adrenals, brain (118–123). Moreover, although the clock is designed to function around a cycle of about 24 hours, its periodicity can be modified by light, activity, or food.

In both the SCN neurons (the master oscillator clock) and peripheral cells (slave clocks), the mechanism of the circadian clock is based on interconnected transcriptional and post-translational feedback loops affecting gene expression in a cell-autonomous fashion. The circadian clock also dictates the rhythmic production of output regulators. These transcription factors, in turn, regulate downstream target genes involved in different biochemical pathways, including glucose, cholesterol, and triglyceride metabolism, the sleeping/waking cycle, thermogenesis, and feeding (124). Pathways downstream from the clock genes include the nuclear receptor peroxisome-proliferator-activated receptor alpha (PPARA). Hepatic PPARA expression is subject to a circadian rhythm directly modulated by the CLOCK and BMLA1 proteins and modulated by glucocorticoids (124,125).

Both the SCN neurons and peripheral cells use epigenetic mechanisms, including histone acetylation and phosphorylation, to generate circadian rhythms in gene expression based on core clock circadian rhythms in H3 acetylation and RNA pol II binding (122,124,126–136). As shown by Etchegaray et al. and by Curtis et al., the transcriptional coactivators and histone acetyltransferases p300/CBP, PCAF, and ACTR associate with the bHLH-PAS proteins, CLOCK and NPAS2, positively regulating clock gene expression (129–131). Transcriptional regulation of the core clock mechanism in mouse liver is accompanied by rhythms in H3 acetylation. The histone acetyltransferase p300 and *Clock* are coprecipitated in a time-dependent manner in vivo, and a complex containing these two molecules is involved in modulating gene expression in response to phase-resetting stimuli (125). Endogenous EZH2, a polycomb group enzyme that methylates lysine 27 on histone H3, coimmunoprecipitates with CLOCK and BMAL1 throughout the circadian cycle in liver nuclear extracts (134). As shown by Doi et al. (131) the *Clock* gene itself encodes a HAT.

Major components of energy homeostasis, including the sleeping-waking cycle, thermogenesis, feeding and glucose metabolism, are subject to circadian regulation, synchronizing energy intake, and expenditure with changes in the external environment imposed by the rising and setting of the sun. Recent epidemiological, clinical, and experimental studies have demonstrated important links between sleep duration and architecture, circadian rhythms, and metabolism, although the genetic pathways connecting these processes remain poorly understood. However, still relatively little is known about epigenetic mechanisms by which genes—cf. PPARA in the liver—are rhythmically induced on a circadian basis (125). For example, CLOCK, which is a HAT, plays an important role in lipid homoeostasis by regulating the transcription of a key protein, PPARA via an

E-box-rich region (125). PPARA is a member of the nuclear receptor superfamily of ligand-activated transcription factors that regulate the expression of genes associated with lipid metabolism. Thus genes induced or inhibited by PPARA can in turn be expressed on a rhythmic pattern. Histone posttranslational modifications and sequence variants regulate genome function. Thus, in addition to specific gene sequence, e.g., E-box-rich regions, there are specific chromatin modifications, histone variants, and histone posttranslational modifications that allow the transcriptional machinery to recognize sequences directly regulated by the clock machinery, e.g., PPARA?

Cells are exposed to a variety of genotoxic insults that constantly threaten genome integrity. Chromatin organization is compromised during the repair of DNA damage. It remains unknown how and to what extent epigenetic information is preserved in vivo. A central question is whether chromatin reorganization involves recycling of parental histones or new histone incorporation. After UV irradiation, new H3.1 histones get incorporated in vivo at repair sites in human cells. H3.1 is not only deposited during S phase but it is also incorporated outside of S phase. This deposition process occurs at a post-repair stage and involves the histone chaperone CAF-1. Thus new histone incorporation at repair sites both challenges epigenetic stability and probably contributes to damage memory (137). Thus maintenance of genome integrity not only involves specific repair pathways that have been characterized in details, however, their coordinated action with factors involved in chromatin modulation remains poorly understood. Genetic variations in the different actors described could contribute to interindividual variation in the rate of accumulation of age- and environment-related accumulation of epimutations.

Lifetime epigenetic alterations occur every day and accumulate over time as a function of age, diet, or disease. Factors such as methionine and TSA modulate histone modification and DNA methylation; Treatment of cellular histones with peptidylarginine deiminase (PAD) results in loss of staining for the histone H4 arginine 3 methyl mark, suggesting that PADs can reverse histone arginine methyl modifications. Are these molecules active on replication-independent events, like TSA? If so it would therefore be interesting to explore their effects on desynchronization (16,87,91).

REFERENCES

1. Waddington C. Canalisation of development and inheritance of acquired characters. Nature 1942; 152:563.
2. Margueron R, Trojer P, Reinberg D. The key to development: interpreting the histone code? Curr Opin Genet Dev 2005; 15(2):163–76.
3. Lippman Z, Martienssen R. The role of RNA interference in heterochromatic silencing. Nature 2004; 431(7006):364–70.
4. Krutzfeldt J, Rajewsky N, Braich R, et al. Silencing of microRNAs in vivo with 'antagomirs'. Nature 2005; 438(7068):685–9.
5. Krutzfeldt J, Stoffel M. MicroRNAs: a new class of regulatory genes affecting metabolism. Cell Metab 2006; 4(1):9–12.
6. Yoder JA, Walsh CP, Bestor TH. Cytosine methylation and the ecology of intragenomic parasites (see comments). Trends Genet 1997; 13(8):335–40.
7. Dokras A, Coffin J, Field L, et al. Epigenetic regulation of maspin expression in the human placenta. Mol Hum Reprod 2006; 12(10):611–7.
8. Rassoulzadegan M, Grandjean V, Gounon P, et al. RNA-mediated non-mendelian inheritance of an epigenetic change in the mouse. Nature 2006; 441(7092):469–74.

9. Bird A. DNA methylation patterns and epigenetic memory. Genes Dev 2002; 16(1):6–21.
10. Weber M, Davies JJ, Wittig D, et al. Chromosome-wide and promoter-specific analyses identify sites of differential DNA methylation in normal and transformed human cells. Nat Genet 2005; 37(8):853–62.
11. Wilson IM, Davies JJ, Weber M, et al. Epigenomics: mapping the methylome. Cell Cycle 2006; 5(2):155–8.
12. Dennis KE, Levitt P. Regional expression of brain derived neurotrophic factor (BDNF) is correlated with dynamic patterns of promoter methylation in the developing mouse forebrain. Brain Res Mol Brain Res 2005; 140(1–2):1–9.
13. Grayson DR, Jia X, Chen Y, et al. Reelin promoter hypermethylation in schizophrenia. Proc Natl Acad Sci U S A 2005; 102(26):9341–6.
14. Champagne FA, Weaver IC, Diorio J, et al. Maternal care associated with methylation of the estrogen receptor-alpha1b promoter and estrogen receptor-alpha expression in the medial preoptic area of female offspring. Endocrinology 2006; 147(6):2909–15.
15. Weaver IC, Cervoni N, Champagne FA, et al. Epigenetic programming by maternal behavior. Nat Neurosci 2004; 7(8):847–54.
16. Weaver IC, Champagne FA, Brown SE, et al. Reversal of maternal programming of stress responses in adult offspring through methyl supplementation: altering epigenetic marking later in life. J Neurosci 2005; 25(47):11045–54.
17. Pogribny IP, Pogribna M, Christman JK, et al. Single-site methylation within the p53 promoter region reduces gene expression in a reporter gene construct: possible in vivo relevance during tumorigenesis. Cancer Res 2000; 60(3):588–94.
18. Lane N, Dean W, Erhardt S, et al. Resistance of IAPs to methylation reprogramming may provide a mechanism for epigenetic inheritance in the mouse. Genesis 2003; 35(2):88–93.
19. Rakyan VK, Chong S, Champ ME, et al. Transgenerational inheritance of epigenetic states at the murine Axin(Fu) allele occurs after maternal and paternal transmission. Proc Natl Acad Sci U S A 2003; 100(5):2538–43.
20. Waterland RA, Jirtle RL. Early nutrition, epigenetic changes at transposons and imprinted genes, and enhanced susceptibility to adult chronic diseases. Nutrition 2004; 20(1):63–8.
21. Druker R, Bruxner TJ, Lehrbach NJ, et al. Complex patterns of transcription at the insertion site of a retrotransposon in the mouse. Nucleic Acids Res 2004; 32(19):5800–8.
22. Morgan HD, Sutherland HG, Martin DI, et al. Epigenetic inheritance at the agouti locus in the mouse. Nat Genet 1999; 23(3):314–8.
23. Bestor TH, Tycko B. Creation of genomic methylation patterns. Nat Genet 1996; 12(4):363–7.
24. Kan PX, Popendikyte V, Kaminsky ZA, et al. Epigenetic studies of genomic retro-elements in major psychosis. Schizophr Res 2004; 67(1):95–106.
25. International Human Genome Sequencing Consortium. Initial sequencing and analysis of the human genome. Nature 2001; 409:860–921.
26. Shen HM, Nakamura A, Sugimoto J, et al. Tissue specificity of methylation and expression of human genes coding for neuropeptides and their receptors, and of a human endogenous retrovirus K family. J Hum Genet 2006; 51(5):440–50.
27. Chen JM, Stenson PD, Cooper DN, et al. A systematic analysis of LINE-1 endonuclease-dependent retrotranspositional events causing human genetic disease. Hum Genet 2005; 117(5):411–27.
28. Waterland RGC. Potential for metabolic imprinting by nutritional perturbation of epigenetic gene regulation. Public Health Issues in Infant and Child Nutrition 2002; 48:317.
29. Waterland RA, Garza C. Potential mechanisms of metabolic imprinting that lead to chronic disease. Am J Clin Nutr 1999; 69(2):179–97.
30. Waterland RA, Lin JR, Smith CA, et al. Post-weaning diet affects genomic imprinting at the insulin-like growth factor 2 (Igf2) locus. Hum Mol Genet 2006; 15(5):705–16.
31. Feinberg AP. Methylation meets genomics. Nat Genet 2001; 27(1):9–10.
32. Zaina S, Nilsson J. Insulin-like growth factor II and its receptors in atherosclerosis and in conditions predisposing to atherosclerosis. Curr Opin Lipidol 2003; 14(5):483–9.

33. Flanagan JM, Popendikyte V, Pozdniakovaite N, et al. Intra- and interindividual epigenetic variation in human germ cells. Am J Hum Genet 2006; 79(1):67–84.
34. Feil R. Environmental and nutritional effects on the epigenetic regulation of genes. Mutat Res 2006; 600(1–2):46–50.
35. Cruz-Correa M, Cui H, Giardiello FM, et al. Loss of imprinting of insulin growth factor II gene: a potential heritable biomarker for colon neoplasia predisposition. Gastroenterology 2004; 126(4):964–70.
36. Jirtle RL. IGF2 loss of imprinting: a potential heritable risk factor for colorectal cancer. Gastroenterology 2004; 126(4): 1190–3.
37. Constancia M, Kelsey G, Reik W. Resourceful imprinting. Nature 2004; 432(7013):53–7.
38. Coan PM, Burton GJ, Ferguson-Smith AC. Imprinted genes in the placenta—a review. Placenta 2005; 26(Suppl. A):S10–20.
39. Wagschal A, Feil R. Genomic imprinting in the placenta. Cytogenet Genome Res 2006; 113(1–4):90–8.
40. Angiolini E, Fowden A, Coan P, et al. Regulation of placental efficiency for nutrient transport by imprinted genes. Placenta 2006; 27(suppl.):98–102.
41. Tycko B. Imprinted genes in placental growth and obstetric disorders. Cytogenet Genome Res 2006; 113(1–4):271–8.
42. Takahashi K, Kobayashi T, Kanayama N. p57(Kip2) regulates the proper development of labyrinthine and spongiotrophoblasts. Mol Hum Reprod 2000; 6(11):1019–25.
43. Plagge A, Gordon E, Dean W, et al. The imprinted signaling protein XL alpha s is required for postnatal adaptation to feeding. Nat Genet 2004; 36(8):818–26.
44. Curley JP, Barton S, Surani A, et al. Coadaptation in mother and infant regulated by a paternally expressed imprinted gene. Proc R Soc Lond B Biol Sci 2004; 271(1545):1303–9.
45. Chen M, Gavrilova O, Liu J, et al. Alternative Gnas gene products have opposite effects on glucose and lipid metabolism. Proc Natl Acad Sci U S A 2005; 102(20):7386–91.
46. Takahashi M, Kamei Y, Ezaki O. Mest/Peg1 imprinted gene enlarges adipocytes and is a marker of adipocyte size. Am J Physiol Endocrinol Metab 2004; 288(1):E117–24.
47. Junien C. L'empreinte parentale: de la guerre des sexes à la solidarité entre généra-tions. Médecine/Sciences 2000; 3:336–44.
48. Keverne EB. Genomic imprinting and the maternal brain. Prog Brain Res 2001; 133:279–85.
49. Plagge A, Isles AR, Gordon E, et al. Imprinted Nesp55 influences behavioral reactivity to novel environments. Mol Cell Biol 2005; 25(8):3019–26.
50. Waterland RA. Assessing the effects of high methionine intake on DNA methylation. J Nutr 2006; 136(Suppl. 6):1706S–10S.
51. Waterland RA, Dolinoy DC, Lin JR, et al. Maternal methyl supplements increase offspring DNA methylation at Axin fused. Genesis 2006; 44(9):401–6.
52. Plagge A, Kelsey G. Imprinting the Gnas locus. Cytogenet Genome Res 2006; 113(1–4):178–87.
53. Williamson CM, Turner MD, Ball ST, et al. Identification of an imprinting control region affecting the expression of all transcripts in the Gnas cluster. Nat Genet 2006; 38(3):350–5.
54. Xie T, Plagge A, Gavrilova O, et al. The alternative stimulatory G protein alpha-subunit XLalphas is a critical regulator of energy and glucose metabolism and sympathetic nerve activity in adult mice. J Biol Chem 2006; 281(28):18989–99.
55. Issa JP, Vertino PM, Boehm CD, et al. Switch from monoallelic to biallelic human IGF2 promoter methylation during aging and carcinogenesis. Proc Natl Acad Sci USA 1996; 93(21):11757–62.
56. Lucifero D, Chaillet JR, Trasler JM. Potential significance of genomic imprinting defects for reproduction and assisted reproductive technology. Hum Reprod Update 2004; 10(1):3–18.
57. Mann MR, Lee SS, Doherty AS, et al. Selective loss of imprinting in the placenta following preimplantation development in culture. Development 2004; 131(15): 3727–35.
58. Dindot SV, Farin PW, Farin CE, et al. Epigenetic and genomic imprinting analysis in nuclear transfer derived Bos gaurus/Bos taurus hybrid fetuses. Biol Reprod 2004; 71(2):470–8.

59. Ma D, Shield JP, Dean W, et al. Impaired glucose homeostasis in transgenic mice expressing the human transient neonatal diabetes mellitus locus, TNDM. J Clin Invest 2004; 114(3):339–48.

60. Delrue MA, Michaud JL. Fat chance: genetic syndromes with obesity. Clin Genet 2004; 66(2):83–93.

61. Rougeulle C, Navarro P, Avner P. Promoter-restricted H3 Lys 4 di-methylation is an epigenetic mark for monoallelic expression. Hum Mol Genet 2003; 12(24):3343–8.

62. Pembrey M. Imprinting and transgenerational modulation of gene expression; human growth as a model. Acta Genet Med Gemellol (Roma) 1996; 45(1–2):111–25.

63. Beaudet AL, Jiang YH. A rheostat model for a rapid and reversible form of imprinting-dependent evolution. Am J Hum Genet 2002; 70(6):1389–97.

64. Young LE. Imprinting of genes and the Barker hypothesis. Twin Res 2001; 4(5):307–17.

65. Pembrey ME, Bygren LO, Kaati G, et al. Sex-specific, male-line transgenerational responses in humans. Eur J Hum Genet 2006; 14(2):159–66.

66. Whitelaw E. Epigenetics: sins of the fathers, and their fathers. Eur J Hum Genet 2006; 14(2):131–2.

67. Dean W, Santos F, Reik W. Epigenetic reprogramming in early mammalian development and following somatic nuclear transfer. Semin Cell Dev Biol 2003; 14(1):93–100.

68. Hajkova P, Erhardt S, Lane N, et al. Epigenetic reprogramming in mouse primordial germ cells. Mech Dev 2002; 117(1–2):15–23.

69. Li E. Chromatin modification and epigenetic reprogramming in mammalian development. Nat Rev Genet 2002; 3(9):662–73.

70. Morgan HD, Santos F, Green K, et al. Epigenetic reprogramming in mammals. Hum Mol Genet 2005; 14(Spec No. 1):R47–58.

71. Reik W, Dean W, Walter J. Epigenetic reprogramming in mammalian development. Science 2001; 293(5532):1089–93.

72. Reik W, Santos F, Dean W. Mammalian epigenomics: reprogramming the genome for development and therapy. Theriogenology 2003; 59(1):21–32.

73. Jaenisch R, Bird A. Epigenetic regulation of gene expression: how the genome integrates intrinsic and environmental signals. Nat Genet 2003; 33(Suppl.):245–54.

74. Li S, Hursting SD, Davis BJ, et al. Environmental exposure, DNA methylation, and gene regulation: lessons from diethylstilbesterol-induced cancers. Ann NY Acad Sci 2003; 983:161–9.

75. Sutherland JE, Costa M. Epigenetics and the environment. Ann NY Acad Sci 2003; 983:151–60.

76. Loukinov DI, Pugacheva E, Vatolin S, et al. BORIS, a novel male germ-line-specific protein associated with epigenetic reprogramming events, shares the same 11-zinc-finger domain with CTCF, the insulator protein involved in reading imprinting marks in the soma. Proc Natl Acad Sci USA 2002; 99(10):6806–11.

77. Yamazaki Y, Mann MR, Lee SS, et al. Reprogramming of primordial germ cells begins before migration into the genital ridge, making these cells inadequate donors for reproductive cloning. Proc Natl Acad Sci USA 2003; 100(21):12207–12.

78. Kelly TL, Trasler JM. Reproductive epigenetics. Clin Genet 2004; 65(4):247–60.

79. Walsh CP, Chaillet JR, Bestor TH. Transcription of intra-cisternal A particle endogenous retroviruses is constrained by cytosine methylation. Nat Genet 1998; 20(2):116–7.

80. Whitelaw NC, Whitelaw E. How lifetimes shape epigenotype within and across generations. Hum Mol Genet 2006; 15(Suppl. 2):R131–7.

81. Blewitt ME, Vickaryous NK, Paldi A, et al. Dynamic reprogramming of DNA methylation at an epigenetically sensitive allele in mice. PLoS Genet 2006; 2(4):e49.

82. Whitelaw E, Martin DI. Retrotransposons as epigenetic mediators of phenotypic variation in mammals. Nat Genet 2001; 27(4):361–5.

83. Rakyan VK, Preis J, Morgan HD, et al. The marks, mechanisms and memory of epigenetic states in mammals. Biochem J 2001; 356(Pt 1):1–10.

84. Rakyan VK, Blewitt ME, Druker R, et al. Metastable epialleles in mammals. Trends Genet 2002; 18(7):348–51.

85. Peaston AE, Whitelaw E. Epigenetics and phenotypic variation in mammals. Mamm Genome 2006; 17(5):365–74.

86. Oates NA, van Vliet J, Duffy DL, et al. Increased DNA methylation at the AXIN1 gene in a monozygotic twin from a pair discordant for a caudal duplication anomaly. Am J Hum Genet 2006; 79(1):155–62.

87. Sarmento OF, Digilio LC, Wang Y, et al. Dynamic alterations of specific histone modifications during early murine development. J Cell Sci 2004; 117(Pt 19):4449–59.

88. Bernstein BE, Mikkelsen TS, Xie X, et al. A bivalent chromatin structure marks key developmental genes in embryonic stem cells. Cell 2006; 125(2):315–26.

89. Polo SE, Almouzni G. Histone metabolic pathways and chromatin assembly factors as proliferation markers. Cancer Lett 2005; 220(1):1–9.

90. Unterberger A, Andrews SD, Weaver IC, et al. DNA methyltransferase 1 knockdown activates a replication stress checkpoint. Mol Cell Biol 2006; 26(20):7575–86.

91. Szyf M, Pakneshan P, Rabbani SA. DNA demethylation and cancer: therapeutic implications. Cancer Lett 2004; 211(2):133–43.

92. Goyal R, Reinhardt R, Jeltsch A. Accuracy of DNA methylation pattern preservation by the Dnmt1 methyltransferase. Nucleic Acids Res 2006; 34(4):1182–8.

93. Vilkaitis G, Suetake I, Klimasauskas S, et al. Processive methylation of hemimethylated CpG sites by mouse Dnmt1 DNA methyltransferase. J Biol Chem 2005; 280(1):64–72.

94. Abdolmaleky HM, Smith CL, Faraone SV, et al. Methylomics in psychiatry: modulation of gene-environment interactions may be through DNA methylation. Am J Med Genet B Neuropsychiatr Genet 2004; 127(1):51–9.

95. Barbot W, Dupressoir A, Lazar V, et al. Epigenetic regulation of an intra-cisternal A particle retrotransposon in the aging mouse: progressive demethylation and de-silencing of the element by its repetitive induction. Nucleic Acids Res 2002; 30(11):2365–73.

96. Chang KT, Min KT. Regulation of lifespan by histone deacetylase. Ageing Res Rev 2002; 1(3):313–26.

97. Friso S, Choi SW. Gene-nutrient interactions and DNA methylation. J Nutr 2002; 132(Suppl. 8):2382S–7S.

98. Fuke C, Shimabukuro M, Petronis A, et al. Age related changes in 5-methylcytosine content in human peripheral leukocytes and placentas: an HPLC-based study. Ann Hum Genet 2004; 68(Pt 3):196–204.

99. Hoal-Van Helden EG, Van Helden PD. Age-related methylation changes in DNA may reflect the proliferative potential of organs. Mutat Res 1989; 219(5–6):263–6.

100. Issa JP. CpG-island methylation in aging and cancer. Curr Top Microbiol Immunol 2000; 249:101–18.

101. Issa JP, Ahuja N, Toyota M, et al. Accelerated age-related CpG island methylation in ulcerative colitis. Cancer Res 2001; 61(9):3573–7.

102. Issa JP, Ottaviano YL, Celano P, et al. Methylation of the oestrogen receptor CpG island links ageing and neoplasia in human colon. Nat Genet 1994; 7(4):536–40.

103. Maier S, Olek A. Diabetes: a candidate disease for efficient DNA methylation profiling. J Nutr 2002; 132(Suppl. 8):2440S–3S.

104. Mays-Hoopes L, Chao W, Butcher HC, et al. Decreased methylation of the major mouse long interspersed repeated DNA during aging and in myeloma cells. Dev Genet 1986; 7(2):65–73.

105. Oakes CC, Smiraglia DJ, Plass C, et al. Aging results in hypermethylation of ribosomal DNA in sperm and liver of male rats. Proc Natl Acad Sci U S A 2003; 100(4):1775–80.

106. Ono T, Uehara Y, Kurishita A, et al. Biological significance of DNA methylation in the ageing process. Age Ageing 1993; 22(1):S34–43.

107. Post WS, Goldschmidt-Clermont PJ, Wilhide CC, et al. Methylation of the estrogen receptor gene is associated with aging and atherosclerosis in the cardiovascular system. Cardiovasc Res 1999; 43(4):985–91.

108. Rath PC, Kanungo MS. Methylation of repetitive DNA sequences in the brain during aging of the rat. FEBS Lett 1989; 244(1):193–8.

109. Singhal RP, Mays-Hoopes LL, Eichhorn GL. DNA methylation in aging of mice. Mech Ageing Dev 1987; 41(3):199–210.

110. Toyota M, Issa JP. CpG island methylator phenotypes in aging and cancer. Semin Cancer Biol 1999; 9(5):349–57.
111. Von Zglinicki T, Burkle A, Kirkwood TB. Stress, DNA damage and ageing: an integrative approach. Exp Gerontol 2001; 36(7):1049–62.
112. Fraga MF, Ballestar E, Paz MF, et al. Epigenetic differences arise during the lifetime of monozygotic twins. Proc Natl Acad Sci USA 2005; 102(30):10604–9.
113. Wu RS, Tsai S, Bonner WM. Patterns of histone variant synthesis can distinguish G0 from G1 cells. Cell 1982; 31(2 Pt 1):367–74.
114. Loyola A, Bonaldi T, Roche D, et al. PTMs on H3 variants before chromatin assembly potentiate their final epigenetic state. Mol Cell 2006; 24(2):309–16.
115. Detich N, Bovenzi V, Szyf M. Valproate induces replication-independent active DNA demethylation. J Biol Chem 2003; 278(30):27586–92.
116. Milutinovic S, D'Alessio AC, Detich N, et al. Valproate induces widespread epigenetic reprogramming which involves demethylation of specific genes. Carcinogenesis 2007; 28(3):560–7.
117. Schibler U. The daily rhythms of genes, cells and organs. Biological clocks and circadian timing in cells. EMBO Rep 2005; 6(Spec No.):S9–13.
118. Kalra SP, Bagnasco M, Otukonyong EE, et al. Rhythmic, reciprocal ghrelin and leptin signaling: new insight in the development of obesity. Regul Pept 2003; 111(1–3):1–11.
119. Boden G, Ruiz J, Urbain JL, et al. Evidence for a circadian rhythm of insulin secretion. Am J Physiol 1996; 271(2 Pt 1):E246–52.
120. Zvonic S, Ptitsyn AA, Conrad SA, et al. Characterization of peripheral circadian clocks in adipose tissues. Diabetes 2006; 55(4):962–70.
121. Ptitsyn AA, Zvonic S, Conrad SA, et al. Circadian clocks are resounding in peripheral tissues. PLoS Comput Biol 2006; 2(3):e16.
122. Oishi K, Amagai N, Shirai H, et al. Genome-wide expression analysis reveals 100 adrenal gland-dependent circadian genes in the mouse liver. DNA Res 2005; 12(3):191–202.
123. Hanai S, Masuo Y, Shirai H, et al. Differential circadian expression of endothelin-1 mRNA in the rat suprachiasmatic nucleus and peripheral tissues. Neurosci Lett 2005; 377(1):65–8.
124. Staels B. When the Clock stops ticking, metabolic syndrome explodes. Nat Med 2006; 12(1):54–5 (discussion 55).
125. Oishi K, Shirai H, Ishida N. CLOCK is involved in the circadian transactivation of peroxisome-proliferator-activated receptor alpha (PPARalpha) in mice. Biochem J 2005; 386(Pt 3):575–81.
126. Turek FW, Joshu C, Kohsaka A, et al. Obesity and metabolic syndrome in circadian Clock mutant mice. Science 2005; 308(5724):1043–5.
127. Rudic RD, McNamara P, Curtis AM, et al. BMAL1 and CLOCK, two essential components of the circadian clock, are involved in glucose homeostasis. PLoS Biol 2004; 2(11):e377.
128. Kreier F, Yilmaz A, Kalsbeek A, et al. Hypothesis: shifting the equilibrium from activity to food leads to autonomic unbalance and the metabolic syndrome. Diabetes 2003; 52(11):2652–6.
129. Curtis AM, Seo SB, Westgate EJ, et al. Histone acetyltransferase-dependent chromatin remodeling and the vascular clock. J Biol Chem 2004; 279(8):7091–7.
130. Etchegaray JP, Lee C, Wade PA, et al. Rhythmic histone acetylation underlies transcription in the mammalian circadian clock. Nature 2003; 421(6919):177–82.
131. Doi M, Hirayama J, Sassone-Corsi P. Circadian regulator CLOCK is a histone acetyltransferase. Cell 2006; 125(3):497–508.
132. Debruyne JP, Noton E, Lambert CM, et al. A clock shock: mouse CLOCK is not required for circadian oscillator function. Neuron 2006; 50(3):465–77.
133. Inoue I, Shinoda Y, Ikeda M, et al. CLOCK/BMAL1 is involved in lipid metabolism via transactivation of the peroxisome proliferator-activated receptor (PPAR) response element. J Atheroscler Thromb 2005; 12(3):169–74.
134. Etchegaray JP, Yang X, DeBruyne JP, et al. The polycomb group protein EZH2 is required for mammalian circadian clock function. J Biol Chem 2006; 281(30):21209–15.

135. Shimba S, Ishii N, Ohta Y, et al. Brain and muscle Arnt-like protein-1 (BMAL1), a component of the molecular clock, regulates adipogenesis. Proc Natl Acad Sci USA 2005; 102(34):12071–6.
136. Oishi K, Kasamatsu M, Ishida N. Gene- and tissue-specific alterations of circadian clock gene expression in streptozotocin-induced diabetic mice under restricted feeding. Biochem Biophys Res Commun 2004; 317(2):330–4.
137. Polo SE, Roche D, Almouzni G. New histone incorporation marks sites of UV repair in human cells. Cell 2006; 127(3):481–93.

8.2 Implications for Obesity and Common Diseases

C. Gallou-Kabani, A. Vigé, M.S. Gross, and C. Junien
INSERM, AP-HP, Université Paris Descartes and Faculté de Médecine, INSERM Unit 781, Clinique Maurice Lamy, Hôpital Necker-Enfants Malades, Paris, France

The various non-Mendelian features of obesity, such as the high degree of discordance between monozygote (MZ) twins, clinical differences between men and women, and fluctuations in the course of the disease, are consistent with epigenetic mechanisms for the influence of fetal environment on adult phenotype (1). Thus, in addition to harboring a number of gene variants conferring susceptibility (2), individuals with metabolic syndrome, obesity, and type 2 diabetes (T2D) may show a lifelong imbalance between energy intake and energy expenditure as well as incorrect "EpiG programming" during their early development as a result of placental insufficiency, inadequate maternal body composition, nutritional imbalance, and metabolic disturbances during critical time windows of development (3,4), which may have a persistent effect on the health of the offspring and may even be transmitted to the next generation. The environment modifies the epigenetic patterns of susceptible genes during development in such a way that key functions, such as appetite control, metabolic balance, and fuel utilization are permanently modified. Moreover, epigenetic alterations occur day after day and accumulate over time, as age-, diet-, and disease-related deteriorations interact with several other processes. The transgenerational effects (TGEs) of incorrectly erased epigenetic marks resulting from the behavior and nutrition of previous generations may complete the picture. Lifetimes shape the multitude of epigenomes not only within but also across generations (5).

The phenotype of an individual is thus the result of complex interactions between genetic background, with its millions of polymorphisms, tissue-, sex-, stage-, and age-specific "epigenome(s)," which result from millions of subtly different epigenetic patterns and environmental factors. Epigenetic information is heritable during cell division but is not contained within the DNA sequence itself. The interaction of an individual's environmental experience with his or her genotype determines the history of his or her multidimensional phenotype, beginning at conception and continuing throughout adulthood. As shown by discordance between MZ twins for a host of common polygenic disorders, the same genotype can give rise to many possible environmental phenotype histories (6–11). The potential to react changes continually, from conception to death (12). Research on obesity and cardiovascular disease (CVD) has identified tens of high-risk environmental agents and hundreds of genes, each with many variations, influencing disease risk. As the number of interacting agents involved increases, the number of cases of disease with the same etiology and associated with a particular multigene genotype decreases (1,2,12).

Unraveling the molecular causes and mechanisms of common forms of obesity and associated disorders remains a major challenge, despite considerable efforts in this area. Now that studies of the organization of the human genome sequence are reaching completion, studies of the epiG control of genomes are required to determine how the same DNA sequence generates different cells, lineages, and organs under the influence of different environmental factors, providing a basic biological knowledge of both normal and disease states (13).

DEVELOPMENTAL ORIGIN OF HEALTH AND ADULT DISEASE

In the last 10 years, a series of studies—notably those by Barker, Hales, and co-workers, who first coined the term "fetal programming" leading to a "thrifty phenotype"—have demonstrated that common disorders, such as obesity, CVD, diabetes, hypertension, asthma, and even schizophrenia take root in early nutrition, during gestation and lactation, hence the new term "developmental origin of health and disease" (DOHaD) (4,14–25). Although our understanding of the fundamental biologic mechanisms underlying such phenomena remains rudimentary, consequences of these fetal alterations persist postnatally and may result in metabolic alterations throughout life (26,27).

A significant and increasing proportion of pregnant women are affected by metabolic syndrome but the effects of these conditions and of an unbalanced diet and metabolic disturbances during pregnancy on the various critical windows of development remain to be explored. Whereas the long-term effects of undernutrition such as the Dutch winter famine in 1944–1945, with the benefit of 60 years hindsight, have clearly demonstrated to result in the development of metabolic syndrome, not enough time has passed and it is therefore too early for us to assess the long-term effects of the impact of the rapidly increasing prevalence of overweight in women during the preconceptual, pregnancy, and lactation periods. Gestational diabetes can occur in these offspring and transmit the effect to the next generation. These alterations in fetal development can be associated with fetal macrosomia (maternal diabetes) or fetal growth-restriction (maternal/fetal malnutrition).

The relation between birth weight and later metabolic disease therefore is U-shaped. Adult metabolic condition is thus to a considerable extent programmed in utero, fetal and neonatal weight being symptoms of disturbed fetal development. Moreover, in addition to genetic background and an abnormal intrauterine environment, germline epigenetic inheritance may also account for these effects on the next generation(s). This concept of intrauterine programming of disease is illustrated by reviews of epidemiological human studies and experimental animal studies (25,28,29).

Human Epidemiological Studies

Some of the strongest evidence of the developmental origin of adult diseases has come from studies on the offspring of mothers exposed to dietary restriction and on MZ twins discordant for T2D (6,7). The repetition, intensity, and duration of famines such as those that affected the Pima Indians (1870–1930), the Irish (1845–1849), and the Finns (1866–1868), have led to the selection of more resistant individuals, who survived thanks to thrifty genes. Conversely, during the nine months of siege in the Netherlands at Amsterdam, Rotterdam, and The Hague, at the end of the Second World War (October 1994–May 1945), despite a doubling in the mortality rate, both adults and fetuses rapidly adapted to restricted calorie intake, without necessarily having to make use of thrifty genes (30,31).

With 60 years of hindsight, we can now analyze the consequences over several generations of the drastic decrease in calorie intake in pregnant women during famines. Fetuses exposed to dietary restrictions have a greater risk of glucose intolerance, insulin resistance, obesity, and diabetes (32,33). This is probably due to disruption of the programming of endocrine systems (34) and of key centers of the central nervous system (35). Moreover, studies of individuals who were in utero during the Dutch famine winter have suggested that the detrimental effects of poor maternal nutrition are transmitted to her grandchildren (36).

A significant and increasing proportion of French women (14–27% OBEPI cohort 2003) are overweight when pregnant. Whereas the long-term effects of gestational diabetes are well documented (37,38), the consequences of overweight and metabolic syndrome in the mother, together with an unbalanced diet and metabolic disturbances during the periconceptual period, gestation, and lactation, for fetal programming, various critical windows of development, and during aging (39) are poorly documented and remain to be explored (28).

Animal Experimental Models

What are the factors influencing this vicious cycle? Fetal development is dependent on maternal supply of fuels and building blocks. Disturbed maternal metabolism or inappropriate maternal nutrition confronts the fetus with an unfavorable intrauterine milieu. A recent review examined animal studies in which the fetal and postnatal environment had been manipulated by changing maternal dietary intake or modifying uterine artery flow (28). Maternal protein restriction (28,40,41), maternal calorie restriction, fetal exposure to glucocorticoids (42–44), intrauterine artery ligation (45), maternal iron restriction (46), maternal and/or postnatal nutritional excess (3,29,47) result in long-term programming of decreased beta-cell mass, blood pressure, diabetes, etc.

Animal studies clearly demonstrate that there is a direct association between nutrient imbalance in fetal life and later disease states, including hypertension, diabetes, obesity, and renal disease. Experimental studies examining the impact of micro- or macronutrient restriction and excess in rodent pregnancy provide clues to the mechanisms that link fetal nutrition to permanent physiological changes that promote disease. Exposure to glucocorticoids in early life appears to be an important consequence of nutrient imbalance and may lead to alterations in gene expression that have major effects on tissue development and function. While these associations have been widely accepted to be the product of nutritional factors operating in pregnancy, evidence from human populations to support this assertion is scarce (48).

Most studies examined the consequences of protein restriction during gestation, conditions not fully matching the features of the current epidemic of the metabolic syndrome. A smaller number of studies have dealt with the consequences of a high-carbohydrate or fat-rich diet, conditions corresponding more closely to the current epidemics of metabolic factors associated with the metabolic syndrome. However, it remains unclear whether metabolic syndrome can be reliably induced by the interventions made, due to differences between protocols, diets (e.g., type of fatty acids), sex, and time periods examined (28). Recent experiments have shown that the features of metabolic syndrome in the adult offspring of fat-fed rats may be acquired antenatally and during suckling. Moreover, exposure during pregnancy confers adaptive protection against endothelial dysfunction—but not against hypertension—due to maternal fat-feeding during suckling (49). However, these data only partially reflect the features of metabolic syndrome because pregnant mothers were not overweight and therefore did not display the metabolic disturbances of metabolic syndrome that could also interfere with fetal/postnatal programming.

Disturbances in the maternal metabolism that may alter the nutrient supply from mother to fetus can induce structural and functional adaptations during fetal development, with lasting consequences for growth and metabolism of the offspring throughout life. This effect has been investigated, by several research groups, in different experimental models where the maternal metabolism during pregnancy was experimentally manipulated (maternal diabetes and maternal malnutrition) and the effect on the offspring was investigated. The altered maternal/fetal metabolism appears to be associated with a diabetogenic effect in the adult offspring, including gestational diabetes. This diabetic pregnancy in the offspring again induces a diabetogenic effect into the next generation, via adaptations during fetal development (50).

The familial predisposition to type 2 diabetes is mediated by both genetic and intrauterine environmental factors. In the normal course of events, maternal genes always develop in the same uterus, thus restricting studies aimed at investigating the relative contribution of these factors. Gill-Randall et al. have developed an embryo transfer paradigm in rats to overcome this difficulty. Interestingly, in GK (GotoKakizaki) rats, a euglycemic intrauterine environment cannot overcome the strong genetic predisposition to diabetes. However, in Wistar rats with a low genetic risk of diabetes, exposure to hyperglycemia in utero significantly increases the risk of diabetes in adult life (51). Thus a control intrauterine environment cannot overcome the effects of genetic predisposition. In contrast, even in animals with a low risk the abnormal uterine milieu becomes detrimental. These experimental data in laboratory animals are confirmed by epidemiological studies on infants of mothers suffering from diabetes or malnutrition during pregnancy (52).

Recent data suggest that an appropriate dietary fatty-acid profile and intake during the periconceptual/gestation/lactation period helps the female offspring to cope with deleterious intrauterine conditions. Gallou-Kabani et al. investigated whether reducing fat intake during the periconceptual/gestation/lactation period, in mothers with high-fat diet–induced obesity, could be used to modify fetal/neonatal metabolic syndrome programming positively, thereby preventing metabolic syndrome. Sensitivity/resistance to the high-fat diet differed significantly between generations and sexes. A similar proportion of the first- and second-generation males (80%) developed hyperphagia, obesity, and diabetes. In contrast, a significantly higher proportion of the female offspring (43%) than of the previous generation (17%) were resistant. Despite having free access to the high-fat diet these female mice were no longer hyperphagic, remained lean, with normal insulin sensitivity and normal glycemia, but mild hypercholesterolemia and glucose intolerance, thus displaying an adapted "satiety phenotype" (53).

It can be concluded that fetal development in an abnormal intrauterine milieu can induce alterations in the fetal metabolism, with lasting consequences for the offspring in adult life. The most marked effect is the development of gestational diabetes, thereby transmitting the diabetogenic tendency to the next generation again. Malnourished fetuses adopt several strategies to optimize their chances of survival during the neonatal period, but these strategies assume that the same type of nutritional conditions will prevail. A selective distribution of nutrients ensures that brain growth is given priority over the growth of other organs such as the liver, muscle, and pancreas.

Disease risk is greater when there is a mismatch between the early developmental environment versus that experienced in mature life and nutritional influences are particularly important (54). The adaptations adopted during fetal programming may prove to be detrimental if food becomes more abundant (55). Alternatively, a fetus that experienced a balanced diet during gestation, despite an overweight mother, appears better-equipped to resist the attractive palatable high-fat diet, instead of becoming hyperphagic, than fetuses raised in a normal womb with a control diet (53). Thus predictive adaptive responses to unbalanced nutrient delivery in utero may be inappropriate for the postnatal conditions experienced (56). In addition, the responses required to cope with environmental challenges in early life may have long-term effects on the adult organism, adverse long-term effects of coping (57). Thus, any change in conditions may have deleterious or beneficial consequences. The concept of fetal origin of adult diabetes therefore is of major significance for public health in the immediate as well as in the far future (52,58–61).

Critical Spatiotemporal Windows

EpiG programming is tightly regulated over time and space during fetal development and lactation. There are therefore critical windows for the supply of specific nutrients by the placenta, demand from the fetus, and circulating hormone levels. In addition to magnitude of exposure, one has to consider also the timing and duration of exposure. For example, leptin appears to play a crucial neurotrophic role in the development of the hypothalamic circuits regulating food intake and adiposity. The neurodevelopmental effects of leptin appear to be restricted to a specific, critical neonatal period—the second week of life—coinciding with a natural upsurge in leptin levels. The timing and amplitude of the postnatal leptin surge has important consequences for normal body-weight regulation and glucose homeostasis later in life. During this period, leptin promotes the formation of projections from the arcuate nucleus through direct effects on the brain and has a trophic effect on these feeding circuits, whereas at other times, it inhibits food intake and increases the rate of metabolism. These early neurotrophic processes presumably require differentiation-dependent epigenetic modifications, although this has yet to be demonstrated experimentally. Failure to develop these structures in due time may result in long-lasting and potentially irreversible effects on adult metabolism (62).

Several studies have shown that the risk of CVD, obesity, hypertension, diabetes, cancer, and schizophrenia later in life depends on the timing of the calorie restriction during pregnancy (16–23). In the Dutch winter famine cohort, children subject to dietary restrictions in utero during the first six months of pregnancy had similar birth weights to other newborns. However, these subjects had a higher incidence of obesity in adulthood in the first generation with higher body mass index (BMI) and waist circumference in 50-year-old women, but not in men. Thus, disturbances in central endocrine regulatory systems established in early gestation may contribute to the development of central obesity in later life (31,63).

Children subjected to dietary restrictions in utero during the third trimester of pregnancy had a lower birth weight (6–10% lower than the birth weights recorded before the famine), due to a direct effect of the mother's dietary restrictions on the fetus. Glucose tolerance was decreased most strongly in subjects exposed during mid- or late-gestation. The effect on glucose tolerance was especially large in people who became obese (31). Individuals exposed to famine in early gestation have a more atherogenic lipid profile than those not exposed to famine in utero. This suggests that maternal malnutrition during early gestation may program lipid metabolism without affecting size at birth (64,65). This may imply that adaptations that enable the fetus to continue to grow may nevertheless have adverse consequences for health in later life. It also implies that the long-term consequences of improved nutrition of pregnant women will be underestimated if they are solely based on the size of the baby at birth (24).

Maternal protein restriction in rats during either pregnancy and/or lactation alters postnatal growth, appetitive behavior, leptin physiology, triglycerides and cholesterol concentrations, and modifies glucose metabolism and insulin resistance in a sex- and time window of exposure-specific manner (60). Long-term programming of postnatal growth and physiology can be induced irreversibly during the preimplantation period of development by maternal protein undernutrition. The mildly hyperglycemic and amino acid-depleted maternal environment generated by undernutrition may act as an early mechanism of programming and initiate conditions of "metabolic stress," restricting early embryonic proliferation and the generation of appropriately sized stem-cell lineages (14). Maternal low-protein diet fed exclusively during the rat preimplantation period induces low birth weight, altered postnatal growth, and hypertension in a gender-specific manner (66). Neonatal exposure to maternal diabetes through the intake of dam's milk in rats leads to a complex malprogramming of hypothalamic orexigenic and anorexigenic circuits that are critically involved in the lifelong regulation of food intake, body weight, and metabolism (67). A post-weaning diet deficient in methyl donors can affect genomic imprinting at the insulin-like growth factor 2 (Igf2) loci in mice suggesting that childhood diet could contribute to IGF2 loss of imprinting in humans (68).

Since these critical windows are obviously different for the developmental processes involved in different tissues/organs, a nutritional insult at a critical period of cell division or differentiation can permanently alter the structure or function of an organ and consequently metabolic processes. The epigenome is most vulnerable to environmental factors during embryogenesis because the DNA synthetic rate is high and the elaborate DNA methylation patterning and chromatin structure required for normal tissue/organ development is established precisely during this period (69).

Environmental Influences on Epigenetic Reprogramming

Since 1999, evidence has accumulated suggesting that epigenetic chromatin remodeling is one of the mechanisms underlying both developmental programming and non-Mendelian transgenerational inheritance in plants and mammals. Environmental factors and nutrition may also affect the fidelity with which patterns of epigenetic modifications are maintained throughout life (1). The human fetus develops along a narrow growth trajectory that must balance the demands of the fetus with the capabilities of the mother (70).

Indisputable proofs of principle have been provided by four outstanding papers (71–74) and many others in the meantime. Embryo culture conditions, nuclear transfer, maternal body composition, stress or behavior, nutrient availability, and dietary interventions—under- or over-nutrition due to litter size, crop abundance during the grandparents' lifetime (75,76), carcinogens and radiation exposure, endocrine disruptors, folate intake/deficiency—may affect IG, transposons, genes, or genome-wide epigenetic marks during a narrow spatiotemporal window (1,73,74,77–117).

The A^{vy} and $Axin^{Fu}$ phenotypes can be influenced by providing the mice with a specific diet (71,72). In the A^{vy} mice, the mouse food was complemented with extra folic acid (folate), vitamin B12, choline, and betaine which are thought to enhance the metabolism of methyl donors in the cell. If nonagouti dams (a/a) are mated with male mice carrying the A^{vy} allele (A^{vy}/a), the proportion of agouti offspring can be increased by feeding the dam a methyl-supplemented diet during pregnancy. Dietary supplementation with a methyl donor during pregnancy increases the proportion of pups carrying a methylated intracisternal A particle (IAP) sequence (72,113,115,118). Moreover, the coat color phenotype and A^{vy} methylation pattern persisted into adulthood (114). Similarly, maternal genistein alters coat color and protects a^{vy} offspring from obesity through modification of the fetal epigenome (119). Thus, an environmental factor increases the probability of methylation upstream from the A^{vy} locus (67,94,114,116–118). Conversely, when mice are fed a methyl-donor-deficient diet (lacking folic acid, vitamin B12, and choline), this led to downregulation of the imprinted gene Igf2. This reduced expression correlated with altered DNA methylation at a differentially methylated region (117). Similarly, maternal genistein alters coat color and protects a^{vy} offspring from obesity through modification of the fetal epigenome (119). Thus, an environmental factor increases the probability of methylation upstream from the A^{vy} locus (67,94,114,116–118).

Another murine metastable epiallele, $Axin^{Fu}$ similarly exhibits epigenetic plasticity to maternal diet. Methyl donor supplementation of female mice before and during pregnancy reduced by half the incidence of tail kinks in $Axin^{Fu}$ offspring, by increasing $Axin^{Fu}$ methylation in tail in a tissue specific manner suggesting a mid-gestation effect. Thus, similar to A^{vy}, epiG metastability at $Axin^{Fu}$ confers lability to early nutrition. Thus nutritional effects on DNA methylation during development may be tissue-specific, occur at diverse ontogenic periods (117). These studies represent a clear demonstration of how nutrition can influence the epigenetic organization of genes and as a consequence, can have long-term effects on gene expression and phenotype. These studies emphasize that dietary supplements may not always be beneficial and can have aberrant effects on the regulation of gene expression.

In mammals, imprinted genes have an important role in feto-placental development. They affect the growth, morphology, and nutrient transfer capacity of the placenta and, thereby, control the nutrient supply for fetal growth. In particular, the reciprocally imprinted Igf2–H19 gene complex has a central role in these processes and matches the placental nutrient supply to the fetal nutrient demands for growth. Comparison of Igf2P0 (Igf2 isoform) and complete Igf2 null mice has shown that interplay between placental and fetal Igf2 regulates both placental growth and nutrient transporter abundance. In turn, epigenetic modification of genes via changes in DNA methylation may provide a mechanism linking environmental cues to placental phenotype, with consequences for development both before and after birth (120). When mice are fed a methyl-donor-deficient diet (lacking folic acid, vitamin B12, and choline), this led to downregulation of the Igf2.

This reduced expression correlated with altered DNA methylation at a differentially methylated region (117).

Uteroplacental insufficiency leads to intrauterine growth retardation and increases the risk of insulin resistance and hypertriglyceridemia in both humans and rats. The altered intrauterine milieu associated with uteroplacental insufficiency affects hepatic one-carbon metabolism—increased levels of S-adenosylhomocysteine, homocysteine, and methionine in association with decreased mRNA levels of methionine adenosyltransferase and cystathionine-beta-synthase—with subsequent genome-wide DNA hypomethylation, and increased levels of acetylated histone H3 which thereby alters chromatin dynamics and leads to persistent changes in hepatic gene expression (106). Rats with intrauterine growth retardation due to bilateral uterine artery ligation showed significantly decreased genome-wide and CpG island methylation, as well as altered histone modifications, and levels of DNMT1, methyl CpG binding protein 2 (MeCP2), HDAC1, and zinc in the hippocampus and periventricular white matter. Thus intrauterine growth retardation results in postnatal changes in cerebral chromatin structure. Moreover, these changes are sex specific (121).

The effect of unbalanced maternal nutrition—protein restriction whether or not supplemented in folic acid—on the methylation status and expression of the glucocorticoid receptor (GR) and peroxisomal proliferator-activated receptor (PPAR) genes was investigated in rat offspring after weaning. The GR gene methylation was increased (20%) and expression was higher in protein restricted compared with control pups. The diet supplemented with folic acid prevented these changes. Thus unbalanced prenatal nutrition induces persistent, gene-specific epigenetic changes that alter mRNA expression (122).

Eukaryotes have hundreds of ribosomal RNA (rRNA) genes whose transcription helps establish the proliferative ability of cells by dictating the pace of ribosome production and protein synthesis. In each cell the rRNA genes exist in two distinct types of chromatin structure: an "open" one corresponding to transcriptionally active genes and a "closed" one representing the silent genes. An epigenetic network—comprising an interplay of DNA methylation/demethylation, histone modification, and chromatin-remodeling activities—mediates the transcriptional state of rDNA. Thus, as an indirect consequence, the transcriptional state of rDNA modulates the level of expression of genes in each cell under a given physiopathological status (123). Brown and Szyf recently showed that the methyl-CpG binding domain protein 3 binds to unmethylated rRNA promoters thereby epigenetically maintaining active rRNA promoters (Brown and Szyf, personal communication). rRNA levels have been linked to cancer. Interestingly, in a transgenerational mouse model of carcinogenesis, it has been shown that the sperm of treated fathers had a significantly higher percentage of undermethylated copies of the 45S rRNA gene. Since offspring of treated fathers were significantly heavier than control, epiG modulation of rRNA genes may contribute to the pathophysiological process of obesity (91).

However, while these models did not show so far whether the diet effects can be perpetuated through generations, the demonstration that chemical effects can be perpetuated over generations was recently provided by endocrine disruptors. The transient exposure of a pregnant female rat to the endocrine disruptors vinclozolin (an anti-androgenic compound) or methoxychlor (an estrogenic compound) during the period of gonadal sex determination resulted in an F1 generation with the adult phenotype of low spermatogenic capacity (cell number and viability) and a high incidence of male infertility. Surprisingly, this low level of fertility was inherited through the male germline by almost all males in subsequent generations (F2–F4). These effects on reproduction were found to be correlated with DNA methylation patterns in the germline, with multiple genes displaying changes in their pattern of DNA methylation. Effects were even observed in the fourth generation. These heritable changes occurred in the absence of further environmental treatment, demonstrating the existence of a long-lasting programmed epigenetic event (73).

Epigenetic programming does not necessarily require the ingestion of an environmental substance. Maternal behavior can direct gene expression in the offspring by transmitting a message concerning the nature of the environment the animal will have to live in, rather than just whether that environment is favorable or unfavorable. Differences in DNA methylation pattern between the offspring of female rats with high and low levels of licking/grooming behavior are associated with changes in DNA methylation, histone acetylation, and transcription factor [nerve-growth factor-induced clone A (NGF1A)] binding to the GR gene in the hippocampus (74). This specific type of maternal behavior during early postnatal development in rodents appears to determine the methylation status of a single CpG dinucleotide within the promoter region of the GR gene in the hippocampus of the offspring and appear to involve the estrogen receptor alpha (ESRRA) (see Chapter 8.1) (93). TGEs are thus cyclic, with mothers having high levels of licking/grooming behavior teaching their female offspring to behave in a similar manner. Methylation can repress gene expression by inhibiting transcription factor binding to the methylated binding site or by promoting the binding of repressors (124). This study also showed that the central infusion of trichostatin A (TSA) or methionine can reverse both epiG states, restoring or impairing the corresponding reactivity to stress in adult offspring (74,89).

These "proofs of concept" all identified the nature of the stimulus—methyl donors defect or supplementation, endocrine disruptors, radiation, cyclophosphamide, maternal under- or over-nutrition behavior—the type/number of sequences (89), the rRNA genes (genes belonging to the epigenetic machinery, and other as yet unidentified genes), the type of epiG alterations involved (gene candidate or genome-wide DNA methylation and/or histone modifications), the developmental windows during which the stimuli could efficiently affect epigenetic patterns, the persistence of these changes in adulthood and TGEs. Programming may influence epigenetic patterns in the target gene(s) within the promoter or within the gene itself or at a distance from the promoter, or in genes encoding factors that regulate the basal target gene(s) expression.

EPIGENETIC CHANGES WITHIN THE LIFETIME

Epigenetic modifications to DNA generate reversible and clonally heritable alterations in transcription state. Errors in the elaborate epigenetic silencing apparatus of higher eukaryotes can lead to "epimutation" and the abnormal silencing of a gene. These epigenetic changes are due to: (1) replication-dependent events; (2) replication-independent events linked to transcription (circadian rhythms). Environmental factors interact with both of these mechanisms and act as reversible switches of gene expression that can lock genes in active or repressive state. Effects are due to circulating hormones and environmental factors (radiations, pesticides, etc.), including events, behavior, oxidative damage to methyl-CpG sequences preventing binding of the methyl-binding domain of methyl-CpG binding protein 2 (MeCP2) (125), and nutritional status (e.g., folate status) (1,5,68).

Age-, Diet-, and Disease-Related Epigenetic Deteriorations

There is compelling evidence to suggest that DNA methylation varies between tissues, individuals and disease conditions in humans and various animals. Intra- and interindividual epigenetic variations have been detected in human germ cells (126). It also varies with aging, with both hyper- and hypomethylation observed. Moreover, epigenetic alterations that occur day after day and accumulate over time, as age-, diet-, and disease-related deteriorations interact with several other processes. Epigenetic changes within the lifetime of the organism are linked to several other processes known to deteriorate during the initiation and progression of metabolic syndrome and associated disorders. These processes include not only incorrect early epigenetic programming of tissues and organs, but also lifelong mitochondrial dysfunction, deteriorations in chromosomal epigenetic patterns with chromosomal instability and telomere shortening. They also comprise the disturbance of oscillatory, circadian, and seasonal rhythms, including the alternation of sleeping and waking, feeding/fasting, and temperature regulation with the rhythmic expression of clock genes, one of which was recently identified as a histone acetyl transferase, a key element of the epigenetic machinery (127). These processes are known to deteriorate during progression to metabolic syndrome, under the influence of oxidative stress, aging and folate status, leading to the relaxation (or silencing) of expression for a number of key genes. Thus epigenetic variation may also help to account for the late onset and progressive nature of most common diseases, the quantitative nature of complex traits, and the role of environment in disease development, particularly in cases where a purely sequence-based approach is inconclusive. At every stage during the cascade of epigenetic fluctuations (during both fetal development and aging), the nutritional balance must be "optimal."

An epigenetic drift is observed during aging, with global hypomethylation and the hyper- or hypomethylation of CpG dinucleotides in the promoters of several genes, leading to major changes in the level of expression of these genes (2–7%). Thus, epiG alterations do occur but are reversed more frequently than genetic changes. Moreover, the rate of mutation at mCpG is 20–40 times higher than for other nucleotides, because of spontaneous deamination events converting 5-mC to T and cytosine to uracil (128). Epimutations often produce mosaic patterns of gene expression or silencing and can be inherited through the germline (1,129) and result in promoting the occurrence of age-related diseases. The intrinsic plasticity of the epigenetic state has been demonstrated through studies of aging, carcinogenesis, psychiatric disorders, diabetes, and atherogenesis in mice and humans twins and suggests that the labile nature of the epigenetic state may facilitate the manipulation of the adult phenotype during development (98,126,130–146).

Beckwith-Wiedemann syndrome (BWS) presents as visceromegaly, macro- glossia, hyperinsulinism, predisposition to tumors and other congenital abnormalities, and is usually associated with imprinting abnormalities of chromosome 11p15. In skin fibroblasts or blood from 10 MZ twin pairs discordant for BWS, the affected twin had an imprinting defect at *KCNQ10T1* on 11p15 in each case, whereas the unaffected twin did not. These epigenetic alterations necessarily occurred after the twinning process, but it remains difficult to assess whether these anomalies result from a deleterious intrauterine milieu or from stochastic events (147).

A progressive loss of epiG integrity has been regarded as a major cause of cancer. Issa et al. (1996) provided evidence of a link between aging, carcinogenesis, and de novo methylation within the promoter of the ESRRA gene in the human colon (102,137,148,149). They then investigated the dynamics of this process for the IG coding the IGF2. Their results demonstrate remarkable changes in the methylation patterns of the imprinted promoter of the *IGF2* gene during aging and carcinogenesis, and provide further evidence for a potential link between aberrant methylation and aging-related diseases (150). The normally silenced intronic IAP retrotransposon has been shown to undergo stochastic activation and demethylation in older mice (131). Similarly, normally silenced murine genes on the inactive X chromosome and in imprinted regions have been shown to undergo age-related, progressive epigenetic derepression (151). These changes, together with rare somatic mutations, may account for the reported increase in heterogeneity of gene expression between cells in aging mice (152).

Circadian Gene Expression

It has been estimated that, depending on the tissue, approximately 10% of our genes display rhythmic modulation with the rhythmic expression of histone acetyl transferase (153–158). Moreover, although the clock is designed to function around a cycle of about 24 hours, its periodicity can be modified by light, activity, or food.

Recent studies have shown that mutation or deletion of the *Clock* and *BMLA1* genes results not only in circadian disturbances but also in metabolic abnormalities of lipid and glucose homeostasis—giving an obesity phenotype (159). The *Clock* gene mutation blunts physiological peaks of activity in the mouse homozygous *Clock* mutant mice. They have a greatly attenuated diurnal feeding rhythm, are hyperphagic and obese, and develop a metabolic syndrome of hyperleptinemia, hyperlipidemia, hepatic steatosis, hyperglycemia, and hypoinsulinemia. They were found to produce lower than normal levels of transcripts encoding selected hypothalamic peptides associated with energy balance (159). The Cre-LoxP (Cre/loxP recombination system) was used to generate whole-animal knockouts of *Clock* and to evaluate the resulting circadian phenotypes. Surprisingly, *Clock*-deficient mice continue to express robust circadian rhythms in locomotor activity, although they do have altered responses to light. CLOCK-deficient animals have lower than normal levels of mRNA and protein in both the master clock in the suprachiasmatic nuclei and a peripheral clock in the liver, although the molecular feedback loops continue to function. These data call into question a central feature of the current mammalian circadian clock model— the need for CLOCK: BMAL1 heterodimers for clock function (160). CLOCK/ BMAL1 plays a role in lipid metabolism, transactivating the peroxisome proliferator-activated receptor (PPAR) response element (161,162). Mutations in the corresponding clock genes influence maintenance of pregnancy, the development of glucose intolerance and insulin resistance, and lipid disturbances, obesity-induced disordered fibrinolysis regulation of adipogenesis, in sleep disorders, and in response to a high-fat diet (160–171).

These results suggest that the circadian clock gene network plays an important role in mammalian energy balance (165,166,168,169,172–184). Future work should help to unveil the position of the epigenetic events within the rhythmic cascade in order to gain more insights into their contribution to the circadian regulation of gene expression.

Mitochondrial Dysfunction

As shown by the cluster of metabolic defects caused by a mutation in a mitochondrial tRNA, mitochondrial defects may play a role in the metabolic syndrome (185,186). Various organisms have no internally methylated cytosine in CCGG sequences in mitochondrial DNA and therefore cannot have defects in DNA methylation (187). However, folate depletion which causes nuclear genetic and epigenetic aberrations in cell culture, also damages mitochondrial DNA in rodents and humans, inducing large-scale deletions due to DNA breakage as a result of the misincorporation of uracil into DNA. Progressive mitochondrial dysfunction therefore results from the age-, tissue-, and folate-dependent accumulation of somatic mutation/deletions in the mitochondrial genome, such mutations being 10 times more frequent than somatic mutations within the nuclear genome, and leading to the production of high levels of reactive oxygen metabolites (188,189).

Deteriorations of Epigenetic Patterns Along the Chromosomes and Telomeres

Epigenetic dysregulation is a key element of cancer development and progression. The changes in epigenetic patterns on chromosomes include hypomethylation, leading to oncogene activation and the hypomethylation of repeated sequences. Transposable elements may cause the uncontrolled proliferation/apoptosis and chromosome instability typical of tumorigenesis, and hypermethylation of the promoters of tumor-suppressor genes may change gene expression profiles either directly, or together with methylation changes (190–193). The central question is how could both processes of hypermethylation (inhibition of tumor suppressors) and hypomethylation (reactivation of oncogenes, chromosome instability, increased metastasis) coexist in the same cell? Could we distinguish the mechanisms responsible for these two processes? This suggests that different enzymes determine them (194).

Telomere length is a crucial factor in chromosome function and senescence. Mean telomere length in humans varies considerably between humans and is largely genetically determined. Heritability has been estimated at 82% in family studies (195), with twin studies providing a narrow heritability estimate of 36% attributable to additive polygenic effects and a large shared familial effect of 49% (196). Telomere shortening, a typical age-related process, can be triggered by environmental or metabolic factors, such as oxidative stress, smoking or obesity, and metabolic syndrome (197,198). By contrast, a lack of DNA methyltransferases increases the frequency of telomeric recombination, leading to telomere elongation in mouse embryonic stem cells (146,199). A lack of histone methyl transferases is also associated with abnormal telomere elongation (200).

TRANSGENERATIONAL EFFECTS

Although it has long been thought that the epigenetic slate is wiped clean in the embryo shortly after fertilization—except for imprinted genes—there are now clear examples of TGEs in mammals. The totipotency of the zygote depends on this clean slate.

Human Epidemiological Studies

Epidemiological data suggesting or demonstrating the existence of TGEs have been obtained for humans (1,25,75,91,201–206).

The Dutch famine is a unique counterpart for animal models that study the effects of restricted maternal nutrition during different stages of gestation using the findings from a cohort study of 2414 people born around the time of the famine. Undernutrition was defined separately for each trimester of pregnancy as an average supply of less than 1000 calories per day from government food rations. Studies of individuals who were exposed in utero to undernutrition during the Dutch winter famine have suggested that the detrimental effects of poor maternal nutrition are transmitted to her grandchildren (36).

Mothers exposed to famine during their first and second trimester in utero (F1) had offspring (F2) with birthweights lower than those of mothers not exposed to famine. The decrease in birthweight was in part due to slower fetal growth rate, in part to shorter gestation. Birthweights in the offspring (F2) of mothers (F1) exposed in their third trimester in utero were, however, not reduced. These findings in mothers exposed to famine in utero are in contrast to the effects of the famine on their mothers (F0) during their pregnancies, where third trimester exposure was associated with a reduction in birthweight in their offspring (F1). The expected usual increase in (F2) offspring birth weights with increasing birth order was not seen after maternal intrauterine exposure in the first trimester of pregnancy. In this group, second born infants weighed, on average, 252 g less at birth than their firstborn siblings and thirdborn infants weighed 419 g less, even after adjustment for trimester of maternal intrauterine exposure, maternal birth weight, smoking during pregnancy, and sex of infants in the sibling pairs. There were no abnormal patterns in offspring birth weights after maternal intrauterine exposure in the second or third trimester of pregnancy. This study suggests that there may be long-term biologic effects, even into the next generation of maternal intrauterine undernutrition which do not correspond to the effects on the mothers' own birth weights (24,207,208).

Pembrey et al. recently suggested that the behavior (or environment) of prepubescent boys may influence the phenotype of their future sons and grand-sons (76,209). Associations have been reported between longevity and food supply during the mid-childhood slow growth period (SGP) in paternal ancestors. Data from the 1890, 1905, and 1920 Overkalix cohorts in northern Sweden have shown that a grandfather "well-nourished" before puberty may transmit a four times higher than normal risk of diabetes to his grandchildren (75). The study of the Overkalix cohorts in northern Sweden on the effects of food supply on offspring and grandchild mortality risk ratios identified sex-specific effects: only the paternal grandfather's food supply was linked to the risk ratio of grandsons, whereas only the paternal grandmother's food supply was associated with the risk ratio of mortality of grand-daughters. These TGEs related to exposure during the SGP (both grandparents) or fetal/infant life (grandmothers), but not during the pubertal period of either grandparent. In another cohort, the Avon Longitudinal Study of Parents and Children (ALSPAC), sex-specific effects were again observed after appropriate adjustment: early paternal smoking was found to be associated with a higher BMI at the age of nine in sons, but not in daughters (76).

Betel nut (*Areca catechu*) consumption has been shown to induce glucose intolerance in adult CD1 mice and in their F1 and F2 offspring, thereby demon-strating the existence of transgenerational metabolic effects. Parents fed on betel nuts were mated with normal controls. Glucose intolerance was detected in male and female F1 progeny, and mean islet areas were greater in the offspring of betel-fed parents than in other mice (210). In humans, in the absence of MetS in either parent and of betel-nut consumption by the offspring, paternal exposure to betel nuts has been shown to increase the risk of early metabolic disease development in children of either sex in a dose-dependent manner, by a factor of 2.53 on average (211).

The involvement of epigenetic processes has not yet been demonstrated in human fetal programming or in either of the examples of possible transmission to subsequent generations cited above. Such demonstrations would require the development of new strategies adapted to humans.

Animal Models

Results obtained for both plants and animals are consistent with an epigenetic and/or gene expression based mechanism for transgenerational inheritance. There is increasing evidence, in both plants and animals, that, following nutritional intervention (caloric, iron, and protein restriction or a fat-rich or carbohydrate-rich diet, betel nut consumption), endocrine disruptors, maternal diabetes, behavioral programming (maternal care), glucocorticoids or exercise stress during pregnancy and lactation that this can affect the following generation(s) (14,25,42,44,53,59–61, 72–74,87,92,210,212–221).

Epigenetic Transmission of TGEs

The molecular basis of these apparently nongenetic TGEs remains unclear, but epigenetic regulation is thought to be involved in fetal programming. Phenomena such as DNA methylation and histone acetylation can result in the static reprogramming of gene transcription by changing chromatin infrastructure. Environmental constraints during early life result in phenotypic changes that may be associated with a higher risk of disease in later life, suggesting that gene transcription is modified in a persistent manner. DNA methylation, which is largely established in utero, provides a causal mechanism by which unbalanced prenatal nutrition could potentially generate such changes in gene expression.

Studies in mice have shown that epigenetic marks are not always cleared between generations. Indisputable proofs of principle have been provided by four outstanding papers (71–74) and many others. These "proofs of principle" all identified the nature of the stimulus, the type/number of sequences, the type of epigenetic alterations involved, the developmental windows during which the stimuli could efficiently affect epigenetic patterns, the persistence of these changes in adulthood and TGEs.

The first two examples of TGEs attributable to epigenetic modifications in mice concerned the A^{vy} and $Axin^{Fu}$ loci (71,72) as described above. The A^{vy} locus displays epigenetic inheritance from the mother but not from the father. The distribution of phenotypes among the offspring depends not only on the phenotype of the dam but also on the phenotype of the grandmother. An A^{vy} dam with the agouti phenotype is more likely to produce agouti offspring than a yellow mother, whereas yellow mothers produce a higher proportion of yellow offspring than agouti mothers (71). The proportion of pups with a phenotype corresponding to a methylated IAP depends on the mother's own phenotype, and therefore on the level of methylation of the mother's own IAP sequence at the A^{vy} locus.

The variable phenotypes of the offspring result from incomplete elimination of the epigenetic modification when allele A is transmitted via the maternal germline (114,222). Consistent with the idea of transgenerational epigenetic inheritance, the methylation status of the *Axin-fused* ($Axin^{Fu}$) allele in mature sperm reflects the methylation status of the allele in the somatic tissue, suggesting that this locus is not subject to epigenetic reprogramming during gametogenesis (72).

Nutrition
Nutrition probably exerts its effects on methylation early in embryonic development, and these effects may concern all tissues or be tissue-specific (117). These effects have already been developed in the preceding section.

Metabolic Imprinting Is Perpetuated Across Generations
Does maternal obesity and/or diet during pregnancy cause metabolic imprinting in the offspring, perpetuating obesity across generations? Waterland et al. compared the offspring of obese A^{vy}/a dams and lean a/a dams. Two separate populations of A^{vy}/a mice were maintained on a control (NIH-31) or a methyl-supplemented diet. The A^{vy} allele was passed through the female germline for several generations, making it possible to assess cumulative effects on the body weight of A^{vy}/a and a/a offspring. Maternal obesity and offspring body weight at weaning were higher in the F1 generation from A^{vy} dams than in that from a/a dams. Mean weight increased with each successive generation in A^{vy}/a offspring only. Furthermore, folate-methyl donor supplementation also had an effect, with higher body weights recorded for F1 than for F2 mice on the control diet (control diet F2<F1) and lower body weights recorded for F1 than for F2 mice on the supplemented diet (supplemented diet F2>F1) (117). Thus maternal obesity during pregnancy can cause metabolic imprinting in the offspring, perpetuating obesity across generations.

Endocrine-Disrupting Chemicals
The indirect demonstration that dietary effects can be perpetuated over generations was recently provided by endocrine disruptors. Endocrine-disrupting chemicals in the environment have been linked to effects on human health and disease. This link is particularly clear for compounds mimicking the effects of estrogens. Exposure to endocrine-disrupting chemicals, such as PCBs, early in life can increase the risk of physical and mental health problems and of altered sex determination (223,224). Epigenetic mechanisms have been implicated in this process. Transgenerational consequences of endocrine-disrupting chemicals exposure may occur and may have evolutionary implications, as suggested by a study showing how such transmission might become incorporated into the genome and subject to selection (225). The transient exposure of a pregnant female rat to the endocrine disruptors vinclozolin (an antiandrogenic compound) or methoxychlor (an estrogenic compound) during the period of gonadal sex determination resulted in an F1 generation with the adult phenotype of low spermatogenic capacity (cell number and viability) and a high incidence of male infertility. Surprisingly, this low level of fertility was inherited through the male germline by almost all males in subsequent generations (F2–F4). These effects on reproduction were found to be correlated with DNA methylation patterns in the germline, with multiple genes displaying changes in their pattern of DNA methylation. Effects were even observed in the fourth generation. These heritable changes occurred in the absence

of further environmental treatment, demonstrating the existence of a long-lasting programmed epigenetic event (73).

The synthetic estrogen diethylstilbestrol is a potent perinatal endocrine disruptor. In humans and experimental animals, exposure to synthetic estrogen diethylstilbestrol during critical periods of reproductive tract differentiation permanently alters estrogen target tissues and results in long-term abnormalities, such as uterine neoplasia, that do not manifest until later in life. In studies with mice exposed to synthetic estrogen diethylstilbestrol during development (DES mice), multiple mechanisms playing a role in the carcinogenic and toxic effects of DES have been identified. Analysis of the uterus in DES mice has revealed changes to gene expression pathways with an estrogen-regulated component. Even low doses of DES increase the incidence of uterine tumors. This greater susceptibility to tumors is passed on via the maternal line to subsequent generations of male and female descendants (226).

Transgenerational Carcinogenesis

Transgenerational carcinogenesis refers to the transmission of cancer risk to the untreated progeny of parents exposed to carcinogens before mating. An increasing body of evidence suggests that the mechanism underlying this process is epigenetic, and might involve hormonal changes and changes in gene expression in the offspring. The exposure of male mice to Cr(III) chloride 2 weeks before mating has been shown to increase significantly the percentage of undermethylated copies of the 45S rRNA in their sperm. The exposure of male mice to Cr(III) chloride 2 weeks before mating affects the incidence of neoplastic and non neoplastic changes in offspring tissues. The sperm of the exposed males had a significantly higher than normal percentage of undermethylated copies of the 45S rRNA gene. One allele of the 45S rRNA spacer promoter was found to be hypomethylated in sperm germ cells after exposure to Cr(III) exposure. This epimutation may increase the risk of tumors in the offspring (227). The offspring of Cr(III)-treated male mice were also found to be significantly heavier than controls, and to have higher serum T3 concentrations. Using microarray analysis of cDNAs from liver, 58 genes, including 25 identified genes, were found to have expression ratios significantly correlated with serum T3 ratios. Thus, epigenetic and/or gene expression-based mechanisms are involved in transgenerational carcinogenesis (91,228–230).

Preconceptional Paternal Exposure to the Anticancer Agent Cyclophosphamide

Preconceptional paternal exposure to cyclophosphamide, a widely used anticancer agent, results in a higher frequency of embryo loss, malformations, and behavioral deficits in the offspring. These abnormalities are transmissible to subsequent generations. Recent studies have shown that paternal exposure to this drug induces aberrant epigenetic programming in early embryos. Zygotes sired by drug-treated males had poor germ cell quality, and displayed disrupted embryo development and the dysregulation of zygotic gene activation, advanced developmental progression, an increase in pronuclear areas, and disruption of the epigenetic programming of both parental genomes. Early postfertilization zygotic pronuclei were hyperacetylated. By mid-zygotic development, male pronuclei were dramatically hypomethylated, whereas female pronuclei were hypermethylated. The number of micronuclei was considerably larger than normal, and histone H4 acetylation and lysine 5 localization to the nuclear periphery were disrupted in two-cell embryos fertilized by spermatozoa from cyclophosphamide-exposed individuals. Thus, disturbances in epigenetic programming may contribute to heritable instabilities later in development, highlighting the importance of epigenetic risk assessment after chemotherapy (231,232).

Behavioral Imprinting Is Perpetuated Across Generations
Maternal effects commonly reflect the quality of the environment and are probably mediated by the quality of maternal provision, which in turn determines growth rates and adult phenotype. In mammals, these effects appear to "program" emotional, cognitive, and endocrine systems, increasing sensitivity to adversity. In highly adverse environments, such effects may be considered adaptive, increasing the chances of the offspring surviving to sexual maturity; however, they have a cost in the form of an increase in the risk of various types of disease in later life (233). Maternal behavior can direct gene expression in the offspring by transmitting a message concerning the nature of the environment the animal will have to live in, rather than just whether that environment is favorable or unfavorable (233). The best example is provided by differences in DNA methylation pattern between the offspring of female rats with high and low levels of licking/grooming behavior as described above (74). Variations in maternal behavior are associated with differences in ESRRA expression and are transmitted across generations. The female offspring of high licking/grooming behavior mothers display high levels of *Essra* expression in the brain and become high licking/grooming mothers themselves when adult (93). TGEs are thus cyclic, with mothers having high levels of licking/grooming behavior teaching their female offspring to behave in a similar manner. Methylation can repress gene expression by inhibiting transcription factor binding to the methylated binding site or by promoting the binding of repressors (124).

Sex-Specific Effects and Modes of Transmission of TGEs
There is compelling epidemiological and experimental evidence to suggest that the adverse consequences of changes in the intrauterine environment or maternal behavior can be passed from mother (F0) to daughter (F1) and on to the next generation (F2). Most of the studies carried out have assumed that these TGEs result from incorrect programming due to an abnormal intrauterine environment/postnatal maternal feeding or behavior of the F1 generation. The high licking/grooming of maternal nutrition and other environmental "exposures" are well recognized, but the possibility of paternal exposure influencing development and health in the subsequent generations is rarely considered. Such effects, if confirmed, would be novel and could have far-reaching implications in the context of chronic diseases.

Modes of Transmission
As already suggested by Campbell and Perkins and supported by data and observations published in 28 papers on TGEs of drug and hormonal treatments in mammals (from 1954 to 1982), there are at least four different possible mechanisms for induced carryover effects: (1) effects transmitted by males and through multiple generations; (2) male transmission through a single generation; (3) transmission through multiple female generations; (4) progressive change while animals are kept under inducing conditions (214).

Transgenerational Persistence and Duration of the Consequences of the Initial Stimulus

Epidemiological studies linking low birth weight and subsequent cardiometabolic disease have given rise to the hypothesis that events in fetal life permanently program subsequent cardiovascular risk. However, the effects of fetal programming may not be limited to the first generation of offspring. Studies in humans and animals have identified programmed intergenerational effects on both birth weight and CVD (220).

The persistence of such programming effects through several generations, with transmission via the maternal or paternal line, indicates the potential importance of epigenetic factors in the intergenerational inheritance of the "programming phenotype" and provides a basis for the inherited association between low birth weight and cardiovascular risk factors. In several rat models, fetal exposure to excess glucocorticoids results in low birth weight with subsequent adult hyperinsulinemia and hyperglycemia. The male offspring of female rats exposed in utero to dexamethasone, but not exposed to this compound during their own pregnancy, also have a low birth weight, glucose intolerance, and high levels of hepatic glucose production. However, these effects have been shown to resolve in the third generation. Similar intergenerational programming was observed in the offspring of male rats exposed in utero to dexamethasone and mated with control females (42).

Endocrine disruptors have been shown to promote an epigenetic transgenerational phenotype involving a number of disease states (e.g., male infertility). The antiandrogenic fungicide vinclozolin was found to act transiently at the time of embryonic sex determination, leading to a spermatogenic cell defect and subfertility in males of the F1 generation. A number of other disease states developed in animals allowed to for up to one year of age. This phenotype was transferred through the male germline to all subsequent generations analyzed (F2–F4). This demonstration of the ability of an environmental factor (e.g., an endocrine disruptor) to cause an epigenetic transgenerational phenotype has implications concerning the potential hazards of environmental toxins, mechanisms of disease etiology, and evolutionary biology (234).

In one study, female rats malnourished during the perinatal period and displaying intrauterine growth retardation at birth were mated at the age of eight months. Early malnutrition impairs the development of the endocrine pancreas, decreasing beta-cell mass in the first generation of offspring and impairing subsequent beta-cell adaptation to pregnancy. This beta-cell alteration is also present in the next generation and involves restricted expansion of the epithelial population expressing pancreatic and duodenal homeobox 1 (Pdx1) (235).

Continued Exposure for Several Generations

In most animal models in which the existence of TGEs has been established only the first-generation animals—males and/or pregnant females—were subjected to the stimulus: endocrine disruptors, low-protein diets, betel-nut chewing, radiotherapy as used for cancer treatment, particular types of maternal behavior, folate-deficient diets, glucocorticoids, etc. Exposure was thus limited to a single generation and little is known about the cumulative effects of exposure over several generations.

In a study carried out two decades ago, Stewart et al. studied colonies of rats that had been maintained for 12 generations on diets with adequate levels of protein or marginally deficient in protein. In the malnourished colony, the proportion of "small-for-gestational-age" offspring was 10 times higher than that for the well-nourished colony. The malnourished colony also grew more slowly and presented a retardation of sexual maturation, particularly in female. The adults of both sexes were significantly lighter and shorter than the adults of the well-nourished colony. The young malnourished rats displayed higher levels of exploratory activity, transient head tremors and a long-lasting, if not permanent, higher level of noise sensitivity. These animals displayed marked differences in behavior and learning patterns when adult and it was difficult to attract and hold their attention. In decision-making situations, the animals became very excited, emitted loud squeals, and tried to escape from what was clearly a stressful situation. A casual examination of the malnourished adults revealed them to be small, badly groomed and excitable, but without gross abnormalities. Thus, changes in malnourished human communities may have a persistent influence, not only on metabolic parameters, but also on the behavior on several subsequent generations (236).

Sex-Specific Effects

Sex specificity may operate at different levels: (1) the sex of the parent transmitting the consequences of exposure to the stimulus; (2) the sex of the offspring displaying the maternal effect or TGEs. Recent studies have shown that maternal or paternal epigenetic inheritance may be influenced by strain background (72). Although our understanding of the fundamental biological mechanisms underlying such phenomena remains rudimentary the effects could be due to cytoplasmic, hormonal or metabolic influences, or preferential influence on gametogenesis in one sex but not in the other or to gender-specific reprogramming of imprinted genes' expression (237).

At fertilization, the paternal genome exchanges protamines for histones, undergoes DNA demethylation, and acquires histone modifications, whereas the maternal genome appears epigenetically more static. Alternatively as shown with two male-specific genes, sex-specific expression in the liver may depend on sexually dimorphic DNA demethylation methylation of a single CpG in a regulatory element, and involve methylation-sensitive transcription factor(s) (238,239). Thus because of these sex-specific differences—not only in timing but also in the mechanisms involved during gametogenesis, postfertilization, in gonadal sex differentiation, and in gonad development and hormonal status—environmental insults can affect differently the mother and the father, but also the female and male offspring.

Sex Specificity of Transmission

Unlike the A^{vy} allele, for which the epigenetic transmission of methylation is limited to the female germline, the $Axin^{Fu}$ locus displays epigenetic inheritance whether transmitted maternally or paternally, but this inheritance depends on the genetic background of the strain concerned (72). While maternal inheritance at the A^{vy} locus could be due to cytoplasmic, hormonal or metabolic influences paternal inheritance at the $Axin^{Fu}$ locus argues against cytoplasmic influences. Indeed, in sharp contrast with the egg, the sperm does not contribute cytoplasm to the zygote. Consistent with the idea of transgenerational inheritance of epigenetic marks, Rakyan et al. showed that the methylation state of $Axin^{Fu}$ in mature sperm reflects the methylation state of the allele in the somatic tissue of the animal, suggesting that it does not undergo epigenetic reprogramming during gametogeneis (72).

Paternal food deprivation consistently decreases serum glucose concentration in both male and female offspring, and may result in changes in corticosterone and insulin-like growth factor-1 concentrations. A male-mediated TGE on metabolism- and growth-related parameters, including glucose concentration, in particular, has been identified (58). The TGE of dexamethasone treatment can be transmitted by either maternal or paternal lines (42).

In another study, the poor fertility—resulting from endocrine disruptor-induced modification of the methylation pattern of a series of genes—was inherited, through the male germline, by almost all the males of the following four generations (73). The anti-androgenic fungicide, vinclozolin, has transient effects at the time of embryonic sex determination, leading to subfertile F1 males with a spermatogenic cell defect (234). These data suggest that environmental factors may have a direct preferential influence on gametogenesis in one sex but not in the other. This is also the case for paternal exposure to the anticancer drug, cyclophosphamide, which has been shown to modify germ cell quality, disrupt embryo development, and dysregulate zygotic gene activation in the rat (232).

Physiological changes in females during aging may affect the growth and reproductive traits not only of the offspring of that female, but also of subsequent generations. Early-adolescent and middle-aged pregnant mice have less testosterone than young-adult pregnant mice. These lower testosterone levels have an effect on the body weight and testicular sperm production of male offspring. A small increase in the levels of estradiol or other estrogens during the fetal development of female mice is also associated with earlier puberty. F2 pups with young adult grandmothers were significantly heavier than pups with grandmothers that were early-adolescent and middle-aged at the time of the pregnancy (240). The effects of maternal age on human offspring have not been investigated in humans, with the exception of genetic abnormalities associated with aging oocytes. With the common shift towards very late pregnancies in human populations, the influence of age-related changes in levels of estradiol and testosterone requires further investigation. Being small for gestational age in both mother and father significantly influences the risk of their offspring being small for gestational age. While previous research has indicated that the birth outcome of the mother is an important determinant of the birth outcome of her offspring, these data indicate that the birth outcome of the father plays an equally critical role in determining fetal growth, strongly suggesting a genetic component (241).

The Vicious Cycle of Mother-to-Daughter Transmission

The diabetic pregnancy in the offspring again induces a diabetogenic effect into the next generation, via adaptations during fetal development (50). The TGE, from the diabetic mother into the third generation, fetuses and adults, is only transmitted via the maternal line: female offspring of diabetic mothers develop gestational diabetes and induce the effect in their fetuses and thereby into the next generation. Male offspring have impaired glucose tolerance, but do not transmit the effect to their offspring (25,52,242–244). In contrast, studies in the offspring of glucocorticoid-treated rats dams, suggest that the effects can also be transmitted through the paternal line (42).

Neonatal female rat pups raised artificially on a high-carbohydrate (HC) milk formula during the suckling period immediately developed hyperinsulinemia, which became chronic during the postweaning period, when these rats were fed a laboratory diet. These rats developed obesity in adulthood. Second-generation pups born to these female rats spontaneously developed chronic hyperinsulinemia and adult-onset obesity (HC phenotype) in the absence of dietary intervention during the suckling period. This metabolic programming, once established, also forms a vicious cycle, because HC female rats spontaneously transmit the HC phenotype to their progeny (212).

What type of epigenetic mechanism can be involved? Variations in maternal behavior are associated with differences in estrogen receptor (ER)-α expression in the medial preoptic area (MPOA) and are transmitted across generations. Thus, the female offspring of high-LG mothers display high levels of ER-α expression in the MPOA and become high-LG mothers themselves when adult (89,93). Cross-fostering studies have confirmed the association between maternal care and ER-α expression in the MPOA. The biological offspring of low-LG mothers fostered at birth by high-LG dams displayed an increase in ER-α expression in the MPOA. Cross-fostering the biological offspring of high-LG mothers with low-LG dams yielded the opposite effect. Levels of cytosine methylation in the ER-α 1b promoter were significantly higher in the adult offspring of low-LG mothers than in the adult offspring of high-LG mothers. These findings suggest that maternal care is associated with cytosine methylation of the ER-α 1b promoter, providing a potential mechanism for the programming of individual differences in ER-α expression and maternal behavior in female offspring (93).

Thus a mother-to-daughter epigenetic transmission can affect somatic tissues, not germline, and result in perpetuating the effect by affecting maternal metabolism or maternal behavior.

Sex Specificity in the Expression of TGE

There are diet, sex, and window-of-exposure–specific effects on offspring. The study of the Overkalix cohorts in northern Sweden on the effects of food supply on offspring and grandchild mortality risk ratios identified sex-specific effects male-line TGEs: only the paternal grandfather's food supply was linked to the risk ratio of grandsons, whereas only the paternal grandmother's food supply was associated with the risk ratio of mortality of grand-daughters. In the ALSPAC, sex-specific effects were again observed after appropriate adjustment: Early paternal smoking was found to be associated with a higher BMI at the age of nine years in sons, but not in daughters (76). Thus sex-specific, male-line transgenerational responses exist in humans, suggesting that the transmission of these effects is mediated by the sex chromosomes, X and Y (76).

In the Dutch winter famine cohort, children subject to dietary restrictions in utero during the first six months of pregnancy had similar birth weights to other newborns. However, despite having normal birth weights, these subjects had a higher incidence of obesity in adulthood in the first generation with higher BMI and waist circumference in 50-year-old women, but not in men (24). Offspring of either sex of males exposed prenatally to dexamethasone mated with control females but only male offspring of female rats which had been exposed prenatally to dexamethasone, but were not manipulated in their own pregnancy, had reduced birth weight (42). The postnatal changes in cerebral chromatin associated with intrauterine growth retardation due to bilateral uterine artery ligation are also sex-specific (121).

A maternal diet low in protein during pregnancy and lactation modifies the growth and metabolism of the progeny (F2) of female offspring (F1) (60,61).

One contributor to the alteration in postnatal growth induced by periconceptional maternal diet low in protein may derive from a gender-specific (male, but not female) programming of imprinted gene (*H19* and *Igf2*) expression originating within the preimplantation embryo itself in response to maternal diet low in protein restricted to the preimplantation period (66).

In mice fed a high-fat diet, a striking difference in sensitivity or resistance to this diet between generations and genders can be observed. Despite ad libitum high-fat diet, a significant proportion of F2 females were resistant to the high-fat diet, since they remained lean, with normal insulin sensitivity and normal glycemia, but mild hypercholesterolemia and glucose intolerance, thus displaying a "satiety phenotype" (53). Conversely feeding a diet rich in lard to pregnant lean rats leads to gender-linked hypertension in offspring (47).

Using a screen based on random *N*-ethyl-*N*-nitrosourea mutagenesis in mice carrying a GFP (green fluorescent protein) transgene displaying variegated expression, Blewitt et al. have identified genes involved in the epigenetic reprogramming of the genome. The behavior of the mutant lines suggests a common underlying mechanism for X inactivation and the silencing of transgenes and retrotransposons. These findings raise the possibility that the presence or absence of the X chromosome in mammals affects the establishment of the epigenetic state at autosomal loci. One explanation for dosage-dependent phenomena is that particular chromosome regions act as sinks for proteins involved in gene silencing, which compete for epigenetic modifiers at unlinked loci and which, conversely, may function as reservoirs providing a ready source of modifier proteins (5,245). However, a role for the Y chromosome, similar to that proposed by Pembrey remains a possibility (76).

These data underscore the importance of studying both sexes in epidemiological protocols or dietary interventions in humans and in experimental models in animals, even though there may be differences in the extent and timing of the processes involved between species (237).

IS THERE A GENETIC BASIS FOR EPIGENETIC INTERINDIVIDUAL VARIABILITY?

In addition to harboring a number of gene variants conferring susceptibility (2), individuals with metabolic syndrome, obesity, and T2D may show a lifelong imbalance between energy intake and energy expenditure associated with incorrect "epigenetic programming" during their early development as a result of placental insufficiency, inadequate maternal nutrition, and metabolic disturbances (3). The various non-Mendelian features of obesity, such as the high degree of discordance between MZ twins, clinical differences between men and women and fluctuations in the course of the disease, are consistent with epigenetic mechanisms for the influence of fetal environment on adult phenotype. Undeniably, genes with their various haplotypes can influence absorption, metabolism, or transport of a bioactive food component or a drug or their site of action and thus influence the overall response to the diet or to the treatment accounting for the great interindividual variability. Likewise, reciprocally, bioactive food components modify the epigenetic patterns and alter the genetic expression of susceptible genes during development in such a way that key functions including a host of cellular events and regulatory processes that attempt to maintain homeostasis and/or survival, such as appetite control, metabolic balance, and fuel utilization are permanently modified and thus influence the outcome for the individual (1). It has long been recognized that nutrients can modify proteins once formed through a variety of processes including phosphorylation or glycatin. Today, with the explosion of new technologies, we can explore on a large scale the level of expression of thousands of expressed genes (nutritional genomics), the corresponding protein products and their post-translationally modified derivatives (proteomics), and the host of metabolites (metabolomics) generated from endogenous metabolic processes or exogenous dietary nutrients and established the relationship between these biological entities and diet, health, or disease (see Section 10).

Epigenetic modifications of DNA produce reversible, clonally heritable alterations in transcription state. Errors in the elaborate epigenetic silencing apparatus of higher eukaryotes can lead to "epimutation," resulting in the abnormal silencing of a gene. Intra- and interindividual epigenetic variations are common, so could there be a genetic origin to epigenetic instability in stochastic events, susceptibility to environment/diets, and susceptibility to replication-dependent and replication-independent events? How much of the epigenetic component is truly independent of genetic changes (246)? In mice a recent study identified a number of genes that, on in vitro mutation, affect epigenetic reprogramming during gametogenesis and early development on a genome-wide level, suggesting a further mechanism by which DNA sequence (mutations) in *trans* can affect the epigenetic state (245).

Developmental Programming and Genetic Background

An adverse fetal environment may permanently modify the effects of specific genes on glucose tolerance, insulin secretion, and insulin sensitivity (24). A significant interaction effect between exposure to famine during midgestation and the PPARG2 Pro12Ala polymorphism was found on the prevalence of impaired glucose tolerance and T2D among 675 term singletons born around the time of 1944–1945 Dutch famine (24). De Rooij et al. recently showed that the effects of the PPARG2 Pro12Ala polymorphism on glucose and insulin metabolism may be modified by prenatal exposure to famine during mid-gestation. The Ala allele of the *PPARG2* gene was associated with a higher prevalence of impaired glucose tolerance and T2D but only in participants who had been prenatally exposed to famine during midgestation (247). Thus the effects of one or several polymorphism(s) may interact not only with prenatal exposure to famine but also with other environmental factors such as diet or behavior.

Stochastic and Age-Related Intra- and Interindividual Epigenetic Variation

Intra- and interindividual epigenetic variation has been detected in human germ cells. The male germline displays locus-, cell-, and age-dependent differences in DNA methylation and differences in DNA methylation between individuals may be significant and much greater than differences in DNA sequence variation. Variation is greatest in promoter CpG islands and pericentromeric satellites in single-copy DNA fragments and repetitive elements, respectively (126).

Significant interindividual variability in the level of CpG methylation has also been detected for specific Alu elements in whole-blood DNA from the members of 48 three-generation families. Surprisingly, some of the elements also displayed quantitative differences in methylation according to the parent of origin. Maternal and paternal elements differ in the likelihood of methylation at particular CpG sites, suggesting that there may be heritable differences between individuals in the fidelity with which allelic DNA methylation differences are established or maintained. The restriction of methylation differences to the centromere/telomere and the absence of such differences in regions of chromosomes known to contain transcriptionally imprinted genes suggest that maternal/paternal epigenetic modifications may also be involved in processes other than transcriptional control (248).

Age-Related and Disease-Specific Epigenetic Alterations

Two types of promoter CpG island methylation are observed in colorectal cancer: age-related and cancer-specific. Cancer-specific methylation at CpG islands occurs mainly in a subset of cases with the CpG island methylator phenotype. The underlying cause of the CpG island methylator phenotype is unknown. A recent study showed that the methylation status of CpG islands is associated with a family history of cancer. The patients with methylation at all four loci studied were 14 times more likely to have a family history of cancer than patients with methylation at none of the four loci. These findings suggest that there may be a genetic component to the CpG island methylator phenotype in colorectal cancer (249). It would be interesting to analyze these families further, for other age-related diseases, such as atherosclerosis, which might also be associated with epigenetic instability. Recent studies have shown that (1) genomic hypomethylation occurs during atherogenesis in human, mouse and rabbit lesions, and is correlated with an increase in transcriptional activity; (2) methyltransferase is expressed in atherosclerotic lesions; and (3) similar levels of hypomethylation occur in advanced lesions and malignant tumors, and this hypomethylation may affect cellular proliferation and gene expression in atherosclerotic lesions (99,250,251). The loss of function of a chromatin protein has been found to accelerate degenerative aging-like phenotypic phenomena in mice (252).

Hereditary nonpolyposis colorectal cancer is caused by heterozygous germline sequence mutations of DNA mismatch repair genes, most frequently *MLH1* or *MSH2* (mutL homolog, colon cancer, nonpolyposis type 2 gene). Individuals with a monoallelic hypermethylation of the *MLH1* gene promoter throughout the soma (implying a germline event) have been identified. These individuals fit the clinical criteria for hereditary nonpolyposis colorectal cancer, which is usually caused by germline mutation of *MLH1*. None of the affected individuals have any genetic abnormality that could account for the presence of the epimutation. Germline *MLH1* epimutations are functionally equivalent to an inactivating mutation and produce a clinical phenotype resembling hereditary nonpolyposis colorectal cancer. This innate epigenetic defect may arise by chance. The heritability of epimutations is low, so family history is not a useful guide for screening (253,254). Epigenetic phenomena tend to be stochastic, reversible, and mosaic. Rules entirely different from those for Mendelian genes, probably govern the occurrence and inheritance of epimutations (255).

Epigenetic events, resulting in changes in gene expression capacity, are important in tumor progression, and variation in genes involved in epigenetic mechanisms might therefore be important in cancer susceptibility. Cebrian et al. found some evidence for association for six SNPs in four genes: DNMT3b [DNA (cytosine-5-)-methyltransferase 3 beta], PRDM2 (PR domain containing 2, with ZNF domain), EHMT1 (EHMT2 euchromatic histone-lysine *N*-methyltransferase 1 and 2). This suggests the possible existence of a functional consequence of harboring these genetic variants in DNA methyl transferase and histone methyltransferases (256). Variants in these genes and in other as yet unidentified genes belonging to the epigenetic machinery could affect epimutation rate and/or susceptibility to environmental factors in other age-related common diseases such as obesity, diabetes, and CVD.

Differential Susceptibility to Methylation of Alleles

DNA methylation profiles may be associated with alleles, including alleles in which the variant nucleotide (C) can itself be methylated, as part of a CpG dinucleotide. Alternatively, the C allele may be part of a haplotype comprising other CpGs within the promoter or within a nearby CpG island. The methylation of specific CpG sites has been reported to be associated with changes in gene expression. A comprehensive screen of chromosome 21q has identified a single CpG island with a C/G SNP displaying methylation of the C allele in peripheral blood DNA, regardless of the parent of origin (257). Moreover, methylated C hypermutability, through deamination, might lead to the replacement of this nucleotide by a T, resulting in the higher frequency of the T allele in some populations. Thus the flexibility of epigenetic patterns under the influence of specific environmental factors could contribute for a large part to the interindividual variability that SNP analysis alone often poorly explains. Only a few studies in humans have reported associations between DNA sequence and epigenetic profile. Thus, genetic approaches to common human diseases should start taking epigenetic variation into account.

Allele-Specific Methylation of 5HT2AR

Based on recent meta-analyses, the C allele of the C102T polymorphism in *HTR2A* [5-hydroxytryptamine (serotonin) receptor 2A] has been implicated in several psychiatric disorders in patients of European but not far Eastern descent, and in abdominal obesity and eating disorders (2,130,258,259). The C allele is hypoactive in normal controls and schizophrenic patients, but displays lower levels of activity in schizophrenic patients than in controls. The *HTR2A* gene displays specific methylation of the C allele not only at the polymorphic site but also at two other CpGs within the promoter, that are in linkage disequilibrium with the C allele (260). The two alleles encode receptor proteins with identical structures, but anti-psychotic treatments increase expression of the C allele in schizophrenic patients, suggesting that this polymorphism may lead to abnormal gene regulation (261,262). Most allele C-specific CpG sites were found to be methylated in human temporal cortex and levels of peripheral leukocytes and methylation were shown to vary between individuals. Levels of promoter methylation are significantly correlated with *HTR2A* expression. The methylation of allele C-specific CpG sites in the first exon are significantly correlated with the expression of DNA methylase 1 (DNMT1) but not S-adenosylhomocysteine hydrolase (AHCY). The higher prevalence of the C allele among schizophrenics may be due to intrinsically low levels of expression of this allele, leading to a lack of *HTR2A* expression in some schizophrenics (263). The simplest model is that allele C is methylated under certain environmental conditions, age, and genetic make-up, thus accounting in parts for differences in susceptibility between populations (260).

Allele-Specific Methylation of DRD2

The *DRD2* (Dopamine receptor D2) gene has several CpG dinucleotide methylation targets (264). DNA methylation may therefore be important for regulation of the expression of this gene (265). The DRD2A1 allele is a regulatory region polymorphism associated with a 30% decrease in *DRD2* expression and linked to Tourette's syndrome, addiction, depression, and obesity/eating disorders (2,259,266,267). In a recent meta-analysis, the C311S *DRD2* polymorphism was found to be associated with schizophrenia (130,268), indicating that *DRD2* is involved in this disorder. In addition, the severity of Tourette's syndrome and the frequency of schizophrenia are higher in twins with a lower birth weight (269,270). A lower birth weight, indicative of undernutrition, may be associated with the methylation of genes such as the *DRD2* gene, resulting in mental illness. Moreover, the level of *DRD2* methylation seems to increase with age (264).

Allele-Specific Changes in Imprinting Patterns
Although the type of mechanism involved is unknown, associations between polymorphisms, in *cis* or *trans*, have been shown to influence the occurrence of imprinting defects associated with BWS and Prader-Willi/Angelman Syndrome (PWS/AS) (see Chapter 5.2), respectively. In BWS, the loss of maternal allele-specific methylation was more common for the G allele, at the T38G SNP (CAGA haplotype) of the differentially methylated region KvDMR1 (271). A common variant (677C T) of the 5′ 10-methylene tetrahydrofolate reductase gene (*MTHFR*) is associated with a higher risk of imprinting defects in the PWS/AS region of 15q (272).

Individuals with colorectal neoplasia were found to have a 5.1-fold increased risk of IGF2 LOI in peripheral blood leucocytes (PBL) than people without CRC. Thus detection of LOI of IGF2 in PBL could possibly be performed early in life, allowing for cancer-preventive measures to be started in high-risk patients before the early stages of CRC are first virtually present (273,274). Whether IGF2 LOI in PBL results from an inherited genetic mutation, and/or an epigenetic alteration induced by an environmental perturbation early in embryogenesis remains to be determined (68,114). Post-weaning diet affects genomic imprinting at the *Igf2* locus in mice suggesting that childhood diet could contribute to IGF2 LOI in humans (68). It would also be interesting to determine if the incidence of other pathologies such as obesity, diabetes, CVD, and even behavioral disorders are higher in individuals with abnormal IGF2 imprinting than in people who do not have this epigenetically induced perturbation in imprinting regulation, or similar abnormalities in other as yet unidentified imprinted domains (274).

Allele-Specific Methylation After Exposure to an Anticancer Drug
Paternal exposure of mice to Cr(III) increases the risk of tumor formation in the offspring. Representational difference analysis of gene methylation in sperm revealed hypomethylation in the 45S rRNA gene after Cr(III) exposure, with the controls used as a reference. The most striking effects were seen in the rRNA spacer promoter, a region in the intergenic region of rRNA gene clusters that can influence transcription. This region has sequence variants (T or G at base -2214). The T allele displays lower levels of DNA methylation than the G allele in control mice. Despite the diversity of sperm DNA methylation patterns, DNA clones from Cr(III)-exposed mice had an average of 19% fewer methylated CpG sites. This difference was limited to the G allele. Strikingly, for nine CpG sites, including the spacer promoter core region, hypomethylation was highly significant in the Cr(III)-treated group. One allele of the 45S rRNA spacer promoter is hypomethylated in sperm germ cells after Cr(III) exposure, potentially increasing the risk of tumors in the offspring (227).

Genetic Basis of Intra- and Interindividual Epigenetic Variation in Circadian Phase Rhythmicity

It has been known for decades that interindividual differences in the amplitude and/or the phase of the body temperature rhythm have been implicated in circadian clock dysfunction associated with affective disorders, chronic forms of insomnia, and intolerance to shiftwork. That the form of overt circadian ($\pm 24\,$hrs) rhythms may vary considerably between individuals may be indicative of the condition of the underlying circadian oscillator (275). The assessment of the phase of the circadian rhythms is of particular relevance because it provides information about the temporal organization of the body's regulatory processes. Morning- and evening-type individuals differ in the phase position of their endogenous circadian oscillator, resulting in differences in the rhythmic expression of histone acetyl transferase and other epigenetic components of the clock (275). Variations in mood over a 24-hour period also differ between morning- and evening-type individuals. Analyses of variance for mood and alertness have shown a significant interaction with time of day for both morning and evening types (276). Significant differences were observed between the two groups of morning-type and evening-type individuals in the circadian phases of body temperature and subjective alertness. During the constant routine, mean between-group differences for these two variables were 2.21 and 4.28 hours, respectively. These findings provide evidence for the endogenous nature of morning- and evening-type behavior.

Twin studies and association studies based on clock gene polymorphisms have shown that these differences are, in part, genetically determined. A genetic analysis of morning/evening preference revealed that the correlation between MZ twins was more than twice as strong as that between dizygotic twins. Genetic effects may therefore operate in a non-additive manner. Biometric model fitting showed no difference between the sexes in the magnitude of genetic and environmental factors. Total heritability—the sum of additive and non-additive genetic influences—for morning/evening preference was 44% for the younger generation and 47% for the older generation (277).

Metabolic syndrome and obesity are associated with a mutation of the *Clock* gene (159). Interestingly, wild type mice show two marked peaks in activity—one occurring just after the lights are switched off and the other just before the lights are switched on. These two peaks are attenuated in Clock mutant mice. Thus disturbances in the alternation of sleeping and waking, feeding and fasting, and thermogenesis may affect the alternation of epigenetic dynamics for the genes involved in these processes. Mouse models for studying the role of different genes in the circadian regulation of gene expression and morning/evening preference have been described: mice with a *Jcl:ICR* genetic background, homozygous for the *Clock* mutation (Cl/Cl on Jcl:ICR). In both wild type mice and Cl/Cl on Jcl:ICR mice, body temperature, activity, waking, and sleeping are completely controlled by the light/dark cycle. However, phases of the rhythm for body temperature, activity, and waking duration in the Cl/Cl on Jcl:ICR mice were about 2 hrs behind those in wild type mice (278). This model may therefore be useful to decipher the genetic bases of interindividual variability.

Association studies using polymorphisms identified in a few clock genes reveal important associations with diurnal preference. A polymorphism in the human *Clock* gene is associated with human diurnal preference, delayed sleep phase syndrome, and extreme diurnal preference. The distribution of scores was clearly shifted towards a preference for evening in subjects carrying one of the two

Clock alleles, 3111C. However, the authors of this study detected no association between a human period gene (*HPER1*) polymorphism diurnal preference in normal adults (279,280). The 3111T/C polymorphism of *hClock* is associated with evening preference and delayed sleep (170). A length polymorphism in the circadian clock gene *Per3* is linked to delayed sleep phase syndrome and extreme diurnal preference (171). Shift work has been associated with metabolic syndrome (281,282). Given the striking differences in expression of some genes (by a factor of up to 10) (157) at different times of day and disease-associated disturbances in the peak expression of rhythmically regulated genes (Ghrelin), it seems likely that the efficacy of drugs—as shown with chronotherapy for cancer—diets, exercise, and certain types of activity differs considerably at different times of day and between individuals. This knowledge should make it possible to increase the efficacy of appropriate dietary/exercise interventions.

Recently, Sakata-Haga et al. observed alterations in circadian rhythm phase shifting ability following ethanol *exposure* during the third trimester brain growth spurt, in the rat (283). Because of possible interactions between the circadian clocks of mother (mature) and fetus (immature), nutritional or environmental insults or disturbances in the circadian rhythms of the mother may also perturb early onset of circadian rhythms in the fetus' physiological activities even before birth (284), cf. alcohol, but also after birth (lactation) during the first year crucial period?

Thus to the question is there a genetic basis for epigenetic variability between individuals in stochastic events, susceptibility to environment/diets, susceptibility to replication-dependent and replication-independent events? The answer is clearly "yes" (192). The finding that, DNA methylation or epigenetic profiles can be associated with particular alleles or with genetically determined circadian variations of histone acetyl transferase expression is of considerable interest. Only a few studies in humans have identified associations between DNA sequence and epigenetic profiles (192,285).

CONCLUSION

The phenotype of an individual—his capacity to react at a given time of his life—is the result of complex interactions between genotype, epigenome, and current, past, and ancestral environment. It is determined by various epigenetic mechanisms involved in developmental programming, circadian deteriorations, lifelong stochastic and environmental deteriorations, TGEs, and, above all, the combined effects of genetics and epigenetics under the influence of a host of environmental factors.

The epidemic of obesity is attributable to a recent and complex change in lifestyle, not just overnutrition and sedentarity but a host of changes in the type and rhythms of activity, leisure, and rest that all interact without our knowing. American's daily sleep has dropped from between eight and nine hours in 1960 to less than seven hours today. A similar trend is thought to have occurred in most industrialized nations. Most people blame television, computers, all-hour supermarkets, and the attitude in some countries that sleep is a superfluous pastime that could more usefully be filled by school, work, or play. And we know that there is overlap between the systems that regulate sleep and those that control appetite in the brain! (286). Owing to these desynchronization shifts, the flexibility of epigenetic changes, the expression of genes do adapt, but unforeseen unwanted effects are also warranted. The task to identify the systems involved and to understand the epigenetic and other mechanisms at stake is immense. Nonetheless, a better knowledge should gradually help us to recognize adapted lifestyle strategies that will help us compensate more intelligently and adapt individually to a rapidly and stealthily changing world.

Can we identify the epigenetic changes—such as those associated with maternal behavior programming (74)—that result from nutritional/metabolic mis-programming? Which genes or sequences are concerned? Which tissues are affected? Does time of day have an effect? Alternatively, the region of the candidate sequence examined might not be the most important one for control by methylation, or the methylation by simply be a consequence rather than a cause of gene inactivity. And above all, other epigenetic modifications that have so far been overlooked such as chromatin remodeling and/or histone modifications, may be responsible (79,81,83,85,87,121,287–294).

The current population-based approach to common diseases relates common DNA sequence variants to either disease status or incremental quantitative traits contributing to disease. Although this purely genetic approach is powerful and general, there is currently no conceptual framework for integrating epigenetic information. A comprehensive epigenetic analysis of SNPs is warranted and this effort may shed new light on rather inconsistent genetic association studies in complex disease. Epialleles and epihaplotypes, combining both DNA sequence and epigenetic information, may be better predictors of the risk of a disease than either of the two components analyzed separately (126,246–249,253–257, 260,263,264,271,272,295). Moreover, epigenotype could potentially be used as a surrogate marker for parental environment, thereby increasing the power of epidemiological studies. This approach might be useful because recent epidemiological studies have suggested that the diet of the grandparents may affect both the birth weight and occurrence of disease in their grandchildren (75,76).

The second challenge will be to determine whether these epigenetic marks are reversible. If they are reversible, we will then need to determine when and how, and whether to use preventive methods or treatments, such as specific diets, drugs, or lifestyle changes. Shall we be able to avoid or slow down, within the fluctuating borders/plasticity of our genetic background, the epigenetic furring up of our genes by an appropriate diet and lifestyle? To be within our grasp in a not too far future, individualized tailoring of obesity and associated disorders' prevention and therapy to optimal epigenetic diets or drugs will require intense efforts to unravel the complexity of epigenetic, genetic, and environment interactions. Optimal "methylation diets" or more broadly speaking "epigenetic diets" should be investigated as part of the prevention and treatment of all these conditions, as well as in disorders such as Rett syndrome, whose primary defects may lie in DNA methylation-dependent gene regulation (112,116). Despite great promises and ongoing clinical trials in cancer epigenetic therapy skeptics might question the real potential of epigenetic treatment, the time required to develop such treatment, its likely specificity and the likelihood of unwanted side effects.

REFERENCES

1. Feil R. Environmental and nutritional effects on the epigenetic regulation of genes. Mutat Res 2006.
2. Rankinen T, Zuberi A, Chagnon YC, et al. The human obesity gene map: the 2005 update. Obesity (Silver Spring) 2006; 14(4):529–644.

3. Gallou-Kabani C, Junien C. Nutritional epigenomics of metabolic syndrome. Diabetes 2005; 54:1899–906.

4. Barker DJ. The fetal origins of diseases of old age. Eur J Clin Nutr 1992; 46(Suppl. 3): S3–9.

5. Whitelaw NC, Whitelaw E. How lifetimes shape epigenotype within and across generations. Hum Mol Genet 2006; 15(Suppl. 2):R131–7.

6. Bo S, Cavallo-Perin P, Ciccone G, et al. The metabolic syndrome in twins: a consequence of low birth weight or of being a twin? Exp Clin Endocrinol Diabetes 2001; 109(3):135–40.

7. Poulsen P, Vaag AA, Kyvik KO, et al. Low birth weight is associated with NIDDM in discordant monozygotic and dizygotic twin pairs. Diabetologia 1997; 40(4):439–46.

8. Petronis A, Gottesman II, Kan P, et al. Monozygotic twins exhibit numerous epigenetic differences: clues to twin discordance? Schizophr Bull 2003; 29(1):169–78.

9. Phillips DI, Hales CN, Barker DJ. Can twin studies assess the genetic component in type 2 (non-insulin-dependent) diabetes mellitus? Diabetologia 1993; 36(5):471–2.

10. Fraga MF, Ballestar E, Paz MF, et al. Epigenetic differences arise during the lifetime of monozygotic twins. Proc Natl Acad Sci U S A 2005; 102(30):10604–9.

11. Petronis A. Epigenetics and twins: three variations on the theme. Trends Genet 2006; 22(7):347–50.

12. Sing CF, Stengard JH, Kardia SL. Genes, environment, and cardiovascular disease. Arterioscler Thromb Vasc Biol 2003; 23(7):1190–6.

13. Mager J, Bartolomei MS. Strategies for dissecting epigenetic mechanisms in the mouse. Nat Genet 2005; 37(11):1194–200.

14. Kwong WY, Wild AE, Roberts P, et al. Maternal undernutrition during the preimplantation period of rat development causes blastocyst abnormalities and programming of postnatal hypertension. Development 2000; 127(19):4195–202.

15. Wynn M, Wynn A. Nutrition around conception and the prevention of low birthweight. Nutr Health 1988; 6(1):37–52.

16. Ravelli GP, Stein ZA, Susser MW. Obesity in young men after famine exposure in utero and early infancy. N Engl J Med 1976; 295(7):349–53.

17. Curhan GC, Chertow GM, Willett WC, et al. Birth weight and adult hypertension and obesity in women. Circulation 1996; 94(6):1310–5.

18. Mckeigue P. Diabetes and insulin action. A life-course approach to chronic disease epidemiology. 1997; 78–100.

19. Frankel S, Gunnell DJ, Peters TJ, et al. Childhood energy intake and adult mortality from cancer: the Boyd Orr Cohort Study. BMJ 1998; 316(7130):499–504.

20. Leon DA. Fetal growth and adult disease. Eur J Clin Nutr 1998; 52(Suppl 1):S72–8; discussion S78–82.

21. Lucas A. Programming by early nutrition: an experimental approach. J Nutr 1998; 128(Suppl 2):401S–6S.

22. Hoek HW, Brown AS, Susser E. The Dutch famine and schizophrenia spectrum disorders. Soc Psychiatry Psychiatr Epidemiol 1998; 33(8):373–9.

23. Waterland RA, Garza C. Potential mechanisms of metabolic imprinting that lead to chronic disease. Am J Clin Nutr 1999; 69(2):179–97.

24. Roseboom T, de Rooij S, Painter R. The Dutch famine and its long-term consequences for adult health. Early Hum Dev 2006; 82(8):485–91.

25. Aerts L, Van Assche FA. Intra-uterine transmission of disease. Placenta 2003; 24(10):905–11.

26. Fall CH, Barker DJ, Osmond C, et al. Relation of infant feeding to adult serum cholesterol concentration and death from ischaemic heart disease. BMJ 1992; 304(6830):801–5.

27. Barker DJ, Gluckman PD, Godfrey KM, et al. Fetal nutrition and cardiovascular disease in adult life. Lancet 1993; 341(8850):938–41.

28. Armitage JA, Khan IY, Taylor PD, et al. Developmental programming of the metabolic syndrome by maternal nutritional imbalance: how strong is the evidence from experimental models in mammals? J Physiol 2004; 561(Pt 2):355–7.

29. Armitage JA, Taylor PD, Poston L. Experimental models of developmental programming: consequences of exposure to an energy rich diet during development. J Physiol 2005; 565(Pt 1):3–8.

30. Grangé G, Dupont JM, Jeanpierre M. Génes et retards de croissance intra-utérins. Médecine/Sciences 1999; 15:82–5.

31. Ravelli AC, van der Meulen JH, Michels RP, et al. Glucose tolerance in adults after prenatal exposure to famine. Lancet 1998; 351(9097):173–7.

32. Martyn CN, Barker DJ, Osmond C. Mothers' pelvic size, fetal growth, and death from stroke and coronary heart disease in men in the UK. Lancet 1996; 348(9037):1264–8.

33. Waterland RA, Garza C. Early postnatal nutrition determines adult pancreatic glucose-responsive insulin secretion and islet gene expression in rats. J Nutr 2002; 132(3):357–64.

34. Hales CN, Barker DJ. Type 2 (non-insulin-dependent) diabetes mellitus: the thrifty phenotype hypothesis. Diabetologia 1992; 35(7):595–601.

35. Levin BE. The obesity epidemic: metabolic imprinting on genetically susceptible neural circuits. Obes Res 2000; 8(4):342–7.

36. Stein AD, Lumey LH. The relationship between maternal and offspring birth weights after maternal prenatal famine exposure: the Dutch Famine Birth Cohort Study. Hum Biol 2000; 72(4):641–54.

37. Plagemann A, Harder T, Franke K, et al. Long-term impact of neonatal breast-feeding on body weight and glucose tolerance in children of diabetic mothers. Diabetes Care 2002; 25(1):16–22.

38. Dabelea D, Hanson RL, Lindsay RS, et al. Intrauterine exposure to diabetes conveys risks for type 2 diabetes and obesity: a study of discordant sibships. Diabetes 2000; 49(12):2208–11.

39. Issa JP. Epigenetic variation and human disease. J Nutr 2002; 132(Suppl. 8):2388S–92S.

40. Remacle C, Bieswal F, Reusens B. Programming of obesity and cardiovascular disease. Int J Obes Relat Metab Disord 2004; 28(Suppl. 3):S46–53.

41. Garofano A, Czernichow P, Breant B. In utero undernutrition impairs rat beta-cell development. Diabetologia 1997; 40(10):1231–4.

42. Drake AJ, Walker BR, Seckl JR. Intergenerational consequences of fetal programming by in utero exposure to glucocorticoids in rats. Am J Physiol Regul Integr Comp Physiol 2004.

43. Drake AJ, Livingstone DE, Andrew R, et al. Reduced adipose glucocorticoid reactivation and increased hepatic glucocorticoid clearance as an early adaptation to high-fat feeding in Wistar rats. Endocrinology 2005; 146(2):913–9.

44. Drake AJ, Walker BR, Seckl JR. Intergenerational consequences of fetal programming by in utero exposure to glucocorticoids in rats. Am J Physiol Regul Integr Comp Physiol 2005; 288(1):R34–8.

45. Simmons RA, Templeton LJ, Gertz SJ. Intrauterine growth retardation leads to the development of type 2 diabetes in the rat. Diabetes 2001; 50(10):2279–86.

46. Lewis RM, Forhead AJ, Petry CJ, et al. Long-term programming of blood pressure by maternal dietary iron restriction in the rat. Br J Nutr 2002; 88(3):283–90.

47. Khan IY, Taylor PD, Dekou V, et al. Gender-linked hypertension in offspring of lard-fed pregnant rats. Hypertension 2003; 41(1):168–75.

48. Langley-Evans SC. Developmental programming of health and disease. Proc Nutr Soc 2006; 65(1):97–105.

49. Khan IY, Dekou V, Hanson M, et al. Predictive adaptive responses to maternal high-fat diet prevent endothelial dysfunction but not hypertension in adult rat offspring. Circulation 2004; 110:1097–102.

50. Pettitt D. Diabetes in subsequent generations. In: Dornhorst A, Hadden DR, eds. Diabetes and Pregancy an International Approach to Diagnosis and Management. Chichester: John Wiley and Sons, 1996:367–76.

51. Gill-Randall R, Adams D, Ollerton RL, et al. Type 2 diabetes mellitus—genes or intrauterine environment? An embryo transfer paradigm in rats. Diabetologia 2004; 47(8):1354–9.

52. Aerts L, Van Assche FA. Animal evidence for the transgenerational development of diabetes mellitus. Int J Biochem Cell Biol 2006; 38(5–6):894–903.

53. Gallou-Kabani C, Vigé A, Gross MS, et al. Resistance to high-fat diet in the female progeny of obese mice fed a control diet during the periconceptual, gestation and lactation periods. Submitted.

54. Gluckman PD, Hanson MA, Morton SM, et al. Life-long echoes: a critical analysis of the developmental origins of adult disease model. Biol Neonate 2005; 87(2):127–39.

55. Ozanne SE, Hales CN. Lifespan: catch-up growth and obesity in male mice. Nature 2004; 427(6973):411–2.

56. Gluckman PD, Hanson MA. Living with the past: evolution, development, and patterns of disease. Science 2004; 305(5691):1733–6.

57. Gluckman PD, Hanson MA, Spencer HG, et al. Environmental influences during development and their later consequences for health and disease: implications for the interpretation of empirical studies. Proc Biol Sci 2005; 272(1564):671–7.

58. Anderson LM, Riffle L, Wilson R, et al. Preconceptional fasting of fathers alters serum glucose in offspring of mice. Nutrition 2006; 22(3):327–31.

59. Pinto ML, Shetty PS. Influence of exercise-induced maternal stress on fetal outcome in Wistar rats: inter-generational effects. Br J Nutr 1995; 73(5):645–53.

60. Zambrano E, Bautista CJ, Deas M, et al. A low maternal protein diet during pregnancy and lactation has sex- and window of exposure-specific effects on offspring growth and food intake, glucose metabolism and serum leptin in the rat. J Physiol 2006; 571(Pt 1):221–30.

61. Zambrano E, Martinez-Samayoa PM, Bautista CJ, et al. Sex differences in transgenerational alterations of growth and metabolism in progeny (F2) of female offspring (F1) of rats fed a low protein diet during pregnancy and lactation. J Physiol 2005; 566(Pt 1):225–36.

62. Bouret SG, Simerly RB. Developmental programming of hypothalamic feeding circuits. Clin Genet 2006; 70(4):295–301.

63. Ravelli AC, Van Der Meulen JH, Osmond C, et al. Obesity at the age of 50 years in men and women exposed to famine prenatally. Am J Clin Nutr 1999; 70(5):811–6.

64. Roseboom TJ, van der Meulen JH, Osmond C, et al. Plasma lipid profiles in adults after prenatal exposure to the Dutch famine. Am J Clin Nutr 2000; 72(5):1101–6.

65. Roseboom TJ, Van der Meulen JH, Ravelli AC, et al. Link between prenatal exposure to the 'Winter of Famine' and long-term medical consequences. Ned Tijdschr Geneeskd 2000; 144(52):2488–91.

66. Kwong WY, Miller DJ, Ursell E, et al. Imprinted gene expression in the rat embryo-fetal axis is altered in response to periconceptional maternal low protein diet. Reproduction 2006; 132(2):265–77.

67. Fahrenkrog S, Harder T, Stolaczyk, E et al. Cross-fostering to diabetic rat dams affects early development of mediobasal hypothalamic nuclei regulating food intake, body weight, and metabolism. J Nutr 2004; 134(3):648–654.

68. Waterland RA, Lin JR, Smith CA, et al. Post-weaning diet affects genomic imprinting at the insulin-like growth factor 2 (*Igf2*) locus. Hum Mol Genet 2006; 15(5):705–16.

69. Dolinoy DC, Weidman JR, Jirtle RL. Epigenetic gene regulation: Linking early developmental environment to adult disease. Reprod Toxicol 2006.

70. Murphy VE, Smith R, Giles WB, et al. Endocrine regulation of human fetal growth: the role of the mother, placenta, and fetus. Endocr Rev 2006; 27(2):141–69.

71. Morgan HD, Sutherland HG, Martin DI, et al. Epigenetic inheritance at the agouti locus in the mouse. Nat Genet 1999; 23(3):314–8.

72. Rakyan VK, Chong S, Champ ME, et al. Transgenerational inheritance of epigenetic states at the murine Axin(Fu) allele occurs after maternal and paternal transmission. Proc Natl Acad Sci U S A 2003; 100(5):2538–2543.

73. Anway MD, Cupp AS, Uzumcu M, et al. Epigenetic transgenerational actions of endocrine disruptors and male fertility. Science 2005; 308(5727):1466–9.

74. Weaver IC, Cervoni N, Champagne FA, et al. Epigenetic programming by maternal behavior. Nat Neurosci 2004; 7(8):847–54.

75. Kaati G, Bygren LO, Edvinsson S. Cardiovascular and diabetes mortality determined by nutrition during parents' and grandparents' slow growth period. Eur J Hum Genet 2002; 10(11):682–8.

76. Pembrey ME, Bygren LO, Kaati G, et al. Sex-specific, male-line transgenerational responses in humans. Eur J Hum Genet 2006; 14(2):159–66.

77. Thompson SL, Konfortova G, Gregory RI, et al. Environmental effects on genomic imprinting in mammals. Toxicol Lett 2001; 120(1–3):143–50.

78. Ogawa H, Ono Y, Shimozawa N, et al. Disruption of imprinting in cloned mouse fetuses from embryonic stem cells. Reproduction 2003; 126(4):549–57.

79. Dean W, Bowden L, Aitchison A et al. Altered imprinted gene methylation and expression in completely ES cell-derived mouse fetuses: association with aberrant phenotypes. Development 1998,125(12),2273-2282.

80. Doherty AS, Mann MR, Tremblay KD, et al. Differential effects of culture on imprinted H19 expression in the preimplantation mouse embryo. Biol Reprod 2000; 62(6):1526–1535.

81. Khosla S, Dean W, Brown D, et al. Culture of preimplantation mouse embryos affects fetal development and the expression of imprinted genes. Biol Reprod 2001; 64(3):918–26.

82. Lucifero D, Chaillet JR, Trasler JM. Potential significance of genomic imprinting defects for reproduction and assisted reproductive technology. Hum Reprod Update 2004; 10(1):3–18.

83. Mann MR, Lee SS, Doherty AS, et al. Selective loss of imprinting in the placenta following preimplantation development in culture. Development 2004; 131(15):3727–735.

84. Farin PW, Piedrahita JA, Farin CE. Errors in development of fetuses and placentas from in vitro-produced bovine embryos. Theriogenology 2005.

85. Humpherys D, Eggan K, Akutsu H, et al. Abnormal gene expression in cloned mice derived from embryonic stem cell and cumulus cell nuclei. Proc Natl Acad Sci U S A 2002; 99(20):12889–94.

86. Li S, Hursting SD, Davis BJ, et al. Environmental exposure, DNA methylation, and gene regulation: lessons from diethylstilbesterol-induced cancers. Ann N Y Acad Sci 2003; 983:161–9.

87. Ruden DM, Xiao L, Garfinkel MD, et al. Hsp90 and environmental impacts on epigenetic states: a model for the trans-generational effects of diethylstibesterol on uterine development and cancer. Hum Mol Genet 2005; 14(Spec No. 1):R149–55.

88. Weaver IC, Champagne FA, Brown SE, et al. Reversal of maternal programming of stress responses in adult offspring through methyl supplementation: altering epigenetic marking later in life. J Neurosci 2005; 25(47):11045–54.

89. Weaver IC, Meaney MJ, Szyf M. Maternal care effects on the hippocampal transcriptome and anxiety-mediated behaviors in the offspring that are reversible in adulthood. Proc Natl Acad Sci U S A 2006; 103(9):3480–5.

90. Szyf M, Weaver IC, Champagne FA, et al. Maternal programming of steroid receptor expression and phenotype through DNA methylation in the rat. Front Neuroendocrinol 2005; 26(3–4):139–62.

91. Cheng RY, Hockman T, Crawford E, et al. Epigenetic and gene expression changes related to transgenerational carcinogenesis. Mol Carcinog 2004; 40(1):1–11.

92. Skinner MK, Anway MD. Seminiferous cord formation and germ-cell programming: epigenetic transgenerational actions of endocrine disruptors. Ann N Y Acad Sci 2005; 1061:18–32.

93. Champagne FA, Weaver IC, Diorio J, et al. Maternal care associated with methylation of the estrogen receptor-alpha1b promoter and estrogen receptor-alpha expression in the medial preoptic area of female offspring. Endocrinology 2006; 147(6):2909–15.

94. Cooney CA, Dave AA, Wolff GL. Maternal methyl supplements in mice affect epigenetic variation and DNA methylation of offspring. J Nutr 2002; 132(Suppl 8):2393S–400S.

95. Davis CD, Uthus EO, Finley JW. Dietary selenium and arsenic affect DNA methylation in vitro in Caco-2 cells and in vivo in rat liver and colon. J Nutr 2000; 130(12):2903–9.

96. Day JK, Bauer AM, DesBordes C, et al. Genistein alters methylation patterns in mice. J Nutr 2002; 132(Suppl. 8):2419S–23S.

97. Dong C, Yoon W, Goldschmidt-Clermont PJ. DNA methylation and atherosclerosis. J Nutr 2002; 132(Suppl. 8):2406S–9S.

98. Friso S, Choi SW. Gene-nutrient interactions and DNA methylation. J Nutr 2002; 132(Suppl. 8):2382S–7S.

99. Hiltunen MO, Turunen MP, Hakkinen TP, et al. DNA hypomethylation and methyl-transferase expression in atherosclerotic lesions. Vasc Med 2002; 7(1):5–11.

100. Hu JF, Nguyen PH, Pham NV, et al. Modulation of *Igf2* genomic imprinting in mice induced by 5-azacytidine, an inhibitor of DNA methylation. Mol Endocrinol 1997; 11(13):1891–8.

101. Ingrosso D, Cimmino A, Perna AF, et al. Folate treatment and unbalanced methyla-tion and changes of allelic expression induced by hyperhomocysteinaemia in patients with uraemia. Lancet 2003; 361(9370):1693–9.

102. Issa JP, Baylin SB, Belinsky SA. Methylation of the estrogen receptor CpG island in lung tumors is related to the specific type of carcinogen exposure. Cancer Res 1996; 56(16):3655–8.

103. Jaenisch R. DNA methylation and imprinting: why bother? (see comments). Trends Genet 1997; 13(8):323–9.

104. Laukkanen MO, Mannermaa S, Hiltunen MO, et al. Local hypomethylation in athero-sclerosis found in rabbit ec-sod gene. Arterioscler Thromb Vasc Biol 1999; 19(9): 2171–8.

105. Lyn-Cook BD, Blann E, Payne PW, et al. Methylation profile and amplification of proto-oncogenes in rat pancreas induced with phytoestrogens. Proc Soc Exp Biol Med 1995; 208(1):116–9.

106. MacLennan NK, James SJ, Melnyk S, et al. Uteroplacental insufficiency alters DNA methylation, one-carbon metabolism, and histone acetylation in IUGR rats. Physiol Genomics 2004; 18(1):43–50.

107. Margison G. A new damage limitation exercise: ironing (Fe(II)) out minor DNA methylation lesions. DNA Repair (Amst) 2002; 1(12):1057–61.

108. Rampersaud GC, Kauwell GP, Hutson AD, et al. Genomic DNA methylation decreases in response to moderate folate depletion in elderly women. Am J Clin Nutr 2000; 72(4):998–1003.

109. Rees WD, Hay SM, Brown DS, et al. Maternal protein deficiency causes hypermethy-lation of DNA in the livers of rat fetuses. J Nutr 2000; 130(7):1821–6.

110. Sapolsky RM. Mothering style and methylation. Nat Neurosci 2004; 7(8):791–2.

111. Shen L, Ahuja N, Shen Y, et al. DNA methylation and environmental exposures in human hepatocellular carcinoma. J Natl Cancer Inst 2002; 94(10):755–61.

112. Van den Veyver IB. Genetic effects of methylation diets. Annu Rev Nutr 2002; 22: 255–82.

113. Waterland RA. Do maternal methyl supplements in mice affect DNA methylation of offspring? J Nutr 2003; 133(1):238 (author reply 239).

114. Waterland RA, Jirtle RL. Transposable elements: targets for early nutritional effects on epigenetic gene regulation. Mol Cell Biol 2003; 23(15):5293–300.

115. Waterland RA, Jirtle RL. Early nutrition, epigenetic changes at transposons and imprinted genes, and enhanced susceptibility to adult chronic diseases. Nutrition 2004; 20(1):63–8.

116. Waterland RA. Assessing the effects of high methionine intake on DNA methylation. J Nutr 2006; 136(Suppl. 6):1706S–10S.

117. Waterland RA, Dolinoy DC, Lin JR, et al. Maternal methyl supplements increase offspring DNA methylation at Axin fused. Genesis 2006; 44(9):401–6.

118. Wolff GL, Kodell RL, Moore SR, et al. Maternal epigenetics and methyl supplements affect agouti gene expression in Avy/a mice. FASEB J 1998; 12(11):949–57.

119. Dolinoy DC, Weidman JR, Waterland RA, et al. Maternal genistein alters coat color and protects Avy mouse offspring from obesity by modifying the fetal epigenome. Environ Health Perspect 2006; 114(4):567–72.

120. Fowden AL, Sibley C, Reik W, et al. Imprinted genes, placental development and fetal growth. Horm Res 2006; 65(Suppl. 3):50–8.
121. Ke X, Lei Q, James S, et al. Uteroplacental insufficiency affects epigenetic determinants of chromatin structure in brains of neonatal and juvenile IUGR rats. Physiol Genomics 2006; 25(1):16–28.
122. Lillycrop KA, Phillips ES, Jackson AA, et al. Dietary protein restriction of pregnant rats induces and folic acid supplementation prevents epigenetic modification of hepatic gene expression in the offspring. J Nutr 2005; 135(6):1382–6.
123. Santoro R. The silence of the ribosomal RNA genes. Cell Mol Life Sci 2005; 62(18):2067–79.
124. Dennis KE, Levitt P. Regional expression of brain derived neurotrophic factor (BDNF) is correlated with dynamic patterns of promoter methylation in the developing mouse forebrain. Brain Res Mol Brain Res 2005; 140(1–2):1–9.
125. Valinluck V, Tsai HH, Rogstad DK, et al. Oxidative damage to methyl-CpG sequences inhibits the binding of the methyl-CpG binding domain (MBD) of methyl-CpG binding protein 2 (MeCP2). Nucleic Acids Res 2004; 32(14):4100–8.
126. Flanagan JM, Popendikyte V, Pozdniakovaite N, et al. Intra- and interindividual epigenetic variation in human germ cells. Am J Hum Genet 2006; 79(1):67–84.
127. Doi M, Hirayama J, Sassone-Corsi P. Circadian regulator CLOCK is a histone acetyltransferase. Cell 2006; 125(3):497–508.
128. Cooper DN, Youssoufian H. The CpG dinucleotide and human genetic disease. Hum Genet 1988; 78(2):151–5.
129. Reik W, Dean W, Walter J. Epigenetic reprogramming in mammalian development. Science 2001; 293(5532):1089–93.
130. Abdolmaleky HM, Smith CL, Faraone SV, et al. Methylomics in psychiatry: modulation of gene-environment interactions may be through DNA methylation. Am J Med Genet B Neuropsychiatr Genet 2004; 127(1):51–9.
131. Barbot W, Dupressoir A, Lazar V, et al. Epigenetic regulation of an IAP retrotransposon in the aging mouse: progressive demethylation and de-silencing of the element by its repetitive induction. Nucleic Acids Res 2002; 30(11):2365–73.
132. Chang KT, Min KT. Regulation of lifespan by histone deacetylase. Ageing Res Rev 2002; 1(3):313–26.
133. Fuke C, Shimabukuro M, Petronis A, et al. Age related changes in 5-methylcytosine content in human peripheral leukocytes and placentas: an HPLC-based study. Ann Hum Genet 2004; 68(Pt 3):196–204.
134. Hoal-Van Helden EG, Van Helden PD. Age-related methylation changes in DNA may reflect the proliferative potential of organs. Mutat Res 1989; 219(5–6):263–6.
135. Issa JP. CpG-island methylation in aging and cancer. Curr Top Microbiol Immunol 2000; 249:101–18.
136. Issa JP, Ahuja N, Toyota M, et al. Accelerated age-related CpG island methylation in ulcerative colitis. Cancer Res 2001; 61(9):3573–7.
137. Issa JP, Ottaviano YL, Celano P, et al. Methylation of the oestrogen receptor CpG island links ageing and neoplasia in human colon. Nat Genet 1994; 7(4):536–40.
138. Maier S, Olek A. Diabetes: a candidate disease for efficient DNA methylation profiling. J Nutr 2002; 132(Suppl. 8):2440S–3S.
139. Mays-Hoopes L, Chao W, Butcher HC, et al. Decreased methylation of the major mouse long interspersed repeated DNA during aging and in myeloma cells. Dev Genet 1986; 7(2):65–73.
140. Oakes CC, Smiraglia DJ, Plass C, et al. Aging results in hypermethylation of ribosomal DNA in sperm and liver of male rats. Proc Natl Acad Sci U S A 2003; 100(4):1775–80.
141. Ono T, Uehara Y, Kurishita A, et al. Biological significance of DNA methylation in the ageing process. Age Ageing 1993; 22(1):S34–43.
142. Post WS, Goldschmidt-Clermont PJ, Wilhide CC, et al. Methylation of the estrogen receptor gene is associated with aging and atherosclerosis in the cardiovascular system. Cardiovasc Res 1999; 43(4):985–91.

143. Rath PC, Kanungo MS. Methylation of repetitive DNA sequences in the brain during aging of the rat. FEBS Lett 1989; 244(1):193–8.

144. Singhal RP, Mays-Hoopes LL, Eichhorn GL. DNA methylation in aging of mice. Mech Ageing Dev 1987; 41(3):199–210.

145. Toyota M, Issa JP. CpG island methylator phenotypes in aging and cancer. Semin Cancer Biol 1999; 9(5):349–57.

146. Von Zglinicki T, Burkle A, Kirkwood TB. Stress, DNA damage and ageing: an integrative approach. Exp Gerontol 2001; 36(7):1049–62.

147. Weksberg R, Shuman C, Caluseriu O, et al. Discordant KCNQ1OT1 imprinting in sets of monozygotic twins discordant for Beckwith-Wiedemann syndrome. Hum Mol Genet 2002; 11(11):1317–25.

148. Issa JP, Baylin SB. Epigenetics and human disease. Nat Med 1996; 2:281–2.

149. Issa JP, Zehnbauer BA, Civin CI, et al. The estrogen receptor CpG island is methylated in most hematopoietic neoplasms. Cancer Res 1996; 56(5):973–7.

150. Issa JP, Vertino PM, Boehm CD, et al. Switch from monoallelic to biallelic human IGF2 promoter methylation during aging and carcinogenesis. Proc Natl Acad Sci U S A 1996; 93(21):11757–62.

151. Bennett-Baker PE, Wilkowski J, Burke DT. Age-associated activation of epigenetically repressed genes in the mouse. Genetics 2003; 165(4):2055–62.

152. Bahar R, Hartmann CH, Rodriguez KA, et al. Increased cell-to-cell variation in gene expression in ageing mouse heart. Nature 2006; 441(7096):1011–4.

153. Kalra SP, Bagnasco M, Otukonyong EE, et al. Rhythmic, reciprocal ghrelin and leptin signaling: new insight in the development of obesity. Regul Pept 2003; 111(1–3):1–11.

154. Boden G, Ruiz J, Urbain JL, et al. Evidence for a circadian rhythm of insulin secretion. Am J Physiol 1996; 271(2 Pt 1):E246–52.

155. Zvonic S, Ptitsyn AA, Conrad SA, et al. Characterization of peripheral circadian clocks in adipose tissues. Diabetes 2006; 55(4):962–70.

156. Ptitsyn AA, Zvonic S, Conrad SA, et al. Circadian clocks are resounding in peripheral tissues. PLoS Comput Biol 2006; 2(3):e16.

157. Oishi K, Amagai N, Shirai H, et al. Genome-wide expression analysis reveals 100 adrenal gland-dependent circadian genes in the mouse liver. DNA Res 2005; 12(3):191–202.

158. Hanai S, Masuo Y, Shirai H, et al. Differential circadian expression of endothelin-1 mRNA in the rat suprachiasmatic nucleus and peripheral tissues. Neurosci Lett 2005; 377(1):65–8.

159. Turek FW, Joshu C, Kohsaka A, et al. Obesity and metabolic syndrome in circadian Clock mutant mice. Science 2005; 308(5724):1043–5.

160. Debruyne JP, Noton E, Lambert CM, et al. A clock shock: mouse CLOCK is not required for circadian oscillator function. Neuron 2006; 50(3):465–77.

161. Oishi K, Shirai H, Ishida N. CLOCK is involved in the circadian transactivation of peroxisome-proliferator-activated receptor alpha (PPARalpha) in mice. Biochem J 2005; 386(Pt 3):575–81.

162. Inoue I, Shinoda Y, Ikeda M, et al. CLOCK/BMAL1 is involved in lipid metabolism via transactivation of the peroxisome proliferator-activated receptor (PPAR) response element. J Atheroscler Thromb 2005; 12(3):169–74.

163. Miller BH, Olson SL, Turek FW, et al. Circadian clock mutation disrupts estrous cyclicity and maintenance of pregnancy. Curr Biol 2004; 14(15):1367–73.

164. Naruse Y, Oh-hashi K, Iijima N, et al. Circadian and light-induced transcription of clock gene Per1 depends on histone acetylation and deacetylation. Mol Cell Biol 2004; 24(14):6278–87.

165. Rudic RD, McNamara P, Curtis AM, et al. BMAL1 and CLOCK, two essential components of the circadian clock, are involved in glucose homeostasis. PLoS Biol 2004; 2(11):e377.

166. Staels B. When the Clock stops ticking, metabolic syndrome explodes. Nat Med 2006; 12(1):54–5 (discussion 55).

167. Doi M, Yujnovsky I, Hirayama J, et al. Impaired light masking in dopamine D2 receptor-null mice. Nat Neurosci 2006; 9(6):732–4.

168. Shimba S, Ishii N, Ohta Y, et al. Brain and muscle Arnt-like protein-1 (BMAL1), a component of the molecular clock, regulates adipogenesis. Proc Natl Acad Sci U S A 2005; 102(34):12071–6.
169. Oishi K, Ohkura N, Wakabayashi M, et al. CLOCK is involved in obesity-induced disordered fibrinolysis in ob/ob mice by regulating PAI-1 gene expression. J Thromb Haemost 2006; 4(8):1774–80.
170. Mishima K, Tozawa T, Satoh K, et al. The 3111T/C polymorphism of hClock is associated with evening preference and delayed sleep timing in a Japanese population sample. Am J Med Genet B Neuropsychiatr Genet 2005; 133(1):101–4.
171. Archer SN, Robilliard DL, Skene DJ, et al. A length polymorphism in the circadian clock gene Per3 is linked to delayed sleep phase syndrome and extreme diurnal preference. Sleep 2003; 26(4):413–5.
172. Kreier F, Yilmaz A, Kalsbeek A, et al. Hypothesis: shifting the equilibrium from activity to food leads to autonomic unbalance and the metabolic syndrome. Diabetes 2003; 52(11):2652–6.
173. Levine AS, Morley JE. Stress-induced eating in rats. Am J Physiol 1981; 241(1):R72–6.
174. Sindelar DK, Palmiter RD, Woods SC, et al. Attenuated feeding responses to circadian and palatability cues in mice lacking neuropeptide Y. Peptides 2005.
175. Facchinetti F, Comitini G, Petraglia F, et al. Reduced estriol and dehydroepiandrosterone sulphate plasma levels in methadone-addicted pregnant women. Eur J Obstet Gynecol Reprod Biol 1986; 23(1–2):67–73.
176. Groh KR, Ehret CF, Peraino C, et al. Circadian manifestations of barbiturate habituation, addiction and withdrawal in the rat. Chronobiol Int 1988; 5(2):153–66.
177. Kugler J, Ruther E. Clinical aspects of sleep disturbances and sleeping drugs. Eur Neurol 1986; 25(Suppl. 2):22–9.
178. Schibler U. The daily rhythms of genes, cells and organs. Biological clocks and circadian timing in cells. EMBO Rep 2005; 6(Spec No):S9–13.
179. Vescovi PP, Coiro V, Volpi R, et al. Diurnal variations in plasma ACTH, cortisol and beta-endorphin levels in cocaine addicts. Horm Res 1992; 37(6):221–4.
180. Yun AJ, Lee PY, Bazar KA. Temporal variation of autonomic balance and diseases during circadian, seasonal, reproductive, and lifespan cycles. Med Hypotheses 2004; 63(1):155–62.
181. Cummings DE, Frayo RS, Marmonier C, et al. Plasma ghrelin levels and hunger scores in humans initiating meals voluntarily without time- and food-related cues. Am J Physiol Endocrinol Metab 2004; 287(2):E297–304.
182. Damiola F, Le Minh N, Preitner N, et al. Restricted feeding uncouples circadian oscillators in peripheral tissues from the central pacemaker in the suprachiasmatic nucleus. Genes Dev 2000; 14(23):2950–61.
183. Dzaja A, Dalal MA, Himmerich H, et al. Sleep enhances nocturnal plasma ghrelin levels in healthy subjects. Am J Physiol Endocrinol Metab 2004; 286(6):E963–7.
184. Karlsson B, Knutsson A, Lindahl B. Is there an association between shift work and having a metabolic syndrome? Results from a population based study of 27,485 people. Occup Environ Med 2001; 58(11):747–52.
185. Hampton T. Mitochondrial defects may play role in the metabolic syndrome. JAMA 2004; 292(23):2823–4.
186. Wilson FH, Hariri A, Farhi A, et al. A cluster of metabolic defects caused by mutation in a mitochondrial tRNA. Science 2004; 306(5699):1190–4.
187. Groot GS, Kroon AM. Mitochondrial DNA from various organisms does not contain internally methylated cytosine in -CCGG- sequences. Biochim Biophys Acta 1979; 564(2):355–7.
188. Trifunovic A. Mitochondrial DNA and ageing. Biochim Biophys Acta 2006; 1757(5–6):611–7.
189. Kumar S, Subramanian S. Mutation rates in mammalian genomes. Proc Natl Acad Sci U S A 2002; 99(2):803–8.
190. Issa JP. The epigenetics of colorectal cancer. Ann N Y Acad Sci 2000; 910:140–153 (discussion 153–45).

191. Jones PA, Baylin SB. The fundamental role of epigenetic events in cancer. Nat Rev Genet 2002; 3(6):415–28.

192. Wilson IM, Davies JJ, Weber M, et al. Epigenomics: mapping the methylome. Cell Cycle 2006; 5(2):155–8.

193. Feinberg AP. The epigenetics of cancer etiology. Semin Cancer Biol 2004; 14(6):427–32.

194. Szyf M, Pakneshan P, Rabbani SA. DNA demethylation and cancer: therapeutic implications. Cancer Lett 2004; 211(2):133–43.

195. Vasa-Nicotera M, Brouilette S, Mangino M, et al. Mapping of a major locus that determines telomere length in humans. Am J Hum Genet 2005; 76(1):147–51.

196. Andrew T, Aviv A, Falchi M, et al. Mapping genetic loci that determine leukocyte telomere length in a large sample of unselected female sibling pairs. Am J Hum Genet 2006; 78(3):480–6.

197. Obana N, Takagi S, Kinouchi Y, et al. Telomere shortening of peripheral blood mononuclear cells in coronary disease patients with metabolic disorders. Intern Med 2003; 42(2):150–3.

198. Valdes AM, Andrew T, Gardner JP, et al. Obesity, cigarette smoking, and telomere length in women. Lancet 2005; 366(9486):662–4.

199. Gonzalo S, Jaco I, Fraga MF, et al. DNA methyltransferases control telomere length and telomere recombination in mammalian cells. Nat Cell Biol 2006; 8(4):416–24.

200. Garcia-Cao M, O'Sullivan R, Peters AH, et al. Epigenetic regulation of telomere length in mammalian cells by the Suv39h1 and Suv39h2 histone methyltransferases. Nat Genet 2004; 36(1):94–9.

201. Jablonka E, Lamb MJ. The changing concept of epigenetics. Ann N Y Acad Sci 2002; 981:82–96.

202. Pembrey M. Imprinting and transgenerational modulation of gene expression; human growth as a model. Acta Genet Med Gemellol (Roma) 1996; 45(1–2):111–25.

203. Junien C, Gallou-Kabani C, Vige A, et al. Nutritional epigenomics of metabolic syndrome. Med Sci (Paris) 2005; 21(4):396–404.

204. Pembrey M. Genomic imprinting and the possible role of epigenetic inheritance in trangenerational effects. International Genomic Imprinting Meeting 1999;17.

205. Junien C. L'empreinte parentale: de la guerre des sexes à la solidarité entre généra-tions. Médecine/Sciences 2000; 3:336–44.

206. Branca F, Lorenzetti S. Health effects of phytoestrogens. Forum Nutr 2005; 57: 100–11.

207. Lumey LH. Decreased birthweights in infants after maternal in utero exposure to the Dutch famine of 1944–1945. Paediatr Perinat Epidemiol 1992; 6(2):240–53.

208. Lumey LH, Stein AD. Offspring birth weights after maternal intrauterine undernutri-tion: a comparison within sibships. Am J Epidemiol 1997; 146(10):810–9.

209. Bygren LO, Kaati G, Edvinsson S. Longevity determined by paternal ancestors' nutrition during their slow growth period. Acta Biotheor 2001; 49(1):53–9.

210. Boucher BJ, Ewen SW, Stowers JM. Betel nut (Areca catechu) consumption and the induction of glucose intolerance in adult CD1 mice and in their F1 and F2 offspring (see comments). Diabetologia 1994; 37(1):49–55.

211. Chen TH, Chiu YH, Boucher BJ. Transgenerational effects of betel-quid chewing on the development of the metabolic syndrome in the Keelung Community-based Integrated Screening Program. Am J Clin Nutr 2006; 83(3):688–92.

212. Srinivasan M, Aalinkeel R, Song F, et al. Programming of islet functions in the progeny of hyperinsulinemic/obese rats. Diabetes 2003; 52(4):984–90.

213. Patel MS, Srinivasan M. Metabolic programming: causes and consequences. J Biol Chem 2002; 277(3):1629–32.

214. Campbell JH, Perkins P. Transgenerational effects of drug and hormonal treatments in mammals: a review of observations and ideas. Prog Brain Res 1988; 73:535–53.

215. Blewitt ME, Vickaryous NK, Paldi A, et al. Dynamic reprogramming of DNA methylation at an epigenetically sensitive allele in mice. PLoS Genet 2006; 2(4):e49.

216. Peaston AE, Whitelaw E. Epigenetics and phenotypic variation in mammals. Mamm Genome 2006; 17(5):365–74.

217. Martin JF, Johnston CS, Han CT, et al. Nutritional origins of insulin resistance: a rat model for diabetes-prone human populations. J Nutr 2000; 130(4):741–4.

218. Reusens B, Remacle C. Intergenerational effect of an adverse intrauterine environment on perturbation of glucose metabolism. Twin Res 2001; 4(5):406–11.

219. Lane N, Dean W, Erhardt S, et al. Resistance of IAPs to methylation reprogramming may provide a mechanism for epigenetic inheritance in the mouse. Genesis 2003; 35(2):88–93.

220. Drake AJ, Walker BR. The intergenerational effects of fetal programming: non-genomic mechanisms for the inheritance of low birth weight and cardiovascular risk. J Endocrinol 2004; 180(1):1–16.

221. Haig D. Altercation of generations: genetic conflicts of pregnancy. Am J Reprod Immunol 1996; 35(3):226–32.

222. Whitelaw E and Martin DI. Retrotransposons as epigenetic mediators of phenotypic variation in mammals. Nat Genet 2001; 27(4):361–5.

223. Kelce WR, Monosson E, Gamcsik MP, et al. Environmental hormone disruptors: evidence that vinclozolin developmental toxicity is mediated by antiandrogenic metabolites. Toxicol Appl Pharmacol 1994; 126(2):276–85.

224. Bergeron JM, Crews D, McLachlan JA. PCBs as environmental estrogens: turtle sex determination as a biomarker of environmental contamination. Environ Health Perspect 1994; 102(9):780–1.

225. Crews D, McLachlan JA. Epigenetics, evolution, endocrine disruption, health, and disease. Endocrinology 2006; 147(Suppl 6):S4–10.

226. Newbold RR, Padilla-Banks E, Jefferson WN. Adverse effects of the model environmental estrogen diethylstilbestrol are transmitted to subsequent generations. Endocrinology 2006; 147(Suppl 6):S11–7.

227. Shiao YH, Crawford EB, Anderson LM, et al. Allele-specific germ cell epimutation in the spacer promoter of the 45S ribosomal RNA gene after Cr(III) exposure. Toxicol Appl Pharmacol 2005; 205(3):290–6.

228. Pogribny I, Raiche J, Slovack M, et al. Dose-dependence, sex- and tissue-specificity, and persistence of radiation-induced genomic DNA methylation changes. Biochem Biophys Res Commun 2004; 320(4):1253–61.

229. Raiche J, Rodriguez-Juarez R, Pogribny I, et al. Sex- and tissue-specific expression of maintenance and de novo DNA methyltransferases upon low dose X-irradiation in mice. Biochem Biophys Res Commun 2004; 325(1):39–47.

230. Schwahn BC, Laryea MD, Chen Z, et al. Betaine rescue of an animal model with methylenetetrahydrofolate reductase deficiency. Biochem J 2004; 382(Pt 3):831–40.

231. Barton TS, Robaire B, Hales BF. Epigenetic programming in the preimplantation rat embryo is disrupted by chronic paternal cyclophosphamide exposure. Proc Natl Acad Sci USA 2005; 102(22):7865–70.

232. Hales BF, Barton TS, Robaire B. Impact of paternal exposure to chemotherapy on offspring in the rat. J Natl Cancer Inst Monogr 2005; (34):28–31.

233. Zhang TY, Bagot R, Parent C, et al. Maternal programming of defensive responses through sustained effects on gene expression. Biol Psychol 2006; 73(1):72–89.

234. Anway MD, Skinner MK. Epigenetic transgenerational actions of endocrine disruptors. Endocrinology 2006; 147(Suppl. 6):S43–9.

235. Blondeau B, Avril I, Duchene B, et al. Endocrine pancreas development is altered in foetuses from rats previously showing intra-uterine growth retardation in response to malnutrition. Diabetologia 2002; 45(3):394–401.

236. Stewart RJ, Preece RF, Sheppard HG. Twelve generations of marginal protein deficiency. Br J Nutr 1975; 33(2):233–53.

237. Morgan HD, Santos F, Green K, et al. Epigenetic reprogramming in mammals. Hum Mol Genet 2005; 14(Spec No 1):R47–58.

238. Yokomori N, Kobayashi R, Moore R, et al. A DNA methylation site in the male-specific P450 (Cyp 2d-9) promoter and binding of the heteromeric transcription factor GABP. Mol Cell Biol 1995; 15(10):5355–62.

239. Yokomori N, Moore R, Negishi M. Sexually dimorphic DNA demethylation in the promoter of the Slp (sex-limited protein) gene in mouse liver. Proc Natl Acad Sci U S A 1995; 92(5):1302–6.

240. Wang MH, Vom Saal FS. Maternal age and traits in offspring. Nature 2000; 407(6803):469–70.

241. Jaquet D, Swaminathan S, Alexander GR, et al. Significant paternal contribution to the risk of small for gestational age. BJOG 2005; 112(2):153–9.

242. Aerts L, Holemans K, Van Assche FA. Maternal diabetes during pregnancy: consequences for the offspring. Diabetes Metab Rev 1990; 6(3):147–67.

243. Gauguier D, Bihoreau MT, Ktorza A, et al. Inheritance of diabetes mellitus as consequence of gestational hyperglycemia in rats. Diabetes 1990; 39(6):734–9.

244. Susa JB, Boylan JM, Sehgal P, et al. Persistence of impaired insulin secretion in infant rhesus monkeys that had been hyperinsulinemic in utero. J Clin Endocrinol Metab 1992; 75(1):265–9.

245. Blewitt ME, Vickaryous NK, Hemley SJ, et al. An N-ethyl-N-nitrosourea screen for genes involved in variegation in the mouse. Proc Natl Acad Sci U S A 2005; 102(21): 7629–34.

246. Bjornsson HT, Fallin MD, Feinberg AP. An integrated epigenetic and genetic approach to common human disease. Trends Genet 2004; 20(8):350–8.

247. de Rooij SR, Painter RC, Phillips DI, et al. The effects of the Pro12Ala polymorphism of the peroxisome proliferator-activated receptor-gamma2 gene on glucose/insulin metabolism interact with prenatal exposure to famine. Diabetes Care 2006; 29(5):1052–7.

248. Sandovici I, Kassovska-Bratinova S, Loredo-Osti JC, et al. Interindividual variability and parent of origin DNA methylation differences at specific human Alu elements. Hum Mol Genet 2005; 14(15):2135–43.

249. Frazier ML, Xi L, Zong J, et al. Association of the CpG island methylator phenotype with family history of cancer in patients with colorectal cancer. Cancer Res 2003; 63(16):4805–8.

250. Hiltunen MO, Yla-Herttuala S. DNA methylation, smooth muscle cells, and atherogenesis. Arterioscler Thromb Vasc Biol 2003; 23(10):1750–3.

251. Lund G, Andersson L, Lauria M, et al. DNA methylation polymorphisms precede any histological sign of atherosclerosis in mice lacking apolipoprotein E. J Biol Chem 2004.

252. Mostoslavsky R, Chua KF, Lombard DB, et al. Genomic instability and aging-like phenotype in the absence of mammalian SIRT6. Cell 2006; 124(2):315–29.

253. Hitchins M, Williams R, Cheong K, et al. MLH1 germline epimutations as a factor in hereditary nonpolyposis colorectal cancer. Gastroenterology 2005; 129(5):1392–9.

254. Suter CM, Martin DI, Ward RL. Germline epimutation of MLH1 in individuals with multiple cancers. Nat Genet 2004; 36(5):497–501.

255. Martin GM. Epigenetic drift in aging identical twins. Proc Natl Acad Sci USA 2005; 102(30):10413–4.

256. Cebrian A, Pharoah PD, Ahmed S, et al. Genetic variants in epigenetic genes and breast cancer risk. Carcinogenesis 2006; 27(8):1661–9.

257. Yamada Y, Watanabe H, Miura F, et al. A comprehensive analysis of allelic methylation status of CpG islands on human chromosome 21q. Genome Res 2004; 14(2): 247–66.

258. Abdolmaleky HM, Faraone SV, Glatt SJ, et al. Meta-analysis of association between the T102C polymorphism of the 5HT2a receptor gene and schizophrenia. Schizophr Res 2004; 67(1):53–62.

259. Rankinen T, Bouchard C. Genetics of food intake and eating behavior phenotypes in humans. Annu Rev Nutr 2006; 26:413–34.

260. Polesskaya OO, Aston C, Sokolov BP. Allele C-specific methylation of the 5-HT2A receptor gene: evidence for correlation with its expression and expression of DNA methylase DNMT1. J Neurosci Res 2006; 83(3):362–73.

261. Ngo V, Gourdji D, Laverriere JN. Site-specific methylation of the rat prolactin and growth hormone promoters correlates with gene expression. Mol Cell Biol 1996; 16(7):3245–54.

262. Attwood JT, Yung RL, Richardson BC. DNA methylation and the regulation of gene transcription. Cell Mol Life Sci 2002; 59(2):241–57.

263. Polesskaya OO, Sokolov BP. Differential expression of the 'C' and 'T' alleles of the 5-HT2A receptor gene in the temporal cortex of normal individuals and schizophrenics. J Neurosci Res 2002; 67(6):812–22.

264. Popendikyte V, Laurinavicius A, Paterson AD, et al. DNA methylation at the putative promoter region of the human dopamine D2 receptor gene. Neuroreport 1999; 10(6):1249–55.

265. Petronis A. The genes for major psychosis: aberrant sequence or regulation? Neuropsychopharmacology 2000; 23(1):1–12.

266. Blum K, Braverman ER, Wood RC, et al. Increased prevalence of the Taq I A1 allele of the dopamine receptor gene (DRD2) in obesity with comorbid substance use disorder: a preliminary report. Pharmacogenetics 1996; 6(4):297–305.

267. Blum K, Braverman ER, Wu S, et al. Association of polymorphisms of dopamine D2 receptor (DRD2), and dopamine transporter (DAT1) genes with schizoid/avoidant behaviors (SAB). Mol Psychiatry 1997; 2(3):239–46.

268. Glatt S, Faraoune S, Tsuang MT. Meta-analysis identifies an association between the dopamine D2 receptor gene and schizophrenia. Mol Psychiatry, in press.

269. Tasman A, Kay J, Lieberman J, eds. Psychiatry. New York: John Wiley & Sons, 2003.

270. Stabenau JR, Pollin W. Heredity and environment in schizophrenia, revisited. The contribution of twin and high-risk studies. J Nerv Ment Dis 1993; 181(5):290–7.

271. Murrell A, Heeson S, Cooper WN, et al. An association between variants in the IGF2 gene and Beckwith-Wiedemann syndrome: interaction between genotype and epigenotype. Hum Mol Genet 2004; 13(2):247–55.

272. Zogel C, Bohringer S, Gross S, et al. Identification of cis- and trans-acting factors possibly modifying the risk of epimutations on chromosome 15. Eur J Hum Genet 2006; 14(6):752–8.

273. Cruz-Correa M, Cui H, Giardiello FM, et al. Loss of imprinting of insulin growth factor II gene: a potential heritable biomarker for colon neoplasia predisposition. Gastroenterology 2004; 126(4):964–70.

274. Jirtle RL. IGF2 loss of imprinting: a potential heritable risk factor for colorectal cancer. Gastroenterology 2004; 126(4):1190–3.

275. Kerkhof GA, Van Dongen HP. Morning-type and evening-type individuals differ in the phase position of their endogenous circadian oscillator. Neurosci Lett 1996; 218(3):153–6.

276. Kerkhof GA. The 24-hour variation of mood differs between morning- and evening-type individuals. Percept Mot Skills 1998; 86(1):264–6.

277. Vink JM, Groot AS, Kerkhof GA, et al. Genetic analysis of morningness and eveningness. Chronobiol Int 2001; 18(5):809–22.

278. Sei H, Oishi K, Morita Y, et al. Mouse model for morningness/eveningness. Neuroreport 2001; 12(7):1461–4.

279. Katzenberg D, Young T, Finn L, et al. A CLOCK polymorphism associated with human diurnal preference. Sleep 1998; 21(6):569–76.

280. Katzenberg D, Young T, Lin L, et al. A human period gene (HPER1) polymorphism is not associated with diurnal preference in normal adults. Psychiatr Genet 1999; 9(2):107–9.

281. Di Lorenzo L, De Pergola G, Zocchetti C, et al. Effect of shift work on body mass index: results of a study performed in 319 glucose-tolerant men working in a Southern Italian industry. Int J Obes Relat Metab Disord 2003; 27(11):1353–8.

282. Nagaya T, Yoshida H, Takahashi H, et al. Markers of insulin resistance in day and shift workers aged 30-59 years. Int Arch Occup Environ Health 2002; 75(8):562–8.

283. Sakata-Haga H, Dominguez HD, Sei H, et al. Alterations in circadian rhythm phase shifting ability in rats following ethanol exposure during the third trimester brain growth spurt. Alcohol Clin Exp Res 2006; 30(5):899–907.

284. Reppert S. Interaction between the circadian clocks of mother and fetus. In: Chadwick DJ, Ackrill K, eds. Circadian Clocks and Their Adjustment. Chichester, UK: Wiley, 1995:198–211, Ciba Foundation Symposium, 183; 1995.

285. Murrell A, Rakyan VK, Beck S. From genome to epigenome. Hum Mol Genet 2005; 14(Spec No. 1):R3–10.

286. Pearson H. Medicine: sleep it off. Nature 2006; 443(7109):261–3.

287. Vadlamudi S, Kalhan SC, Patel MS. Persistence of metabolic consequences in the progeny of rats fed a HC formula in their early postnatal life. Am J Physiol 1995; 269(4 Pt 1):E731–8.

288. McKay JA, Williams EA, Mathers JC. Folate and DNA methylation during in utero development and aging. Biochem Soc Trans 2004; 32(Pt 6):1006–7.

289. Young LE, Fernandes K, McEvoy TG, et al. Epigenetic change in IGF2R is associated with fetal overgrowth after sheep embryo culture. Nat Genet 2001; 27(2):153–4.

290. Baqir S, Smith LC. Growth restricted in vitro culture conditions alter the imprinted gene expression patterns of mouse embryonic stem cells. Cloning Stem Cells 2003; 5(3):199-212.

291. Pantoja C, de Los Rios L, Matheu A, et al. Inactivation of imprinted genes induced by cellular stress and tumorigenesis. Cancer Res 2005; 65(1):26–33.

292. McLachlan JA, Burow M, Chiang TC, et al. Gene imprinting in developmental toxicology: a possible interface between physiology and pathology. Toxicol Lett 2001; 120(1–3):161–4.

293. O'Neil JS, Burow ME, Green AE, et al. Effects of estrogen on leptin gene promoter activation in MCF-7 breast cancer and JEG-3 choriocarcinoma cells: selective regulation via estrogen receptors alpha and beta. Mol Cell Endocrinol 2001; 176(1–2):67–75.

294. Li S, Hansman R, Newbold R, et al. Neonatal diethylstilbestrol exposure induces persistent elevation of c-fos expression and hypomethylation in its exon-4 in mouse uterus. Mol Carcinog 2003; 38(2):78–84.

295. Paz MF, Wei S, Cigudosa JC, et al. Genetic unmasking of epigenetically silenced tumor suppressor genes in colon cancer cells deficient in DNA methyltransferases. Hum Mol Genet 2003; 12(17):2209–19.

9.1 Genes Regulating Adipose-Tissue Development and Function

Sven Enerbäck

Medical Genetics, Department of Medical Biochemistry, Göteborg University, Göteborg, Sweden

In times of excess caloric intake, adipose tissue serves as an energy buffer. Superfluous calories are stored as triglycerides (TGs), ready to satisfy future needs. To perform this seemingly simple task, the adipose tissue needs to be well connected. It needs to know the general energy status of the organism, including present demand, storage capacity, size of present energy store, etc. At yet another level of integration, energy, in the form of free fatty acids (FFA), can be redistributed, for example, from adipose tissue to meet the demands of other cell types (e.g., myocytes). An elaborate system of endocrine and paracrine functions as well as neuronal signaling makes sure that the adipose tissue is well integrated into the general energy network described in greater detail elsewhere in this book. The importance of adipose tissue in this context is illustrated by the dramatic metabolic consequences that are induced by lack of it. Lipodystrophy both in man and mouse leads to, among other things, steatosis, hepatomegaly, and insulin resistance. In mice, transplanting adipose tissue back to lipodystrophic mice has been used as a way to treat this condition (1). This approach leads to a more or less complete reversal of the metabolic disturbances. Thus, supplying ample TG storage capacity to mice that lack it can cure many obesity-linked symptoms such as fatty liver and insulin resistance.

Genes that affect number of available adipocytes, both those that are ready to be used and those that can be induced to differentiate from precursor cells, would be of interest in terms of total adipocyte storage capacity. Another set of interesting genes in this context are genes that affect the efficiency by which TGs are stored and maintained in adipocytes. For instance if uptake of FFA by adipocytes is enhanced this might lead to a more efficient allocation of TG to adipocytes and hence an increase in adipose-tissue size. On the other hand, in a situation with constant flow of FFA to adipocytes the efficiency of the conversion of FFA to TG will affect adipose-tissue mass. Finally, the total TG mass in adipocytes could be utilized within the adipocyte by, for instance, uncoupling of oxidative phosphorylation, e.g., uncoupling protein 1 (UCP1), and as a result some of the energy stored will be dissipated as heat. An interesting consequence is that an increase of UCP1-expressing brown adipocytes would promote a decrease in the total pool of TG that is stored in adipose tissue, including both brown and white adipocytes. This is extreme in patients with pheochromocytoma, a catecholamine-producing tumor originating form the medulla of the suprarenal gland; here, increased circulating levels of epinephrine and norepinephrine induce brown adipose-tissue (BAT) hyperplasia. Typically such patients, prior to treatment, display increased BAT around the tumor, where the catecholamine levels most likely are the highest. The increased BAT stores might very well contribute to the lean phenotype associated with this condition.

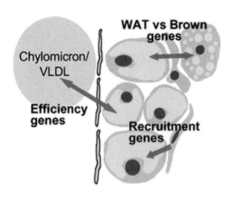

FIGURE 1 A schematic representation of three adipose-tissue functions and corresponding genes.

While focus is on three sets of adipose-tissue genes as potential candidates for adipose-tissue expressed genes related to obesity (as depicted in Fig. 1), both negative and positive regulators of adipose-tissue compartment size will be discussed:

1. Recruitment genes: regulate number of adipocytes, including genes regulating recruitment of adipocytes form precursor cells.
2. Efficiency genes: regulate the efficiency by which FFA are taken up and stored as TGs by adipocyte, including the efficiency by which lipolysis acts on stored TGs within the adipocyte.
3. BAT versus WAT genes: regulate uncoupling and other similar mechanisms that enable adipose tissue to dissipate some of its energy content as heat.

RECRUITMENT GENES

In times of positive energy-balance surplus, energy is stored as TG in adipocytes. Some of the physiological responses to a positive energy balance, such as high insulin levels, also serve as inducers of adipocyte differentiation. In this way the total adipocyte storage capacity will be maintained at a level that will meet metabolic demand. "Lipogenic" genes like CCAAT/enhancer-binding protein (C/EBPs) and peroxisome proliferator-activated receptors (PPARs) are of fundamental importance for adipogenesis and their activity will regulate the TG storage capacity of the adipose tissue (2). The extreme case of total or partial lack of adipose tissue (lipodystrophy) has been linked to mutations in the *LMNA* gene encoding lamin A/C and the seipin (*BSCL2*) gene as well as in the *AGPAT* (2 1-acylglycerol-3-phosphate *O*-acyltransferase 2 (lysophosphatidic acid acyltransferase, beta)). While altered function of lamin A/C appears to be part of more generalized multiorgan laminopathies *AGPAT2* encodes an enzyme involved in triacylglycerol synthesis (3). Decreased number of adipocyte and hence a concomitant reduced capacity to store TGs leads to ectopic TG depositions in liver and muscle, the first step toward insulin resistance and the metabolic syndrome. Genes that influence the number of adipocytes will thus also regulate the total TG storage capacity in adipose tissue. A good ability to recruit adipocytes will postpone the onset of ectopic TG depositions. To some extent obesity will delay the onset of insulin resistance, only when the recruitment fails excess TGs are rerouted to other sites (4). In mice models, it has been established that *PPARG* expression is necessary for proper development of adipose tissue (5,6). Humans with mutations that prevent ligand activation of PPARG, due to mutations in the ligand-binding domain, develop partial lipodystrophy, insulin resistance and hepatic steatosis as part of a PPARG ligand resistance syndrome (7). On the other hand, other mutations in PPARG2 such as the Pro12Ala might be associated with increased adipose tissue (8). Thus, there are several examples of genes that will influence the size of adipose tissue and hence affect the susceptibility for developing obesity.

EFFICIENCY GENES

Altered uptake and/or mobilization (lipolysis) of TGs in adipocytes constitute a possible mechanism contributing to development obesity. While genes that lead to increased uptake will act to preserve an ample TG store, genes that enhance lipolysis will do the opposite. For instance, mice lacking the adipose TG lipase (ATGL)—the major enzyme responsible for breakdown of cellular fat stores— display increased adipose mass. Such mice show a phenotype with decreased ability to mobilize TG stores leading to an accumulation of TGs in WAT and BAT (9). In humans there is an association between polymorphic markers in the *ATGL* gene and levels of TG and FFA, some markers also show association to serum glucose levels and risk of type 2 diabetes (10).

BROWN ADIPOSE-TISSUE VS. WHITE ADIPOSE-TISSUE GENES

Brown adipocytes offer a unique possibility to dissipate energy as heat through uncoupling of respiration and oxidative phosphorylation via UCP1. The proton gradient over the inner mitochondrial membrane will be short-circuited by the action of, UCP1, and instead of ATP heat, will be produced, a process referred to as *adaptive thermogenesis*. Genetic ablation of the nuclear receptor corepressor RIP140 (nuclear receptor interacting protein 1) results in a lean phenotype resistant to diet-induced obesity. Even though the molecular mechanism underlying this phenotype to some extent remains unknown it is likely that expression of *UCP1* in WAT depots of *Rip140 −/−* mice is important in terms of explaining the phenotype (11). Similar phenotype is seen in mice with ectopic expression of *Ucp1* in WAT. In such mice the fat specific aP2 promoter drives *Ucp1* expression. When crossed with genetically obese mice like A^{vy} a reduction of total body weight and sub-cutaneous fat stores was observed. This demonstrates that *Ucp1* expression, when induced in white adipocytes, protects from both diet as well as genetically induced obesity (12).

Brown adipocytes are present in human adipose tissue under normal conditions (13,14) and known to expand in response to adrenergic stimuli. As is the case in patients with pheochromocytoma, in such patient there is an expansion of UCP1-positive BAT cells (15), the uncoupling of which most likely contributes to the lean phenotype typically seen in such patients. Thus, BAT is normally present and can be induced and function in terms of *adaptive thermogenesis* in humans. Thus, promoting brown fat differentiation offers an attractive way to counteract both diet-induced and genetically acquired obesity. Forkhead box C2 (FOXC2) is a forkhead transcription factor, when its overexpressed in adipose tissue there is a significant increase of the BAT compartment. Such mice are also refractory to diet-induced obesity and insulin resistance (16). In humans, lower levels of *FOXC2* mRNA have been reported in insulin-resistant subjects as compared with healthy controls (17), as well as genetically linked to insulin resistance (18). FOXC2 appears to be upstream of another important brown fat agonist of peroxisome proliferator-activated receptor gamma, coactivator 1 alpha and beta (PPARGC1A and B) that acts as a master regulator of brown fat mitochondrogenesis (19) since even in the absence of PPARGC1A and B FOXC2 is still inducible by protein kinase A (PKA) as opposed to other PKA-inducible genes e.g., iodothyronine, type 2 (deiodinase D2), and C/EBP beta. Increased levels of FOXC2 and inhibition of retinoblastoma protein is part of a phenotypic switch that enhances brown over white adipocyte differentiation (20). In response to induced hyperleptinemia white adipocytes greatly increase their fat oxidation to the extent that they deplete their TG stores. Of genes measured the most prominent increase was noted for FOXC2, a more than four-fold increase (21). Recently, it was demonstrated that the alternative stimulatory G-protein alpha-subunit XL alpha is a critical regulator of energy and glucose metabolism and sympathetic nerve activity both these activities are to some extent dependent on induction of FOXC2 (22). Thus, genes enhancing an expansion of BAT might prove to be interesting drug targets for antiobesity therapies. On the other hand mutations in these genes could also be associated with obesity.

REFERENCES

1. Gavrilova O, Marcus-Samuels B, Graham D, et al. Surgical implantation of adipose tissue reverses diabetes in lipoatrophic mice. J Clin Invest 2000; 105:271–8.
2. Wu Z, Rosen ED, Brun R, et al. Cross-regulation of C/EBP alpha and PPAR gamma controls the transcriptional pathway of adipogenesis and insulin sensitivity. Mol Cell 1999; 3:151–8.
3. Capeau J, Magre J, Lascols O, et al. Diseases of adipose tissue: genetic and acquired lipodystrophies. Biochem Soc Trans 2005; 33:1073–7.
4. Unger RH, Orci L. Lipotoxic diseases of nonadipose tissues in obesity. Int J Obes Relat Metab Disord 2000; 24(Suppl. 4):S28–32.
5. Barak Y, Nelson MC, Ong ES, et al. PPAR gamma is required for placental, cardiac, and adipose tissue development. Mol Cell 1999; 4:585–95.
6. Rosen ED, Sarraf P, Troy AE, et al. PPAR gamma is required for the differentiation of adipose tissue in vivo and in vitro. Mol Cell 1999; 4:611–7.
7. Semple RK, Chatterjee VK, O'Rahilly S. PPAR gamma and human metabolic disease. J Clin Invest 2006; 116:581–9.
8. Valve R, Sivenius K, Miettinen R, et al. Two polymorphisms in the peroxisome proliferator-activated receptor-gamma gene are associated with severe overweight among obese women. J Clin Endocrinol Metab 1999; 84:3708–12.
9. Haemmerle G, Lass A, Zimmermann R, et al. Defective lipolysis and altered energy metabolism in mice lacking adipose triglyceride lipase. Science 2006; 312:734–7.
10. Schoenborn V, Heid IM, Vollmert C, et al. The ATGL gene is associated with free fatty acids, triglycerides, and type 2 diabetes. Diabetes 2006; 55:1270–5.
11. Leonardsson G, Steel JH, Christian M, et al. Nuclear receptor corepressor RIP140 regulates fat accumulation. Proc Natl Acad Sci USA 2004; 101:8437–42.
12. Kopecky J, Clarke G, Enerback S, et al. Expression of the mitochondrial uncoupling protein gene from the aP2 gene promoter prevents genetic obesity. J Clin Invest 1995; 96:2914–23.
13. Krief S, Lonnqvist F, Raimbault S, et al. Tissue distribution of beta 3-adrenergic receptor mRNA in man. J Clin Invest 1993; 91:344–9.
14. Zancanaro C, Carnielli VP, Moretti C, et al. An ultrastructural study of brown adipose tissue in pre-term human new-borns. Tissue Cell 1995; 27:339–48.

15. Bouillaud F, Villarroya F, Hentz E, et al. Detection of brown adipose tissue uncoupling protein mRNA in adult patients by a human genomic probe. Clin Sci (Lond) 1988; 75:21–7.

16. Cederberg A, Gronning LM, Ahren B, et al. FOXC2 is a winged helix gene that counteracts obesity, hypertriglyceridemia, and diet-induced insulin resistance. Cell 2001; 106:563–73.

17. Yang X, Enerback S, Smith U. Reduced expression of FOXC2 and brown adipogenic genes in human subjects with insulin resistance. Obes Res 2003; 11:1182–91.

18. Ridderstrale M, Carlsson E, Klannemark M, et al. FOXC2 mRNA expression and a 5′ untranslated region polymorphism of the gene are associated with insulin resistance. Diabetes 2002; 51:3554–60.

19. Uldry M, Yang W, St-Pierre J, et al. Complementary action of the PGC-1 coactivators in mitochondrial biogenesis and brown fat differentiation. Cell Metab 2006; 3:333–41.

20. Hansen JB, Jorgensen C, Petersen RK, et al. Retinoblastoma protein functions as a molecular switch determining white versus brown adipocyte differentiation. Proc Natl Acad Sci USA 2004; 101:4112–7.

21. Orci L, Cook WS, Ravazzola M, et al. Rapid transformation of white adipocytes into fat-oxidizing machines. Proc Natl Acad Sci USA 2004; 101:2058–63.

22. Xie T, Plagge A, Gavrilova O, et al. The alternative stimulatory G protein alpha-subunit XLalphas is a critical regulator of energy and glucose metabolism and sympathetic nerve activity in adult mice. J Biol Chem 2006; 281:18989–99.

9.2 Genetics of Adipose-Tissue Development and Function in Humans

Ingrid Dahlman and Peter Arner
Karolinska Institutet, Department of Medicine, Karolinska University Hospital–Huddinge, Stockholm, Sweden

It is attractive to speculate that important obesity genes express in the tissue that is most affected by obesity, namely the adipose tissue. Adipose tissue contains the largest store of energy in the body and plays important roles in regulating energy homeostasis. A number of adipocyte-specific events could be subjected to genetic modification causing obesity (Fig. 1):

- Adipogenesis: Although less well-documented in man than in rodents, there is a continuous formation of fat cells throughout life.
- Lipid turnover: More than 95% of the fat cell volume consists of lipids, which constantly are turned over due to new synthesis and breakdown (lipolysis).
- Mitochondria function: Although brown fat, which has high fatty acid oxidation capacity, is sparse in adult humans, it is possible to demonstrate some in vivo functional activity of such adipocytes in adulthood by, for example, treatment with so-called beta 3-agonists. In addition, the mitochondria activity of white fat cells has recently been recognized to be more important than considered before.
- Permissive hormone effects: Several hormones have pleiotrophic effects on human fat cells, such as insulin and steroid hormones, and in particular, sex hormones.
- Endocrine/autocrine function: Besides their role in energy homeostasis, fat cells have an important endocrine/paracrine role. Adipocytes secrete a number of hormones, enzymes, inflammatory proteins, and other factors that control peripheral organs and the brain and also adipose-tissue function in an autocrine fashion.

These various functions and pathways highlight that adipocyte-expressed genes can influence obesity either by local effects in adipose tissue, such as adipogenesis and mitochondria energy expenditure, or via secretion of various factors such as hormones and free fatty acids (FFA) that have peripheral effects.

Human adipose tissue is in many ways differently regulated than in rodents, which provide widely studied experimental models of obesity (1). Therefore the adipose genes causing human obesity might be quite different from those anticipated by studies in rodents. This chapter describes what is known about adipose tissue–expressed genes in genetic predisposition to common human obesity. Thus, our starting point is fat cell biology and specific genes will be discussed in their specific biological context; starting with adipogenesis, we subsequently discuss pathways regulating lipid storage, energy expenditure, insulin signaling, and finally adipose tissue–secreted molecules (Table 1). To the extent that human studies of adipose-tissue genes have been guided by results obtained in experimental models, some of these results will be mentioned. Obesity is strongly

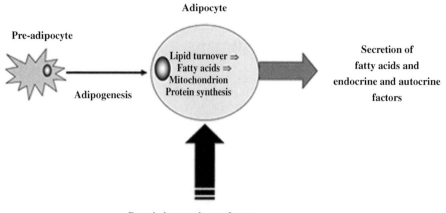

FIGURE 1   Genetic variance in human adipocyte formation, regulation, and function may cause or prevent obesity.

associated with insulin resistance, and there is evidence of shared susceptibility alleles, which is briefly discussed below.

Before initiating a detailed discussion about genes regulating obesity and fat mass in adipose tissue, we must ask, what evidence is there that such genes exist? First, there are rare monogenic disorders, i.e., deficiency of the adipocyte-secreted hormone leptin causes morbid obesity (see Chapter 5.4), whereas mutations in other adipose tissue–expressed genes causes lack of adipose tissue as observed in lipodystrophy. Second, similar weight gain in, as opposed to large differences between, twin-pairs following a period of controlled excess food intake support a genetic impact on metabolic pathways (2), see Chapter 2.4. For common obesity, the evidence for a role of specific adipose tissue–expressed genes in obesity is so far incomplete, i.e., initial claims of significant associations between alleles and obesity have been difficult to confirm. Thus, genes discussed below are so far candidates for obesity, of which some looks promising.

ADIPOGENESIS

Adipogenesis, or the formation of new adipocytes, is orchestrated by the transcription factors Peroxisome proliferator-activated receptor gamma (PPARG) and CCAAT/enhancer-binding protein alpha (C/EBPA) (3,4). In particular the PPARG gene is a strong candidate gene for regulating fat mass and obesity. PPARG is a lipid sensor and acts as a master regulator of fat cell function and energy homeostasis by inducing expression of genes promoting uptake of fatty acids, triglyceride (TG) synthesis, and insulin sensitivity (review in (5)). PPARG exists in three isoforms differing in their 5' sequence. PPARG2 is the most abundant isoform in human adipose tissue and it is the only isoform that is exclusively expressed in this organ. Obesity has been reported to increase, or to have no impact on, PPARG2 expression in subcutaneous adipose tissue (6,7).

In humans, rare, dominant, negative mutations in the ligand-binding domain of PPARG gene cause partial lipodystrophy as well as severe hepatic and

TABLE 1 Candidate Genes for Obesity in Human Adipose Tissue

Chromosome	Gene
Adipogenesis	
1q21.2	*LMNA*
2p21	*Lipin*
3p25-p2	***PPARG***
5q31.3	*GR*
17p11.2	*SREBP1*
Lipid turnover	
5q32-q3	***ADRB2***
8p12-p11.2	***ADRB3***
10q24-q26	*ADRB1*
10	*GB3*
15q26	*PLIN*
19q13	***HSL***
Mitochondrion and energy expenditure	
4p15.1	*PGC1A*
4q28-q31	*UCP1*
5q32	*PGC1B*
11q13	***UCP2***
11q13	*UCP3*
11q13	*ESRRA*
18p11.2	*CIDEA*
Insulin signaling	
3q27	*AHSG*
6q22-q2	***ENPP1***
10q23.3-q24.1	*SORBS1*
Adipokines	
1q21	*IL6R*
3q27	*ADIPOQ*
6p21.3	***TNFA***
7p21	*IL6*
7q21.3-q22	*PAI*
19p13.2	*RETN1*

Note: Bold denotes strong candidate genes for obesity based on established function in adipocytes and/or strong evidence of genetic association.

peripheral insulin resistance, which have been linked to the inability of adipose tissue to trap and store FFA (8). The most extensively studied common *PPARG* variant is Pro2Ala, which is specific for the PPARG2 5'-region. The Ala12 allele is according to a meta-analysis of several studies associated with higher body mass index (BMI) in subjects with BMI > 27 kg/m^2 (9) and, consistent with the impact of PPARG agonists thiazolidinediones, has in repeated studies been reported to protect against type 2 diabetes (T2DM) (8). These findings are difficult to functionally link with the observation that the Ala12 allele exhibits reduced DNA binding and transactivation (10). Interestingly, the impact of Pro2Ala on obesity has been reported to be modified by composition of fatty acid intake (see Chapter 8.3) (11).

The transcription factor sterol regulatory element–binding protein 1C (SREBP1C) stimulates expression of genes, including PPARG, promoting adipogenesis and TG storage in experimental systems (12,13). *SREBP1C* is encoded by the same gene (sterol regulatory element–binding transcription factor 1, SREBF1) as *SREBP1A*, which primarily regulates cholesterol metabolism, by the use of different promoters. *SREBP1C* adipose-tissue expression is down regulated in human obesity (14). One haplotype in the *SREBP1* gene has been associated with morbid obesity, T2DM, and dyslipidemia in French Caucasian cohorts (15). This haplotype carries single-nucleotide polymorphisms (SNPs) in the 5' untranslated region that could affect mRNA processing hereby regulating protein levels.

Recently, other transcription factors and coregulators that modify PPARG activity in experimental models have emerged as candidate genes for obesity. The transcription factor Forkhead box C2 (FOXC2) blocks adipogenesis by interfering with PPARG promotion of gene expression (16) and protects against adiposity in experimental animals (17). One allele at a SNP in the putative promoter has been associated with susceptibility to as well as protection against obesity (18,19). No function has been associated with this SNP and human adipose-tissue *FOXC2* expression is not associated with obesity (20) leaving us with limited support for an impact of this gene on obesity.

The adipose tissue–expressed gene lipin (*LPIN1*) acts upstream of PPARG in adipocyte differentiation, and promotes fat storage and obesity in the mouse by as yet not fully understood mechanisms (21). Human adipose-tissue expression of lipin has recently been shown to correlate inversely with insulin resistance but not obesity, and one intronic SNP associates with obesity in Finns (22). The impact of the lipin gene on obesity should be investigated in additional populations before any definitive conclusions can be made regarding the impact on this gene on obesity. Lamin A/C (LMNA) is an element of the nuclear lamina. Mutations in this gene are one cause of partial lipodystrophy, indicating a role in human adipogenesis. A silent mutation in *LMNA* is associated with obesity in two Canadian populations (23,24).

Glucocorticoid hormone potentates the early steps of preadipocyte differentiation and promote visceral obesity and insulin resistance (25,26). Adipose-tissue expression of the glucocorticoid receptor is down regulated, and expression of hydroxysteroid (11-beta) dehydrogenase 1 (*HSD11B1*), a regulator of glucocorticoid bioavailability, is increased in human obesity (27,28). SNPs in the glucocorticoid receptor have been associated with glucocorticoid sensitivity and in some, but not all, studies changes in body composition (29). SNPs in *HSD11B1* are unlikely to predispose to common obesity (28).

PATHWAYS CONTROLLING LIPID STORAGE IN ADIPOCYTES

Lipid storage in adipocytes is governed by the balance between TG synthesis versus lipolysis with subsequent fatty acid release. Insulin and glucocorticoid hormones are the physiological stimulators of extracellular lipoprotein lipase (LPL), which hydrolyzes TGs in lipoproteins to provide FFA to tissues for deposit as TG. Acylation-stimulating protein (ASP), a cleavage product from complement factor C3, is secreted by adipocytes and acts as a paracrine signal to stimulate the enzyme diacylglycerol acyltransferase, which is responsible for the synthesis of TG. Available data does not support an independent impact of LPL or ASP SNPs on obesity (30). Various transport proteins facilitate fatty acid transport through the plasma membrane and in the cell for subsequent biosynthesis of TG. These genes have not been investigated for an impact on human obesity (31).

During lipolysis TGs are broken down in a stepwise fashion to FFA and glycerol. In humans, lipolysis is modulated by the sympathetic nervous system, insulin, and atrial natriuretic peptide (ANP) (32) and is markedly influenced by fat depot, sex, and adiposity. Among obese subjects, basal lipolysis is increased in all fat depots, whereas the lipolytic response to catecholamines is decreased in subcutaneous fat and increased in visceral fat. This has been associated with region-specific changes in expression of adrenoreceptors and downstream molecules, i.e., hormone-sensitive lipase (HSL). The resulting increased release of FFA from adipose observed in obesity affect systemic insulin resistance (31).

Catecholamines are the most potent regulators of lipolysis in human adipocytes and act through stimulatory beta 1 (ADRB1), beta 2 (ADRB2), and beta 3 (ADRB3) adrenoreceptors or inhibitory alpha 2 (ADRA2) adrenoreceptors (31). ADRB3 is functionally active principally in omental adipocytes. Alleles at nonsynonymous *ADRB2* polymorphisms that affect receptor function in vitro (33,34) have been associated with increased lipolysis and obesity, although this has not been confirmed in all subsequent studies (35,36). More recently, the impact of variations in the *ADRB2* gene on gene expression, in vivo function, and obesity has been associated with specific gene haplotypes that cannot be predicted from individual SNPs (37–39). Furthermore, a coding allele, Arg64, in the *ADRB3* genes has been associated with weight gain and reduced basal metabolic rate (40,41), as well as obesity and decreased lipolysis (42,43). However, the impact on obesity is not confirmed in all studies (44). In the *ADRB1* gene, the Gly389Arg SNP, which affect coupling of the receptor to downstream targets, has been associated with obesity (45,46). Surprisingly, this polymorphism has no apparent impact on fat cell lipolysis in vivo (47).

Beta adrenoreceptors signal via G stimulatory proteins that activate adenylate cyclase, leading to increased cyclic AMP and protein kinase A, which phosphorylates and activates HSL (31). A polymorphism in exon 10 of the gene encoding the beta 3 subunit of heterodimeric G-proteins (GB3), C825T, regulates protein levels and splicing (48). The 825T allele displays enhanced signaling (48) but, surprisingly, reduced catecholamine-induced lipolysis (49), and is associated with obesity in some (50) but not all studied populations (49,51). HSL is the rate-limiting step in lipolysis, hydrolyzing TG to diglycerides and subsequently monoglycerides (31). One HSL promoter SNP has been identified that regulate gene expression (52). This SNP has been reported to have opposite effect on adiposity in different populations (52,53). Furthermore, an allele of an intronic repeat in the HSL gene has been reported to be associated with obesity, T2DM, and decreased lipolysis (54–56). Perilipin (PLIN) is a phosphoprotein that coats the surfaces of intracellular lipid droplets in adipocytes and protects them against hydrolysis. *PLIN* expression is increased in adipose tissue of obese subjects (57). One intronic *PLIN* SNP is associated with lower gene expression and increased lipolysis (58). Additional SNPs in the *PLIN* gene have been reported to be associated with obesity phenotypes in women (59,60).

There are no genetic studies of the ANP signaling pathway in human obesity.

THE MITOCHONDRION AND ENERGY EXPENDITURE IN ADIPOSE-TISSUE

Animal models have highlighted adipose-tissue mitochondria and energy expenditure as key risk factors for obesity. For example, development of obesity in ob/ob mice is accompanied by decreased expression of nuclear-encoded mitochondria genes (61).

Uncoupling protein 1 (UCP1), 2 (UCP2), and 3 (UCP3) are mitochondria membrane transporters that are involved in dissipating the proton electrochemical gradient, thereby releasing stored energy as heat (62–64). This implies a major role for UCPs in energy expenditure and possibly adiposity. UCP1 is induced by cold and catecholamines, and is primarily expressed in brown adipocytes, which are rare in adult humans (65). However, *UCP1* mRNA has been detected at low levels in human white adipose tissue and is reported to be decreased in intra-abdominal adipose tissue of obese subjects (66). The G allele at the *UCP1* gene promoter SNP, A-3826G, has been associated with reduced gene expression (67) and weight gain, but the latter has not been confirmed by other investigators (68–70).

Whereas *UCP2* is widely expressed, *UCP3* is restricted to skeletal muscle and adipose tissue (71). Visceral fat *UCP2* expression is decreased in obese subjects (72). Otherwise, expression of these genes displays no major dependence on BMI, but both are increased in individuals undergoing fasting suggesting a role in metabolic adaptation to fasting (71). Genetic analysis supports a role for the *UCP2* gene in common human obesity. Thus, a SNP at −866 in the promoter of *UCP2* affects mRNA expression in vitro, is associated with mRNA levels in visceral fat, and obesity in independent populations (73). Furthermore, a *UCP2* exon 4 SNP has been reported to be associated with basal metabolic rate but not obesity, and an exon 8 SNP with obesity (74,75). Regarding UCP3, rare mutations affecting the amino acid sequence have been associated with decreased respiratory quotient and fat oxidation (76). In addition, a *UCP3* promoter SNP and an intronic repeat have been associated with obesity (77–79). These associations between UCP3 gene polymorphisms have not been confirmed in other studies (summarized by Damcott et al. (79).

Some insights have been obtained, primarily in experimental models, on the transcriptional regulation of mitochondria beta oxidation. PPARG, coactivator 1 alpha (PGC1A) is induced by cold and exercise in muscle and promotes mitochondria biogenesis and, when ectopically expressed in adipocytes, expression of UCP1 and key mitochondria enzymes of the respiratory chain (80). *PGC1A* is expressed at low levels in human adipose tissue (81). Adipose-tissue expression of *PGC1A* is reduced in morbid obesity (82) and insulin-resistant states, as well as correlated to *UCP1* expression (83). *PGC1A* SNPs have been reported to be associated with obesity in Austrian women (84).

It has been shown in mice that PGC1A induced expression of mitochondria respiratory chain genes is partly mediated by the estrogen-related receptor alpha (ESRRA) (85). A polymorphism in the 5'-flanking region of the *ESRRA* gene has been reported to be associated with obesity in a Japanese population (86). PPARG, coactivator 1 beta (PGC1B) is a recently discovered homolog of PGC1A which, like PGC1A, in experimental animals induces expression of genes involved in oxidative phosphorylation (87). Its expression in human adipose tissue relative to obesity has to our knowledge not been investigated. One coding *PGC1B* SNP, Ala203Pro, has in a Danish population been reported to protect against obesity but not T2DM (88).

A recently discovered candidate gene for obesity and for regulation of energy expenditure in human adipocytes is cell death-inducing DFFA-like effector a (CIDEA). Although the molecular function of CIDEA is unknown, available data are compatible with an impact on mitochondria respiratory function. The PPARG agonists thiazolidinediones induce mitochondria biogenesis and expression of mitochondria genes as well as CIDEA (61). Mice deficient in CIDEA display increased oxygen consumption (89) and adipose-tissue gene expression is strongly reduced in obese humans (90). A coding *CIDEA* SNP has been associated with obesity in female and male Swedes (91).

INSULIN SIGNALING IN ADIPOCYTES

Insulin signaling in adipose tissue can have a dramatic impact on adiposity as shown in the adipocytes-specific insulin receptor (INSR) defect mouse, which is lean and displays increased oxidative phosphorylation (92). Polymorphisms in the INSR or INSR substrate genes do not seem to affect human adiposity (93), but there is some evidence that other modifiers of insulin signaling may do.

Sorbin and SH3-domain-containing-1 (SORBS1) is the human homolog of c-Cbl-associated protein (CAP), which is highly expressed in adipocytes and through interaction with the INSR regulates glucose uptake (94). A nonsynonymous *SORBS1* SNP has been associated with obesity and T2DM (95). Mice deficient in the alpha(2)-Heremans–Schmid glycoprotein (*AHSG*) gene, which inhibits insulin-induced INSR autophosphorylation and tyrosine kinase activity in vitro, display improved insulin sensitivity and resistance to weight gain (96). SNPs in the human *AHSG* gene have been reported to be associated with adipocyte insulin action (97) and obesity (98). Ectonucleotide pyrophosphatase/phosphodiesterase 1 (ENPP1) is an inhibitor of insulin-receptor tyrosine kinase. One *ENPP1* haplotype is associated with obesity and T2DM in several populations, as well as with increased circulating ENPP1 (99). Expression of a long *ENPP1* mRNA isoform, which includes one of the SNPs defining the risk haplotype, is specific for pancreatic islet beta cells, adipocytes, and liver. In addition, one ENPP1 SNP may impair insulin binding to the INSR (99). These associations with obesity phenotypes were not always confirmed (see Chapters 6.2 and 6.3).

SEX HORMONES, ADIPOSE TISSUE, AND OBESITY

An increased adipose mass is seen in women after menopause when estrogen levels decrease, while estrogen replacement therapy decreases adipose mass. Estrogen increases HSL and reduces LPL enzyme activity in humans and animals, which is expected to lead to a decrease in TG deposition. *ESRA* mRNA and protein expression and *ESRB* mRNA expression have been detected in human adipose tissue (100). Adipose-tissue *ESRA* mRNA levels are increased following weight reduction (101). Intronic ESRA SNPs have been associated with sex-specific effects on obesity in women (102) and men (103). These results are unconfirmed.

ENDOCRINE AND PARACRINE ACTION OF ADIPOCYTES

Human adipose tissue secretes several hormones and cytokines, together termed adipokines, which, besides local effects, through release into circulation participate in regulation of whole body metabolism and insulin action.

Adiponectin (ADIPOQ) is a hormone exclusively expressed in differentiated adipocytes, primarily implicated in insulin sensitivity but also a candidate for obesity. In animal models ADIPOQ increases insulin sensitivity (104) and circulating ADIPOQ levels in humans are associated with higher glucose disposal and energy expenditure (105). *ADIPOQ* expression is reduced in human obesity and insulin-resistant states, and up regulated following weight loss and by thiazolidinediones treatment (106). One *ADIPOQ* allele at a synonymous SNP in exon 2, as well as a haplotype that carries this allele, has been associated with obesity and circulating ADIPOQ levels in several populations (107,108). In addition, *ADIPOQ* polymorphisms have in repeated studies been associated with T2DM (106). ADIPOQ receptor polymorphisms have to our knowledge not been investigated for association with obesity (109).

Plasminogen activator inhibitor (PAI) is a regulator of the fibrinolytic system implicated in human ischemic heart disease. Mice deficient in PAI are resistant to diet-induced obesity, display increased metabolic rate, and promoted adipocyte differentiation in vitro (110,111) implying a role in body weight regulation as well. Human adipose tissue secretion of PAI is enhanced by tumor necrosis factor-α (TNF-α) (112) and increased in obesity (113). One functional promoter SNP in the *PAI* gene has been reported to be associated with obesity, but this has not been confirmed by others (114,115).

Human obesity is associated with macrophage infiltration in adipose tissue (116) and enhanced adipose-tissue expression of proinflammatory mediators including TNF-α (117), monocyte chemoattractant protein 1 (MCP1), and interleukin-6 (IL-6). The secretion of proinflammatory factors from adipose tissue are reduced following weight reduction (118). The obesity-associated proinflammatory state in adipose tissue can contribute to insulin resistance and thus, potentially, to the metabolic complications of obesity (119,120). The role of TNF-α in adipocytes has been investigated in several studies. TNF-α has been shown to increase lipolysis in humans in vivo and in primary cultures of preadipocytes (31). TNF-α treatment downregulates *PLIN* (31) and *ADIPOQ* expression (Table 2) (106). The TNFA locus has been linked to obesity (121). Subsequent studies have focused on the impact of a –308 promoter SNP that influences gene transcription (122). In a recent meta-analysis, this polymorphism was associated with a modest increased risk of developing obesity, odds ratio 1:23 (123). The impact of IL-6 on adipose tissue is less clear. However, at a polymorphic site in the IL-6 promoter, the –174G

TABLE 2   Adipose-Tissue Genes with Possible Influence on Human Obesity

Gene	Findings with polymorphism
PPARG	Meta-analysis suggests linkage between polymorphism and BMI. Obesity-associated polymorphisms lead to amino acid functional changes.
ADRB2	Association with obesity in many studies. Obesity-associated polymorphisms lead to amino acid changes that are functional in transfected cells and in human fat cells (lipolysis).
ADRB3	Association with obesity in many studies. The obesity-associated polymorphism leads to amino acid changes that are functional in transfected cells and in human fat cells (lipolysis).
HSL	Association with obesity in many studies. Obesity-associated polymorphism is associated with low lipolysis in human fat cells.
UCP2	Association with obesity in independent samples. The obesity-associated polymorphism in promoter leads to altered promoter function and influences gene expression in adipose tissue
ENPP1	Association with obesity in independent samples. The obesity-associated polymorphism is functional (impairs insulin binding to the insulin receptor)
TNFA	Meta-analysis suggests linkage between polymorphism and BMI. The obesity associated polymorphism in the promoter is functional

allele has in different populations been shown to protect against obesity (124,125). A polymorphic CA repeat in the IL-6 gene has in two independent populations been reported to be associated with obesity (126). Furthermore, polymorphisms in the IL-6 receptor (IL-6R) have been reported to be associated with obesity in Pima Indians and a Spanish population (127,128).

Adipose tissue infiltrating macrophages are the source of resistin, which in experimental models is implicated in insulin resistance (106,129). Adipose tissue expression of resistin is increased in human obese subjects (129). One resistin 5'-flanking SNP has been reported to be associated with obesity in a Canadian, but not in a Swedish population (130).

CONCLUSIONS

It is an attractive hypothesis that some obesity genes have a primary role in regulating fat cell function (131). Expanding knowledge about adipose tissue cell and molecular biology has guided geneticists into analyzing specific adipose tissue expressed genes in human obesity. So far, established function in adipocytes and/ or strong evidence of genetic association has implied a handful of adipocyte genes in obesity. In this regard, the authors consider *PPARG*, *ADRB2*, *ADRB3*, *HSL*, *UCP2*, *ENPP1*, and *TNFA* of particular interest. The function of these genes imply that the primary place of action of some alleles predisposing to obesity is in adipocytes; by regulating adipogenesis (*PPARG*), as well as adipocyte lipolysis (*ADRB2*, *ADRB3*, *HSL*) and energy expenditure (*UCP2*). On the other hand, some of these genes are directly or indirectly involved in the secretory function of adipocytes. Besides *TNFA* modulators of lipolysis affect levels of circulating FFA, which can act as signaling molecules in metabolism. This suggests that alleles in adipocyte genes via peripheral effects regulate body weight potentially by effect on energy expenditure or food intake. The best described example of the latter is adipocytes-secreted leptin regulating food intake.

Due to a complex etiology of obesity and underpowered genetic studies it has proven difficult to unambiguously demonstrate association between gene alleles and obesity. If candidate genes are located in obesity-linked chromosomal regions this provides additional support, increasing the probability, that the genes have a role in obesity. On the other hand, true obesity-allele association does not require linkage to the chromosomal region. With the rapid development in human genome research, including new tools such as dense whole genome maps of common polymorphisms and high throughput genotyping allowing complete analysis of multiple genes in large materials of patients and controls, we predict that much of current controversies will be solved in the coming years. In addition, expanding knowledge in the field of adipocyte molecular biology provides new obesity candidates, for example transcription factors and cofactors, which should be analyzed for impact on human obesity. These development converge in the coanalysis of adipose tissue gene-expression profiles and gene alleles in obese and nonobese subjects.

REFERENCES

1. Arner P. The adipocyte in insulin resistance: key molecules and the impact of the thiazolidinediones. Trends Endocrinol Metab 2003; 14:137–45.
2. Bouchard C, Tremblay A, Despres JP, et al. The response to long-term overfeeding in identical twins. N Engl J Med 1990; 322:1477–82.

3. Tontonoz P, Hu E, Spiegelman BM. Stimulation of adipogenesis in fibroblasts by PPAR gamma 2, a lipid-activated transcription factor. Cell 1994; 79:1147–56.
4. Wu Z, Rosen ED, Brun R, et al. Cross-regulation of C/EBP alpha and PPAR gamma controls the transcriptional pathway of adipogenesis and insulin sensitivity. Mol Cell 1999; 3:151–8.
5. Lehrke M, Lazar MA. The many faces of PPARgamma. Cell 2005; 123:993–9.
6. Vidal-Puig AJ, Considine RV, Jimenez-Linan M, et al. Peroxisome proliferator-activated receptor gene expression in human tissues. Effects of obesity, weight loss, and regulation by insulin and glucocorticoids. J Clin Invest 1997; 99:2416–22.
7. Rieusset J, Andreelli F, Auboeuf D, et al. Insulin acutely regulates the expression of the peroxisome proliferator-activated receptor-gamma in human adipocytes. Diabetes 1999; 48:699–705.
8. Gurnell M. Peroxisome proliferator-activated receptor gamma and the regulation of adipocyte function: lessons from human genetic studies. Best Pract Res Clin Endocrinol Metab 2005; 19:501–23.
9. Masud S, Ye S. Effect of the peroxisome proliferator activated receptor-gamma gene Pro12Ala variant on body mass index: a meta-analysis. J Med Genet 2003; 40:773–80.
10. Deeb SS, Fajas L, Nemoto M, et al. A Pro12Ala substitution in PPARgamma2 associated with decreased receptor activity, lower body mass index and improved insulin sensitivity. Nat Genet 1998; 20:284–7.
11. Luan J, Browne PO, Harding AH, et al. Evidence for gene-nutrient interaction at the PPARgamma locus. Diabetes 2001; 50:686–9.
12. Kim JB, Spiegelman BM. ADD1/SREBP1 promotes adipocyte differentiation and gene expression linked to fatty acid metabolism. Genes Dev 1996; 10:1096–107.
13. Fajas L, Schoonjans K, Gelman L, et al. Regulation of peroxisome proliferator-activated receptor gamma expression by adipocyte differentiation and determination factor 1/sterol regulatory element binding protein 1: implications for adipocyte differentiation and metabolism. Mol Cell Biol 1999; 19:5495–503.
14. Kolehmainen M, Vidal H, Alhava E, et al. Sterol regulatory element binding protein 1c (SREBP-1c) expression in human obesity. Obes Res 2001; 9:706–12.
15. Eberle D, Clement K, Meyre D, et al. SREBF-1 gene polymorphisms are associated with obesity and type 2 diabetes in French obese and diabetic cohorts. Diabetes 2004; 53:2153–7.
16. Davis KE, Moldes M, Farmer SR. The forkhead transcription factor FoxC2 inhibits white adipocyte differentiation. J Biol Chem 2004; 279:42453–61.
17. Cederberg A, Gronning LM, Ahren B, et al. FOXC2 is a winged helix gene that counteracts obesity, hypertriglyceridemia, and diet-induced insulin resistance. Cell 2001; 106:563–73.
18. Kovacs P, Lehn-Stefan A, Stumvoll M, et al. Genetic variation in the human winged helix/forkhead transcription factor gene FOXC2 in Pima Indians. Diabetes 2003; 52:1292–5.
19. Carlsson E, Almgren P, Hoffstedt J, et al. The FOXC2 C-512T polymorphism is associated with obesity and dyslipidemia. Obes Res 2004; 12:1738–43.
20. Di Gregorio GB, Westergren R, Enerback S, et al. Expression of FOXC2 in adipose and muscle and its association with whole body insulin sensitivity. Am J Physiol Endocrinol Metab 2004; 287:E799–803.
21. Phan J, Reue K. Lipin, a lipodystrophy and obesity gene. Cell Metab 2005; 1:73–83.
22. Suviolahti E, Reue K, Cantor RM, et al. Cross-species analyses implicate Lipin 1 involvement in human glucose metabolism. Hum Mol Genet 2006; 15:377–86.
23. Hegele RA, Cao H, Harris SB, et al. Genetic variation in LMNA modulates plasma leptin and indices of obesity in aboriginal Canadians. Physiol Genomics 2000; 3:39–44.
24. Hegele RA, Huff MW, Young TK. Common genomic variation in LMNA modulates indexes of obesity in Inuit. J Clin Endocrinol Metab 2001; 86:2747–51.
25. Peeke PM, Chrousos GP. Hypercortisolism and obesity. Ann NY Acad Sci 1995; 771:665–76.

26. Grunfeld C, Baird K, Van Obberghen E, et al. Glucocorticoid-induced insulin resistance in vitro: evidence for both receptor and postreceptor defects. Endocrinology 1981; 109:1723–30.

27. Boullu-Ciocca S, Paulmyer-Lacroix O, Fina F, et al. Expression of the mRNAs coding for the glucocorticoid receptor isoforms in obesity. Obes Res 2003; 11:925–9.

28. Tomlinson JW, Walker EA, Bujalska IJ, et al. 11beta-hydroxysteroid dehydrogenase type 1: a tissue-specific regulator of glucocorticoid response. Endocr Rev 2004; 25:831–66.

29. van Rossum EF, Lamberts SW. Polymorphisms in the glucocorticoid receptor gene and their associations with metabolic parameters and body composition. Recent Prog Horm Res 2004; 59:333–57.

30. Martin LJ, Cianflone K, Zakarian R, et al. Bivariate linkage between acylation-stimulating protein and BMI and high-density lipoproteins. Obes Res 2004; 12:669–78.

31. Large V, Peroni O, Letexier D, et al. Metabolism of lipids in human white adipocyte. Diabetes Metab 2004; 30:294–309.

32. Moro C, Crampes F, Sengenes C, et al. Atrial natriuretic peptide contributes to physiological control of lipid mobilization in humans. FASEB J 2004; 18:908–10.

33. Green SA, Turki J, Bejarano P, et al. Influence of beta 2-adrenergic receptor genotypes on signal transduction in human airway smooth muscle cells. Am J Respir Cell Mol Biol 1995; 13:25–33.

34. McGraw DW, Forbes SL, Kramer LA, et al. Polymorphisms of the 5' leader cistron of the human beta2-adrenergic receptor regulate receptor expression. J Clin Invest 1998; 102:1927–32.

35. Large V, Hellstrom L, Reynisdottir S, et al. Human beta-2 adrenoceptor gene polymorphisms are highly frequent in obesity and associate with altered adipocyte beta-2 adrenoceptor function. J Clin Invest 1997; 100:3005–13.

36. Rosmond R. Association studies of genetic polymorphisms in central obesity: a critical review. Int J Obes Relat Metab Disord 2003; 27:1141–51.

37. Drysdale CM, McGraw DW, Stack CB, et al. Complex promoter and coding region beta 2-adrenergic receptor haplotypes alter receptor expression and predict in vivo responsiveness. Proc Natl Acad Sci USA 2000; 97:10483–8.

38. Eriksson P, Dahlman I, Ryden M, et al. Relationship between beta-2 adrenoceptor gene haplotypes and adipocyte lipolysis in women. Int J Obes Relat Metab Disord 2004; 28(2):185–90.

39. Jiao H, Dahlman I, Eriksson P, et al. A common beta2-adrenoceptor gene haplotype protects against obesity in Swedish women. Obes Res 2005; 13:1645–50.

40. Clement K, Vaisse C, Manning BS, et al. Genetic variation in the beta 3-adrenergic receptor and an increased capacity to gain weight in patients with morbid obesity. N Engl J Med 1995; 333:352–4.

41. Sipilainen R, Uusitupa M, Heikkinen S, et al. Polymorphism of the beta3-adrenergic receptor gene affects basal metabolic rate in obese Finns. Diabetes 1997; 46:77–80.

42. Kadowaki H, Yasuda K, Iwamoto K, et al. A mutation in the beta 3-adrenergic receptor gene is associated with obesity and hyperinsulinemia in Japanese subjects. Biochem Biophys Res Commun 1995; 215:555–60.

43. Hoffstedt J, Poirier O, Thorne A, et al. Polymorphism of the human beta3-adrenoceptor gene forms a well-conserved haplotype that is associated with moderate obesity and altered receptor function. Diabetes 1999; 48:203–5.

44. Gagnon J, Mauriege P, Roy S, et al. The Trp64Arg mutation of the beta3-adrenergic receptor gene has no effect on obesity phenotypes in the Quebec Family Study and Swedish Obese Subjects cohorts. J Clin Invest 1996; 98:2086–93.

45. Mason DA, Moore JD, Green SA, et al. A gain-of-function polymorphism in a G-protein coupling domain of the human beta1-adrenergic receptor. J Biol Chem 1999; 274:12670–4.

46. Dionne IJ, Garant MJ, Nolan AA, et al. Association between obesity and a polymorphism in the beta(1)-adrenoceptor gene (Gly389Arg ADRB1) in Caucasian women. Int J Obes Relat Metab Disord 2002; 26:633–9.

47. Ryden M, Hoffstedt J, Eriksson P, et al. The Arg 389 Gly beta1-adrenergic receptor gene polymorphism and human fat cell lipolysis. Int J Obes Relat Metab Disord 2001; 25:1599–603.

48. Siffert W, Rosskopf D, Siffert G, et al. Association of a human G-protein beta3 subunit variant with hypertension. Nat Genet 1998; 18:45–8.

49. Ryden M, Faulds G, Hoffstedt J, et al. Effect of the (C825T) Gbeta(3) polymorphism on adrenoceptor-mediated lipolysis in human fat cells. Diabetes 2002; 51:1601–8.

50. Siffert W, Forster P, Jockel KH, et al. Worldwide ethnic distribution of the G protein beta3 subunit 825T allele and its association with obesity in Caucasian, Chinese, and Black African individuals. J Am Soc Nephrol 1999; 10:1921–30.

51. Benjafield AV, Lin RC, Dalziel B, et al. G-protein beta3 subunit gene splice variant in obesity and overweight. Int J Obes Relat Metab Disord 2001; 25:777–80.

52. Talmud PJ, Palmen J, Walker M. Identification of genetic variation in the human hormone-sensitive lipase gene and 5' sequences: homology of 5' sequences with mouse promoter and identification of potential regulatory elements. Biochem Biophys Res Commun 1998; 252:661–8.

53. Garenc C, Perusse L, Chagnon YC, et al. The hormone-sensitive lipase gene and body composition: the HERITAGE Family Study. Int J Obes Relat Metab Disord 2002; 26:220–7.

54. Magre J, Laurell H, Fizames C, et al. Human hormone-sensitive lipase: genetic mapping, identification of a new dinucleotide repeat, and association with obesity and NIDDM. Diabetes 1998; 47:284–6.

55. Hoffstedt J, Arner P, Schalling M, et al. A common hormone-sensitive lipase i6 gene polymorphism is associated with decreased human adipocyte lipolytic function. Diabetes 2001; 50:2410–3.

56. Lavebratt C, Ryden M, Schalling M, et al. The hormone-sensitive lipase i6 gene polymorphism and body fat accumulation. Eur J Clin Invest 2002; 32:938–42.

57. Kern PA, Di Gregorio G, Lu T, et al. Perilipin expression in human adipose tissue is elevated with obesity. J Clin Endocrinol Metab 2004; 89:1352–8.

58. Mottagui-Tabar S, Ryden M, Lofgren P, et al. Evidence for an important role of perilipin in the regulation of human adipocyte lipolysis. Diabetologia 2003; 46:789–97.

59. Qi L, Shen H, Larson I, et al. Gender-specific association of a perilipin gene haplotype with obesity risk in a white population. Obes Res 2004; 12:1758–65.

60. Qi L, Corella D, Sorli JV, et al. Genetic variation at the perilipin (PLIN) locus is associated with obesity-related phenotypes in White women. Clin Genet 2004; 66:299–310.

61. Wilson-Fritch L, Nicoloro S, Chouinard M, et al. Mitochondrial remodeling in adipose tissue associated with obesity and treatment with rosiglitazone. J Clin Invest 2004; 114:1281–9.

62. Boss O, Samec S, Paoloni-Giacobino A, et al. Uncoupling protein-3: a new member of the mitochondrial carrier family with tissue-specific expression. FEBS Lett 1997; 408:39–42.

63. Cassard AM, Bouillaud F, Mattei MG, et al. Human uncoupling protein gene: structure, comparison with rat gene, and assignment to the long arm of chromosome 4. J Cell Biochem 1990; 43:255–64.

64. Gimeno RE, Dembski M, Weng X, et al. Cloning and characterization of an uncoupling protein homolog: a potential molecular mediator of human thermogenesis. Diabetes 1997; 46:900–6.

65. Bouillaud F, Ricquier D, Mory G, et al. Increased level of mRNA for the uncoupling protein in brown adipose tissue of rats during thermogenesis induced by cold exposure or norepinephrine infusion. J Biol Chem 1984; 259:11583–6.

66. Oberkofler H, Dallinger G, Liu YM, et al. Uncoupling protein gene: quantification of expression levels in adipose tissues of obese and non-obese humans. J Lipid Res 1997; 38:2125–33.

67. Esterbauer H, Oberkofler H, Liu YM, et al. Uncoupling protein-1 mRNA expression in obese human subjects: the role of sequence variations at the uncoupling protein-1 gene locus. J Lipid Res 1998; 39:834–44.

68. Clement K, Ruiz J, Cassard-Doulcier AM, et al. Additive effect of A→G (−3826) variant of the uncoupling protein gene and the Trp64Arg mutation of the beta 3-adrenergic receptor gene on weight gain in morbid obesity. Int J Obes Relat Metab Disord 1996; 20:1062–6.

69. Urhammer SA, Fridberg M, Sørensen TIA, et al. Studies of genetic variability of the uncoupling protein 1 gene in Caucasian subjects with juvenile-onset obesity. J Clin Endocrinol Metab 1997; 82:4069–74.

70. Urhammer SA, Hansen T, Borch-Johnsen K, et al. Studies of the synergistic effect of the Trp/Arg64 polymorphism of the beta3-adrenergic receptor gene and the −3826 A→G variant of the uncoupling protein-1 gene on features of obesity and insulin resistance in a population-based sample of 379 young Danish subjects. J Clin Endocrinol Metab 2000; 85:3151–4.

71. Millet L, Vidal H, Andreelli F, et al. Increased uncoupling protein-2 and -3 mRNA expression during fasting in obese and lean humans. J Clin Invest 1997; 100:2665–70.

72. Oberkofler H, Liu YM, Esterbauer H, et al. Uncoupling protein-2 gene: reduced mRNA expression in intraperitoneal adipose tissue of obese humans. Diabetologia 1998; 41:940–6.

73. Esterbauer H, Schneitler C, Oberkofler H, et al. A common polymorphism in the promoter of UCP2 is associated with decreased risk of obesity in middle-aged humans. Nat Genet 2001; 28:178–83.

74. Walder K, Norman RA, Hanson RL, et al. Association between uncoupling protein polymorphisms (UCP2–UCP3) and energy metabolism/obesity in Pima Indians. Hum Mol Genet 1998; 7:1431–5.

75. Cassell PG, Neverova M, Janmohamed S, et al. An uncoupling protein 2 gene variant is associated with a raised body mass index but not Type II diabetes. Diabetologia 1999; 42:688–92.

76. Argyropoulos G, Brown AM, Willi SM, et al. Effects of mutations in the human uncoupling protein 3 gene on the respiratory quotient and fat oxidation in severe obesity and type 2 diabetes. J Clin Invest 1998; 102:1345–51.

77. Lanouette CM, Giacobino JP, Perusse L, et al. Association between uncoupling protein 3 gene and obesity-related phenotypes in the Quebec Family Study. Mol Med 2001; 7:433–41.

78. Otabe S, Clement K, Dina C, et al. A genetic variation in the 5' flanking region of the UCP3 gene is associated with body mass index in humans in interaction with physical activity. Diabetologia 2000; 43:245–9.

79. Damcott CM, Feingold E, Moffett SP, et al. Genetic variation in uncoupling protein 3 is associated with dietary intake and body composition in females. Metabolism 2004; 53:458–64.

80. Puigserver P, Wu Z, Park CW, et al. A cold-inducible coactivator of nuclear receptors linked to adaptive thermogenesis. Cell 1998; 92:829–39.

81. Larrouy D, Vidal H, Andreelli F, et al. Cloning and mRNA tissue distribution of human PPARgamma coactivator-1. Int J Obes Relat Metab Disord 1999; 23:1327–32.

82. Semple RK, Crowley VC, Sewter CP, et al. Expression of the thermogenic nuclear hormone receptor coactivator PGC-1alpha is reduced in the adipose tissue of morbidly obese subjects. Int J Obes Relat Metab Disord 2004; 28:176–9.

83. Hammarstedt A, Jansson PA, Wesslau C, et al. Reduced expression of PGC-1 and insulin-signaling molecules in adipose tissue is associated with insulin resistance. Biochem Biophys Res Commun 2003; 301:578–82.

84. Esterbauer H, Oberkofler H, Linnemayr V, et al. Peroxisome proliferator-activated receptor-gamma coactivator-1 gene locus: associations with obesity indices in middle-aged women. Diabetes 2002; 51:1281–6.

85. Mootha VK, Handschin C, Arlow D, et al. Erralpha and Gabpa/b specify PGC-1alpha-dependent oxidative phosphorylation gene expression that is altered in diabetic muscle. Proc Natl Acad Sci USA 2004; 101:6570–5.

86. Kamei Y, Lwin H, Saito K, et al. The 2.3 genotype of ESRRA23 of the ERR alpha gene is associated with a higher BMI than the 2.2 genotype. Obes Res 2005; 13:1843–4.

87. Meirhaeghe A, Crowley V, Lenaghan C, et al. Characterization of the human, mouse and rat PGC1 beta (peroxisome-proliferator-activated receptor-gamma co-activator 1 beta) gene in vitro and in vivo. Biochem J 2003; 373:155–65.
88. Andersen G, Wegner L, Yanagisawa K, et al. Evidence of an association between genetic variation of the coactivator PGC-1beta and obesity. J Med Genet 2005; 42:402–7.
89. Zhou Z, Yon Toh S, Chen Z, et al. Cidea-deficient mice have lean phenotype and are resistant to obesity. Nat Genet 2003; 35:49–56.
90. Nordstrom EA, Ryden M, Backlund EC, et al. A human-specific role of cell death-inducing DFFA (DNA Fragmentation Factor-{alpha})-like effector a (CIDEA) in adipocyte lipolysis and obesity. Diabetes 2005; 54:1726–34.
91. Dahlman I, Kaaman M, Jiao H, et al. The CIDEA gene V115F polymorphism is associated with obesity in Swedish subjects. Diabetes 2005; 54:3032–4.
92. Bluher M, Michael MD, Peroni OD, et al. Adipose tissue selective insulin receptor knockout protects against obesity and obesity-related glucose intolerance. Dev Cell 2002; 3:25–38.
93. Stumvoll M, Haring H. Insulin resistance and insulin sensitizers. Horm Res 2001; 55(Suppl. 2):3–13.
94. Baumann CA, Ribon V, Kanzaki M, et al. CAP defines a second signalling pathway required for insulin-stimulated glucose transport. Nature 2000; 407:202–7.
95. Lin WH, Chiu KC, Chang HM, et al. Molecular scanning of the human sorbin and SH3-domain-containing-1 (SORBS1) gene: positive association of the T228A polymorphism with obesity and type 2 diabetes. Hum Mol Genet 2001; 10:1753–60.
96. Mathews ST, Singh GP, Ranalletta M, et al. Improved insulin sensitivity and resistance to weight gain in mice null for the Ahsg gene. Diabetes 2002; 51:2450–8.
97. Dahlman I, Eriksson P, Kaaman M, et al. alpha2-Heremans–Schmid glycoprotein gene polymorphisms are associated with adipocyte insulin action. Diabetologia 2004; 47:1974–9.
98. Lavebratt C, Wahlqvist S, Nordfors L, et al. AHSG gene variant is associated with leanness among Swedish men. Hum Genet 2005; 117:54–60.
99. Meyre D, Bouatia-Naji N, Tounian A, et al. Variants of ENPP1 are associated with childhood and adult obesity and increase the risk of glucose intolerance and type 2 diabetes. Nat Genet 2005; 37:863–7.
100. Mizutani T, Nishikawa Y, Adachi H, et al. Identification of estrogen receptor in human adipose tissue and adipocytes. J Clin Endocrinol Metab 1994; 78:950–4.
101. Dahlman I, Linder K, Arvidsson Nordstrom E, et al. NUGENOB: changes in adipose tissue gene expression by energy-restricted diets in obese women. Am J Clin Nutr 2005; 81:1275–85.
102. Okura T, Koda M, Ando F, et al. Association of polymorphisms in the estrogen receptor alpha gene with body fat distribution. Int J Obes Relat Metab Disord 2003; 27:1020–7.
103. Fox CS, Yang Q, Cupples LA, et al. Sex-specific association between estrogen receptor-alpha gene variation and measures of adiposity: the Framingham Heart Study. J Clin Endocrinol Metab 2005; 90:6257–62.
104. Berg AH, Combs TP, Du X, et al. The adipocyte-secreted protein Acrp30 enhances hepatic insulin action. Nat Med 2001; 7:947–53.
105. Salmenniemi U, Zacharova J, Ruotsalainen E, et al. Association of adiponectin level and variants in the adiponectin gene with glucose metabolism, energy expenditure, and cytokines in offspring of type 2 diabetic patients. J Clin Endocrinol Metab 2005; 90:4216–23.
106. Koerner A, Kratzsch J, Kiess W. Adipocytokines: leptin—the classical, resistin—the controversical, adiponectin—the promising, and more to come. Best Pract Res Clin Endocrinol Metab 2005; 19:525–46.
107. Menzaghi C, Ercolino T, Di Paola R, et al. A haplotype at the adiponectin locus is associated with obesity and other features of the insulin resistance syndrome. Diabetes 2002; 51:2306–12.
108. Bouatia-Naji N, Meyre D, Lobbens S, et al. ACDC/adiponectin polymorphisms are associated with severe childhood and adult obesity. Diabetes 2006; 55:545–50.

109. Kadowaki T, Yamauchi T. Adiponectin and adiponectin receptors. Endocr Rev 2005; 26:439–51.
110. Ma LJ, Mao SL, Taylor KL, et al. Prevention of obesity and insulin resistance in mice lacking plasminogen activator inhibitor 1. Diabetes 2004; 53:336–46.
111. Liang X, Kanjanabuch T, Mao SL, et al. Plasminogen activator inhibitor-1 modulates adipocyte differentiation. Am J Physiol Endocrinol Metab 2006; 290:E103–3.
112. Pandey M, Loskutoff DJ, Samad F. Molecular mechanisms of tumor necrosis factor-alpha-mediated plasminogen activator inhibitor-1 expression in adipocytes. FASEB J 2005; 19:1317–9.
113. Eriksson P, Reynisdottir S, Lonnqvist F, et al. Adipose tissue secretion of plasminogen activator inhibitor-1 in non-obese and obese individuals. Diabetologia 1998; 41:65–71.
114. Hoffstedt J, Andersson IL, Persson L, et al. The common –675 4G/5G polymorphism in the plasminogen activator inhibitor-1 gene is strongly associated with obesity. Diabetologia 2002; 45:584–7.
115. Freeman MS, Mansfield MW, Hoffstedt J, et al. The common –675 4G/5G polymorphism in the plasminogen activator inhibitor-1 gene is strongly associated with obesity. Diabetologia 2002; 45:1602–3 [author reply 1604].
116. Weisberg SP, McCann D, Desai M, et al. Obesity is associated with macrophage accumulation in adipose tissue. J Clin Invest 2003; 112:1796–808.
117. Hotamisligil GS, Arner P, Caro JF, et al. Increased adipose tissue expression of tumor necrosis factor-alpha in human obesity and insulin resistance. J Clin Invest 1995; 95:2409–15.
118. Arvidsson E, Viguerie N, Andersson I, et al. Effects of different hypocaloric diets on protein secretion from adipose tissue of obese women. Diabetes 2004; 53:1966–71.
119. Hotamisligil GS, Murray DL, Choy LN, et al. Tumor necrosis factor alpha inhibits signaling from the insulin receptor. Proc Natl Acad Sci USA 1994; 91:4854–8.
120. Sartipy P, Loskutoff DJ. Monocyte chemoattractant protein 1 in obesity and insulin resistance. Proc Natl Acad Sci USA 2003; 100:7265–70.
121. Norman RA, Bogardus C, Ravussin E. Linkage between obesity and a marker near the tumor necrosis factor-alpha locus in Pima Indians. J Clin Invest 1995; 96:158–62.
122. Wilson AG, Symons JA, McDowell TL, et al. Effects of a polymorphism in the human tumor necrosis factor alpha promoter on transcriptional activation. Proc Natl Acad Sci USA 1997; 94:3195–9.
123. Sookoian SC, Gonzalez C, Pirola CJ. Meta-analysis on the G-308A tumor necrosis factor {alpha} gene variant and phenotypes associated with the metabolic syndrome. Obes Res 2005; 13:2122–31.
124. Berthier MT, Paradis AM, Tchernof A, et al. The interleukin 6-174G/C polymorphism is associated with indices of obesity in men. J Hum Genet 2003; 48:14–9.
125. Wernstedt I, Eriksson AL, Berndtsson A, et al. A common polymorphism in the interleukin-6 gene promoter is associated with overweight. Int J Obes Relat Metab Disord 2004; 28:1272–9.
126. Huang QY, Shen H, Deng HY, et al. Linkage and association of the CA repeat polymorphism of the IL6 gene, obesity-related phenotypes, and bone mineral density (BMD) in two independent Caucasian populations. J Hum Genet 2003; 48:430–7.
127. Wolford JK, Colligan PB, Gruber JD, et al. Variants in the interleukin 6 receptor gene are associated with obesity in Pima Indians. Mol Genet Metab 2003; 80:338–43.
128. Escobar-Morreale HF, Calvo RM, Villuendas G, et al. Association of polymorphisms in the interleukin 6 receptor complex with obesity and hyperandrogenism. Obes Res 2003; 11:987–96.
129. Savage DB, Sewter CP, Klenk ES, et al. Resistin/Fizz3 expression in relation to obesity and peroxisome proliferator-activated receptor-gamma action in humans. Diabetes 2001; 50:2199–202.
130. Engert JC, Vohl MC, Williams SM, et al. 5' flanking variants of resistin are associated with obesity. Diabetes 2002; 51:1629–34.
131. Arner P. Obesity—a genetic disease of adipose tissue? Br J Nutr 2000; 83(Suppl. 1): S9–16.

Nutritional Regulation of Adipocyte Differentiation

Lise Madsen, Rasmus Koefoed Petersen, and Karsten Kristiansen
Eukaryotic Gene Expression and Differentiation Group, Department of Biochemistry and Molecular Biology, University of Southern Denmark, Odense, Denmark

Today's dietary problems of excessive energy intake and obesity are relatively new phenomena in evolutionary history. As man evolved, the ability to store excess energy as body fat was a favorable evolutionary strategy for survival in periods with limited food availability. Although humans evolved under fundamentally different environmental conditions, at the genetic level, we are still essentially the same as we were at the end of Paleolithic Era some 10,000 years ago. Thus, the human genome has hardly adapted to the profound dietary and environmental changes that were ushered in by the agricultural revolution some 10,000 years ago, a fairly recent development in evolutionary terms. Boyd Eaton and colleagues at Emory University have spent several decades reconstructing prehistoric diets from anthropological evidence and observations of surviving hunter-gatherer societies and several overview articles on the matter have been published.

Prior to the agricultural revolution, carbohydrate sources primarily consisted of wild plants, fruits, and vegetables. These contain far more complex and far less energy-dense carbohydrates than the cereal grains that gradually would dominate as carbohydrate sources after the agricultural revolution (1–3). Furthermore, the macronutrient composition in the preagricultural diet was high in protein and fat at the expense of carbohydrates (1–3). The Industrial Revolution some 200 years ago introduced further dietary pressures, placing a further burden on our genetic background.

Today, clinicians have few tools for fighting obesity efficiently. As dietary fat contains more calories than protein and carbohydrates, limiting the intake of fat has been recommended as a prophylactic by several official institutions, including the World Health Organization and the American Heart Association. As a result of this almost exclusive focus on dietary fat, food companies have removed fat and/or reduced the fat content of a wide variety of their products. During the last decade, however, this approach has come under increasing scrutiny, as there seems to be no direct relationship between fat-intake and obesity. In United States, energy intake from dietary fats dropped from 40% to 33% from the 1960s to 1995. In the same period, the number of obese adults (BMI 25 kg/m^2) steadily increased, reaching 56% in the early 1990s and 65% at present (4–6). Thus, action from the government has not been effective but, rather, counterproductive.

To a large extent, dietary fats have been substituted by refined carbohydrates. Furthermore, during the last decades, the intake of refined sugars from sources such as soft-drinks has increased dramatically. Soft-drinks, as well as other common products, such as cereals, contain refined sugars with high glycemic-index ratings that would have contributed little or no energy to the typical preagricultural diet prevailing during human evolution. Additionally, with an excess availability of food, our diets and lifestyle have become progressively more divergent from those of our ancient ancestors, as we no longer have to spend as much energy to obtain our food. On a macronutrient level, a number of the various alternative high-protein/low-carbohydrate diets of today, the Atkins Diet and the Zone Diet being the most popular, are more in line with the Stone Age diet. According to recent trials, several of these high-protein/low-carbohydrate diets are reported to induce weight loss in several trials recently reviewed (7), but the efficacy of such diets compared to traditional low-fat diets and the safety of their use are matters of dispute.

The dietary effects on adipose tissue development can be divided into effects on cell size and cell number. Formation of new adipocytes is a critical event in development of obesity, as mature adipocytes do not proliferate. Differentiation of multipotent mesenchymal stem cells or preadipocytes into lipid accumulating adipocytes is a physiological process induced by hormonal stimulation and sequential activation of key transcription factors. Here we focus on how macronutrients and dietary factors directly affect adipose tissue mass and development of obesity by targeting a set of key regulatory transcription factors involved in both adipocyte differentiation and lipid homeostasis in mature adipocytes. Fundamentally, adipocyte differentiation follows identical routes in man and rodents. As most experimental work has been performed using rodent models, including numerous informative transgenic models, this review primarily focuses on data obtained from studies on rodents.

ADIPOCYTE DIFFERENTIATION

The differentiation of preadipocytes into mature adipocytes is a rather well-characterized process whereby precursor cells are transformed into lipid-loaded mature fat cells. Three major classes of transcriptional regulators play pivotal roles in the differentiation process: peroxisome proliferator-activated receptors (PPARs), the CCAAT/enhancer–binding proteins (C/EBPs), and the adipocyte determination and differentiation-dependent factor-1 (ADD1)/sterol regulatory element-binding proteins (SREBPs). More recently, members of the liver X receptor (LXR) family were also suggested to play a role in adipocyte differentiation and function. Each of these transcription factors are potential sites for nutritional control. The role of these transcription factors in adipogenesis is discussed below (Fig. 1).

The Peroxisome Proliferator-Activated Receptors

The peroxisome proliferator-activated receptors (PPARs) comprise a subfamily of three nuclear receptors: peroxisome proliferator-activated receptor alpha (PPARA), peroxisome proliferator-activated receptor delta (PPARD), and peroxisome proliferator-activated receptor gamma (PPARG). The PPARs heterodimerize with members of the retinoid X receptor (RXR) subfamily and bind to PPAR-responsive elements in the regulatory regions of target genes. Ligands of both PPARs and RXRs enhance dimerization and DNA binding and induce expression of responsive genes. All three PPARs are involved in regulation of lipid metabolism, but each has a distinctive role. Although all three PPAR subtypes have been detected in adipose tissue, the key role in adipocyte development is orchestrated by PPARG, and the adipocyte differentiation process is strictly dependent on activation of this receptor (8–11). PPARG knockouts are embryonic lethal due to placental dysfunction (8,10,11). Embryo lethality can be circumvented by adipose tissue– targeted knockout of PPARG, which results in

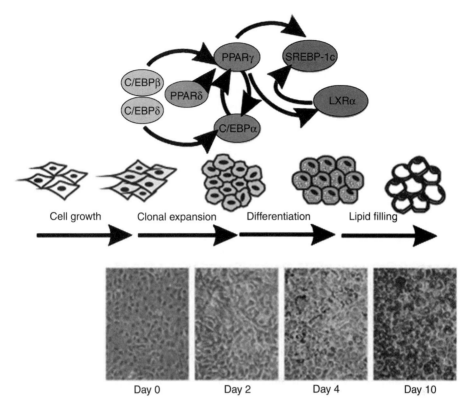

FIGURE 1 (*See color insert.*) The differentiation of preadipocytes into mature adipocytes is a highly regulated, multistep process that requires a coordinated program of transcriptional events leading to changes in gene expression. When confluent 3T3-L1 preadipocytes are treated with differentiation inducers, CEBPD and CEBPB are rapidly induced; the cells synchronously reenter the cell cycle and undergo approximately two rounds of cell division, a process termed "mitotic clonal expansion". Toward the end of the mitotic clonal expansion phase, CEBPB and CEBPD contribute to the induction of PPARG expression, which may also be promoted by activation of PPARD. CEBPB and CEBPD, together with PPARG, also induce expression of CEBPA. At this point, the cells round up and change phenotype. Once induced, CEBPA and PPARG2 are able to reciprocally induce expression of each other via a positive-feedback loop, which promotes and maintains the differentiated state. CEBPA cooperates with PPARG to induce additional target genes, such as the transcription factors SREBP and LXR, controlling expression of lipogenic genes, and the cells become lipid loaded.

severely lipodystrophic animals lacking adipose tissue (9). Heterozygous *Pparg*-deficient mice are reported to have decreased fat mass and smaller sized adipocytes (10,12,13).

PPARD is expressed in preadipocytes and may be induced during the initial stages of adipocyte differentiation (14). However, the role of PPARD in the differentiation process has been a matter of debate. A role for PPARD in development of adipose tissue is corroborated by the fact that adipose tissue stores are reduced in PPARD null mice (15,16). Recently, it was also demonstrated that adipocyte differentiation of *Ppard*-deficient cells is impaired even in the presence of a PPARG agonist (17). Overexpression of PPARD is insufficient to stimulate differentiation of fibroblasts (17,18) and 3T3-L1 cells (19). The lack of effect in these experiments may, however, be due to the lack of a cAMP-elevating agent. We have demonstrated that addition of a cAMP-elevating agent is crucial for the ability of PPARD ligands to induce expression of PPARG and induce adipocyte differentiation in PPARD expressing NIH-3T3 cells (20). Also, forced expression of PPARD has been reported to enhance the responsiveness of preadipocytes to PPARD ligands in terms of maximal response and sensitivity and to promote terminal differentiation by inducing *PPARG* expression (21). A second possible role for PPARD in adipogenesis is modulation of clonal expansion, as ligand activation of PPARD causes increased cell proliferation (21). Moreover, enforced expression of PPARD also renders the nonadipogenic 3T3-C2 cell-line capable of resuming cell proliferation in response to administration of fatty acids (22).

The last subtype, PPARA, is also expressed at low levels in preadipocytes, and expression is induced during adipocyte differentiation (23). However, PPARA is dispensable for adipocyte differentiation, as white adipose tissue develops normally in PPARA knockout mice. Nevertheless, larger adipose stores and increased body weight are reported in aged PPARA-deficient mice (24,25). This effect might be due to a decreased capacity of β-oxidation of fatty acids, as activation of PPARA is reported to increase fatty acid oxidation accompanied by increased mRNA levels of *UCP2* and *UCP3* (26). Feeding rodents PPARA activators is indeed known to reduce fat depots (27) and enhance mRNA levels and activity of enzymes involved in β-oxidation in adipose tissue (26,28).

CCAAT/Enhancer–Binding Protein (C/EBP)

CCAAT/EBPs constitute a family comprising six transcription factors of which four, CCAAT/EBP, alpha (CEBPA), beta (CEBPB), and delta (CEBPD) and, CHOP10 (approved name DNA-damage-inducible transcript 3) are expressed in preadipocytes/adipocytes (29–32). They all contain a highly conserved, basic leucine zipper domain at the C-terminus that is involved in dimerization and DNA binding. CEBPA, −B, and −D can form homo- and heterodimers with each other and are positively involved in adipocyte differentiation where the resulting different combinations of activator and repressor domains allow fine-tuning of the transcriptional response. CHOP10 is unable to form homodimers, and heterodimers involving CHOP10 are due to substitutions in the basic DNA binding region of CHOP10 unable to bind to canonical C/EBP responsive elements. Hence, CHOP10 functions as a negative regulator of C/EBP activity (31). Expression of *CHOP10* is induced by hypoxia (33) and very low glucose levels (34,35). Interestingly, the soy component genistein was shown to induce expression of *CHOP10* and inhibit adipocyte differentiation of 3T3-L1 preadipocytes (36). However, it remains to be established whether such mechanisms affect adipocyte function *in vivo*.

The expression of CEBPB and CEBPD is transiently induced during the early phases of differentiation, whereas CEBPA is induced later and remains expressed at high levels in mature adipocytes. CEBPB is reported to be important for clonal expansion (37), whereas CEBPA is important for growth arrest (38) and insulin sensitivity (39,40). Several lines of evidence indicate that CEBPB and CEBPD induce the expression of CEBPA and PPARG2 (30,40,41). Early studies indicated that binding of CEBPB to CEBP responsive elements were prevented during the early stages of differentiation (42), and it was suggested that this delay was caused by the high levels of CHOP10 present at the beginning of the differentiation process (43). However, later studies using ChIP have revealed that binding of CEBPB and CEBPD to regulatory elements in the CEBPA and PPARG2 promoters occurred with no delay and closely mirrored the accumulation of CEBPB and CEBPD in the differentiating cells (44). Still, it is clear that the transcription of the *PPARG2* and the *CEBPA* gene is first initiated once the cells have passed the G_1-S checkpoint of the mitotic clonal expansion process, an induction that may be dependent on a shift from CEBPB/CEBPD occupancy to CEBPA occupancy (44). Once induced, CEBPA and PPARG2 are then able to reciprocally induce expression of each other via a positive-feedback loop, which then promotes and maintains the differentiated state (45). For this reason, CEBPA and PPARG2 are considered key components for terminal differentiation. Mice lacking either the *Cebp* or *Cebpd* genes exhibit minor alteration in adipose tissue, but adipose tissue mass are severely decreased in mice lacking both (46). Mice with total *Cebpa* knockout lack adipose tissue and die a few hours after birth (47). Impaired liver gluconeogenesis and the resulting hypoglycemia appear to be major causes for the early death. Interestingly, transgenic expression of *Cebpa* in the liver of the knockout mice improves survival, but these mice are devoid of white adipose tissue, except for the mammary fat pad, whereas brown adipose tissue developed almost normally, suggesting that *Cebpa* is required for development of most white adipose tissue depots but not for brown adipose tissue (48).

Sterol Regulatory Element–Binding Proteins

Sterol regulatory element–binding proteins (SREBPs) or SREBF constitute a family of transcription factors involved in regulation of intracellular lipid homeostasis. Three SREBP isoforms exist, SREBP1A, SREBP1C, and SREBP2, that all have different roles in lipid synthesis. All SREBP transcription factors are synthesized as inactive precursors bound to the endoplasmic reticulum membranes. Upon activation, the precursor translocates to the Golgi, where it is proteolytically cleaved. The released active domain travels to the nucleus and activates transcription. The SREBP1C isoform mainly controls genes involved in fatty acid synthesis, whereas SREBP2 predominantly regulates genes involved in cholesterol synthesis. The SREBP1A isoform seems to be implicated in both pathways. SREBP1C is the predominant SREBP1 isoform expressed in adipose tissue (49). During adipocyte differentiation, SREBP1mRNA is highly induced (50), and the transcription factor is proteolytically activated (51). Several lines of evidence have suggested a role for SREBP1C in adipocyte differentiation, thereby its alternative name, ADD1 (50). The suggested roles for SREBP1C in adipocyte differentiation are activation of the CEBPB promoter (52) and induction of PPARG expression (53), as well as stimulation of the synthesis of an endogenous PPARG ligand (54). Although these findings strongly suggest a role for SREBP1C in adipocyte differentiation, SREBP1C knockout mice have normal adipose tissue (55,56), and mice that lack both the SREBP1C and −1A isoforms also have normal amounts of adipose tissue and fully differentiated adipocytes expressing normal levels of adipocyte-specific markers (57). Whereas adipocyte-specific overexpression of *Srebp1c* in mice surprisingly inhibits adipocyte differentiation in a severe manner and renders the mice lipodystrophic (58), adipocyte-specific transgenic expression of *Srebp1a* in mice led to massively enlarged adipocytes with increased expression of lipogenic genes and increased rates of de novo fatty acid synthesis (59).

The Nuclear Receptors

Liver X Receptors (LXRs) (approved gene name nuclear receptor subfamily 1, group H, member 2) exist in two subtypes, LXR alpha (LXR-α) and LXR beta (LXR-β), both being highly expressed in adipose tissue (60–62). Moreover, LXR-α expression is induced during adipocyte differentiation (63), and it was demonstrated that PPARG is a LXR-α target-gene in adipocytes (64). However, LXR is apparently dispensable as *Lxr*-α/-β double knockout mice develop adipose tissue (65,66). Older double knockout mice exhibit reduced adipose-tissue stores (65), but the basis for this phenotype is not yet known. The role of LXR as a modulator of adipogenesis has been a matter of debate, as different laboratories have obtained different results. Activation of LXR has been reported to increase differentiation (65) or to have no effect (63). Moreover, activation of ectopically expressed LXR-α was shown to inhibit differentiation (63), whereas suppression of LXR-α by siRNA in 3T3-L1 cells was reported to impair adipocyte differentiation (64).

CARBOHYDRATES

Types of Carbohydrates and Carbohydrate Sources

With the emergence of agriculture, grains such as corn, wheat, and rice became important nutritional sources providing a considerable amount of our daily energy intake. Today's diet includes these grains in the form of highly glycemic carbohydrates such as bread, cereals, and pasta where they contribute to monopolize a large percentage of our daily intake. Whatever the form, such carbohydrates contributed little or no energy to the typical preagricultural diet. During the last few centuries the intake of refined sugar has also increased tremendously. In England, the average annual intake of refined sucrose rose from 6.8 kg in 1815 to 54.5 kg in 1970, and similar trends are reported for Sweden, Norway, and Denmark (1,67). Over the last three decades, the increased consumption of refined sugar from soda and other soft-drinks has only escalated this trend. In Norway, the average intake of soda per year increased from 41 L in 1970 to 127 L (representing 9 kg refined sugar) in 2001 (68).

Maintenance of blood glucose within the normal range of 4.4 to 6.0 mmol/L requires a precise balance between peripheral tissue glucose uptake and hepatic glucose release. Intake of a meal containing carbohydrates elevates blood glucose and thereby triggering insulin secretion. The rise in insulin facilitates the insulin-dependent uptake of glucose by peripheral tissues, although this process is in balance with an insulin-independent uptake mechanism. In this respect, the type of carbohydrates in the meal is of great importance, as different types of carbohydrates have different glycemic index values (the glycemic index being an indicator of the ability of different carbohydrates to raise the blood glucose levels within 2 hrs). Generally, simple carbohydrates and refined grain carbohydrates produce high postprandial levels of blood glucose, whereas more complex carbohydrates have a lower glycemic index. Recently, it was demonstrated that obesity-prone C57BL/6J mouse fed a high glycemic-index diet after 9 weeks had 93% more body fat of those fed a low-glycemic-index diet (69).

A diet enriched in sucrose is able to induce glucose intolerance and insulin resistance in rodents both with (70–73) and without a concomitant induction of obesity (70,71). During absorption, sucrose is hydrolyzed into equal quantities of fructose and glucose. Blood glucose is then delivered to the adipocytes via insulin dependent and noninsulin dependent uptake. Fructose is, on the other hand, largely metabolized in an insulin-independent manner, but it appears that the fructose component is the primary nutrient mediator of sucrose-induced glucose intolerance and insulin resistance (74).

Increased blood levels of glucose and insulin render the body in an anabolic state that favors hepatic lipogenic activity and thus promotes postprandial carbohydrate oxidation at the expense of fat oxidation. Consequently, fuel partitioning is altered in a way that may be conducive to body fat gain. Under normal conditions, lipids are not stored in the liver, but transferred to peripheral tissues by chylomicroms and lipoproteins. The fatty acids are then released from the lipoproteins by increased adipocyte lipoprotein lipase activity from adipocytes. Under such circumstances, the glucose uptake in adipocytes is also enhanced due to upregulation of GLUT1 (solute carrier family 2 (facilitated glucose transporter), member 1) and GLUT4 (solute carrier family 2 (facilitated glucose transporter), member 4), the latter being predominant after a carbohydrate-rich meal. High glucose levels in the plasma thus render the body in a perfect condition for uptake and storage of lipids in adipose tissue.

Effect of Feeding Status (Blood Glucose) on Transcriptional Activity in Adipose Tissue

Feeding status may not only affect adipose tissue by controlling the number of adipose cells but may very well determine the amount of lipid in each cell. It is clear that insulin signaling in adipose tissue plays an important role in lipid storage and regulation of glucose homeostasis (75). Indeed, mice that have a fat-specific disruption of the insulin receptor gene have low fat mass (75). The expression of SREBP1 is altered concomitant with the two key genes of energy homeostasis, fatty acid synthase and leptin during fasting and refeeding of mice (76). The expression of lipogenic genes is controlled by the transcription factors SREBP1A and −1C (49,77,78), but the nutritional induction of genes involved in lipogenesis is mainly controlled by the SREBP1C isoform. When blood glucose and insulin levels are low, expression of SREBP1C and lipogenic genes is reduced dramatically in both liver (79) and adipose tissue (76). Interestingly, refeeding fasted animals a fat-free, high carbohydrate diet induces de novo fatty acid synthesis and expression of SREBP1C and lipogenic genes to levels significantly higher than those observed in the normal fed state in both liver (79) and adipose tissue (76). Insulin activates the rat SREBP1C promoter through the combined actions of SREBP, LXR, Sp-1, and NF-Y *cis*-acting elements.

The role of LXR-α in mediating the insulin response of lipogenic gene expression has received attention during recent years. As the increased expression of lipogenic genes in mice treated with LXR agonists is blunted in SREBP1C knockout mice, the role of SREBP1C in the LXR response appears to be essential (55). Also, LXR -α/-β-deficient mice have reduced expression of SREBP1C and lipogenic genes (80,81), and insulin regulation of several important lipogenic enzymes in liver is dependent on LXRs (82). Moreover, lipogenesis in adipocytes requires glucose that is supplied by transport through the insulin-responsive glucose transporter GLUT4 that is also directly regulated by the LXRs (83).

FAT
Dietary Fat

Several dieters consider the seemingly large amount of fat in our diet as the main culprit when it comes to the problems of obesity. The amount of fat in the modern

Western diet is, however, comparable to the moderate to high amount associated with Paleolitic nutrition (84). It is worth noting that the fatty acid composition of the preagricultural dietary fat was quite different. A modern Western diet contains little fish, and thus less n–3 PUFAs. On the other hand, today's diet is abundant in n–6 fatty acids from vegetable oils (corn, sunflower, safflower, cottonseed, and soybeans) that are used in industrially prepared food. In addition, industrially produced animal feed is also rich in grains containing n–6 PUFAs, leading to meat enriched in n–6 PUFAs at the expense of n–3 fatty acids (85). Whereas the ratio of n–6 to n–3 PUFAs in the Stone Age was 1:1, the ratio in the current Western diet is with a few exceptions 20 to 30 to 1 (84). Thus, it is the composition and nature of the fatty acids rather than the mere quantity of ingested fats that have undergone fundamental changes. Moreover, new manufacturing procedures have introduced fatty acids with atypical structural characteristics in vegetable oils. For instance, margarine is produced by partially solidifying vegetable oils via hydrogenation. The hydrogenation process produces novel *trans* fatty acid isomers that rarely, if ever, are found in natural food sources. *Trans* fatty acids are found in processed foods like commercial baked products such as cookies, cakes, and crackers, and even in bread, all of which benefit from a longer shelf life due to their inclusion. *Trans* fat is also used for frying and is found in large quantities in popular fast foods (86).

Feeding rodents a high-fat diet generally induces proliferation and differentiation of preadipocytes as well as adipose-tissue hypertrophy (87–93). The type of fat, however, is important since feeding fish oil enriched in n–3 PUFAs actually decreases body weight and fat mass in a dose-dependent manner (94). n–3 PUFAs are generally able to limit hyperplasia as well as hypertrophy in high fat fed rats (87,95–99). Concerning a diet enriched in n–6 PUFAs, a few studies demonstrate decreased adipose-tissue growth (100,101), but n–6 PUFAs are often associated with an increased propensity for obesity (102–104).

Dietary Fatty Acids as Modulators of Transcription Factors Involved in Adipocyte Differentiation

High fat feeding leads to increased levels of expression of the transcription factors CEBPA and PPARG and a number of PPARG-target genes involved in adipocyte differentiation and lipid storage (105). Most fatty acids are able to activate all three members of the PPAR family at micromolar concentrations (106–109). However, their ability to activate PPARG does not correlate to their ability to induce adipocyte differentiation (110). PUFAs are generally better activators of the PPARs than saturated fatty acids (110). On the other hand, whereas saturated fatty acids are weak stimulators of adipocyte differentiation, PUFAs have rather strong inhibitory effects (110). In contrast to the effect of n–6 versus n–3 PUFAs on adipose-tissue development in rodents, n–6 PUFAs have a stronger inhibitory effect than n–3 PUFAs on differentiation of 3T3-L1 cells (110).

PUFAs are activators of PPARA and they therefore are able to increase β-oxidation in mature adipocytes (110). Furthermore, there appears to be a good correlation between decreased amount of white adipose tissue and hepatic PPARA activation (94). Activation of PPARA by n–3 PUFAs increases hepatic β-oxidation and energy expenditure and thereby decreases the output of very low-density lipoprotein (VLDL) particles from the liver and limits triacylglycerol supply to adipose tissue. As triacylglycerol stores in fat cells are largely derived from circulating triacylglycerols, increased hepatic β-oxidation and decreased apolipo-protein expression and release of VLDL particles results in a repartitioning of fatty acids, which then are drained from blood and extrahepatic tissues.

Fatty acids are able to activate PPARD in transfection assays, but less is known about fatty acid–induced activation of PPARD in vivo. Similar to PPARD-agonists, dietary PUFAs, especially of the *n*–3 family, activate genes involved in β-oxidation in skeletal muscle as well as in brown and white adipose tissue (99,111–115). Thus, in addition to its role in adipocyte differentiation, PPARD seems to act as a key metabolic regulator of fat burning in peripheral tissues. Accordingly, adipose-tissue targeted expression of a constitutively active form of PPARD was shown to reduce adiposity (116). These transgenic animals have increased expression of genes required for fatty acid oxidation and energy dissipa-tion. Furthermore, treatment with PPARD agonists caused severe lipid depletion (116). Activation of PPARD in adipose tissue also reverses obesity in the leptin receptor deficient *Lepr*$^{db/db}$ mice (116).

PUFAs are also well-known to alter expression of lipogenic genes by interfer-ing with SREBP1 expression at different levels in mouse liver. Dietary PUFAs are able to both lower *SREBP1C* mRNA levels (117–119) as well as to inhibit the proteolytic maturation that is necessary for SREBP to exert transcriptional activity (94,120,121). Dietary PUFAs are also known to repress the expression of lipogenic genes in adipose tissue (97,122), but far less is known concerning the underlying mechanism in this tissue. During differentiation, de novo fatty acid synthesis also increases tremendously, but the rate of de novo fatty acid syntheses and triacylgly-cerol accumulation are severely decreased in the presence of PUFAs (110,123). Similar to the effect of PUFAs on differentiation and triacylglycerol accumulation, *n*–6 PUFAs are more effective than *n*–3 PUFAs in inhibiting de novo fatty acid synthesis (110). PUFAs of the *n*–6 family inhibit differentiation more efficiently than PUFAs of the *n*–3 family (110), and arachidonic acid reduces the rate of de novo fatty acid synthesis in both a prostaglandin-dependent and -independent manner. Part of the inhibitory action of arachidonic acid on fatty acid synthesis is probably due to its polyunsaturated nature as eicosapentaenoic acid (EPA) and docosahex-aenoic acid (DHA) of the *n*–3 PUFA family were also able to inhibit de novo fatty acid synthesis in a cyclooxygenase-independent manner (110,123).

LXR-α is a potent activator of SREBP1C expression and thereby expression of several lipogenic genes in both liver and adipose tissue (64,66). The increased expression of lipogenic genes in mice treated with LXR agonists is blunted in SREBP1C knockout mice, indicating an essential role for SREBP1C in the LXR response (55), and LXR α/β-deficient mice have reduced expression of SREBP1C and lipogenic genes (80,81). Two groups have suggested that LXR-α is responsible for mediating the PUFA effect on SREBP1 (124,125). Activation of the SREBP1C promoter by LXR-α is suppressed by PUFAs (125). *n*–6 PUFAs are more potent LXR antagonists than *n*–3 PUFAs, whereas monounsaturated and saturated fatty acids have little effect (125). Thus, it appears that PUFAs downregulate lipogenic gene expression by serving as antagonists for LXR in the liver. In differentiating 3T3-L1 cells, however, the inhibitory effect of PUFAs on de novo fatty acid synthesis and triacylglycerol accumulation was similar in both the absence and presence of the LXR-agonist (110).

In conclusion, it is evident that the type of dietary fat is of a great importance when it comes to development of obesity in rodents. Whereas a high fat diet enriched in saturated fat induces obesity, a diet enriched in PUFAs, in particular of the *n*–3 family, decreases adipose-tissue mass and suppresses the development of obesity in rodents. The precise underlying mechanism is, however, still not elucidated. One specific transcription factor may theoretically be responsible for mediating the action of PUFAs alone, but as a number of key regulatory transcription factors involved in adipogenesis are clearly targeted by PUFAs it is more likely that more than one is implicated.

PROTEINS
Dietary Protein and Effect on Metabolism
The primitive man consumed far more animal proteins than we do today. It is estimated that the average dietary protein intake constituted 37% of the total caloric intake (2). Currently, recommended daily protein intake is set at minimal levels necessary to prevent deficiency and to maintain nitrogen balance. The role of protein in diets is currently receiving considerably more interest. Although controversial, high-protein, low-carbohydrate diets are reported to increase weight loss and reduce loss of lean body mass in humans (126–132).

The precise effects of dietary proteins and amino acids have not yet been elucidated, as earlier studies have been focused on defining a minimum requirement to maintain nitrogen balance. The primary obvious role of dietary protein is of course to provide amino acids for endogenous protein synthesis, but amino acids also participate in a number of metabolic processes. Thus, intake of certain specific amino acids appears to have specific metabolic roles and potentially specific actions. One example is dietary tryptophan and tyrosine that may accumulate in the brain as precursors to neurotransmitters, potentially influencing appetite regulatory neurotransmitters (133). A second example is the well-known effect of branched chain amino acids (leucine, valine, and isoleucine) on the insulin signaling pathway and protein synthesis that will be discussed below.

Furthermore, an interrelationship between amino acid and glucose metabolism exists via the glucos-alanine cycle. After a meal, blood glucose is maintained within the normal homeostatic limits by insulin-stimulated glucose uptake in peripheral tissues. However, after an overnight fast, amino acids are the primary carbon source for gluconeogenesis and hepatic glucose release (134). In a similar manner, a low-carbohydrate and high-protein diet would theoretically reduce the role of insulin in managing acute changes in blood glucose and thus increase the role of the liver in supporting the maintenance of blood glucose. Although the mechanism is not yet elucidated, increased dietary protein at the expense of carbohydrate has been shown to stabilize blood glucose during the nonabsorptive periods and reduce postprandial insulin response (135).

Direct Effects of Amino Acids on Adipocytes
Whereas a diet enriched in sucrose and fat induces adipose-tissue mass in rodents, a diet enriched in protein is on the other hand reported to delay the development of adiposity and to improve glucose homeostasis in the obesity prone C57BL/6J mice (136). The underlying mechanisms for the effects of dietary protein are not yet understood and interpretations of the different published studies is complicated by the fact that the dietary protein sources differ in their amino acids profiles. Studies using dietary supplement of selective amino acids are scarce. So far, reduced body weight and obesity are observed by dietary supplementation of L-glutamine (137) and arginine (138).

Arginine and Nitric Oxide

Dietary arginine supplementation markedly reduces body weight as well as the weights of abdominal and epididymal adipose tissues (138). This effect was followed by increased nitric oxide synthesis, lipolysis, and oxidation of both glucose and octanoate in abdominal and epididymal adipose tissues (138). Nitric oxide, produced from arginine by nitric oxide synthase, plays an important role in fat metabolism. Nitric oxide is able to induce mitochondrial biogenesis by acting on PPARG coactivator-1A (PGC1A) expression (139–141) in diverse cell types, including adipocytes. Thus, nitric oxide may stimulate the oxidation of fatty acid in several organs, as well as adipocytes. This theory is supported by the fact that inhibition of systemic nitric oxide synthesis inhibits fatty acid β-oxidation and increase body fat mass in rats (142).

Leucine and Modulation of Insulin and mTOR Signaling

The metabolic effects of dietary-branched chain amino acids (leucine, valine, and isoleucine) have also received much attention during the last decade. In particular, leucine is described as a direct acting nutrient signal in adipocytes.

Branched chain amino acids are well known to stimulate secretion of insulin, glucagon, growth hormone, and insulin-like growth factor 1, but leucine also appears to regulate protein synthesis in adipose tissue by mechanisms that are independent of insulin (143). The effects of leucine on protein synthesis in adipocytes involve activation of the mammalian target of rapamycin (mTOR). In addition to protein synthesis, mTOR-signaling appears to be essential for differentiation of preadipocytes, adipose-tissue morphogenesis, hypertrophic growth, and leptin secretion. All of these functions are also reported to be regulated by leucine. For example, it has been shown that leucine regulates the organization of adipocytes into tissue-like structures (144), adipose tissue leptin synthesis/secretion (145), and protein synthesis (143,146).

The targets of the mTOR serine/threonine protein kinase pathway include several components of the translation machinery. In particular, a substrate of mTOR, the eukaryotic initiation factor 4E-binding protein-1 (EIF4EBP1), is of great interest, as this factor appears to be a novel regulator of adipogenesis and metabolism (147). Phosphorylation of EIF4EBP1 leads to its release from the eukaryotic initiation factor eIF4E, which then can interact with eIF4G and induce translation of a number of proteins. EIF4EBP1 is highly induced during differentiation of adipocytes and phosphorylated in response to insulin (148), and mice lacking this translational inhibitor have less white adipose tissue (147).

In isolated adipocytes, leucine stimulates phosphorylation of EIF4EBP1 and decreases its association with eIF-4E (149). As inhibition of mTOR by rapamycin is known to inhibit differentiation of adipocytes (150), the effect of leucine on EIF4EBP1phosphorylation would imply a stimulatory effect of leucine on adipocyte differentiation. However, the mTOR signaling pathway is also demonstrated to control the ratio of CEBPA isoforms in differentiating adipocytes. When eIF-4E is constitutively activated, CEBPA is expressed mainly in its truncated form (151). Growth arrest, contact inhibition and thereby terminal differentiation are prevented (151). The effect of a leucine-enriched diet on adipose tissue development and function would thus be interesting to evaluate.

In conclusion, it is evident that both the amount of protein in the diet, as well as the amino acid profile of the dietary protein is able to influence adipose tissue development and function. Further studies are, however, necessary to elucidate the underlying mechanisms.

MACRONUTRIENT INTERACTION

Macronutrients can regulate transcriptional activity and gene expression in adipocytes both directly and indirectly. It is well known that transcriptional activity and gene expression are regulated by major feeding hormone, insulin, as well as the classical hormones that are secreted in the fasted state, catecholamines and glucagon and their second messenger, cAMP. The amount of carbohydrates relative to the amount of protein and fat in the diet will influence the secretion of these hormones, and the relative composition of macronutrients in the diet will thus indirectly regulate transcriptional activity. In addition, different types of carbohydrates differ in their ability to regulate the secretion of both insulin and glucagons, and therefore the type of carbohydrate in the diet may profoundly affect the insulin/glucagon ratio. The types of protein and fat in the diet are also of both quantitative and qualitative importance, as certain amino acids and fatty acids can directly influence transcriptional activity in adipose tissue (Fig. 2).

While the knowledge concerning specific effects of certain macronutrients on transcriptional activity and gene expression is increasing, several unanswered questions remain, and some results seem to contradict each other. The indirect effect of macronutrients on the hormonal status of the animals might explain some of these findings. As an example, the effects of PUFAs are normally studied in animals fed a standard laboratory chow diet. Thus, plasma glucose and insulin levels are within the normal range, and the expression of LXR-α and SREBP1 are moderate. To unmask the inhibitory effects of PUFAs on SREBP-target genes, experiments must be performed where animals are refed after an overnight fast. Unfortunately, such experimental conditions may mask any effect of PUFAs on PPARA activation, as the expression of PPARA after fasting is low and the effect of PPARA activators are blunted (152,153).

This may be of particular importance concerning the effect of PUFAs of the n–6 family, as fundamentally opposite effects of n–6 fatty acids are reported on adipose-tissue development in animals and adipocyte differentiation in vitro (110). In vitro, the inhibitory effect of arachidonic acid requires elevation of cellular cAMP. In the absence of elevated cAMP levels, arachidonic acid acts proadipogenic, an effect that is potentiated by insulin. One could therefore postulate that the adipogenic effect of arachidonic acid on adipose tissue development in animals and possible also in humans, would be particular marked if a high arachidonic intake is combined with a high intake of carbohydrates.

CONCLUSION

Nutritional regulation of transcriptional activity and gene expression is an important mechanism in the adaptation of mammals to their nutritional environment, and a number of key regulatory transcription factors involved in adipogenesis are targeted by macronutrients. Although several factors, such as a large variety of different feeding regimes, complicate interpretation of the available published results, some general conclusions may be made.

When man evolved, both the qualitative and quantitative composition of macronutrients was very different from our modern diet. Prior to the agricultural revolution, the amount of carbohydrates in the diet was far lower than today and the available carbohydrate sources contained far more complex carbohydrates and far less energy-dense carbohydrates than carbohydrate sources that would

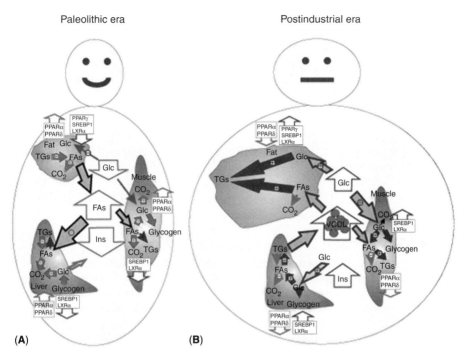

FIGURE 2   A simplified scheme of lipid homeostasis in the fed and fasted states. The size of the arrows indicates the magnitude of the flux of fatty acid and fatty acid metabolites. Potential stimulatory or inhibitory effects of (**A**) a Stone Age diet and (**B**) a modern diet on transcription factors are indicated with arrows. A Stone Age diet enriched in protein and fat would compare to a typical modern diet and lead to a lower plasma levels of insulin and glucose. Thus, the expression and activity of SREBP1 and LXR-a, and thereby of lipogenic genes, would be low. On the other hand, the expression and activity of transcription factors controlling fatty acid catabolism, PPARA and PPARD, would be high. Dietary fat might therefore be burned in the liver and in muscle. Moreover, free fatty acids from lipolysis in adipose tissue might be delivered to the liver where they can be burned. Conversely, a modern diet more enriched in carbohydrates, with a high glycemic index, leads to an increased plasma level of glucose and insulin. Thus, expression and activity of SREBP1 and LXR-α will be high, whereas expression and activity of PPARD and PPARA will be low. Under such circumstances, when lipogenesis is high and fatty acid β-oxidation in liver and muscle are low, both dietary and de novo synthesized fat are transported from the liver into the bloodstream within VLDL particles. Fatty acids are then taken up by peripheral tissues, where they can be stored.

dominate after the agricultural revolution. Frequent meals rich in protein and fat, such as those that dominated the diet of primitive man, would beneficially regulate both the hormonal status and transcriptional activity of several factors involved in adipogenesis. In contrast, a constant ingestion of sugar results in a chronically elevated level of blood sugar and insulin and thus renders the body in a constant lipogenic state. Under such conditions, fatty acid synthesis is high, whereas fatty acid oxidation and expression of PPARA and PPARD are low. Fatty acids are secreted from the liver into circulation and taken up by adipose tissue. Adding fat to such a diet would then increase fat storage in the adipose tissue.

In contrast to high glycemic carbohydrates, dietary proteins does not elevate plasma insulin and glucose levels. Indeed, increasing amounts of protein or low glycemic carbohydrates in the diet reduces the expression of LXR-α and SREBP1 while increasing expression of PPARA and PPARD. Under these conditions, fatty acids are mobilized from adipose tissue and fatty acid oxidation in both liver and peripheral tissue is high. Dietary fatty acids, especially PUFAs, can then via activation of PPARA and PPARD target genes contribute to activate genes that would contribute to their own catabolism.

Studies of macronutrient energy proportions in the diet of hunter-gatherer societies, analogous to those of our initial human ancestors, show a relatively high protein intake of 19% to 35%, a highly variable fat intake of 28% to 47% and low carbohydrate level of 22% to 40%. Current dietary guidelines advocate a daily intake of macronutrients with carbohydrates accounting for ≥55% of dietary energy, fats limited to ≤30% of dietary energy, and protein at ≤15% of energy. From a transcriptional activity point of view this is perhaps a shortsighted recommendation.

ACKNOWLEDGMENT

We wish to thank Christopher Chailland for helpful comments and suggestions during preparation of this manuscript. Work in the authors' laboratory has been supported by The Danish Biotechnology Program, The Danish Natural Science Research Council, and the European Community (contract QLK1-CT-2001-00183).

REFERENCES

1. Cordain L, Eaton SB, Sebastian A, et al. Origins and evolution of the Western diet: health implications for the 21st century. Am J Clin Nutr 2005; 81:341–54.
2. Eaton S, Eaton SB, Konner MJ, et al. An evolutionary perspective enhances understanding of human nutritional requirements. J Nutr 1996; 126:1732–40.
3. Cordain L, Miller JB, Eaton SB, et al. Plant-animal subsistence ratios and macronutrient energy estimations in worldwide hunter-gatherer diets. Am J Clin Nutr 2000; 71:682–92.
4. Connor WE, Connor SL, Katan MB, et al. Should a low-fat, high-carbohydrate diet be recommended for everyone? N Engl J Med 1997; 337:562–7.
5. Hill JO, Wyatt HR, Reed GW, et al. Obesity and the environment: where do we go from here? Science 2003; 299:853–5.
6. Weinberg SL. The diet-heart hypothesis: a critique. J Am Coll Cardiol 2004; 43:731–3.
7. Schoeller A, Buchholz AC. Energetics of obesity and weight control: does diet composition matter? J Am Diet Assoc 2005; 105:24–8.
8. Barak Y, Nelson MC, Ong ES, et al. PPARγ is required for placental, cardiac, and adipose tissue development. Mol Cell 1999; 4:585–95.
9. Koutnikova H, Cock TA, Watanabe M, et al. Compensation by the muscle limits the metabolic consequences of lipodystrophy in PPARγ hypomorphic mice. PNAS 2003; 100:14457–62.
10. Kubota N, Terauchi Y, Miki H, et al. PPARγ Mediates high-fat diet-induced adipocyte hypertrophy and insulin resistance. Mol Cell 1999; 4:597–609.
11. Rosen ED, Sarraf P, Troy AE, et al. PPARγ is required for the differentiation of adipose tissue in vivo and in vitro. Mol Cell 1999; 4:611–7.
12. Kadowaki T, Hara K, Kubota N, et al. The role of PPARgamma in high-fat diet-induced obesity and insulin resistance. J Diabetes Complications 2002; 16:41–5.
13. Yamauchi T, Kamon J, Waki H, et al. The mechanisms by which both heterozygous peroxisome proliferator-activated receptor gamma (PPARgamma) deficiency and PPARgamma agonist improve insulin resistance. J Biol Chem 2001; 276:41245–54.
14. Amri EZ, Bonino F, Ailhaud G, et al. Cloning of a protein that mediates transcriptional effects of fatty acids in preadipocytes. J Biol Chem 1995; 270:2367–71.

15. Barak Y, Liao D, He W, et al. Effects of peroxisome proliferator-activated receptor delta on placentation, adiposity, and colorectal cancer. PNAS 2002; 99:303–8.
16. Peters JM, Lee SST, Li W, et al. Growth, adipose, brain, and skin alterations resulting from targeted disruption of the mouse peroxisome proliferator-activated receptor beta (delta). Mol Cell Biol 2000; 20:5119–28.
17. Matsusue K, Peters JM, Gonzalez FJ. PPARβ/δ potentiates PPARγ-stimulated adipocyte differentiation. FASEB J 2004; 18:1477–9.
18. Brun RP, Tontonoz P, Forman BM, et al. Differential activation of adipogenesis by multiple PPAR isoforms. Genes Dev 1996; 10:974–84.
19. Berger J, Leibowitz MD, Doebber TW, et al. Novel peroxisome proliferator-activated receptor (PPAR) gamma and PPARdelta ligands produce distinct biological effects. J Biol Chem 1999; 274:6718–25.
20. Hansen JB, Zhang H, Rasmussen TH, et al. Peroxisome proliferator-activated receptor delta (PPARdelta)-mediated regulation of preadipocyte proliferation and gene expression is dependent on cAMP signaling. J Biol Chem 2001; 276:3175–82.
21. Bastie C, Luquet S, Holst D, et al. Alterations of peroxisome proliferator-activated receptor delta activity affect fatty acid-controlled adipose differentiation. J Biol Chem 2000; 275:38768–73.
22. Jehl-Pietri C, Bastie C, Gillot I, et al. Peroxisome-proliferator-activated receptor delta mediates the effects of long-chain fatty acids on post-confluent cell proliferation. Biochem J 2000; 350:93–8.
23. Chawla A, Lazar MA. Peroxisome proliferator and retinoid signaling pathways co-regulate preadipocyte phenotype and survival. PNAS 1994; 91:1786–90.
24. Poynter ME, Daynes RA. Peroxisome proliferator-activated receptor alpha activation modulates cellular redox status, represses nuclear factor-kappa B signaling, and reduces inflammatory cytokine production in aging. J Biol Chem 1998; 273: 32833–41.
25. Costet P, Legendre C, More J, et al. Peroxisome proliferator-activated receptor alpha-isoform deficiency leads to progressive dyslipidemia with sexually dimorphic obesity and steatosis. J Biol Chem 1998; 273:29577–85.
26. Cabrero A, Alegret M, Sanchez RM, et al. Bezafibrate reduces mRNA levels of adipocyte markers and increases fatty acid oxidation in primary culture of adipocytes. Diabetes 2001; 50:1883–90.
27. Cabrero A, Llaverias G, Roglans N, et al. Uncoupling protein-3 mRNA levels are increased in white adipose tissue and skeletal muscle of bezafibrate-treated rats. Biochem Biophys Res Commun 1999; 260:547–56.
28. Vazquez M, Roglans N, Cabrero A, et al. Bezafibrate induces acyl-CoA oxidase mRNA levels and fatty acid peroxisomal beta-oxidation in rat white adipose tissue. Mol Cell Biochem 2001; 216:71–8.
29. Cao Z, Umek R, McKnight S. Regulated expression of three C/EBP isoforms during adipose conversion of 3T3-L1 cells. Genes Dev 1991; 5:1538–52.
30. Christy RJ, Kaestner KH, Geiman DE, et al. CCAAT/enhancer binding protein gene promoter: binding of nuclear factors during differentiation of 3T3-L1 preadipocytes. PNAS 1991; 88:2593–7.
31. Ron D, Habener JF. CHOP, a novel developmentally regulated nuclear protein that dimerizes with transcription factors C/EBP and LAP and functions as a dominant-negative inhibitor of gene transcription. Genes Dev 1992; 6:439–53.
32. Christy RJ, Yang VW, Ntambi JM, et al. Differentiation-induced gene expression in 3T3-L1 preadipocytes: CCAAT/enhancer binding protein interacts with and activates the promoters of two adipocyte-specific genes. Genes Dev 1989; 3:1323–35.
33. Carriere A, Carmona MC, Fernandez Y, et al. Mitochondrial reactive oxygen species control the transcription factor CHOP-10/GADD153 and adipocyte differentiation: a mechanism for hypoxia-dependent effect. J Biol Chem 2004; 279:40462–9.
34. Batchvarova N, Wang XZ, Ron D. Inhibition of adipogenesis by the stress-induced protein CHOP (Gadd153). EMBO J 1995; 14:4654–61.
35. Carlson SG, Fawcett TW, Bartlett JD, et al. Regulation of the C/EBP-related gene gadd153 by glucose deprivation. Mol Cell Biol 1993; 13:4736–44.

36. Harmon AW, Patel Y, Harp JB. Genistein inhibits CCAAT/enhancer-binding protein beta (C/EBPbeta) activity and 3T3-L1 adipogenesis by increasing C/EBP homologous protein expression. Biochem J 2002; 367:203–8.

37. Tang C, Cho HP, Nakamura MT, et al. Regulation of human delta-6 desaturase gene transcription: identification of a functional direct repeat-1 element. J Lipid Res 2003; 44:686–95.

38. Tao H, Umek RM. C/EBPalpha is required to maintain postmitotic growth arrest in adipocytes. DNA Cell Biol 2000; 19:9–18.

39. El Jack AK, Hamm JK, Pilch PF, et al. Reconstitution of INSULIN-sensitive glucose transport in fibroblasts requires expression of both PPARgamma and C/EBPalpha. J Biol Chem 1999; 274:7946–51.

40. Wu Z, Rosen ED, Brun R, et al. Cross-regulation of C/EBP alpha and PPAR gamma controls the transcriptional pathway of adipogenesis and insulin sensitivity. Mol Cell 1999; 3:151–8.

41. Wu X, Xie Y, Bucher NL, et al. Conditional ectopic expression of C/EBP beta in NIH-3T3 cells induces PPAR gamma and stimulates adipogenesis. Genes Dev 1995; 9:2350–63.

42. Tang QQ, Jiang MS, Lane MD. Repressive effect of Sp1 on the C/EBPalpha gene promoter: role in adipocyte differentiation. Mol Cell Biol 1999; 19:4855–65.

43. Tang QQ, Lane MD. Role of C/EBP homologous protein (CHOP-10) in the programmed activation of CCAAT/enhancer-binding protein-beta during adipogenesis. PNAS 2000; 97:12446–50.

44. Salma N, Xiao H, Imbalzano AN. Temporal recruitment of CCAAT/enhancer-binding proteins to early and late adipogenic promoters in vivo. J Mol Endocrinol 2006; 36:139–51.

45. Rosen ED, Walkey CJ, Puigserver P, et al. Transcriptional regulation of adipogenesis. Genes Dev 2000; 14:1293–307.

46. Tanaka T, Yoshida N, Kishimoto T, et al. Defective adipocyte differentiation in mice lacking the C/EBPbeta and/or C/EBPdelta gene. EMBO J 1997; 16:7432–43.

47. Wang ND, Finegold MJ, Bradley A, et al. Impaired energy homeostasis in C/EBP alpha knockout mice. Science 1995; 269:1108–12.

48. Linhart HG, Ishimura-Oka K, DeMayo F, et al. C/EBPalpha is required for differentiation of white, but not brown, adipose tissue. PNAS 2001; 98:12532–7.

49. Shimomura I, Shimano H, Horton JD, et al. Differential expression of exons 1a and 1c in mRNAs for sterol regulatory element binding protein-1 in human and mouse organs and cultured cells. J Clin Invest 1997; 99:838–45.

50. Tontonoz P, Kim JB, Graves RA, et al. ADD1: a novel helix-loop-helix transcription factor associated with adipocyte determination and differentiation. Mol Cell Biol 1993; 13:4753–9.

51. Inoue J, Kumagai H, Terada T, et al. Proteolytic activation of SREBPs during adipocyte differentiation. Biochem Biophys Res Commun 2001; 283:1157–61.

52. Lay SL, Lefrere I, Trautwein C, et al. Insulin and sterol-regulatory element-binding protein-1c (SREBP1C) regulation of gene expression in 3T3-L1 adipocytes. Identification of ccaat/enhancer-binding protein beta as an srebp-1c target. J Biol Chem 2002; 277:35625–34.

53. Fajas L, Schoonjans K, Gelman L, et al. Regulation of peroxisome proliferator-activated receptor gamma expression by adipocyte differentiation and determination factor 1/sterol regulatory element binding protein 1: implications for adipocyte differentiation and metabolism. Mol Cell Biol 1999; 19:5495–503.

54. Kim JB, Wright HM, Wright, et al. ADD1/SREBP1 activates PPARgamma through the production of endogenous ligand. PNAS 1998; 95:4333–7.

55. Liang G, Yang J, Horton JD, et al. Diminished hepatic response to fasting/refeeding and liver X receptor agonists in mice with selective deficiency of sterol regulatory element-binding protein-1c. J Biol Chem 2002; 277:9520–8.

56. Shimano H, Horton JD, Shimomura I, et al. Isoform 1c of sterol regulatory element binding protein is less active than isoform 1a in livers of transgenic mice and in cultured cells. J Clin Invest 1997; 99:846–54.

57. Shimano H, Shimomura I, Hammer RE, et al. Elevated levels of SREBP-2 and cholesterol synthesis in livers of mice homozygous for a targeted disruption of the SREBP-1 gene. J Clin Invest 1997; 100:2115–24.
58. Shimomura I, Hammer RE, Richardson JA, et al. Insulin resistance and diabetes mellitus in transgenic mice expressing nuclear SREBP-1c in adipose tissue: model for congenital generalized lipodystrophy. Genes Dev 1998; 12:3182–94.
59. Horton JD, Shimomura I, Ikemoto S, et al. Overexpression of sterol regulatory element-binding protein-1a in mouse adipose tissue produces adipocyte hypertrophy, increased fatty acid secretion, and fatty liver. J Biol Chem 2003; 278:36652–60.
60. Willy PJ, Umesono K, Ong ES, et al. LXR, a nuclear receptor that defines a distinct retinoid response pathway. Genes Dev 1995; 9:1033–45.
61. Annicotte J-S, Schoonjans K, Auwerx J. Expression of the liver X receptor α and β in embryonic and adult mice. Anat Rec Part A 2004; 277A:312–6.
62. Steffensen KR, Nilsson M, Schuster GU, et al. Gene expression profiling in adipose tissue indicates different transcriptional mechanisms of liver X receptors α and β respectively. Biochem Biophys Res Commun 2003; 310:589–93.
63. Ross SE, Erickson RL, Gerin I, et al. Microarray analyses during adipogenesis: understanding the effects of Wnt signaling on adipogenesis and the roles of liver X receptor α in adipocyte metabolism. Mol Cell Biol 2002; 22:5989–99.
64. Seo JB, Moon HM, Kim WS, et al. Activated liver X receptors stimulate adipocyte differentiation through induction of peroxisome proliferator-activated receptor γ expression. Mol Cell Biol 2004; 24:3430–44.
65. Juvet L, Andersen SM, Schuster GU, et al. On the role of liver X receptors in lipid accumulation in adipocytes. Mol Endocrinol 2003; 17:172–82.
66. Cleave TL. The Saccharine Disease. Bristol, UK: John Wright & Sons, 1974:6–27.
67. Schultz JR, Tu H, Luk A, et al. Role of LXRs in control of lipogenesis. Genes Dev 2000; 14:2831–8.
68. Sosial og helsedirektoratet. Utviklingen i Norsk kosthold 2002. 2003.
69. Pawlak DB, Kushner JA, Ludwig DS. Effects of dietary glycaemic index on adiposity, glucose homoeostasis, and plasma lipids in animals. Lancet 2004; 364:778–85.
70. Pagliassotti MJ, Prach PA, Koppenhafer TA, et al. Changes in insulin action, triglycerides, and lipid composition during sucrose feeding in rats. Am J Physiol Regul Integr Comp Physiol 1996; 271:R1319–26.
71. Storlien LH, Kraegen EW, Jenkins AB, et al. Effects of sucrose vs starch diets on in vivo insulin action, thermogenesis, and obesity in rats. Am J Clin Nutr 1998; 47:420–7.
72. Fukuchi S, Hamaguchi K, Seike M, et al. Role of fatty acid composition in the development of metabolic disorders in sucrose-induced obese rats. Exp Biol Med 2004; 229:486–93.
73. Flatt PR, Bailey CJ, Kwasowski P, et al. Effects of diets rich in sucrose, coconut fat and safflowerseed oil on the development of the obese hyperglycaemic (ob/ob) syndrome in mice. Diabetes Res 1990; 13:23–8.
74. Thresher JS, Podolin DA, Wei Y, et al. Comparison of the effects of sucrose and fructose on insulin action and glucose tolerance. Am J Physiol Regul Integr Comp Physiol 2000; 279:R1334–40.
75. Bluher M, Michael MD, Peroni OD, et al. Adipose tissue selective insulin receptor knockout protects against obesity and obesity-related glucose intolerance. Develop Cell 2002; 3:25–38.
76. Kim JB, Sarraf P, Wright M, et al. Nutritional and insulin regulation of fatty acid synthetase and leptin gene expression through ADD1/SREBP1. J Clin Invest 1998; 101:1–9.
77. Hua X, Wu J, Goldstein JL, et al. Structure of the human gene encoding sterol regulatory element binding protein-1 (SREBF1) and localization of SREBF1 and SREBF2 to chromosomes 17p11.2 and 22q13. Genomics 1995; 25:667–73.
78. Yokoyama C, Wang X, Briggs MR, et al. SREBP-1, a basic-helix-loop-helix-leucine zipper protein that controls transcription of the low density lipoprotein receptor gene. Cell 1993; 75:187–97.

79. Horton JD, Bashmakov Y, Shimomura I, et al. Regulation of sterol regulatory element binding proteins in livers of fasted and refed mice. PNAS 1998; 95:5987–92.

80. Peet DJ, Turley SD, Ma W, et al. Cholesterol and bile acid metabolism are impaired in mice lacking the nuclear receptor LXR. Cell 1998; 93:693–704.

81. Stulnig TM, Steffensen KR, Gao H, et al. Novel roles of liver X receptors exposed by gene expression profiling in liver and adipose tissue. Mol Pharmacol 2002; 62:1299–305.

82. Tobin KAR, Ulven SM, Schuster GU, et al. Liver X receptors as insulin-mediating factors in fatty acid and cholesterol biosynthesis. J Biol Chem 2002; 277:10691–7.

83. Dalen KT, Ulven SM, Bamberg K, et al. Expression of the insulin-responsive glucose transporter GLUT4 in adipocytes is dependent on liver X receptor α. J Biol Chem 2003; 278:48283–91.

84. Eaton SB, Eaton S3. Paleolithic vs. modern diets—selected pathophysiological implications. Eur J Nutr 2000; 39:67–70.

85. Crawford M. Fatty acids in free-living and domestic animals. Lancet 1968; 1:1333.

86. Stender S, Dyerberg J, Astrup A. High levels of industrially produced trans fat in popular fast foods. N Engl J Med 2006; 354:1650–2.

87. Belzung F, Raclot T, Groscolas R. Fish oil *n*–3 fatty acids selectively limit the hypertrophy of abdominal fat depots in growing rats fed high-fat diets. Am J Physiol 1993; 246:R1111–8.

88. Berger JJ, Barnard RJ. Effect of diet on fat cell size and hormone-sensitive lipase activity. J Appl Physiol 1999; 87:227–32.

89. Ellis RJ, McDonald RB, Stern JS. A diet high in fat stimulates adipocyte proliferation in older (22 month) rats. Exp Gerontol 1990; 25:141–8.

90. Klyde BJ, Hirsch J. Increased cellular proliferation in adipose tissue of adult rats fed a high-fat diet. J Lipid Res 1979; 20:705–15.

91. Miller WH, Faust IM, Hirsch J. Demonstration of de novo production of adipocytes in adult rats by biochemical and radioautographic techniques. J Lipid Res 1984; 25:336–47.

92. Roberts CK, Barnard RJ, Liang KH, et al. Effect of diet on adipose tissue and skeletal muscle VLDL receptor and LPL: implications for obesity and hyperlipidemia. Atherosclerosis 2002; 161:133–41.

93. Shillabeer G, Lau DC. Regulation of new fat cell formation in rats: the role of dietary fats. J Lipid Res 1994; 35:592–600.

94. Nakatani T, Kim HJ, Kaburagi Y, et al. A low fish oil inhibits SREBP-1 proteolytic cascade, while a high-fish-oil feeding decreases SREBP-1 mRNA in mice liver: relationship to anti-obesity. J Lipid Res 2003; 44:369–79.

95. Hill JO, Peters JC, Lin D, et al. Lipid accumulation and body fat distribution is influenced by type of dietary fat fed to rats. Int J Obes Relat Metab Disord 1993; 17:223–36.

96. Parrish CC, Pathy DA, Angel A. Dietary fish oils limit adipose tissue hypertrophy in rats. Metabolism 1990; 39:217–9.

97. Raclot T, Groscolas R, Langin D, et al. Site-specific regulation of gene expression by *n*–3 polyunsaturated fatty acids in rat white adipose tissues. J Lipid Res 1997; 38:1963–72.

98. Rustan AC, Hustvedt BE, Drevon CA. Dietary supplementation of very long-chain *n*–3 fatty acids decreases whole body lipid utilization in the rat. J Lipid Res 1993; 34:1299–309.

99. Ukropec J, Reseland JE, Gasperikova D, et al. The hypotriglyceridemic effect of dietary *n*–3 FA is associated with increased beta-oxidation and reduced leptin expression. Lipids 2003; 38:1023–9.

100. Matsuo T, Takeuchi H, Suzuki H, et al. Body fat accumulation is greater in rats fed a beef tallow diet than in rats fed a safflower or soybean oil diet. Asia Pac J Clin Nutr 2002; 11:302–8.

101. Okuno M, Kajiwara K, Imai S, et al. Perilla oil prevents the excessive growth of visceral adipose tissue in rats by down-regulating adipocyte differentiation. J Nutr 1997; 127:1752–7.

102. Cleary M, Phillips F, Morton R. Genotype and diet effects in lean and obese Zucker rats fed either safflower or coconut oil diets. Proc Soc Exp Biol Med 1999; 220:153–61.
103. Massiera F, Saint-Marc P, Seydoux J, et al. Arachidonic acid and prostacyclin signaling promote adipose tissue development: a human health concern? J Lipid Res 2003; 44:271–9.
104. Prentice AM. Overeating: the health risks. Obes Res 2001; 9:234S–8.
105. Lopez IP, Marti A, Milagro FI, et al. DNA Microarray analysis of genes differentially expressed in diet-induced (Cafeteria) obese rats. Obes Res 2003; 11:188–94.
106. Forman BM, Chen J, Evans RM. Hypolipidemic drugs, polyunsaturated fatty acids, and eicosanoids are ligands for peroxisome proliferator-activated receptors alpha and delta. PNAS 1997; 94:4312–7.
107. Johnson TE, Holloway MK, Vogel R, et al. Structural requirements and cell-type specificity for ligand activation of peroxisome proliferator-activated receptors. J Steroid Biochem Mol Biol 1997; 63:1–18.
108. Kliewer SA, Sundseth SS, Jones SA, et al. Fatty acids and eicosanoids regulate gene expression through direct interactions with peroxisome proliferator-activated receptors alpha and gamma. PNAS 1997; 94:4318–23.
109. Yu K, Bayona W, Kallen CB, et al. Differential activation of peroxisome proliferator-activated receptors by eicosanoids. J Biol Chem 1995; 270:23975–83.
110. Madsen L, Petersen RK, Kristiansen K. Regulation of adipocyte differentiation and function by polyunsaturated fatty acids. Biochim Biophys Acta—Mol Basis Disease 2005; 1740:266–86.
111. Power GW, Newsholme EA. Dietary fatty acids influence the activity and metabolic control of mitochondrial carnitine palmitoyltransferase I in rat heart and skeletal muscle. J Nutr 1997; 127:2142–50.
112. Totland GK, Madsen L, Klementsen B, et al. Proliferation of mitochondria and gene expression of carnitine palmitoyltransferase and fatty acyl-CoA oxidase in rat skeletal muscle, heart and liver by hypolipidemic fatty acids. Biol Cell 2000; 92:317–29.
113. Cha SH, Fukushima A, Sakuma K, et al. Chronic docosahexaenoic acid intake enhances expression of the gene for uncoupling protein 3 and affects pleiotropic mRNA levels in skeletal muscle of aged C57BL/6NJcl mice. J Nutr 2001; 131:2636–42.
114. Baillie RA, Takada R, Nakamura M, et al. Coordinate induction of peroxisomal acyl-CoA oxidase and UCP-3 by dietary fish oil: a mechanism for decreased body fat deposition. Prostaglandin Leukot Essent Fatty Acids 1999; 60:351–6.
115. Hun CS, Hasegawa K, Kawabata T, et al. Increased uncoupling protein2 mRNA in white adipose tissue, and decrease in leptin, visceral fat, blood glucose, and cholesterol in KK-Ay mice fed with eicosapentaenoic and docosahexaenoic acids in addition to linolenic acid. Biochem Biophys Res Commun 1999; 259:85–90.
116. Wang YX, Lee CH, Tiep S, et al. Peroxisome-proliferator-activated receptor δ activates fat metabolism to prevent obesity. Cell 2003; 113:159–70.
117. Mater MK, Thelen AP, Pan DA, et al. Sterol response element-binding protein 1c (SREBP1c) is involved in the polyunsaturated fatty acid suppression of hepatic S14 gene transcription. J Biol Chem 1999; 274:32725–32.
118. Xu J, Nakamura MT, Cho HP, et al. Sterol regulatory element binding protein-1 expression is suppressed by dietary polyunsaturated fatty acids. A mechanism for the coordinate suppression of lipogenic genes by polyunsaturated fats. J Biol Chem 1999; 274:23577–83.
119. Kim HJ, Takahashi M, Ezaki O. Fish oil feeding decreases mature sterol regulatory element-binding protein 1 (SREBP-1) by down-regulation of SREBP-1c mRNA in mouse liver. A possible mechanism for down-regulation of lipogenic enzyme mRNAs. J Biol Chem 1999; 274:25892–98.
120. Hannah VC, Ou J, Luong A, et al. Unsaturated fatty acids down-regulate SREBP isoforms 1a and 1c by two mechanisms in HEK-293 cells. J Biol Chem 2001; 276: 4365–72.
121. Thewke DP, Panini SR, Sinensky M. Oleate potentiates oxysterol inhibition of transcription from sterol Regulatory element-1-regulated promoters and maturation of sterol regulatory element-binding proteins. J Biol Chem 1998; 273:21402–7.

122. Shillabeer G, Hornford J, Forden JM, et al. Hepatic and adipose tissue lipogenic enzyme mRNA levels are suppressed by high fat diets in the rat. J Lipid Res 1990; 31:623–31.

123. Petersen RK, Jorgensen C, Rustan AC, et al. Arachidonic acid-dependent inhibition of adipocyte differentiation requires PKA activity and is associated with sustained expression of cyclooxygenases. J Lipid Res 2003; 44:2320–30.

124. Ou J, Tu H, Shan B, et al. Unsaturated fatty acids inhibit transcription of the sterol regulatory element-binding protein-1c (SREBP-1c) gene by antagonizing ligand-dependent activation of the LXR. PNAS 2001; 98:6027–32.

125. Yoshikawa T, Shimano H, Yahagi N, et al. Polyunsaturated fatty acids suppress sterol regulatory element-binding protein 1c promoter activity by inhibition of liver X receptor (LXR) binding to LXR response elements. J Biol Chem 2002; 277:1705–11.

126. Farnsworth E, Luscombe ND, Noakes M, et al. Effect of a high-protein, energy-restricted diet on body composition, glycemic control, and lipid concentrations in overweight and obese hyperinsulinemic men and women. Am J Clin Nutr 2003; 78:31–9.

127. Foster GD, Wyatt HR, Hill JO, et al. A randomized trial of a low-carbohydrate diet for obesity. N Engl J Med 2003; 348:2082–90.

128. Layman DK, Baum JI. Dietary protein impact on glycemic control during weight loss. J Nutr 2004; 134:968S–73.

129. Layman DK, Boileau RA, Erickson DJ, et al. A reduced ratio of dietary carbohydrate to protein improves body composition and blood lipid profiles during weight loss in adult women. J Nutr 2003; 133:411–7.

130. Parker B, Noakes M, Luscombe N, et al. Effect of a high-protein, high-monounsaturated fat weight loss diet on glycemic control and lipid levels in type 2 diabetes. Diabetes Care 2002; 25:425–30.

131. Piatti PM, Monti F, Fermo I, et al. Hypocaloric high-protein diet improves glucose oxidation and spares lean body mass: comparison to hypocaloric high-carbohydrate diet. Metabolism 1994; 43:1481–7.

132. Skov A, Toubro S, Ronn B, et al. Randomized trial on protein vs carbohydrate in ad libitum fat reduced diet for the treatment of obesity. Int J Obes 1999; 23:528–36.

133. Fernstrom MH, Fernstrom JD. Brain tryptophan concentrations and serotonin synthesis remain responsive to food consumption after the ingestion of sequential meals. Am J Clin Nutr 1995; 61:312–9.

134. Waterhouse C, Keilson J. The contribution of glucose to alanine metabolism in man. J Lab Clin Med 1978; 92:803–12.

135. Layman DK, Shiue H, Sather C, et al. Increased dietary protein modifies glucose and insulin homeostasis in adult women during weight loss. J Nutr 2003; 133:405–10.

136. Klaus S. Increasing the protein:carbohydrate ratio in a high-fat diet delays the development of adiposity and improves glucose homeostasis in mice. J Nutr 2005; 135:1854–8.

137. Opara EC, Petro A, Tevrizian A, et al. L-glutamine supplementation of a high fat diet reduces body weight and attenuates hyperglycemia and hyperinsulinemia in C57BL/6J mice. J Nutr 1996; 126:273–9.

138. Fu WJ, Haynes TE, Kohli R, et al. Dietary L-arginine supplementation reduces fat mass in Zucker diabetic fatty rats. J Nutr 2005; 135:714–21.

139. Lehman JJ, Barger PM, Kovacs A, et al. Peroxisome proliferator-activated receptor {gamma} coactivator-1 promotes cardiac mitochondrial biogenesis. J Clin Invest 2000; 106:847–56.

140. Wu Z, Puigserver P, Andersson U, et al. Mechanisms controlling mitochondrial biogenesis and respiration through the thermogenic coactivator PGC-1. Cell 1999; 98:115–24.

141. Nisoli E, Clementi E, Paolucci C, et al. Mitochondrial biogenesis in mammals: the role of endogenous nitric oxide. Science 2003; 299:896–9.

142. Khedara A, Goto T, Morishima M, et al. Elevated body fat in rats by the dietary nitric oxide synthase inhibitor, L-N omega nitroarginine. Biosci Biotechnol Biochem 1999; 63:698–702.

143. Lynch CJ, Patson BJ, Anthony J, et al. Leucine is a direct-acting nutrient signal that regulates protein synthesis in adipose tissue. Am J Physiol Endocrinol Metab 2002; 283:E503–13.

144. Fox HL, Kimball SR, Jefferson LS, et al. Amino acids stimulate phosphorylation of p70S6k and organization of rat adipocytes into multicellular clusters. Am J Physiol Cell Physiol 1998; 274:C206–13.

145. Roh C, Han J, Tzatsos A, et al. Nutrient-sensing mTOR-mediated pathway regulates leptin production in isolated rat adipocytes. Am J Physiol Endocrinol Metab 2003; 284: E322–30.

146. Lynch CJ, Hutson SM, Patson BJ, et al. Tissue-specific effects of chronic dietary leucine and norleucine supplementation on protein synthesis in rats. Am J Physiol Endocrinol Metab 2002; 283:E824–35.

147. Tsukiyama-Kohara K, Poulin F, Kohara M, et al. Adipose tissue reduction in mice lacking the translational inhibitor 4E-BP1. Nat Med 2001; 7:1128–32.

148. Lin TA, Kong X, Saltiel AR, et al. Control of PHAS-I by insulin in 3T3-L1 adipocytes. J Biol Chem 1995; 270:18531–8.

149. Fox HL, Pham PT, Kimball SR, et al. Amino acid effects on translational repressor 4E-BP1 are mediated primarily by L-leucine in isolated adipocytes. Am J Physiol Cell Physiol 1998; 275:C1232–8.

150. Yeh W, Bierer BE, McKnight SL. Rapamycin inhibits clonal expansion and adipogenic differentiation of 3T3-L1 cells. PNAS 1995; 92:11086–90.

151. Calkhoven CF, Muller C, Leutz A. Translational control of C/EBPalpha and C/EBPbeta isoform expression. Genes Dev 2000; 14:1920–32.

152. Inoue I, Takahashi K, Katayama S, et al. Effect of troglitazone (CS-045) and bezafibrate on glucose tolerance, liver glycogen synthase activity, and beta-oxidation in fructose-fed rats. Metabolism 1995; 44:1626–30.

153. Skorve J, Berge RK. The hypocholesterolemic effect of sulfur-substituted fatty acid analogues in rats fed a high carbohydrate diet. Biochim Biophys Acta 1993; 1167:175–81.

9.4 Genes Involved in Muscle Function

Béatrice Morio and Stéphane Walrand
INRA, UMR 1019, Unité de Nutrition Humaine, Clermont-Ferrand, France

Yves Boirie
INRA, UMR 1019, Université de Clermont-Ferrand, Auvergne and Unité de Nutrition Humaine, Clermont-Ferrand, France

Skeletal muscle represents an important component and a key determinant of energy and substrate metabolism in the body. Because of its relatively low resting energy metabolism, skeletal muscle has often been neglected in explaining inter-individual differences in metabolic rate, while it is the largest tissue mass and can account for 30% of the total resting energy expenditure. If the metabolic rate of other organs, such as the brain, heart, liver, or kidney, is constantly sustained and varies very little during the course of the day, skeletal muscle metabolism can change dramatically from resting to maximal physical activity during; this muscle oxygen consumption can account for up to 90% of the whole-body oxygen uptake. It is thus suggested that a major part of the variability between subjects in whole body metabolic rate and energy balance is related to differences in skeletal muscle metabolism. In addition to its contribution to energy metabolism, skeletal muscle is the main site of lipid oxidation in the body through mitochondrial oxidative systems in the fasting state as well as during exercise. Hence, disturbances in fat oxidation may promote the development of increased adipose-tissue stores and obesity but also increased triacylglycerol storage in muscle and skeletal-muscle insulin resistance. Beyond muscle involvement in energy expenditure, reduced muscle fat oxidation may be a primary factor leading to obesity and/or insulin resistance. However, the precise sequence of events leading to increased adiposity and insulin resistance in obesity and type 2 diabetes is yet to be determined. Several factors may influence the variation in muscle energy expenditure and substrate metabolism, such as thyroid hormone, insulin, muscle fiber types, muscle tone, sympathetic innervation, and catecholamines levels. More knowledge on skeletal muscle metabolism is required to understand how the muscle contributes to the development of obesity and fat deposition and to know how skeletal muscle utilization may help prevent obesity and its related metabolic disorders across all human ages. This chapter focuses on the involvement of physical activity (i.e., muscle functioning-related energy expenditure) in the etiology of obesity. Thereafter, the involvement of muscle "genetics" is examined.

INVOLVEMENT OF SKELETAL MUSCLE IN ENERGY BALANCE
Muscle Energy Expenditure
Skeletal muscle is essential for posture maintenance and performance during physical activity. In the resting human, muscle energy expenditure averages 13 kcal/kg/day, which is approximately 19-fold lower than the metabolic activity of the liver and brain, and 34-fold lower than that of heart and kidneys. Due to its mass, which contributes for 30% to 40% of body weight, resting muscle energy

expenditure can account for up to 20% to 30% of basal metabolic rate (1). Muscle energy expenditure dramatically increases during exercise. Exercise such as brisk walking is associated with increase in whole body energy expenditure of about three- to five-fold resting value [usually expressed as metabolic equivalent (MET), see Chapter 1.1 for definition]. For very high-intensity exercise such as marathon running, the increase in energy expenditure reaches 18 to 20 METs. Physical activity–related energy expenditure is the most variable component of daily energy expenditure. Muscle "functioning" is thus a critical player in day-to-day energy balance and its role might be envisaged as in the pathophysiology of human obesity.

A Paleolithic Inheritance

During human evolution, and especially in the recent decades, decreased physical activity parallels the increase in the prevalence of obesity, although a potential causal association between these two phenomena remains a matter of debate. Booth et al. (2,3) have proposed that *Homo sapiens'* inherited genes evolved to support a physically active lifestyle, the result of which is an inability to face chronic physical inactivity. A disadapted genome has been therefore suggested to result in abnormal gene expression, which in turn exhibits as clinically overt diseases such as obesity.

Role of Nonexercise Activity Thermogenesis in Obesity

Nonexercise activity thermogenesis (NEAT), which is the cumulative energy expended during maintenance of posture, fidgeting, and other physical activities of daily life that are not formal and voluntary sport exercise, such as walking [(5), see definitions in Chapter 1.1)]. Three components of NEAT are considered and might be discerned in studies evaluating the role of nonexercise activity in obesity; first is the energy expenditure of body posture (energy expanded while sitting, standing, and changing from one position to another), second is the energy expenditure of movement (while walking, for example), third is the amount of other movement, such as fidgeting. NEAT is highly variable among individuals (4). It has, therefore, been proposed as a contributor of fat mass accumulation when individual's environment changes. NEAT is likely to be regulated through a central mechanism that integrates NEAT with energy intake and energy stores. NEAT is activated with overfeeding and suppressed with underfeeding (5), and might also depend on education, age, body composition, gender, and possibly genetics. Most studies have shown a decrease in NEAT or NEAT component (such as fidgeting) in obese patients (6). In longitudinal studies in Pima Indians, NEAT components measured in calorimetric chambers was found to be a familial trait, and a low NEAT component was associated with subsequent weight gain in males (7). Recent evidences have demonstrated that NEAT is critical in determining a subject's susceptibility to gain body fat during periods of overfeeding (8). Changes in NEAT after 8 weeks of overfeeding accounted for the 10-fold interindividual differences in fat storage.

Role of Physical Activity to Prevent Weight Gain

Beside NEAT, physical activities at a MET level of 4 or higher (i.e., sports-like exercises) are also proposed to play an important role in weight maintenance (9). The evidence of an inverse relationship between daily physical activity and weight gain remains inconclusive (9). Regarding weight regain and maintenance after weight loss, studies in postobese women have demonstrated that around 77% of weight regain at 1 year was explained by low physical activity. Weight maintainers spent 79 min/day practicing 4 MET intensity activities whereas weight gainers spent only 16 min/day (10). According to these observations, a recent consensus (11) proposed that 60 to 90 min/day of moderate intensity activity, or smaller amounts of vigorous exercises, were necessary to prevent weight regain after weight loss in obese subjects.

Beta Adrenergic Activity

Brain dopaminergic pathways are crucial for the control of movement. Three missense substitutions have been identified in the dopamine D2 receptor (DRD2). The prevalence of the variant Ser311Cys has been shown to greatly vary among individuals and studies in genetically heterogeneous human populations have associated this variant to higher body mass index (BMI) (12–16). However, Tataranni and colleagues have found that Pima Indians with a Cys311-encoding allele, despite a higher BMI, showed only a tendency for lower physical activity-related energy expenditure and no significant differences in NEAT compared to individuals homozygous for the Ser311-encoding allele (16). These data therefore suggested a limited effect of the Ser311Cys mutation on body weight and composition.

Role of Muscle Genetics and Functioning in Obesity

It is conceivable that endurance capacity and muscle strength can influence the aptitude for physical activity, thus determining the inclination to be active or sedentary and the predisposition to maintain or gain weight.

Studies in young male twins showed very high heritability (>85%) for arm anthropometric and strength (17) and for muscle response to resistance training (18). Several genes involved in the myostatin pathway, but not the myostatin gene itself (which deficiency is known to result in a hypermuscular phenotype) have been shown to be important quantitative trait loci for human muscle strength (19,20). However, another study performed in an heterogeneous population has not confirmed significant association between myostatin polymorphism and muscle mass and strength at baseline or in response to resistance training (21).

It is well known in athletes that high maximal aerobic capacity (VO_{2max}) is associated with decreased exercise difficulty and increased performance. This appears to apply to the whole population in which high heritability in VO_{2max} has been described (22). Hence, significant racial differences for VO_{2max} and difficulty in doing submaximum exercises have been evidenced between African American and Caucasian American women (23). The augmented exercise difficulty in African American women was suggested to contribute to decreased physical activity and increased predisposition to obesity. Furthermore in the same populations, Larew and colleagues (24) have demonstrated the existence of a trilogy between muscle strength, muscle aerobic capacity, and long-term weight management. These findings pointed toward a direct role of muscle aerobic and anaerobic metabolism in body weight regulation and questioned the involvement of genetic determinism of muscle metabolic function.

Muscle Typology and Metabolic Activity

Combined data from the literature suggest that about 45% of the phenotype variance is heritable, the remaining variance being mainly influenced by environmental factors (25,26). Furthermore, the overfeeding study in young identical twin males from Bouchard et al. has evidenced significant involvement of genetic factors in the determinism of weight gain (27) and that part of these adaptations were determined by differences in muscle fiber types and metabolic activity (28). In that respect, several studies have found low proportions of slow-twitch oxidative (Type I) muscle fibers (29–32) and high proportions of fast-twitch glycolytic (Type IIb) fibers (29–31) in individuals with high body fat stores.

Racial differences (33) and significant family aggregation (34,35) have been described for maximal activities of enzymes of muscle energy production pathways (for both glycolytic and oxidative pathways). Low muscle mitochondrial activity has been proposed to participate to a decreased fat oxidation and increased fat storage (36). To support this hypothesis, low mitochondrial enzyme oxidative capacity has been reported among individuals with greater weight gain after overfeeding (28,37) and in obese patients compared to lean adults (38).

Muscle UCPs and Predisposition to Obesity

Uncoupling proteins (UCP) are carriers expressed in the mitochondrial inner membrane that uncouple oxygen consumption by the respiratory chain from ATP synthesis. Possible functions of UCPs include control of ATP synthesis, regulation of fatty acid metabolism, and control of reactive oxygen species production. UCP2 is expressed in a wide range of tissues and organs. Its expression in tissues involved in lipid and energy metabolism and mapping of the gene to a region linked to obesity have suggested its implication in obesity (39). However, several studies have evidenced that variants in UCP2 may play a role in energy metabolism, but slightly contributes to obesity in Pima Indians (40,41) if not in Danish subjects (42).

UCP3 is mainly expressed in skeletal muscle although it is also expressed in white and brown adipose tissues. Physiological role of UCP3 remains yet to be elucidated. It may not be involved in mitochondrial uncoupling, but uncoupling may occur as a side effect of a more pivotal role played by UCP3. Association between variants in UCP3 and BMI and fat mass has been described in different ethnicities, i.e., Pima Indians (43), French Canadians (44), and South-Indian and European women (45). Furthermore, variants in UCP3 were shown to be involved in the regulation of body composition changes after regular exercise in African and Caucasian Americans (46). Therefore, combined data strongly suggest that some alleles of UCP3 might be involved in the etiology of obesity.

GENE EXPRESSION PROFILING IN SKELETAL MUSCLE FROM OBESE PATIENTS

Obesity is accompanied by complex changes in the expression of thousands of genes across various functional categories in skeletal muscle. In the present part, we will focus on genes associated with the metabolic activity of skeletal muscle and their modification in obese people.

Fat Storage

Numerous processes and factors are known to regulate fuel partitioning and fat deposition in adipose tissue and skeletal muscle, including substrate competition, hormonal milieu and the expression of genes whose products play active roles in tissue energy homeostasis, such as fatty acid translocase (FAT/CD36), fatty acid-binding protein (FABP), UCP, and respiratory chain complexes.

The rate of fatty acid uptake by skeletal muscle together with *fat/cd36* and *fabp* gene expressions have been measured in obese and lean Zucker rats (47). With obesity there is an increased fatty acid uptake of up to 1.8-fold in muscle. Although FAT/CD36 transcript level and protein content were not modified in skeletal muscle cells of obese rats, the plasma membrane FAT/CD36, and FABP proteins were significantly increased. Thus, in obesity, alteration of fatty acid transport in muscle cell is not associated with changes in fatty acid transporter mRNAs, but with the increased abundance of the proteins at the plasma membrane. It is postulated that in obesity fatty acid transporters are relocated from an intracellular pool to the plasma membrane in skeletal muscle (47). The effect of increased availability of lipids in blood on fatty acid transporter gene expressions was also evaluated in rats. Lipoprotein lipase (*Lpl*), *Fat/cd36*, and fatty acid transporter (*Fatp1*) gene expressions were not changed by a hypercaloric fat diet in skeletal muscle from nonobese rats (48). By contrast, an increase in blood free fatty acid after a 3 to 24 h lipid infusion is associated with a marked increase in skeletal muscle and adipose tissue *Fat/cd36* mRNA levels in lean Zucker rats (49). Interestingly in this study, *Slc2A4* (*Glut4*) mRNA level significantly decreased in red fiber type muscle and increased in visceral adipose tissue. These data suggest that the in vivo gene expression of *Fat/cd36* and *Slc2A4* in visceral fat and red fiber type muscle are differently regulated by circulating lipids and that selective insulin resistance seems to favor, at least in part, a prevention of fat accumulation in tissues not primarily destined for fat storage, thus contributing to increased adiposity (49).

As previously mentioned, mitochondrial UCPs are involved in heat loss by generating a dissipation of the proton electrochemical gradient across the inner mitochondrial membrane in skeletal muscle. An increase in muscle *Ucp3* mRNA levels was found in rats after 30 days of a high-fat and high-calorie feeding in a nongenetically obese animal strain (50). Some authors have proposed that an increased *Ucp3* expression after a high-fat feeding may be seen as a mean to uncouple mitochondria and increase fat oxidation to limit fat deposition in skeletal muscle.

Recent evidence suggests that once inside the muscle cell, fatty acids derived from the uptake of nonesterified fatty acids, act as signaling molecules. They bind to and activate the peroxisome proliferators-activated receptor (PPAR) protein family, in particular PPARG, which modulates the expression of genes involved in lipid storage and metabolism. An increase in the mRNA and protein levels of PPARG, which can stimulate the expression of *FAT/CD36* and *FABP*, has been described in obese women (51). Studies have also focused on assessing a potential regulatory role for *Pparg2* in the muscle *Ucp* mRNA expression in rats. These results showed that high-energy diet intake lowered muscle *Pparg2* mRNA levels and a significant negative relation was found between *Pparg2* expression with muscle *Ucp3*. These observations suggest that muscle *Ucp3* mRNA expression may be negatively affected by PPARG2 in fat-feeding rats (50). By contrast, gastrocnemius muscle *Ucp3* mRNA levels were significantly reduced in obese rats when compared with lean strain (52). It was suggested that the downregulation of *Ucp3* gene expression together with a mitochondrial oxygen consumption observed in obese rats may be linked to lower fat oxidation, which would promote triglyceride accumulation in skeletal muscle.

Metabolic Capacity

Inefficient skeletal muscle lipid utilization may relate to the development of obesity. There is evidence of impaired muscle fatty acid utilization in the obese state, and studies indicate that differences in muscle fatty acid oxidative capacity might play a role in the pathogenesis of obesity (53). Underlying mechanisms for disturbed fatty acid handling may be associated to impaired muscle fatty acid uptake and a reduced ability to oxidize fat.

Mitochondria play fundamental roles in intermediary metabolism, such as fatty acid oxidation. Mitochondria possess a distinct DNA but the vast majority of mitochondrial proteins are encoded by the nuclear DNA. Skeletal muscle mitochondria-related genetic and functional defects have been reported in association with decreased fatty acid oxidation and obesity. The reduction in electron transport chain activity in muscle of obese subjects could be caused by reduced mitochondrial content or reduced functional capacity of mitochondria. To address this issue, Kelley's group (54) has measured mitochondrial DNA (mtDNA) content in muscle biopsies from lean and obese subjects. Assessment of mtDNA is regarded as a quantitative index of mitochondrial content in tissues, including skeletal muscle. Compared with the findings in muscle from lean healthy volunteers, these authors did find a significant decrease in mtDNA in muscle in obesity. This indicates that decreased mitochondrial content at least partly explains reduced electron transport chain activity in obese subjects (25,26). However, the decrement in electron transport chain activity was greater than the corresponding decrement in mtDNA content (54). These findings suggest that functional impairments in electron transport chain activity in obesity are not fully accounted for by reduced mitochondrial content.

The molecular basis for the decreased mitochondrial content of skeletal muscle in obese subjects may be represented by a decrease in the expression and/ or activity of peroxisome proliferator-activated receptor gamma (PPARG), coactivator 1 alpha (PGC1A) (55). PGC1A was first characterized as a transcriptional coactivator which interacted with PPARG to enable expression of its protranscriptional activity. Subsequent research revealed that PGC1A acts as a coactivator for a range of other transcriptional factors (56). In particular, PGC1A is essential to the transcriptional activity of nuclear respiratory factors 1 and 2 (NRF-1, NRF-2), which stimulate the expression of numerous genes required for the expansion and replication of mitochondria (57). For example, PGC1A has a positive impact on expression of the muscle isoform of carnitine palmitoyltransferase-I, often considered rate-limiting for mitochondrial fatty acid oxidation (58). There is now evidence that underexpression and/or diminished activity of PGC1A in skeletal muscle is common in obese subjects. Not surprisingly, this downregulation of PGC1A is associated with decreased expression of the range of mitochondrial genes which are targets for the transcriptional activity of NRF-1 and NRF-2. Furthermore, a chromosomal locus (4p15.1) which appears to strongly influence BMI in Mexican-Americans is where the *PGC1* gene resides. These considerations suggest that there are marked genetically determined variations in the expression and/or activity of PGC1a in skeletal muscle, which appear to modulate the oxidative capacity of skeletal muscle and consequently risk for obesity.

It was also proposed that PGC1A enables muscle mitochondria to better cope with a high lipid load (59). *Pgc1A* expression and muscle mitochondrial efficiency is compromised by diet-induced obesity in rodents. Hence, chronic high fat under conditions of low PGC1A expression, caused accelerated rates of incomplete fatty acid oxidation and accumulation of beta-oxidative intermediates (59). The use of oligonucleotide microarray analysis in human subjects under high fat diet revealed around 300 muscle genes which were differentially regulated by the high fat diet (60). Expression of *PGC1A* gene and of genes involved in mitochondrial oxidative phosphorylation, e.g., members of mitochondrial complexes I and II and mitochondrial carrier proteins, decreased. In another study (61), a triglyceride emulsion was infused in healthy volunteers to increase plasma-free fatty acid and microarray analysis was performed in muscle biopsies. *PGC1A* mRNA, along with mRNAs for a number of nuclear-encoded mitochondrial genes, were reduced by lipid infusion. These data were confirmed by separate experiments in rats (62) and mice (60) fed a high fat diet for several weeks. Combined, these results suggest a mechanism whereby high fat diet downregulates genes necessary for beta-oxidation, oxidative phosphorylation, and mitochondrial biogenesis. These changes mimic those observed in obesity and, if sustained, may result in mitochondrial dysfunction in the prediabetic/insulin-resistantstate.

CONCLUSION

Skeletal muscle is a key factor for the development of obese phenotype since it is involved in both energy and substrate metabolism, especially in fat metabolism. There is accumulating evidence that a disturbed muscle function including inactivity-induced positive energy balance or a reduced mitochondrial fat oxidative capacity results in the accumulation of fat and lipid intermediates in many tissues, which may interfere with insulin signaling and induce an impaired insulin-mediated glucose uptake. Genetic and metabolic predispositions for a reduced fatty acid handling, including not only adipose tissue metabolic disturbances but also abnormal muscle fatty acid uptake and a reduced ability to oxidize fat, represent a major explanation for interindividual variability of fat storage. More is to identify about the molecular mechanisms involved in these processes.

REFERENCES

1. Elia M. Organ and tissue contribution to metabolic rate. In: Kinney JM, Tucker HN, eds. Energy Metabolism: Tissue Determinants and Cellular Corollaries. New York: Raven Press, 1992:61–79.
2. Booth FW, Chakravarthy MV, Gordon SE, et al. Waging war on physical inactivity: using modern molecular ammunition against an ancient enemy. J Appl Physiol 2002; 93:3–30.
3. Booth FW, Chakravarthy MV, Spangenburg EE. Exercise and gene expression: physiological regulation of the human genome through physical activity. J Physiol 2002; 543(Pt 2):399–411.
4. Donahoo WT, Levine JA, Melanson EL. Variability in energy expenditure and its components. Curr Opin Clin Nutr Metab Care 2004; 7:599–605.
5. Levine JA, Kotz CM. NEAT—non-exercise activity thermogenesis—egocentric & geocentric environmental factors vs. biological regulation. Acta Physiol Scand 2005; 184: 309–18.
6. Ravussin E, Bogardus C. Energy balance and weight regulation: genetics versus environment. Br J Nutr 2000; 83(Suppl. 1):S17–20.
7. Zurlo F, Ferraro RT, Fontvielle AM, et al. Spontaneous physical activity and obesity: cross-sectional and longitudinal studies in Pima Indians. Am J Physiol 1992; 263(2 Pt 1): E296–300.

8. Levine JA, Eberhardt NL, Jensen MD. Role of nonexercise activity thermogenesis in resistance to fat gain in humans. Science 1999; 283:212–4.
9. Hunter GR, Byrne NM. Physical activity and muscle function but not resting energy expenditure impact on weight gain. J Strength Cond Res 2005; 19:225–30.
10. Weinsier RL, Hunter GR, Desmond RA, et al. Free-living activity energy expenditure in women successful and unsuccessful at maintaining a normal body weight. Am J Clin Nutr 2002; 75:499–504.
11. Saris WH, Blair SN, Van Baak MA, et al. How much physical activity is enough to prevent unhealthy weight gain? Outcome of the IASO 1st Stock Conference and consensus statement. Obes Rev 2003; 4:101–14.
12. Comings DE, Flanagan SD, Dietz G, et al. The dopamine D2 receptor (DRD2) as a major gene in obesity and height. Biochem Med Metab Biol 1993; 50:176–85.
13. Comings DE, Gade R, MacMurray JP, et al. Genetic variants of the human obesity (OB) gene: association with body mass index in young women, psychiatric symptoms, and interaction with the dopamine D2 receptor (DRD2) gene. Mol Psychiatry 1996; 1: 325–35.
14. Noble EP, Noble RE, Ritchie T, et al. D2 dopamine receptor gene and obesity. Int J Eat Disord 1994; 15:205–17.
15. Blum K, Braverman ER, Wood RC, et al. Increased prevalence of the Taq I A1 allele of the dopamine receptor gene (DRD2) in obesity with comorbid substance use disorder: a preliminary report. Pharmacogenetics 1996; 6:297–305.
16. Tataranni PA, Baier L, Jenkinson C, et al. A Ser311Cys mutation in the human dopamine receptor D2 gene is associated with reduced energy expenditure. Diabetes 2001; 50:901–4.
17. Thomis MA, Beunen GP, Van Leemputte M, et al. Inheritance of static and dynamic arm strength and some of its determinants. Acta Physiol Scand 1998; 163:59–71.
18. Thomis MA, Beunen GP, Maes HH, et al. Strength training: importance of genetic factors. Med Sci Sports Exerc 1998; 30:724–31.
19. Huygens W, Thomis MA, Peeters MW, et al. Quantitative trait loci for human muscle strength: linkage analysis of myostatin pathway genes. Physiol Genomics 2005; 22:390–7.
20. Huygens W, Thomis MA, Peeters MW, et al. Linkage of myostatin pathway genes with knee strength in humans. Physiol Genomics 2004; 17:264–70.
21. Thomis MA, Huygens W, Heuninckx S, et al. Exploration of myostatin polymorphisms and the angiotensin-converting enzyme insertion/deletion genotype in responses of human muscle to strength training. Eur J Appl Physiol 2004; 92:267–74.
22. Perusse L, Gagnon J, Province MA, et al. Familial aggregation of submaximal aerobic performance in the HERITAGE family study. Med Sci Sports Exerc 2001; 33: 597–604.
23. Hunter GR, Weinsier RL, Zuckerman PA, et al. Aerobic fitness, physiologic difficulty and physical activity in Black and White women. Int J Obes Relat Metab Disord 2004; 28:1111–7.
24. Larew K, Hunter GR, Larson-Meyer DE, et al. Muscle metabolic function, exercise performance, and weight gain. Med Sci Sports Exerc 2003; 35:230–6.
25. Simoneau JA, Colberg SR, Thaete FL, et al. Skeletal muscle glycolytic and oxidative enzyme capacities are determinants of insulin sensitivity and muscle composition in obese women. FASEB J 1995; 9:273–8.
26. Simoneau JA, Bouchard C. Genetic determinism of fiber type proportion in human skeletal muscle. FASEB J 1995; 9:1091–5.
27. Bouchard C, Tremblay A, Despres JP, et al. The response to long-term overfeeding in identical twins. N Engl J Med 1990; 322:1477–82.
28. Sun G, Ukkola O, Rankinen T, et al. Skeletal muscle characteristics predict body fat gain in response to overfeeding in never-obese young men. Metabolism 2002; 51:451–6.
29. Krikekos AD, Pan DA, Lillioja S, et al. Interrelationships between muscle morphology, insulin action, and adiposity. Am J Physiol 1996; 270:R1332–9.
30. Kriketos AD, Baur LA, O'Conner J, et al. Muscle fiber type composition in infant and adult populations and relationships with obesity. Int J Obes 1997; 21:796–801.

31. Lillioja S, Young AA, Culter CL, et al. Skeletal muscle capillary density and fiber type are possible determinants of in vivo insulin resistance in man. J Clin Invest 1987; 80: 415–24.

32. Ama PF, Simoneau JA, Boulay MR, et al. Skeletal muscle characteristics in sedentary black and Caucasian males. J Appl Physiol 1986; 61:1758–61.

33. Wade AJ, Marbut MM, Round J. Muscle fiber type and aetiology of obesity. Lancet 2001; 335:805–8.

34. Rico-Sanz J, Rankinen T, Joanisse DR, et al. HERITAGE Family Study. Familial resemblance for muscle phenotypes in the HERITAGE Family Study. Med Sci Sports Exerc 2003; 35:1360–6.

35. Petersen KF, Dufour S, Befroy D, et al. Impaired mitochondrial activity in the insulin-resistant offspring of patients with type 2 diabetes. N Engl J Med 2004; 350:664–71.

36. Kelley DE, Goodpaster BH, Storlien L. Muscle triglyceride and insulin resistance. Annu Rev Nutr 2002; 22:325–46.

37. Simoneau JA, Tremblay A, Theriault G, et al. Relationships between the metabolic profile of human skeletal muscle and body fat gain in response to overfeeding. Med Sports Sci Exerc 1994; 26:S159.

38. Petersen KF, Shulman GI. Etiology of insulin resistance. Am J Med 2006; 119(5 Suppl. 1): S10–6.

39. Comuzzie AG, Allison DB. The search for human obesity genes. Science 1998; 280: 1374–7.

40. Kovacs P, Ma L, Hanson RL, et al. Genetic variation in UCP2 (uncoupling protein-2) is associated with energy metabolism in Pima Indians. Diabetologia 2005; 48:2292–5.

41. Walder K, Norman RA, Hanson RL, et al. Association between uncoupling protein polymorphisms (UCP2–UCP3) and energy metabolism/obesity in Pima Indians. Hum Mol Genet 1998; 7:1431–5.

42. Dalgaard LT, Andersen G, Larsen LH, et al. Mutational analysis of the UCP2 core promoter and relationships of variants with obesity. Obes Res 2003; 11:1420–7.

43. Schrauwen P, Xia J, Walder K, et al. A novel polymorphism in the proximal UCP3 promoter region: effect on skeletal muscle UCP3 mRNA expression and obesity in male non-diabetic Pima Indians. Int J Obes Relat Metab Disord 1999; 23:1242–5.

44. Lanouette CM, Giacobino JP, Perusse L, et al. Association between uncoupling protein 3 gene and obesity-related phenotypes in the Quebec Family Study. Mol Med 2001; 7: 433–41.

45. Cassell PG, Saker PJ, Huxtable SJ, et al. Evidence that single nucleotide polymorphism in the uncoupling protein 3 (UCP3) gene influences fat distribution in women of European and Asian origin. Diabetologia 2000; 43:1558–64.

46. Lanouette CM, Chagnon YC, Rice T, et al. Uncoupling protein 3 gene is associated with body composition changes with training in HERITAGE study. J Appl Physiol 2002; 92:1111–8.

47. Luiken JJ, Arumugam Y, Dyck DJ, et al. Increased rates of fatty acid uptake and plasmalemmal fatty acid transporters in obese Zucker rats. J Biol Chem 2001; 276: 40567–73.

48. Ferrer-Martinez A, Marotta M, Turini M, et al. Effect of sucrose and saturated-fat diets on mRNA levels of genes limiting muscle fatty acid and glucose supply in rats. Lipids 2006; 41:55–62.

49. Fabris R, Nisoli E, Lombardi AM, et al. Preferential channeling of energy fuels toward fat rather than muscle during high free fatty acid availability in rats. Diabetes 2001; 50: 601–8.

50. Margareto J, Marti A, Martinez JA. Changes in UCP mRNA expression levels in brown adipose tissue and skeletal muscle after feeding a high-energy diet and relationships with leptin, glucose and PPAR gamma. J Nutr Biochem 2001; 12:130–7.

51. Bower JF, Davis JM, Hao E, et al. Differences in transport of fatty acids and expression of fatty acid transporting proteins in adipose tissue of obese black and white women. Am J Physiol Endocrinol Metab 2006; 290:E87–91.

52. Corbalan MS, Margareto J, Martinez JA, et al. High-fat feeding reduced muscle uncoupling protein 3 expression in rats. J Physiol Biochem 1999; 55:67–72.

53. Blaak EE. Metabolic fluxes in skeletal muscle in relation to obesity and insulin resistance. Best Pract Res Clin Endocrinol Metab 2005; 19:391–403.

54. Ritov VB, Menshikova EV, He J, et al. Deficiency of subsarcolemmal mitochondria in obesity and type 2 diabetes. Diabetes 2005; 54:8–14.

55. McCarty MF. Up-regulation of PPARgamma coactivator-1alpha as a strategy for preventing and reversing insulin resistance and obesity. Med Hypotheses 2005; 64: 399–407.

56. Puigserver P. Tissue-specific regulation of metabolic pathways through the transcriptional coactivator PGC1-alpha. Int J Obes (Lond) 2005; 29(Suppl. 1):S5–9.

57. Patti ME, Butte AJ, Crunkhorn S, et al. Coordinated reduction of genes of oxidative metabolism in humans with insulin resistance and diabetes: potential role of PGC1 and NRF1. Proc Natl Acad Sci USA 2003; 100:8466–71.

58. Napal L, Marrero PF, Haro D. An intronic peroxisome proliferator-activated receptor-binding sequence mediates fatty acid induction of the human carnitine palmitoyltransferase 1A. J Mol Biol 2005; 354:751–9.

59. Koves TR, Li P, An J, et al. Peroxisome proliferator-activated receptor-gamma co-activator 1alpha-mediated metabolic remodeling of skeletal myocytes mimics exercise training and reverses lipid-induced mitochondrial inefficiency. J Biol Chem 2005; 280:33588–98.

60. Sparks LM, Xie H, Koza RA, et al. A high-fat diet coordinately downregulates genes required for mitochondrial oxidative phosphorylation in skeletal muscle. Diabetes 2005; 54:1926–33.

61. Richardson DK, Kashyap S, Bajaj M, et al. Lipid infusion decreases the expression of nuclear encoded mitochondrial genes and increases the expression of extracellular matrix genes in human skeletal muscle. J Biol Chem 2005; 280:10290–7.

62. Sreekumar R, Unnikrishnan J, Fu A, et al. Effects of caloric restriction on mitochondrial function and gene transcripts in rat muscle. Am J Physiol Endocrinol Metab 2002; 283: E38–43.

9.5 Genes Involved in Gut and Brain Dialogue

Philip Just Larsen
Rheoscience, Rødovre, Denmark

Jens Juul Holst
Faculty of Health Sciences, Institute of Biomedicine, The Panum Institute, University of Copenhagen, Copenhagen, Denmark

Humans and most other living creatures have evolved in environments where food has only been occasionally available. In this context it is understandable that evolutionary selection pressure has favored those individuals who have been able to eat and store as much energy as possible once available. Vast energy stores founded during periods of plenty subsequently served as supplementary calories during periods where food was scarce, enabling women of childbearing age to sustain both pregnancy periods and breast-feeding. Such evolutionary advantages are detrimental in environments where food is never scarce and our current fight against obesity is to a large extent a result of genetic background. Hence it should come as little surprise that a thorough understanding of the expression regulation and function of gene products involved in energy homeostasis is fundamental in our mapping of pathways governing body weight. The brain has a central role as homeostatic device integrating external and internal sensory information for the purpose of keeping physiological variables within narrow limits. Body energy depots are among such regulated variables, and the major central nervous system (CNS) sites involved in this regulation are hypothalamus and lower brainstem areas receiving visceral sensory afferents.

Except for the identification of mutations in the gene encoding the MC4 receptor as a frequent cause of early onset obesity in humans (see Chapter 5.6) exhaustive analyses of candidate genes as well as the entire human genome have been disappointingly unsuccessful in identifying genes linked to increased obesity risk. It is likely that a number of the methodological problems encountered in the early studies of obesity associated candidate genes can be eliminated (standardized genotyping, larger populations, reduced genetic variation, etc.). However, the polygenic nature of obesity and related metabolic complications comprise a much larger challenge for the identification of individual genes responsible for emergence of an obese phenotype. Obesity arises in individuals who carry a cluster of genes each of which generates only a minor tendency to accumulate energy (i.e., fat). Thus, the challenge lies in understanding why human genetics in the current environmental context promotes obesity rather than leanness. In less than a generation, the prevalence of obesity has risen dramatically in most areas of the world. For instance among adults in the United States, obesity is the rule rather than the exception. Thus, it is obvious that our genetic blueprint already harness a combination of genes promoting obesity. In addition to such almost universal predisposition for obesity come ethnic variations, but genetic panmixing between various ethnic groups has probably been quite modest during the last 30 years and hence cannot explain the surge in prevalence of obesity. The interesting question to address is what events may trigger permanent changes of obesity promoting gene functions.

Conceptually, the hunt for genetic variation exerting major impact on obesity may be more fruitful in subjects who in spite of obesigenic environment remain lean. Unfortunately, almost all of today's studies searching for obesity-related genetic polymorphisms are based on populations characterized by various obesity pathologies (weight, childhood obesity, abnormal feeding pattern, insulin resistance, and the likes) (1).

The challenge is to identify the genes, which in the current environmental context are of importance for the regulation of energy storage at large and ectopic triglyceride accumulation in particular. As previously mentioned, obesity is rarely caused by monogenic defects (http://obesitygene.pbrc.edu), but in those rare cases, the functional cause is essentially always to be explained by dysfunctional appetite regulation (http://obesitygene.pbrc.edu/cgi-bin/ace/sgd_table.cgi). Essentially all examined animals from fish to humans are equipped with a robust homeostatic device ensuring relatively stable depots are maintained throughout life. However, in the light of the current obesity epidemic it is obvious that such energy or body weight set point device is not tightly secured against upward drift. From analyses of human and animal feeding behavior it has become evident that most organisms are incapable of correctly assessing energy density of ingested food once it exceeds a critical threshold around 500 to 600 kcal/100 g (2,3). Evidence from epidemiological observations as well as well-controlled animal experiments suggests that early genes-environment interactions cause dysfunctional appetite regulation, which contribute to elevated and perhaps even drifting body weight set point (4,5). Hence, the challenge is to identify which of thousands of genes expressed in neuroendocrine appetite regulating pathways are responsible for fixation and defense of normal (low) energy depot incapable of inducing dysmetabolic syndrome. As previously alluded to such answers may be found among the 10% to 20% "diet-resistant" individuals, who despite exposure to energy-dense diets do not overeat (10–20%) and hence maintain a stable body weight set point throughout life (3,6).

As there is evidence to support that the current obesity epidemic is ascribable to gene-environment interactions on appetite regulation and body-weight set point adjustment, a survey of obesity-promoting genes should direct its attention to genes involved in normal appetitive behavior and adjustment of body-weight set point. Hunger and satiety are primarily determined by intricate interplay between digestive portions of the gastrointestinal tract and integrative homeostatic centers of the brain, including the hypothalamus and the caudal brainstem. In addition, endocrine signals from energy storing depots, such as adipocytes and hepatocytes, are also integrated in the CNS, but as these signals are described in other chapters of this volume, we refer to those for further details. A simple diagram summarizing current knowledge about neuroendocrine pathways involved in appetite regulation is presented in Figure 1.

In the present chapter we have included a few human single-gene obesity disorders, but as they are rare, we have mostly concentrated on obesity-promoting genes, which have been identified via evidence gathered from a variety of genetically manipulated murine models subsequently substantiated by human genetic linkage analysis in a variety of obesity-related phenotypes. In the most recent version of the obesity gene map, 248 genes that, when mutated or expressed in excess as transgenes, result in phenotypes characterized by altered body fat mass and distribution (1). Obviously, not all of these genes are pivotal in appetite regulation, but the abundance of genes, which, when dysfunctional, cause

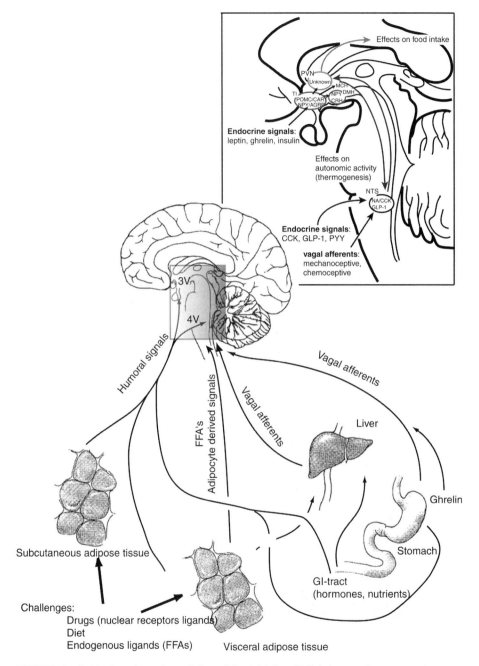

FIGURE 1 Gut-brain axis and regulation of food intake. GLP-1 (preproglucagon, prohormone convertase); PYY (and Y2 receptors), Ghrelin (and GHS receptors), CCK (and CCK receptors), hepatic signals (fatty acid oxidation), gastrointestinal mechanosensory nerves. Central signals: POMC-derived peptides (and MC4 MC3 receptors), leptin receptors, leptin, orexins; CART, NPY and galanin, DMH genes (hibernating etc.); GABA; SLC-1; dopamine, clock. *Abbreviations*: CART, cocaine amphetamine-regulated transcript; CCK, cholecystokinin; FFA, free fatty acids; GI, gastrointestinal; MCH, melanin-concentrating hormone; NPY, neuropeptide Y; POMC, proopiomelanocortin.

jeopardized body fat accumulation, mirrors quite well the complexity of energy homeostasis.

The neuroanatomical circuitry defining a central homeostatic device enabling maintenance of relatively constant sizes of energy depots is far from understood. The sensory components of such energy depot set point device includes leptin-sensitive neurons in the arcuate, ventromedial and dorsomedial hypothalamic nuclei, but as leptin is not the only variable reflecting energy status. Neurons responding to such diverse stimuli as fluctuations in insulin levels, endocrine signals from the digestive tract as well as nutrients are bound to be involved. As both seasonal variation and endocrine status like those appearing in connection with pregnancy has major impact on body weight set point, the gain of the system is subject to adjustment governed by hypothalamic neurons sensitive to light and sex steroids. Short-term signals to the hypothalamic neurons involved in maintenance of energy arise during digestion, and are ultimately integrated in the lower brainstem before being conveyed into the hypothalamus. That, however, is not to say that brainstem circuits are not sensitive to long-term perturbations of energy homeostasis.

It is fully recognized that gastrointestinally released hormones either before onset of a meal or in the postprandial wake of nutrient absorption have an impact on feeding and metabolism. A long-favored idea claimed that peripherally released gastrointestinal tract hormones would mediate their actions via sensory afferents innervating the gastrointestinal tract. However, the prevailing idea of how ghrelin and peptideYY[3-36], two peptide hormones released from the stomach and the gut respectively, influence neural circuits involved in regulation of energy homeostasis propose that both hormones gain access to the hypothalamic arcuate and ventromedial nuclei. Both of these nuclei are shielded from the general circulation by the blood-brain barrier. In the mouse, ghrelin is actively transported across the blood-brain barrier by saturable transporters both from the brain to the blood and from the blood to the cerebrospinal fluid (7). The situation is slightly different for PYY[3-36] as the bidirectional transport across the blood-brain barrier is nonsaturable, albeit of similar magnitude as other important gastrointestinal tract hormones known to impact hypothalamic functions (8).

Mechanical distension of the stomach comprises a powerful anorectic signal once the tension of the gastric wall exceeds certain threshold. Based on anatomical topographic criteria it is possible to classify vagal afferents in three distinct categories, interganglionic laminar endings (IGLEs), intramuscular arrays (IMAs), and mucosal terminals (MTs). Physiological property of IGLEs and IMAs is mainly mechanosensitive because they respond to changes in intramural tension and similar mechanical distortion. The MTs are sensitive to changes in pH and humoral substances released by enteroendocrine cells as well as mechanical distortion (9). Not long ago it was shown that mice deficient for neurotrophin-4 (NT4) have basically no IGLEs in the duodenum, jejunum, and ileum (10). These small intestine IGLEs deficient mice are phenotypically characterized by increased meal durations and increased meal sizes. However, because of compensatory counterregulator mechanisms NT4-deficient mice do not develop obesity suggesting that this type of vagal mechanosensory fibers are not essential in defending a fixed body weight set point. Similarly, mice lacking the IMAs due to a mutation in the c-Kit receptor do not develop an obese phenotype (11). The underlying mechanism of how the mouse $W/W^v/c\text{-}Kit$ mutation leads to loss of IMAs is probably ascribed to the impaired development of intramuscular type of interstitial cells of Cajal (ICC-IMs). The ICC-IMs apparently provide trophic support for IMAs. In contrast to NT4-deficient mice, c-Kit receptor mutant mice eat smaller meals of shorter duration but with increased frequency. Despite distinctly altered pattern of short-term feeding, *c-Kit* mutant mice compensate adequately with resulting normal defense of body weight set point (11). However, *c-Kit* receptor mutant mice display enhanced anorectic response to cholecystokinin A receptor (CCKAR) activation suggesting that postprandial CCK-mediated suppression of further feeding is mediated preferentially via IGLEs within the myenteric plexus of the stomach and small intestine and/or free nerve ending in the mucosal lamina of the gastrointestinal tract. Both IGLEs and IMAs mediate anorectic actions of gastric distension to the nucleus of the solitary tract (NTS). Interestingly, the purely mechanical stimulus of gastric balloon distension has now been shown to preferentially activate preproglucagon synthesizing neurons of the NTS (12). In contrast, gastric balloon distension had no impact on catecholaminergic neurons of the NTS (12).

The chemosensory vagal afferents also terminate in the NTS but mainly via synapses on ascending catecholaminergic neurons and NTS interneurons. The vagal chemosensory afferents express functional receptors activated by postprandially released gastrointestinal tract hormones such as CCK, PYY$^{3-36}$, and glucagon-like peptide 1 (GLP-1) (13,14, and author's own unpublished PJL). So, in summary, mechanosensory vagal afferents synapse with brainstem GLP-1/GLP-2 synthesizing neurons, while chemosensory vagal afferents target catecholaminergic neurons. The gain of both of these ascending NTS pathways is likely to be influenced by longer term fluctuations of energy status as both catecholaminergic and preproglucagon expressing NTS neurons coexpress the long Ob-Rb form of the leptin receptor (15). In the following paragraphs, evidence of genetic variation leading to obesity or other metabolic perturbations is presented for some of the important signaling components in the pathways conveying information about prandial events and size of energy status to hypothalamic and brainstem areas involved in energy homeostasis.

PERIPHERAL SIGNALS
Leptin and Leptin Receptors

The adipocyte derived hormone leptin is synthesized and secreted in amounts directly correlated to intracellular triglyceride accumulation. The story of how meticulous search for a single-gene mutation in ob/ob mice led to the identification of leptin is well known as is also the subsequent identification of dysfunctional leptin receptor function as the cause of similar obesity syndromes in db/db mice and Zucker rats. When leptin is absent, mice and human develop a characteristic phenotype of voracious overeating and morbid obesity and replacement therapy completely reverses this phenotype to that of normal appetite regulation and normal body weight (16). By nature, the downstream localization of leptin receptors, render the obesity syndrome of subjects with mutated leptin receptors insensitive to leptin replacement therapy (see Chapter 5.5). In the CNS, leptin receptors are expressed by neurons in several limbic areas most of which serve integrative roles in regulation of diverse neuroendocrine functions like energy homeostasis, thermoregulation, reproduction, bone formation, appetitive behavior, and autonomic output. With respect to regulation of energy homeostasis, leptin receptors in the arcuate, dorsomedial and ventromedial hypothalamic nuclei as well as in lower brainstem nuclei are considered of highest importance. Impact of leptin on energy homeostasis is mediated via neurons in the hypothalamic arcuate (equivalent to the human tuberoinfundibular nucleus) nucleus, the ventromedial nucleus and the dorsomedial nucleus. Thus, these regions of the brain serve a role as "energy sensor" measuring an important long-term feedback to body weight set point device. In the ventral portion of the arcuate nucleus, two populations of neurons are located, a medial group characterized by their content of both neuropeptide Y (NPY) and Agouti-related peptide (AgRP), and a lateral group characterized by their content of proopiomelanocortin (POMC) derived peptides as well as cocaine amphetamine-regulated transcript (CART) peptides. Medial NPY/AgRP neurons are inhibited by leptin whereas lateral POMC/CART neurons are stimulated by leptin. Hence it is obvious to propose that NPY and AgRP are anabolic neutrotransmitters favoring positive energy balance via stimulation of feeding and inhibition of energy expenditure, whereas POMC and CART derived peptides are catabolic neurotransmitters decreasing food intake and increasing energy expenditure (17).

Interestingly, selective silencing of leptin receptor expression in arcuate neurons have only mild impact on body weight homeostasis suggesting that other areas like the ventromedial and dorsomedial nuclei are of importance with respect to long-term body weight set point maintenance (see Chapter 3.2) (18,19). The ventral portion of the arcuate nucleus projects to several hypothalamic nuclei including the paraventricular nucleus and the lateral hypothalamic area. These areas contain effector neurons which upon stimulation cause altered autonomic output and feeding behavior. A wide variety of transmitters with ascribed functions on energy homeostasis are synthesized in neurons of these hypothalamic sites.

Ghrelin and Growth Hormone Secretagogue Receptors

Ghrelin is an acylated gastrointestinal peptide synthesized in endocrine cells in the mucosal lining of the gut and released in proportion to energy deficits. Administration of exogenous ghrelin to both man and rodents acutely increases food intake and leads to persistent positive energy balance (20,21). Consistent with its pattern of release and plasma fluctuations, ghrelin is likely to be a major factor initiating feeding but it is currently unknown what precisely triggers ghrelin bouts before meals. In a cohort of obese Swedish people, some evidence has been gathered to propose that ghrelin mutations may influence appetite, but as one would be looking for gain of function mutations, ghrelin single-nucleotide polymorphisms (SNPs) are probably more likely to occur among lean subjects. Ghrelin accesses the brain via specific transport mechanism and activates hypothalamic neurons expressing the growth hormone secretagogue receptor (GHSR). In the hypothalamus this receptor is expressed by neurons of the arcuate and the ventromedial nuclei. There is evidence that common SNPs and haplotypes within the genetic region encoding the GHSR are involved in the pathogenesis of human obesity (22), but it has also been shown that missense mutations of the GHSR segregate with short stature and no apparent impact on body weight (23).

Peptide YY[3–36]

Secretion of PYY[3–36] and its costored peptides derived from postprandial processing of preproglucagon from enteroendocrine L-cells is triggered by luminal nutrients. Plasma levels of both PYY$^{3-36}$ and GLP-1 rise after a meal and concomitant administration of the two peptides synergistically inhibit food intake in humans (24). The mechanisms via which sugars activate L-cells involve closure of ATP-sensitive K$^+$ (K(ATP)) channels as well as entry of electrogenic sugars via a sodium-glucose cotransporter (25). It was also recently proposed that a specific fatty acid sensing G-protein coupled receptor GPR120 when activated by unsaturated long-chain free fatty acids triggered PYY$^{3-36}$ and GLP-1 secretion (26).

Since the advent of the first report showing that PYY$^{3-36}$ exerts acute anorectic effects in humans (27), a number of studies providing confirmatory evidence of this initial observation have been published. Thus as seen for GLP-1, obese humans have significantly lower postprandial levels of PYY$^{3-36}$ (28). Also, the therapeutic success of gastric bypass surgery for as a mean to reduce body weight correlates nicely with postsurgical elevation of circulating and postprandial levels of PYY$^{3-36}$ (29). Genetic variation of the gene encoding peptide YY has been observed and in some instances SNPs have been associated with increased obesity and diabetes prevalence among carriers of specific variants further substantiating the importance of PYY$^{3-36}$ as an anorectic gastrointestinal hormone (30–32). Batterham and colleagues propose that postprandially released PYY$^{3-36}$ exerts its anorectic action via interference with Y2 receptor expressing neurons of the arcuate nucleus, although other possible scenarios exist. Thus, it is equally possible that Y2 receptors expressed in neurons of the dorsal vagal complex as well as the vagal afferents mediate anorectic actions of peripheral PYY$^{3-36}$. A human genetic variation of the Y2 receptor has been associated with increased probability of lean phenotype among Swedish men. This observation obviously needs broader confirmation, but it is interesting as it would indicate a clear gain of function mutation.

Glucagon-Like Peptide-1 (GLP-1)

In L-cells of the intestine, the peptide GLP-1 is derived from post-translational processing of preproglucagon, whereas processing proglucagon in the pancreas leads to formation of mainly glucagon. The two processing pathways rely on prohormone convertases 1 and 2 (PC1 and PC2) of which PC1 is primarily active in L-cells, while PC2 is primarily active in pancreatic α-cells. However, PC1 is also involved in processing of proinsulin and POMC rendering subjects with loss of function mutations of this gene susceptible to multiple endocrine perturbations (33). Evidence gathered from use of metabolically stable GLP-1 receptor agonist strongly supports that both peripheral and central GLP-1 receptors mediate lasting anorexia and when constantly stimulated promote negative energy balance (34). However deletion of the GLP-1 receptor in mice has no impact on body weight phenotype, but does cause mild impairment of meal-induced satiety suggesting that genetic defects of this receptor is unlikely to have major impact on body weight homeostasis. This may simply reflect the large degree of redundancy rather than minuscule functional importance of the GLP-1 receptor in body weight regulation as many pharmacological agents have shown their lasting efficacy on body weight.

CENTRAL SIGNALS
Proopiomelanocortin (POMC)

In the forebrain, this gene product is exclusively expressed in the arcuate nucleus. Post-translational processing leads to formation of α-melanocyte-stimulating hormone (α-MSH), β-MSH, γ-MSH, and β-endorphin. Both α-MSH and β-MSH are endogenous ligands for MC3 and MC4 receptors expressed in the brain. Activation of hypothalamic MC4 receptors leads to decreased appetite and increased energy expenditure. Candidate gene analyses have confirmed that defects in POMC processing and/or β-MSH are associated with childhood obesity (see Chapter 5.5) (35,36).

Prohormone Convertase 1 (PC1)
This enzyme catalyzes posttranslational processing of several peptide hormones including POMC and proinsulin. Hence, dysfunctional PC1 action leads to decreased synthesis of α-MSH in hypothalamic neurons as well as decreased insulin secretion (33). Genetically modified mice with ablated PC1 function show same characteristics but are also growth deficient.

Melanocortin 4 Receptor (MC4R)
Central actions of α-MSH are primarily mediated via two G-protein coupled receptors, MC3R and MC4R. In humans, several SNPs have been described for the MC4R gene and various degrees of loss of function are associated with these mutations giving rise to early onset of obesity. Similarly, mice carrying homozygous deletion of the MC4R gene develop an obesity syndrome, which is most marked in male subjects. The human relevance of MC4R mutations for development of obesity has been validated in several populations with different ethnic backgrounds (see Chapter 5.6) (37).

Melanocortin 3 Receptor (MC3R)
The MC3R is expressed in POMC/CART neurons of the arcuate nucleus and serves as an inhibitory autoreceptor when upon stimulation with α-MSH decrease activity of these neurons. Strangely, mutations of the MC3R in humans are associated with obesity syndromes, and mice carrying a homozygous deletion of the *MC3R* gene have increased fat mass and decreased energy expenditure. Thus, more studies are required to fully understand the involvement of this receptor in appetite regulation and energy homeostasis.

Cocaine Amphetamine-Regulated Transcript (CART)
Together with α-MSH, CART derived peptides are the principal neurotransmitters of arcuate POMC containing neurons. However, CART is expressed in many more neurons of the brain rendering functional analysis of this neuropeptide more complicated (38). From the precursor peptide CART55-102 is synthesized, and this peptide elicits anorexia when administered into the brain of a variety of animals (39). In contrast to α-MSH, the putative endogenous CART receptor remains to be identified. In some populations, amino acid substitutions of the coding region of the peptide is associated with hereditary obesity (40), whereas other population analyses have been unable to demonstrate CART mutations associated with obesity (41).

Neuropeptide Y (NPY)
The gene encoding NPY was among to be deleted in a knock out mouse model and it came as a great surprise that absence of the most orexigenic neuropeptide

was without a phenotype. Not only did this observation emphasize the redundancy of energy homeostasis regulating pathways, but also the shortcomings of simplistic reductionist approaches in design of biological experiments. Subsequent studies have shown that lack of both *Npy* and galanin (*Gal*) genes in mice yields an unexpected obesity syndrome. A few SNPs giving rise to gain of function mutations in humans have been associated with increased obesity but these observations remain to be verified in larger populations.

Neuropeptide Y Receptors

Four receptor genes have been identified in this family of G-protein coupled receptors, all of which are negatively coupled to cAMP. In mice deletion of NPY receptors Y1 and Y5 (NPY1R and NPY5R) have been described to cause late onset obesity, and hence these receptors have been recognized as mediators of NPY induced feeding. However, pharmacological characterization of the role of various Y-receptors and regulation of energy homeostasis is somewhat complicated as Y2 and Y4 receptors mediate anorexia. Therefore, nonselective Y-receptor ligands may have highly unpredictable impact on energy homeostasis. In humans, various Y-receptor SNPs have been described for NPY1R and NPYR5 but again these observations need to be confirmed in wider populations.

Agouti-Related Peptide (AgRP)

In the brain, this peptide is expressed exclusively in the NPY neurons of the arcuate nucleus. It represents a unique example of an endogenous antagonist of the MC3R and MC4R (42). Genetically engineered mice that constantly overexpress Agrp develop early onset obesity (43), and mice with postembryonic ablation of the Agrp gene develop a lean hypophagic phenotype (44,45). From human genetic studies evidence has been gathered to support that gain of function SNPs are associated with obesity (46).

Glutamate Decarboxylase 2 (GAD2)

Gammabutyric acid (GABA) is one of the most abundant neurotransmitters of the brain. In the arcuate nucleus, GABA is colocalized with NPY/AgRP. A common side effect of some GABAergic neurotransmitters like antiepileptic agents vigabatrin and valproic acid is weight gain. Therefore, it has been speculated that increased hypothalamic GABA function leads to positive energy balance. Recently, a genome wide scan identified the obesity associated microsatellite D10S197 within the GAD2 gene (47). Subsequent SNP analysis confirmed that exon 7 contains an obesity associated SNP (−239A>G), leading to increased expression of CNS GAD2 and hence promotes increased GABA synthesis in the brain. However, the pertinence of such genetic association is still a matter of debate since it has not been confirmed in independent populations (see Chapter 6.2).

Melanin-Concentrating Hormone (MCH) and MCH-1 Receptors

POMC/CART and NPY/AgRP neurons of the arcuate nucleus synapse with neurons in the lateral hypothalamic area expressing the orexigenic neuropeptide MCH. Rodent studies with genetically manipulated mice have convincingly shown that deletion of both the peptide and or the receptor yields skinny mice whereas transgenic overexpression of *Mch* gives rise to obese mice. Also physiological and pharmacological evidence support the role of MCH as an anabolic neurotransmitter, which increases its activity during states of negative energy balance to compensate for this.

Solute Carrier Family 6 Member 14 (SLC6A14)

In a recent microsatellite analysis of a cohort of obese Finnish individuals a locus on chromosome Xq24 was shown to be strongly associated with obesity (48). Subsequent SNP analysis confirmed that *SLC6A14* gene, which codes for a sodium/potassium-dependent transporter of neutral and basic amino acids, constitute the obesity associated gene (49). The *SLC6A14* gene is expressed in capillary endothelium of the CNS and is responsible for uptake of amino acids like the serotonin precursor amino acid tryptophan. Therefore, dysfunctional SLC6A14 is likely to be associated with reduced substrate availability for serotonin synthesis.

CONCLUSION

As evidenced by the vast list of genes involved in body weight homeostasis presented annually by Bouchard and colleagues the present chapter is but a glimpse of all of the involved molecular pathways involved in maintenance of body energy homeostasis (1). However, it is the hope that a didactical presentation will enable the reader to find inspiration for further reading about this fascinating topic to which there seems no satiation.

REFERENCES

1. Rankinen T, Zuberi A, Chagnon YC, et al. The human obesity gene map: the 2005 update. Obesity (Silver Spring) 2006; 14:529–644.
2. Prentice AM, Poppitt SD. Importance of energy density and macronutrients in the regulation of energy intake. Int J Obes Relat Metab Disord 1996; 20(Suppl. 2):S18–23.
3. Levin BE, Dunn-Meynell AA, Balkan B, et al. Selective breeding for diet-induced obesity and resistance in Sprague–Dawley rats. Am J Physiol 1997; 273:R725–30.
4. Vickers MH, Breier BH, Cutfield WS, et al. Fetal origins of hyperphagia, obesity, and hypertension and postnatal amplification by hypercaloric nutrition. Am J Physiol Endocrinol Metab 2000; 279:E83–7.
5. Bendixen H, Holst C, Sørensen TIA, et al. Major increase in prevalence of overweight and obesity between 1987 and 2001 among Danish adults. Obes Res 2004; 12:1464–72.
6. Blundell JE, Lawton CL, Cotton JR, et al. Control of human appetite: implications for the intake of dietary fat. Annu Rev Nutr 1996; 16:285–319.
7. Banks WA, Tschop M, Robinson SM, et al. Extent and direction of ghrelin transport across the blood–brain barrier is determined by its unique primary structure. J Pharmacol Exp Ther 2002; 302:822–7.
8. Nonaka N, Shioda S, Niehoff ML, et al. Characterization of blood–brain barrier permeability to PYY3–36 in the mouse. J Pharmacol Exp Ther 2003; 306:948–53.
9. Berthoud HR, Lynn PA, Blackshaw LA. Vagal and spinal mechanosensors in the rat stomach and colon have multiple receptive fields. Am J Physiol Regul Integr Comp Physiol 2001; 280:R1371–81.
10. Fox EA, Phillips RJ, Baronowsky EA, et al. Neurotrophin-4 deficient mice have a loss of vagal intraganglionic mechanoreceptors from the small intestine and a disruption of short-term satiety. J Neurosci 2001; 21:8602–15.
11. Chi MM, Powley TL. c-Kit mutant mouse behavioral phenotype: altered meal patterns and CCK sensitivity but normal daily food intake and body weight. Am J Physiol Regul Integr Comp Physiol 2003; 285:R1170–83.

12. Vrang N, Phifer CB, Corkern MM, et al. Gastric distension induces c-Fos in medullary GLP1/2 containing neurons. Am J Physiol Regul Integr Comp Physiol 2003; 285:R470–8.
13. Corp ES, McQuade J, Moran TH, et al. Characterization of type A and type B CCK receptor binding sites in rat vagus nerve. Brain Res 1993; 623:161–6.
14. Zhang X, Shi T, Holmberg K, et al. Expression and regulation of the neuropeptide Y Y2 receptor in sensory and autonomic ganglia. Proc Natl Acad Sci USA 1997; 94:729–34.
15. Hay-Schmidt A, Helboe L, Larsen PJ. Leptin receptor immunoreactivity is present in ascending serotonergic and catecholaminergic neurons of the rat. Neuroendocrinology 2001; 73:215–26.
16. O'Rahilly S, Farooqi IS, Yeo GSH, et al. Minireview: human obesity—lessons from monogenic disorders. Endocrinology 2003; 144:3757–64.
17. Schwartz MW, Woods SC, Porte D, et al. Central nervous system control of food intake. Nature 2000; 404:661–71.
18. Balthasar N, Coppari R, McMinn J, et al. Leptin receptor signaling in POMC neurons is required for normal body weight homeostasis. Neuron 2004; 42:983–91.
19. Dhillon H, Zigman JM, Ye C, et al. Leptin directly activates SF1 neurons in the VMH, and this action by leptin is required for normal body-weight homeostasis. Neuron 2006; 49:191–203.
20. Wren AM, Seal LJ, Cohen MA, et al. Ghrelin enhances appetite and increases food intake in humans. J Clin Endocrinol Metab 2001; 86:5992.
21. Tschöp M, Smiley DL, Heiman ML. Ghrelin induces adiposity in rodents. Nature 2000; 407:908–13.
22. Baessler A, Hasinoff MJ, Fischer M, et al. Genetic linkage and association of the growth hormone secretagogue receptor (ghrelin receptor) gene in human obesity. Diabetes 2005; 54:259–67.
23. Pantel J, Legendre M, Cabrol S, et al. Loss of constitutive activity of the growth hormone secretagogue receptor in familial short stature. J Clin Invest 2006; 116:760–8.
24. Neary NM, Small CJ, Druce MR, et al. Peptide YY3–36 and glucagon-like peptide-17-36 inhibit food intake additively. Endocrinology 2005; 146(12):5120–27.
25. Gribble FM, Williams L, Simpson AK, et al. A novel glucose-sensing mechanism contributing to glucagon-like peptide-1 secretion from the GLUTag cell line. Diabetes 2003; 52:1147–54.
26. Hirasawa A, Tsumaya K, Awaji T, et al. Free fatty acids regulate gut incretin glucagon-like peptide-1 secretion through GPR120. Nat Med 2005; 11:90–4.
27. Batterham RL, Cowley MA, Small CJ, et al. Gut hormone PYY(3–36) physiologically inhibits food intake. Nature 2002; 418:650–4.
28. Batterham RL, Cohen MA, Ellis SM, et al. Inhibition of food intake in obese subjects by peptide YY3–36. N Engl J Med 2003; 349:941–8.
29. Naslund E, Gryback P, Hellstrom PM, et al. Gastrointestinal hormones and gastric emptying 20 years after jejunoileal bypass for massive obesity. Int J Obes Relat Metab Disord 1997; 21:387–92.
30. Ma L, Tataranni PA, Hanson RL, et al. Variations in peptide YY and Y2 receptor genes are associated with severe obesity in Pima Indian men. Diabetes 2005; 54:1598–602.
31. Torekov SS, Larsen LH, Glumer C, et al. Evidence of an association between the Arg72 allele of the peptide YY and increased risk of type 2 diabetes. Diabetes 2005; 54:2261–5.
32. Ahituv N, Kavaslar N, Schackwitz W, et al. A PYY Q62P variant linked to human obesity. Hum Mol Genet 2006; 15:387–91.
33. Jackson RS, Creemers JW, Ohagi S, et al. Obesity and impaired prohormone processing associated with mutations in the human prohormone convertase 1 gene. Nat Genet 1997; 16:303–6.
34. Larsen PJ, Holst JJ. Glucagon-related peptide 1 (GLP-1): hormone and neurotransmitter. Regul Pept 2005; 128:97–107.
35. Krude H, Biebermann H, Luck W, et al. Severe early-onset obesity, adrenal insufficiency and red hair pigmentation caused by POMC mutations in humans. Nature Genetic 1998; 19:155–7.
36. Challis BG, Pritchard LE, Creemers JW, et al. A missense mutation disrupting a dibasic prohormone processing site in pro-opiomelanocortin (POMC) increases susceptibility

to early-onset obesity through a novel molecular mechanism. Hum Mol Genet 2002; 11:1997–2004.

37. Farooqi IS, Keogh JM, Yeo GS, et al. Clinical spectrum of obesity and mutations in the melanocortin 4 receptor gene. N Engl J Med 2003; 348:1085–95.

38. Vrang N, Larsen PJ, Clausen JT, et al. Neurochemical characterization of hypothalamic cocaine-amphetamine-regulated transcript neurons. J Neurosci 1999; 19:RC5,1–8.

39. Kristensen P, Judge M, Thim L, et al. The hypothalamic peptide CART is regulated by leptin and counteracts NPY induced feeding. Nature (London) 1998; 393:72–6.

40. del Giudice EM, Santoro N, Cirillo G, et al. Mutational screening of the cart gene in obese children: identifying a mutation (leu34phe) associated with reduced resting energy expenditure and cosegregating with obesity phenotype in a large family. Diabetes 2001; 50:2157–60.

41. Echwald SM, Sørensen TIA, Andersen T, et al. Sequence variants in the human cocaine and amphetamine-regulated transcript (CART) gene in subjects with early onset obesity. Obes Res 1999; 7:532–6.

42. Barsh GS, He L, Gunn TM. Genetic and biochemical studies of the Agouti-attracting system. J Recept Signal Transduct Res 2002; 22:63–77.

43. Ellacott KL, Cone RD. The central melanocortin system and the integration of short- and long-term regulators of energy homeostasis. Recent Prog Horm Res 2004; 59:395–408.

44. Bewick GA, Gardiner JV, Dhillo WS, et al. Post-embryonic ablation of AgRP neurons in mice leads to a lean, hypophagic phenotype. FASEB J 2005; 19:1680–2.

45. Wortley KE, Anderson KD, Yasenchak J, et al. Agouti-related protein-deficient mice display an age-related lean phenotype. Cell Metab 2005; 2:421–7.

46. Argyropoulos G, Rankinen T, Neufeld DR, et al. A polymorphism in the human Agouti-related protein is associated with late-onset obesity. J Clin Endocrinol Metab 2002; 87:4198–202.

47. Boutin P, Dina C, Vasseur F, et al. GAD2 on chromosome 10p12 is a candidate gene for human obesity. PLOS Biol 2003; 1:001–11.

48. Ohman M, Oksanen L, Kaprio J, et al. Genome-wide scan of obesity in Finnish sibpairs reveals linkage to chromosome Xq24. J Clin Endocrinol Metab 2000; 85:3183–90.

49. Suviolahti E, Oksanen LJ, Ohman M, et al. The SLC6A14 gene shows evidence of association with obesity. J Clin Invest 2003; 112:1762–72.

10.1 Introduction to Omics Platforms

Martin Kussmann, Frédéric Raymond, and Michael Affolter

Functional Genomics Group, Bioanalytical Science Department, Nestlé Research Center, Lausanne, Switzerland

Proteomics, the comprehensive analysis of a protein complement in a cell, tissue, or biological fluid at a given time, has been enabled by quantum leaps in mass spectrometric technology, which allowed identification of large, involatile biomolecules. Over the last two decades, this discipline evolved from the sole delivery of protein identities to a platform that reveals clues to function through quantitative proteomics, i.e., the global comparison of protein amounts between two defined biological states, and the characterization of protein modifications and interactions.

Proteomics is an integral part and key player in the family of omic disciplines as there are genomics (gene analysis), transcriptomics (gene expression analysis), metabonomics (metabolite profiling), and proteomics (1). Considering complexity, dynamics, and protein concentration range of any given proteome, proteomics is the most challenging omic discipline and requires the most sophisticated analysis pipeline encompassing sample preparation, analyte preseparation and the tools for protein detection, identification, characterization and quantitation. Apart from addressing the most complex "ome," proteomics represents the only platform that delivers not only markers for disposition and efficacy but also targets of intervention (2).

Metabonomics is a diagnostic tool for metabolic classification of individuals. The great asset of this platform is the quantitative, noninvasive analysis of easily accessible human body fluids like urine, blood, and saliva. Metabonomics has been employed in preclinical and clinical research, for environmental, biomedical application, and in toxicology (3). Moreover, it has gained a strong impact in nutritional research (4).

With many genomes sequenced, their respective transcriptomes can be predicted with certain accuracy. Genome-wide gene expression analysis (transcriptomics) can therefore deliver a comprehensive view on all genes active at a given time in a given sample. This degree of completeness in terms of analysis can neither be achieved with proteomics not with metabonomics, simply because neither the (e.g., human) proteome nor the metabolome are known (yet).

TRANSCRIPTOMICS

The comprehensive study of active and regulated genes through transcriptomic techniques, such as microarrays, has created molecular insight into health and disease mechanisms. The molecular description of health is a greater challenge than that of disease, as health encompasses a wider biological "bandwidth." The analysis of gene expression deepens the understanding of pathways and regulatory networks, helps identifying diagnostic and prognostic biomarkers as well as potential targets for intervention. Moreover, transcriptomic studies have improved the understanding of the complex interaction between genetic and environmental factors, such as lifestyle and nutrition (1,5) and have enabled the assessment of nutritional interventions at global gene expression level.

Genome-Wide Expression Analysis

Today, mainly two platforms for paralleled multiple gene expression analysis are employed: serial analysis of gene expression (SAGE) and DNA microarrays. The latter consist of a predefined arrangement of many probe sequences, which serve as hybridization templates for RNA or DNA fragments generated from the sample. This technology allows for parallel monitoring of gene expression levels, and has been extended to the study of gene regulation and interaction at whole-genome level. The platform features high-density arrays of probe sequences, multicolour fluorescent labeling, fluorescent signal detection, and complex software for data analysis and interpretation. DNA microarrays either use one- or two-color fluorescent tagging allowing for direct transcript profile comparisons of, e.g., different tissue types (6), normal versus diseased sample (7), and time-course monitoring of cell cultures subjected to different treatments and conditions (8). They either rely on polymerase chain reaction (PCR)-amplified cDNAs (100–3000 bp), short oligonucleotides (15–25 mers), or long oligonucleotides (50–120 mers) as array elements.

Microarrays have become a reference technology for gene expression profiling with broad application areas like genetic screening for mutations (9), safety assessment of food products (10), detection of allele-specific gene expression (11), and disease diagnostics (12). This said, microarrays are "closed systems" as they are limited to measuring transcript abundances with preselected, known probe sequences. Moreover, technology standardization in order to achieve inter-platform and inter-laboratory comparability (13) is challenging.

More recent multiplexed technologies offer alternatives to microarrays, such as SAGE (14), massively parallel signature sequencing (MPSS) (15), and total gene expression analysis (TOGA) (16). These platforms represent "open systems," can go beyond a known preselection of probes and are therefore suited for gene discovery. In addition, they offer linear gene expression quantitation over a wide dynamic range. SAGE offers the attractive feature of analyzing the expression pattern of thousands of genes in a quantitative manner without prior sequence information. Moreover, SAGE-based quantitation of gene expression relies on fluorescence readout of tagged sequences, which covers a wider linear dynamic range than hybridization-based quantitation (17). These advantages have already been exploited in several applications such as the study of brain diseases (18); the identification of targets of oncogenes and tumor suppressor genes (19); and the gene expression response to cardiovascular diseases such as atherosclerosis (20). The major limitation of SAGE is the expensive and time-consuming purification and sequencing of a large number of clones and associated constraints to throughput.

Microarray Platform Comparison

Despite a 10-year history of DNA microarray analysis, the specific sample and data processing methods differ significantly between platforms and laboratories.

Due to this lack of standardization, inter-laboratory and inter-platform comparisons of microarray-derived data sets have to date been difficult: studies interrogating gene regulation in similar contexts have often resulted in poorly overlapping lists of regulated genes (21). This limited inter-platform correspondence may be deduced both to complementarity of the latter and delivery of false-positives (specificity issue) and false-negatives (sensitivity issue). While custom-made microarrays have generally delivered less reproducible results between experimental repeats than commercial microarrays, variances associated with measurement errors within an experiment are comparable between both, custom and commercial, platforms. Moreover, inter-platform correlation is greater when excluding low-abundant genes, especially because of the different levels of background signal (due to nonspecific binding) between platforms (22).

The difficulties in comparing gene expression data between microarray platforms is in parts caused by a missing standard format for exchanging microarray data between laboratories and, most importantly, the absence of rules for description and execution of microarray experiments. In order to address this need for standardization of RNA sample preparation, on-chip hybridization, data acquisition, processing and documentation, the minimal information about a microarray experiment (MIAME) working group defined how to generate, collect, and describe gene expression data (23).

With similar objectives in mind, the Association of Biomolecular Research Facilities (ABRF) performed an inter-platform comparison, in which they outsourced a standardized gene expression study to several laboratories, all of which had in-depth expertise with the respective platform under scrutiny (24). The microarray platforms of Affymetrix, Amersham, and Agilent as well as custom-spotted arrays from whole-genome oligonucleotide sets from Operon, ClonTech, and MWG were compared in terms of reproducibility and consistency. Independent validation of accuracy and sensitivity was provided by assaying the same samples by large-scale quantitative RT-PCR (qRT-PCR) and SAGE on the 100 genes most discordant between platforms.

Nature methods recently dedicated a series of articles to the comparability of microarray data. In one of the studies, 10 experienced laboratories teamed up to compare data from three widely used platforms using identical RNA samples (25). The performance of Affymetrix gene chips was compared to that of two-color spotted cDNA arrays and two-color long oligonucleotide arrays. Whereas generally relatively large differences were observed between facilities using the same platform, the results from the best performing laboratories agreed rather well. Another comparison in the same context considered Affymetrix mouse chips and murine-spotted cDNA arrays and aligned these results with those from qRT-PCR (26). For almost 12,000 genes present on both chips and arrays, the relative impact of experimental procedure and platform choice on measured gene expression was assessed. For more than 90% of the genes, biological treatment has a far greater influence on measured expression than platform use and this overall result was validated by qRT-PCR. In the few cases of inter-platform discrepancies, qRT-PCR generally did not confirm either set of data, suggesting these differences as being due to sequence-specific effects and difficult to compensate for with any platform. The Toxicogenomics Research Consortium contributed a third paper to these investigations (27): RNA expression data were generated in seven laboratories, which compared two standard RNA samples using 12 microarray platforms. Reproducibility for most platforms within any facility was typically good, while reproducibility between laboratories and across platforms was generally poor. Inter-laboratory reproducibility improved significantly with standardized protocols being applied to RNA labeling and hybridization, microarray processing, data acquisition, and normalization.

Summarizing, while technological differences may influence gene expression measurements, standardized procedures, high-quality microarrays and appropriate data collection and transformation are able to generate reproducible and comparable results across laboratories, especially when a common platform and a joint set of procedures are used. Details regarding microarray analysis are provided in Chapter 10.2.

PROTEOMICS

The word "proteome" was coined in late 1994 at the Siena 2D electrophoresis meeting (28) and implies since then the total protein complement present in a cell, tissue, or body fluid at a given time. Consequently, proteomics stands for the comprehensive analysis of this protein complement.

Mass Spectrometry

The impact of mass spectrometry (MS) on proteomics and other fields was acknowledged by the award of the Nobel Prize to John B. Fenn and Koichi Tanaka for the development of electrospray ionization (ESI) and matrix-assisted laser desorption/ionization (MALDI) MS, respectively (29,30). In the ESI mode, peptides and proteins are multiply protonated and then gently transferred from solution to gas phase yielding multiply charged ions (31). The MALDI technique puts molecules straight from solid to gas phase with the help of laser irradiation and the so-called matrix (32). The MALDI process yields predominantly singly charged ions. With these tools at hand, it became feasible to identify proteins on the basis of sets of peptide masses (peptide mass fingerprints [PMF]), generated by a specific protease like trypsin. However, as protein databases grew, as did the interest in identifying proteins through direct interrogation of genomic databases, the need of more specific information became evident. This limitation was overcome by the introduction of the tandem MS (MS/MS) approach, i.e., by fragmenting peptides selectively isolated in the mass spectrometer in order to readout the amino acid sequence. In the ESI operation, sequencing is typically performed by collision of peptides with gas atoms (collision-induced dissociation [CID]) (33,34). The MALDI mode allows for both CID and spontaneous decay, the latter simply giving the peptides enough time to break up, as they carry a lot of energy from the ionization process (35). The combination of MS/MS with increasing mass accuracy (to date: low ppm range) both in MS and MS/MS mode has rendered modern mass spectrometers powerful tools for protein identification.

Today, almost any ion source can be combined with almost any analyser leading to a variety of (hybrid) mass spectrometers. Quadrupole (Q) analysers are scanning mass separators, which enable selected-ion, selected-reaction, and multiple-reaction monitoring (SIM, SRM, and MRM) (36). These acquisition modes deliver information on diagnostic fragment ions and are in particular useful for high-throughput analysis of posttranslational modifications (PTMs) (37). The ion trap (IT) can be repeatedly filled with ions of a given mass and allows for sensitive MS/MS and multiple-stage (MS^n) experiments (38,39). Time-of-flight (ToF) analysers convince by great sensitivity (no scanning, all ions generated are analyzed) and, since the introduction of reflectron analysers (40) and delayed-extraction (also known as pulsed-ion extraction or time-lag focussing) (41) by high mass accuracy (low ppm range) and resolution (10,000+). These three major types of mass analysers can be combined to triple-Q, Q-IT, Q-ToF, IT-ToF, and ToF-ToF tandem mass spectrometers. A fundamentally new way of looking at peptide and protein ions is the so-called Fourier-transform ion cyclotron resonance (FT-ICR) technique (42,43): ions are analyzed by their mass-dependent frequency, with which they resonate in an electromagnetic field. This nondestructive analysis can be done over a long period of time and provides unsurpassed mass accuracy (low ppm) and resolution (100,000+), which allow for so-called top-down protein analysis (44): proteins are identified and analyzed directly, without previous proteolytic digestion or other chemical processing. FT-ICR is particularly powerful for peptide sequencing when combined with electron-capture dissociation (ECD) (45), an electron-induced peptide backbone fragmentation mechanism generating clean c- and z-ion series (46). This fragmentation method generates different and often complementary fragmentation patterns when compared to CID. The generation of clean ion series only revealing one or two types of ions is nowadays also possible by electron-transfer dissociation (ETD), which can be combined with standard ITs (47) and hence bypasses the necessity of an investment into a FT-ICR machine. Moreover, the recently developed OrbiTrap mass spectrometer (48) also determines peptide and protein molecular masses by measuring their frequencies in electromagnetic fields, and offers mass accuracy equivalent to FT-ICR combined with high resolution (80,000) at a significantly lower price compared to FT-ICR instruments.

Proteomic Concepts and Strategies

The complexity of a proteome is overwhelming. While the human genome "only" comprises 25,000+ genes (49,50), the human proteome is estimated to encompass several 100,000 proteins and an order of magnitude more protein forms and variants (due to gene and protein splicing, PTMs, etc.). In addition to this complexity, the overall dynamic range of individual protein levels spans six orders of magnitude in a cell and even 10 in the human body, for example, in plasma (51–53). At present, MS-based proteomic pipelines cover a dynamic range of typically 10^3 in a single spectrum and 10^4 to 10^6 if one takes on-line preseparations into account (54). This circumstance is of utmost importance, because protein analysis lacks the equivalent of PCR amplification (55). However, recent progress has been made in developing such an amplification approach by redirecting self-splicing protein inteins to create so-called "tadpoles," i.e., chimeric molecules composed of a protein head and an oligonucleotide tail (56).

Proteomics addresses three categories of biological interest: protein expression, protein structure, and protein function. While the first category is nowadays approachable at global level and large scale, structure and function studies are rather applied to classes of proteins and subproteomes.

In order to meet all these challenges, several a priori considerations about the sample have to be made: (a) ex vivo proteomics: biological fluid (plasma, urine, saliva, tears, cerebrospinal fluid) versus tissue (e.g., heart, liver, kidney, gut, brain); (b) in vitro proteomics: cells and bacteria; (c) sample pooling for deep analysis of a representative proteome versus many individual sample to assess biological variability (57); (d) total proteome versus subproteomes (e.g., glycoproteins/phosphoproteins); (e) fractionation (to address complexity and dynamic range) (58), depletion (of most abundant proteins) (53), and enrichment (of low-abundant proteins). The separation of proteomes into subsets can be based either on tissue or (sub-) cellular localization, physical protein properties, or temporal expression differences.

Two principal approaches toward global protein display and identification have emerged: (a) the "gel approach" (2DE-MS/MS), i.e., protein display on a two-dimensional gel (2DE, separation by mass and isoelectric point, pI), likely preceded by chromatographic protein preseparation, followed by protein spot excision, in-spot protein digestion and protein identification by (tandem) MS (59); (b) "shotgun proteomics" or multidimensional protein identification technology (MudPIT) (2DLC-MS/MS) (60,61), i.e., early digestion of the protein mixture and multidimensional (e.g., SCX-RP) chromatographic separation of the peptides followed by on-line mass spectrometric peptide detection and sequencing.

The gel strategy offers the advantage of visualization of proteins and, to some extent, their modifications and of preserving the protein context. Given the fact that the two-dimensional gel technique is not easily converted into high-throughput mode, a more automated system, the so-called molecular scanner combining 2DE, transmembrane digestion and blotting with peptide mass finger-printing was described (62). In contrast to the gels, early digestion policies generate peptides upstream in the analysis workflow, because peptides are more easily amenable to separation and analysis and behave more uniformly than proteins. Since proteins with extreme properties, i.e., very small, very large, very hydrophobic, and very acidic/basic proteins tend to give poor 2DE results, one-dimensional gels (mass separation only, no pI focusing) and multidimensional chromatography are alternatively employed (63). In the same light of overcoming intrinsic 2DE limitations but with the objective of preserving the superior iso-electric focusing (IEF) separation power, continuous-flow liquid-phase IEF, or free flow electrophoresis (FFE) (64) and multicompartment off-gel IEF (65) have been developed, the latter also being applied to peptide level (66). IEF nowadays precedes LC separation steps, a trend pointing toward the merger of gel- and the LC-centered strategies. Overall, both the gel-related and the shotgun strategies have shown to complement each other in terms of proteomic coverage.

The complementarity also applies to the major ionization techniques applied today in proteomics and introduced in the preceding chapter, namely ESI and MALDI (67). While LC preseparation couples almost naturally to ESI MS due to the possibility of continuous sample infusion into the ES ion source (68), paralleled MS and MS/MS on a chromatography timescale puts, however, constraints in terms of comprehensive analysis of an eluting peak. Improved preseparation and data acquisition refinements like mass exclusion lists (every peptide only sequenced once), ultrahigh resolution LC (UPLC) plus total MS/MS per chromatographic peak (69), and gas-phase fractionation (70) can alleviate but not resolve the peak capacity problem (71). In view of these intrinsic LC-MS/MS limitations, MALDI MS has been coupled to preceding LC separation in an automated, but off-line mode (72): LC is now timewise uncoupled from MS and the latter is, in acquisition terms, independent of MS/MS. Comparative proteomic studies employing LC-ESI-MS/MS and LC-MALDI-MS/MS reveal complementary results (73).

Protein Modifications

Once a protein profile has been established and proteins of interest have been selected, issues like protein quantitation, protein structure, PTMs, protein interactions (complex components, stoichiometry, contact interfaces), protein localization, and protein dynamics are likely to be addressed in a follow-up study. When it comes to analyzing PTMs, enrichment of modified peptides and proteins is a key prerequisite, because these analytes are often low in abundance and they tend to yield poorer mass spectrometric signals due to inferior ionization and enhanced fragmentation compared to "naked" peptides.

Protein phosphorylation is one of the most abundant and relevant PTMs and quite advanced in terms of global mass spectrometric analysis, which is based on several complementary approaches (74). Commonly, phosphoproteins and peptides are enriched using e.g., affinity-based methods such as immobilized-metal affinity chromatography (IMAC) (75) and, since recently, titanium dioxide material (76). Alternatively, MS-based scanning modes to selectively detect and identify phosphorylated peptides by SIM and SRM are employed. These techniques allow for large-scale phosphoproteome exploration (77) not only in qualitative but also in quantitative aspects, especially if combined with isotope labeling (78).

Glycoprotein enrichment and analysis is more complicated due to the immense variety of natural protein glycosylation: there are N- and O-linked sugars, the latter being relatively simple but often transient like phosphorylation, the first being large assemblies (complex, high-mannose, and hybrid chains with variably extended antennae) but less regulated on the same timescale. Lectins (79,80) and phenylboronates (81,82) are common chemical ways for enriching glycoproteins and peptides. The more transient but structurally simpler O-glycosylation can be addressed in a fashion similar to the phosphopeptide analysis, i.e., through detection of diagnostic mass losses and identification of peptides, which carried the corresponding sugar moieties (83,84). The much more complex N-glycans need to be addressed either by top-down MS (i.e., FT-ICR-MS analysis of intact glycoproteins) (43,85) or by combining sequential exoglycosidase digestion of the glycopeptides or glycans with MS monitoring of the truncated structures (86), or by hyphenation of biochemical and MS methodologies to increase sensitivity and specificity (87).

Quantitative Proteomics

Current approaches toward quantitative proteomics split into four categories: (a) differential protein labeling with dyes, two-dimensional gel electrophoresis (2DE), and *relative* quantitation by imaging (88,89); (b) differential isotope-coded tagging (ICT), chromatography and *relative* quantitation by MS (90–92); (c) *relative* peptide and protein quantitation by direct comparison of LC-MS/MS data (label-free) (93); and (d) *absolute* protein quantitation by spiking "proteotypic" peptides representative of each protein of interest as internal standards (e.g., absolute quantitation [AQUA] technology) (94).

1. The most widely applied approach is "differential imaging gel electrophoresis" (DIGE) (95). This strategy offers differential fluorescence readout, a wide dynamic range and a high information content resulting from two-dimensional protein patterns. However, gel-based techniques reveal their limitations when it comes to the analysis of proteins at the extremes of the p*I* or MW range and if the

proteins are very hydrophobic, like it is the case for membrane proteins (96,97). Moreover, the technique is costly and automation is limited (98).

2. This category splits further into (i) metabolic labeling, i.e., incorporation of isotopically labeled amino acids (e.g., stable isotope labeling of amino acids in cell culture [SILAC]), (examples provided in Chapter 10.5) and (ii) derivatization of proteins and peptides after recovery and/or digestion (isotope-coded affinity tag, ICAT, iTRAQ, ICPL, etc.; for a review see (71)). Isotope-coded labeling (ICL)-related procedures and subsequent MS-based quantitation rely on "early" digestion of the protein mixture and separation at peptide level (shotgun proteomics, MudPIT) (99,100). While gel-associated drawbacks can be circumvented, also ICL approaches have their limitations: multistep chemical derivatization and peptide isolation incorporate the risk of insufficient yields and the alteration of the sample composition. Moreover, ICL approaches are often compromised by a protein bias due to tagging postdigestion, amino acid-targeted reagents (101), or chromatographic separation of heavy and light label (91,102). In view of the need for complementary protein quantitation techniques, our laboratory has developed a differential tagging strategy, which combines protein identification with quantitation (103,104): proteins are specifically labeled at both their N- and C-terminus prior to digestion and the resulting proteolytic terminal peptides can be enriched and/or specifically detected. The tag can furthermore generate simplified fragmentation patterns and hence can facilitate protein identification based on terminal protein sequences.

3. LC-MS/MS-based relative protein quantitation without any labeling at protein or peptide level must necessarily rely on high resolution and high retention time reproducibility of the chromatography (105). In this context, a continuous and rapid alternation between MS and MS/MS mode switching between high- and low-energy collision has been proposed and further explored to study PTMs such as phosphorylation (106) or acetylation and glycosylation (107). The averaged LC-MS/MS intensities of the three most abundant tryptic peptides of a given protein seem to correlate with the absolute amount of this protein and may therefore be useful not only for relative but also for

4. *Absolute quantitation* of proteins in complex mixtures (108). Apart from this possibly useful correlation, absolute protein quantitation in mixtures is—as most other MS-related quantitation technique—to date predominantly based on internal standards. In the "classical" AQUA approach, the most promising peptide in terms of MS amenability of a given protein is synthesized with an isotope tag and spiked into the sample (109). This strategy was proposed at global scale by Aebersold et al. under the name of "proteotypic" peptides (110): it is envisaged to make such a "best flying," labeled peptide for any protein predicted from the human genome sequence. Following the QCAT variant of quantitative proteomics, a set of such tagged proteotypic peptides is designed and incorporated into an artificial, chemically synthesized protein, which is subsequently spiked into the sample and codigested with the unknown proteins, giving rise to defined tryptic peptides of known concentrations (111). Two further absolute protein quantitation methods without internal standards are the so-called visible ICAT approach (VICAT, biotin-containing ICAT reagent providing LC-traceability and quantitation by non-MS techniques) (112), and a combination of acid hydrolysis and amino acid analysis by MALDI-MS (113).

METABONOMICS
Nuclear Magnetic Resonance Spectroscopy and Mass Spectrometry

Nuclear magnetic resonance (NMR) spectroscopy (114) and MS (115) dominate the metabolic profiling strategies employed to date. MS is more generally and NMR is increasingly coupled upfront to LC (116) or GC preseparation of the analytes. Apart from "classical" MALDI- and ESI-based techniques, FT-ICR MS (117,118) has advanced metabonomic analysis due to its superior mass accuracy (low ppm) and resolution (100,000+). Due to this sensitivity and resolution power, FT-ICR nowadays enables deciphering complex metabolite mixtures without extensive preseparation (119).

NMR usually relies on measuring proton resonances (^{1}H-NMR), mainly because this classical one-dimensional measurement is the most sensitive NMR experiment. But also other nuclei are used in NMR-based metabonomics, such as ^{19}F (120).

Both MS and NMR are complementary technologies and therefore often used in parallel in metabonomic laboratories. Modern metabonomic platforms typically consist of some LC preseparation followed by a sample split: the major part of the sample is trapped and preconcentrated for NMR purposes and a smaller amount is directly passed on to MS. While MS is superior in terms of speed, sensitivity and compound identification, NMR offers other specific advantages: the technique is per se quantitative and the axis of the chemical shift (ppm) is more stable and reproducible than the LC-MS typical coordinate of retention time. Consequently, NMR facilitates inter-platform and/or inter-laboratory comparison (121). The sensitivity limitation of NMR-based metabonomics can partially be circumvented by sample preconcentration through reversed-phase capture and by utilization of NMR cryoprobes. A particularly advantageous NMR feature is the option of profiling metabolites in intact tissues by magic angle spinning (MAS) (122). This is important, since any extraction procedure may bias the original sample composition as present in the original tissue material. In order to perform MAS-NMR, a few milligrams of tissue are placed in a special rotor and spun rapidly at 54.7° relative to the applied magnetic field within the bore of the magnet. Doing so, the line broadening, characteristic of solid-state NMR, can be dramatically reduced and, consequently, resolution is greatly enhanced.

Chemometrics

Chemometrics can be understood as a statistical and mathematical toolbox for chemistry (123) and differs in that sense from bioinformatics, which means storage, retrieval, and analysis of computer-derived information (rather than raw data) in a biological context (124). In the context of NMR- and MS-based metabolomics, chemometrics encompasses spectral processing, peak alignment, outlier detection, normalization, and so forth. Chemometrics started as a discipline with the effort to use any entire spectrum as source of information rather than only the assignable peaks (125,126). Today, the interpretation of Omics-derived spectra involves both pattern recognition and peak-to-molecule assignment.

Principal component analysis (PCA) has become a central statistical method to process omic data (127): large amounts of mass spectral or NMR spectroscopic data are in the PCA context understood as a multivariate statistical problem and the metabolite or protein concentrations represent the true variables. Spectra are divided into "bins" of discrete spectral width (ppm in the case of NMR, m/z in the case of MS) and the areas under the curve in these "bins" are integrated and serve as pseudovariables. PCA therefore reduces a large number of (usually correlated) "true" variables into a smaller number of (uncorrelated) variables, the so-called principal components (PC). PCA results in the decomposition of raw data into "scores," which reveal the relationship between samples, and into "loadings" that show the relationships between the variables. The first PC explains the greatest variability in the data, the second PC (independent of/orthogonal to the first) explains it second best and so on. If ones thinks of a data space reduced to a cube, PCA resembles to turning the cube in different angles and to identifying planes in the data space, which separate the groups (typically control and case) investigated and compared.

Applied Metabonomics

An advantage of global metabolite profiling is—besides the complementary use of NMR and MS for the sake of quantitation and sensitivity—the noninvasive nature of monitoring metabolic endpoints in humans (128). Metabonomics has been employed in preclinical and clinical research, for environmental, biomedical application, and in toxicology (129). Moreover, it has gained a strong impact in nutritional research (130). As valid for other Omics disciplines, metabolite profiling, identification and quantitation face the challenge of pronounced interindividual variability. In addition, metabolite profiles vary significantly over time and strongly depend on dietary intake and physical activity. The inter-platform and inter-laboratory variability of NMR-based studies is generally lower compared to MS-based (metabonomic or proteomic) or chip-based (transcriptomic) profiling techniques. In this perspective, recommendations for standardization and reporting of metabolic analyses have been recently published by the standard metabolic reporting structures (SMRS) working group (131).

Earlier metabonomic studies of inborn metabolic errors focused on pathway identification. Lindon et al. have reviewed NMR-based analyses of 40 human inborn errors in metabolism (132). Brindle et al. reported on a rapid and non-invasive metabonomic assessment of the severity of coronary heart disease (133) and on the relationship between serum metabolic profiles and hypertension (134). Mayr et al. chose a combined strategy of proteomics and metabonomics to assess metabolic changes linked to cardiovascular disorders (135).

Beyond disease diagnosis, metabonomics has been successfully used to identify lifestyle-related biomarkers of health, especially influenced by nutritional variation (128,136,137). Metabonomic applications have been furthermore extended from clinical aspects to biomedical research: metabolic profiles of cancer cells have advanced the understanding of tumor development and progression (138). In feasibility studies, MS and NMR-driven metabolic assessment allowed for the biochemical differentiation of commonly used laboratory rat strains (139) and of white and black mice (114,140).

CONCLUSIONS

Gene expression profiling has a long standing but was increasingly confronted with the criticism of difficult inter-platform and inter-study comparability. This issue has been addressed through standardization of sample preparation, data generation, and analysis (MIAME working group (141), details are provided in Chapter 10.2).

The major challenge for proteomics is the complexity and dynamic range of proteomes, which are—in contrast to genomes—hypothetical entities since they are not known. Enhanced resolution and reproducibility of protein separation and improved accuracy of mass spectrometric protein identification have led to more complete proteome coverage, i.e., to more low-abundant proteins identified. Standardization efforts analogous to those in the transcriptomics community are being undertaken, such as Minimal Information About a Proteomics Experiment (MIAPE), guidelines proposed by the Proteomics Standards Initiative of the Human Proteome Organization (142).

Apart from delivering a complementary platform powerful for noninvasive diagnostics, metabonomics has contributed to chemometric approaches to Omics data analysis. Metabonomic platforms now typically integrate NMR spectroscopy (mainly for being quantitative per se) and MS (mainly for its assets in terms of sensitivity and structure elucidation). The SMRS working group (131) takes care of the harmonization of metabonomic data generation, processing, and exchange.

Complementary use of tools is (almost) everything in the Omics business. The Omics technologies are analytical platforms for mechanism, biomarker, and target discovery in health and life sciences. Key for future successful Omics applications is the combined and integrative application of these platforms in the search of causality and correspondence between genes, proteins, and metabolites regulated under a certain condition. Also within one Omics platform, simultaneous application of different analytical strategies yields a more complete picture than relying on one sole technique: in transcriptomics for example, whole-genome chips should be complemented by focused arrays and single gene validation. In proteomics, the "old-fashioned" gels deliver protein images still complementary to "shotgun" (early digestion and peptide separation) policies, and the employment of different mass spectrometers and acquisition modes usually adds value to the data. In metabonomics, NMR complements MS and vice versa, when it comes to quantitation and sensitivity issues.

ACKNOWLEDGMENT

Dr. Laurent-Bernard Fay, head of the Bioanalytical Science Department at NRC, is thankfully acknowledged for scientific advice, critical reading, and support with the bibliography.

TECHNICAL ABBREVIATIONS USED IN THIS CHAPTER AND CHAPTER 10.4

AQUA   absolute quantitation
CID   collision-induced dissociation
2DE   two-dimensional gel electrophoresis
DIGE   differential imaging gel electrophoresis
DPD   differential peptide display
ECD/ETD   electron-capture/transfer dissociation
ESI   electrospray ionization
FFE   free flow electrophoresis
FT-ICR   Fourier-transform ion cyclotron resonance
GC   gas chromatography

GSEA   gene set enrichment analysis
HPLC   liquid chromatography
IC(A)T   isotope-coded (affinity) tag
IC(P)L   isotope-coded (protein) labeling
iTRAQ   isobaric tag for relative and absolute quantitation
IEF   isoelectric focusing
IMAC   immobilized-metal affinity chromatography
IT   ion trap
LC   liquid chromatography
MALDI   matrix-assisted laser desorption/ionization
MES   maximum enrichment score
MIAME   minimal information about a microarray experiment
MIAPE   minimal information about a proteomics experiment
NMR   nuclear magnetic resonance
MPSS   massively parallel signature sequencing
MRM   multiple reaction monitoring
MS   mass spectrometry; multiple sclerosis
MS/MS, MS^2 tandem mass spectrometry
MS^n multiple-stage mass spectrometry
MudPIT   multi-dimensional protein identification technology
NMR   nuclear magnetic resonance
PAGE   poly acrylamide gel electrophoresis
PC(A)   principal component (analysis)
pI   isolelectric point
PMF   peptide mass fingerprint
ppm   parts per million
PTM   posttranslational modification
Q   quadrupole
qRT-PCR   quantitative real-time polymerase chain reaction
RP   reversed phase
SAGE   serial analysis of gene expression
SCX   strong cation exchange
SILAC   stable-isotope labelling with amino acids in cell culture
SIM   selected-ion monitoring
SMRS   standard metabolic reporting structures
SRM   selected-reaction monitoring
ToF   time-of-flight
TOGA   total gene expression analysis
UPLC   ultra performance/pressure liquid chromatography

REFERENCES

1. Kussmann M, Raymond F, Affolter M. OMICS-driven biomarker discovery in nutrition and health. J Biotechnol 2006; 124:758–87.
2. Kussmann M, Affolter M, Fay LB. Proteomics in nutrition and health. Comb Chem High Throughput Screen 2005; 8:679–96.
3. Robertson DG. Metabonomics in toxicology: a review. Toxicol Sci 2005; 85:809–22.
4. Whitfield PD, German AJ, Noble PJ. Metabonomics: an emerging post-genomic tool for nutrition. Br J Nutr 2004; 92:549–55.

5. Hocquette JF. Where are we in genomics? J Physiol Pharmacol 2005; 56(Suppl. 3): 37–70.
6. Sok JC, Kuriakose MA, Mahajan VB, et al. Tissue-specific gene expression of head and neck squamous cell carcinoma in vivo by complementary DNA microarray analysis. Arch Otolaryngol Head Neck Surg 2003; 129:760–70.
7. Li X, Rao S, Wang Y, et al. Gene mining: a novel and powerful ensemble decision approach to hunting for disease genes using microarray expression profiling. Nucleic Acids Res 2004; 32:2685–94.
8. Buchholz M, Braun M, Heidenblut A, et al. Transcriptome analysis of microdissected pancreatic intraepithelial neoplastic lesions. Oncogene 2005; 24:6626–36.
9. Xu N, Podolsky RH, Chudgar P, et al. Screening candidate genes for mutations in patients with hypogonadotropic hypogonadism using custom genome resequencing microarrays. Am J Obstet Gynecol 2005; 192:1274–82.
10. Miraglia M, Berdal KG, Brera C, et al. Detection and traceability of genetically modified organisms in the food production chain. Food Chem Toxicol 2004; 42: 1157–80.
11. Ronald J, Akey JM, Whittle J, et al. Simultaneous genotyping, gene-expression measurement, and detection of allele-specific expression with oligonucleotide arrays. Genome Res 2005; 15:284–91.
12. Napoli C, de Nigris F, Sica V. New advances in microarrays: finding the genes causally involved in disease. Methods Mol Med 2004; 108:215–34.
13. Irizarry RA, Warren D, Spencer F, et al. Multiple-laboratory comparison of microarray platforms. Nat Methods 2005; 2:345–50.
14. Velculescu VE, Zhang L, Vogelstein B, et al. Serial analysis of gene expression. Science 1995; 270:484–7.
15. Brenner S, Johnson M, Bridgham J, et al. Gene expression analysis by massively parallel signature sequencing (MPSS) on microbead arrays. Nat Biotechnol 2000; 18: 630–4.
16. Sutcliffe JG, Foye PE, Erlander MG, et al. TOGA: an automated parsing technology for analyzing expression of nearly all genes. Proc Natl Acad Sci USA 2000; 97: 1976–81.
17. Ye SQ, Usher DC, Zhang LQ. Gene expression profiling of human diseases by serial analysis of gene expression. J Biomed Sci 2002; 9:384–94.
18. Colantuoni C, Purcell AE, Bouton CM, et al. High throughput analysis of gene expression in the human brain. J Neurosci Res 2000; 59:1–10.
19. Polyak K, Riggins GJ. Gene discovery using the serial analysis of gene expression technique: implications for cancer research. J Clin Oncol 2001; 19:2948–58.
20. Beauchamp NJ, van Achterberg TA, Engelse MA, et al. Gene expression profiling of resting and activated vascular smooth muscle cells by serial analysis of gene expression and clustering analysis. Genomics 2003; 82:288–99.
21. Jarvinen AK, Hautaniemi S, Edgren H, et al. Are data from different gene expression microarray platforms comparable? Genomics 2004; 83:1164–8.
22. Shippy R, Sendera TJ, Lockner R, et al. Performance evaluation of commercial short-oligonucleotide microarrays and the impact of noise in making cross-platform correlations. BMC Genomics 2004; 5:61.
23. Brazma A, Hingamp P, Quackenbush J, et al. Minimum information about a microarray experiment (MIAME)-toward standards for microarray data. Nat Genet 2001; 29:365–71.
24. Merriman B. A comparison of multiple microarray platforms for gene expression. Abstract from ABRF 2004. Integrating Technologies in Proteomics and Genomics. February 28–March 2, 2004, Portland, Oregon, USA. J Biomol Tech 2004; 15:88.
25. Irizarry RA, Warren D, Spencer F, et al. Multiple-laboratory comparison of microarray platforms. Nat Methods 2005; 2:345–50.
26. Larkin JE, Frank BC, Gavras H, et al. Independence and reproducibility across microarray platforms. Nat Methods 2005; 2:337–44.
27. Bammler T, Beyer RP, Bhattacharya S, et al. Standardizing global gene expression analysis between laboratories and across platforms. Nat Methods 2005; 2:351–6.

28. Wilkins MR, Sanchez JC, Gooley AA. Progress with proteome projects: why all proteins expressed by a genome should be identified and how to do it. Biotechnol Genet Eng Rev 1996; 13:19–50.

29. Fenn JB. Electrospray wings for molecular elephants (Nobel lecture). Angew Chem Int Ed Engl 2003; 42:3871–94.

30. Tanaka K. The origin of macromolecule ionization by laser irradiation (Nobel lecture). Angew Chem Int Ed Engl 2003; 42:3860–70.

31. Fenn JB, Mann M, Meng CK, et al. Electrospray ionization for mass spectrometry of large biomolecules. Science 1989; 246:64–71.

32. Karas M, Hillenkamp F. Laser desorption ionization of proteins with molecular masses exceeding 10,000 daltons. Anal Chem 1988; 60:2299–301.

33. Shevchenko A, Wilm M, Vorm O, et al. Mass spectrometric sequencing of proteins silver-stained polyacrylamide gels. Anal Chem 1996; 68:850–8.

34. Wilm M, Neubauer G, Mann M. Parent ion scans of unseparated peptide mixtures. Anal Chem 1996; 68:527–33.

35. Medzihradszky KF, Campbell JM, Baldwin MA, et al. The characteristics of peptide collision-induced dissociation using a high-performance MALDI-TOF/TOF tandem mass spectrometer. Anal Chem 2000; 72:552–8.

36. Cox DM, Zhong F, Du M, et al. Multiple reaction monitoring as a method for identifying protein posttranslational modifications. J Biomol Techniq 2004; 15:29–30.

37. Mann M, Jensen ON. Proteomic analysis of post-translational modifications. Nat Biotechnol 2003; 21:255–61.

38. Cooks RG, Glish GL, McLuckey SA, et al. Ion trap mass spectrometry. Chem Eng News 1991; 69:26–41.

39. Cox KA, Williams JD, Cooks RG, et al. Quadrupole ion trap mass spectrometry: current applications and future directions for peptide analysis. Biol Mass Spectrom 1992; 21:226.

40. Cotter RJ. Time-of-flight mass spectrometry for the structural analysis of biological molecules. Anal Chem 1992; 64:1027A–39.

41. Brown RS, Lennon JJ. Mass resolution improvement by incorporation of pulsed ion extraction in a matrix-assisted laser desorption/ionization linear time-of-flight mass spectrometer. Anal Chem 1995; 67:1998–2003.

42. Buchanan MV, Hettich RL. Fourier transform mass spectrometry of high-mass biomolecules. Anal Chem 1993; 65:245A–59.

43. McIver RT Jr, Li Y, Hunter RL. High-resolution laser desorption mass spectrometry of peptides and small proteins. Proc Natl Acad Sci USA 1994; 91:4801–5.

44. Ge Y, Lawhorn BG, ElNaggar M, et al. Top down characterization of larger proteins (45 kDa) by electron capture dissociation mass spectrometry. J Am Chem Soc 2002; 124:672–8.

45. Zubarev RA, Horn DM, Fridriksson EK, et al. Electron capture dissociation for structural characterization of multiply charged protein cations. Anal Chem 2000; 72: 563–73.

46. Roepstorff P, Fohlman J. Proposal for a common nomenclature for sequence ions in mass spectra of peptides. Biomed Mass Spectrom 1984; 11:601.

47. Syka JE, Coon JJ, Schroeder MJ, et al. Peptide and protein sequence analysis by electron transfer dissociation mass spectrometry. Proc Natl Acad Sci USA 2004; 101: 9528–33.

48. Hu Q, Noll RJ, Li H, et al. The Orbitrap: a new mass spectrometer. J Mass Spectrometry 2005; 40:430–43.

49. Lander ES, Linton LM, Birren B, et al. Initial sequencing and analysis of the human genome. Nature 2001; 409:860–921.

50. Venter JC, Adams MD, Myers EW, et al. The sequence of the human genome. Science 2001; 291:1304–51.

51. Anderson NL, Anderson NG. The human plasma proteome: history, character, and diagnostic prospects. Mol Cell Proteomics 2002; 1:845–67.

52. Kettman JR, Coleclough C, Frey JR, et al. Clonal proteomics: one gene—family of proteins. Proteomics 2002; 2:624–31.

53. Rose K, Bougeleret L, Baussant T, et al. Industrial-scale proteomics: from litres of plasma to chemically synthesized proteins. Proteomics 2004; 4:2125–51.

54. Jacobs JM, Adkins JN, Qian WJ, et al. Utilizing human blood plasma for proteomic biomarker discovery. J Proteome Res 2005; 4:1073–85.

55. Domon B, Broder S. Implications of new proteomics strategies for biology and medicine. J Proteome Res 2004; 3:253–60.

56. Burbulis I, Yamaguchi K, Gordon A, et al. Using protein-DNA chimers to detect and count small numbers of molecules. Nat Methods 2005; 2:31–7.

57. Rose K. Industrialization of proteomics: scaling up proteomic processes. Nat Encyclopedia Human Genome 2003; 435–9.

58. Righetti PG, Castagna A, Herbert BR, et al. Prefractionation techniques in proteome analysis. Proteomics 2003; 3:1397–407.

59. Görg A. Advances in 2D gel techniques. Trends Biotechnol 2004; 19:3–6.

60. Wolters DA, Washburn MP, Yates JR. An automated multidimensional protein identification technology for shotgun proteomics. Anal Chem 2001; 73:5683–90.

61. Washburn MP, Yates JR. New methods for proteome analysis: multidimensional chromatography and mass spectrometry. Trends Biotechnol 2001; 19:27–30.

62. Müller M, Gras R, Appel RD. Visualisation and analysis of molecular scanner peptide mass spectra. J Am Soc Mass Spectrom 2002; 13:221–31.

63. Wu CC, Yates JR III. The application of mass spectrometry to membrane proteomics. Nat Biotechnol 2003; 21:262–7.

64. Weber G, Bocek P. Recent developments in preparative free flow isoelectric focusing. Electrophoresis 1998; 19:1649–53.

65. Michel PE, Reymond F, Arnaud IL, et al. Protein fractionation in a multicompartment device using Off-Gel isoelectric focussing. Electrophoresis 2004; 24:3–11.

66. Heller M, Ye M, Michel PE, et al. Added value for tandem mass spectrometry shotgun proteomics data validation through isoelectric focusing of peptides. J Proteome Res 2005; 4:2273–82.

67. Kussmann M, Roepstorff P. Characterisation of the covalent structure of proteins from biological material by MALDI mass spectrometry—possibilities and limitations. Spectroscopy 1998; 14:1–27.

68. Emmett MR, Caprioli RM. Micro-electrospray mass spectrometry: ultra-high-sensitivity analysis of peptides and proteins. J Am Soc Mass Spectrom 1994; 5:605–13.

69. McKenna T, Campuzano I, Ritchie M, et al. The Waters Protein Expression System for Qualitative and Quantitative Proteomics. Waters Technical Note 2004, June: Library No. 720000910EN.

70. Yi EC, Marelli M, Lee H, et al. Approaching complete peroxisome characterization by gas-phase fractionation. Electrophoresis 2002; 23:3205–16.

71. Julka S, Regnier F. Quantification in proteomics through stable isotope coding: a review. J Proteome Res 2004; 3:350–63.

72. Zhen Y, Xu N, Richardson B, et al. Development of an LC-MALDI method for the analysis of protein complexes. J Am Soc Mass Spectrom 2004; 15:803–22.

73. Barofsky DF, Martin S, LaRotta A. Roundtable on MALDI-ToF-ToF. J Biomol Techniques 2004; 15:89–90.

74. Reinders J, Sickmann A. State-of-the-art in phosphoproteomics. Proteomics 2005; 5: 4052–61.

75. Nuhse TS, Stensballe A, Jensen ON, et al. Large-scale analysis of in vivo phosphorylated membrane proteins by immobilized metal ion affinity chromatography and mass spectrometry. Mol Cell Proteom 2003; 2:1234–43.

76. Pinkse MWH, Uitto PM, Hilhorst MJ, et al. Selective isolation at the femtomole level of phosphopeptides from proteolytic digests using 2D-nanoLC-ESI-MS/MS and titanium oxide. Anal Chem 2004; 76:3935–43.

77. Beausoleil SA, Jedrychowski M, Schwartz D, et al. Large-scale characterization of HeLa cell nuclear phosphoproteins. Proc Natl Acad Sci USA 2004; 101: 12130–5.

78. Gruhler A, Olsen JV, Mohammed S, et al. Quantitative phosphoproteomics applied to the yeast pheromone signaling pathway. Mol Cell Proteom 2005; 4:310–27.

79. Kobata A, Endo T. Immobilized lectin columns: useful tools for the fractionation and structural analysis of oligosaccharides. J Chromatogr 1992; 597:111–22.

80. West I, Goldring O. Lectin affinity chromatography. Meth Mol Biol 1996; 59: 177–85.

81. Gould BJ, Hall PM. m-Aminophenylboronate affinity ligands distinguish between nonenzymically glycosylated proteins and glycoproteins. Clin Chim Acta 1987; 163: 225–30.

82. Jack CM, Sheridan B, Kennedy L, et al. Non-enzymatic glycosylation of low-density lipoprotein. Results of an affinity chromatography method. Diabetologia 1988; 31: 126–7.

83. Carr SA, Huddleston MJ, Bean MF. Selective identification and differentiation of N- and O-linked oligosaccharides in glycoproteins by liquid chromatography-mass spectrometry. Protein Sci 1993; 2:183–96.

84. Huddleston MJ, Bean MF, Carr SA. Collisional fragmentation of glycopeptides by electrospray ionization LC/MS and LC/MS/MS: methods for selective detection of glycopeptides in protein digests. Anal Chem 1993; 65:877–84.

85. Zubarev RA, Horn DM, Fridriksson EK, et al. Electron capture dissociation for structural characterization of multiply charged protein cations. Anal Chem 2000; 72: 563–73.

86. Kuster B, Krogh TN, Mortz E, et al. Glycosylation analysis of gel-separated proteins. Proteomics 2001; 1:350–61.

87. Novotny MV, Mechref Y. New hyphenated methodologies in high-sensitivity glycoprotein analysis. J Sep Sci 2005; 28:1956–68.

88. Görg A, Obermaier C, Boguth G, et al. The current state of two-dimensional electrophoresis with immobilized pH gradients. Electrophoresis 2000; 21:1037–53.

89. Quadroni M, James P. Proteomics and automation. Electrophoresis 1999; 20: 664–77.

90. Gygi S, Rist B, Gerber S, et al. Quantitative analysis of complex protein mixtures using isotope-coded affinity tags. Nat Biotechnol 1999; 17:994–9.

91. Zhang R, Sioma C, Wang S, et al. Fractionation of isotopically labeled peptides in quantitative proteomics. Anal Chem 2001; 73:5142–9.

92. Han D, Eng J, Zhou H, et al. Quantitative profiling of differentiation-induced microsomal proteins using isotope-coded affinity tags and mass spectrometry. Nat Biotechnol 2001; 19:946–51.

93. Higgs RE, Knierman MD, Gelfanova V, et al. Comprehensive label-free method for the relative quantification of proteins from biological samples. J Proteome Res 2005; 4: 1442–50.

94. Gerber SA, Rush J, Stemman O, et al. Absolute quantification of proteins and phosphoproteins from cell lysates by tandem MS. Proc Natl Acad Sci USA 2003; 100: 6940–5.

95. Tonge R, Shaw J, Middleton B, et al. Validation and development of fluorescence two-dimensional differential gel electrophoresis proteomics technology. Proteomics 2001; 1: 377–96.

96. Henningsen R, Gale BL, Straub KM, et al. Application of zwitterionic detergents to the solubilization of integral membrane proteins for two-dimensional gel electrophoresis and mass spectrometry. Proteomics 2002; 2:1479–88.

97. Wu CC, MacCoss MJ, Howell KE, et al. A method for the comprehensive proteomic analysis of membrane proteins. Nat Biotechnol 2003; 21:532–8.

98. Nordhoff E, Egelhofer V, Giavalisco P, et al. Large-gel two-dimensional electrophoresis-matrix assisted laser desorption/ionization-time of flight-mass spectrometry: an analytical challenge for studying complex protein mixtures. Electrophoresis 2001; 22: 2844–55.

99. Wu CC, MacCoss MJ. Shotgun proteomics: tools for the analysis of complex biological systems. Curr Opin Mol Ther 2002; 4:242–50.

100. Liu H, Lin D, Yates JR. Multidimensional separations for protein/peptide analysis in the post-genomic era. Biotechniques 2002; 32:898–902.

101. Haynes PA, Yates JR. Proteome profiling—pitfalls and progress. Yeast 2000; 17:81–7.

102. Zhang R, Regnier F. Minimizing resolution of isotopically coded peptides in comparative proteomics. J Proteome Res 2002; 1:139–47.
103. Guillaume E, Panchaud A, Affolter M, et al. Differentially isotope-coded N-terminal protein sulphonation: combining protein identification and quantification. Proteomics 2006; 6:2338–49.
104. Panchaud A, Guillaume E, Affolter M, et al. Combining protein identification and quantification: C-terminal isotope-coded tagging using sulfanilic acid. Rapid Commun Mass Spectrom 2006; 20:1585–94.
105. Wiener MC, Sachs JR, Deyanova EG, et al. Differential mass spectrometry: a label-free LC-MS method for finding significant differences in complex peptide and protein mixtures. Anal Chem 2004; 76:6085–96.
106. Bateman RH, Carruthers R, Hoyes JB, et al. A novel precursor ion discovery method on a hybrid quadrupole orthogonal acceleration time-of-flight (Q-TOF) mass spectrometer for studying protein phosphorylation. J Am Soc Mass Spectrom 2002; 13: 792–803.
107. Niggeweg R, Kocher T, Gentzel M, et al. A general precursor ion-like scanning mode on quadrupole-TOF instruments compatible with chromatographic separation. Proteomics 2006; 6:41–53.
108. Silva JC, Gorenstein MV, Li GZ, et al. Absolute quantification of proteins by LCMSE: a virtue of parallel MS acquisition. Mol Cell Proteom 2006; 5:144–56.
109. Gerber SA, Rush J, Stemman O, et al. Absolute quantification of proteins and phosphoproteins from cell lysates by tandem MS. Proc Natl Acad Sci USA 2003; 100: 6940–5.
110. Kuster B, Schirle M, Mallick P, et al. Scoring proteomes with proteotypic peptide probes. Nat Rev Mol Cell Biol 2005; 6:577–83.
111. Beynon RJ, Doherty MK, Pratt JM, et al. Multiplexed absolute quantification in proteomics using artificial QCAT proteins of concatenated signature peptides. Nat Methods 2005; 2:587–9.
112. Lu Y, Bottari P, Turecek F, et al. Absolute quantification of specific proteins in complex mixtures using visible isotope-coded affinity tags. Anal Chem 2004; 76: 4104–11.
113. Mirgorodskaya OA, Korner R, Novikov A, et al. Absolute quantitation of proteins by a combination of acid hydrolysis and matrix-assisted laser desorption/ionization mass spectrometry. Anal Chem 2004; 76:3569–75.
114. Gavaghan CL, Holmes E, Lenz E, et al. An NMR-based metabonomic approach to investigate the biochemical consequences of genetic strain differences: application to the C57BL10J and Alpk:ApfCD mouse. FEBS Lett 2000; 484:169–74.
115. Glassbrook N, Ryals J. A systematic approach to biochemical profiling. Curr Opin Plant Biol 2001; 4:186–90.
116. Watkins SM, German JB. Toward the implementation of metabolomic assessments of human health and nutrition. Curr Opin Biotechnol 2002; 13:512–6.
117. Buchanan MV, Hettich RL. Fourier transform mass spectrometry of high-mass biomolecules. Anal Chem 1993; 65:245A–59.
118. McIver RT Jr, Li Y, Hunter RL. High-resolution laser desorption mass spectrometry of peptides and small proteins. Proc Natl Acad Sci USA 1994; 91:4801–5.
119. Aharoni A, Ric de Vos CH, Verhoeven HA, et al. Nontargeted metabolome analysis by use of Fourier transform ion cyclotron mass spectrometry. Omics 2002; 6:217–34.
120. Nishikawa Y, Dmochowska B, Madaj J, et al. Vitamin C metabolomic mapping in experimental diabetes with 6-deoxy-6-fluoro-ascorbic acid and high resolution ^{19}F-nuclear magnetic resonance spectroscopy. Metabolism 2003; 52:760–70.
121. Keun HC, Beckonert O, Griffin JL, et al. Cryogenic probe ^{13}C NMR spectroscopy of urine for metabonomic studies. Anal Chem 2002; 74:4588–93.
122. Shockcor JP, Holmes E. Metabonomic applications in toxicity screening and disease diagnosis. Curr Top Med Chem 2002; 2:35–51.
123. Lavine B, Workman JJ Jr. Chemometrics. Anal Chem 2004; 76:3365–71.
124. Bains W. Company strategies for using bioinformatics. Trends Biotechnol 1996; 14: 312–7.

125. Stoyanova R, Nicholson JK, Lindon JC, et al. Sample classification based on Bayesian spectral decomposition of metabonomic NMR data sets. Anal Chem 2004; 76:3666–74.
126. Holmes E, Antti H. Chemometric contributions to the evolution of metabonomics: mathematical solutions to characterising and interpreting complex biological NMR spectra. Analyst 2002; 127:1549–57.
127. Robertson DG. Metabonomics in toxicology: a review. Toxicol Sci 2005; 85:809–22.
128. German JB, Roberts MA, Watkins SM. Genomics and metabonomics as markers for the interaction of diet and health: lessons from lipids. J Nutr 2003; 133:2078S–83.
129. Robertson DG. Metabonomics in toxicology: a review. Toxicol Sci 2005; 85:809–22.
130. Whitfield PD, German AJ, Noble PJ. Metabonomics: an emerging post-genomic tool for nutrition. Br J Nutr 2004; 92:549–55.
131. Lindon JC, Nicholson JK, Holmes E, et al. Summary recommendations for standardization and reporting of metabolic analyses. Nat Biotechnol 2005; 23:833–8.
132. Lindon JC, Holmes E, Bollard ME, et al. Metabonomics technologies and their applications in physiological monitoring, drug safety assessment and disease diagnosis. Biomarkers 2004; 9:1–31.
133. Brindle JT, Antti H, Holmes E, et al. Rapid and noninvasive diagnosis of the presence and severity of coronary heart disease using ^{1}H-NMR-based metabonomics. Nat Med 2002; 8:1439–44.
134. Brindle JT, Nicholson JK, Schofield PM, et al. Application of chemometrics to ^{1}H NMR spectroscopic data to investigate a relationship between human serum metabolic profiles and hypertension. Analyst 2003; 128:32–6.
135. Mayr M, Mayr U, Chung YL, et al. Vascular proteomics: linking proteomic and metabolomic changes. Proteomics 2004; 4:3751–61.
136. Noguchi Y, Sakai R, Kimura T. Metabonomics and its potential for assessment of adequacy and safety of amino acid intake. J Nutr 2003; 133:2097S–100.
137. Teague C, Holmes E, Maibaum E, et al. Ethyl glucoside in human urine following dietary exposure: detection by ^{1}H NMR spectroscopy as a result of metabonomic screening of humans. Analyst 2004; 129:259–64.
138. Griffin JL, Shockcor JP. Metabolic profiles of cancer cells. Nat Rev Cancer 2004; 4: 551–61.
139. Holmes E, Nicholson JK, Tranter G. Metabonomic characterization of genetic variations in toxicological and metabolic responses using probabilistic neural networks. Chem Res Toxicol 2001; 14:182–91.
140. Plumb R, Granger J, Stumpf C, et al. Metabonomic analysis of mouse urine by liquid-chromatography-time of flight mass spectrometry (LC-TOFMS): detection of strain, diurnal and gender differences. Analyst 2003; 128:819–23.
141. Brazma A, Hingamp P, Quackenbush J, et al. Minimum information about a microarray experiment (MIAME)-toward standards for microarray data. Nat Genet 2001; 29:365–71.
142. Orchard S, Taylor CF, Hermjakob H, et al. Advances in the development of common interchange standards for proteomic data. Proteomics 2004; 4:2363–5.

10.2 Analysis and Data Integration

R. Keira Curtis and Antonio Vidal-Puig
Department of Clinical Biochemistry, University of Cambridge, Cambridge, U.K.

Matej Orešič
VTT Technical Research Centre of Finland, Espoo, Finland

Systems biology is a modern approach to understanding global processes, analogous to looking at the "big picture" of biology. This approach is helpful for describing simple cause-and-effect biological responses to specific stimuli but also allows the identification of further secondary and tertiary interactions forming biologically relevant networks. Such an ambitious goal requires a multidisciplinary strategy involving different techniques, which generate heterogeneous types of data that need to be integrated with new emerging knowledge in order to describe the whole system. This was an unrealistic goal until recently but with modern high throughput methodologies and sophisticated computational techniques it is becoming possible to integrate new experimental information with current biological knowledge to address the most complex biological questions. The challenge of the systems biology approach is to integrate heterogeneous information across different spatial and temporal scales of the biological systems. This represents a change in research style from a hypothesis driven to a data-driven approach. In some ways a systems biology approach requires a change of mentality, in order to feel comfortable with a degree of uncertainty while waiting for the data required to solve the problem.

Obesity results from a failure of mechanisms that control energy balance. This may involve genetic defects in the mechanisms controlling food intake, energy expenditure, expandability of the adipose tissue, partition of nutrients toward specific organs, or genetically inherited traits leading to inactivity (detailed in previous chapters). Since obesity is a relatively new problem of the last 40 years, we need to consider also the effect of environmental factors interacting with genetically determined traits. Another layer of complexity is determined by the concept of biological redundancy. Since energy homeostasis is so important for survival, the system has evolved toward a very tightly regulated redundant system characterized by: (a) similar responses induced by different pathways and (b) compensatory mechanisms systems restoring, at least partially, the steady state of energy homeostasis.

For these reasons a systems biology approach is, in our opinion, suited to the identification not only of what mechanisms may lead to obesity, but also the compensatory biological strategies that are found in vivo. Indeed some of these compensatory mechanisms may be targeted to increase the success rate of current strategies to lose weight. Furthermore, a systems biology approach may be used to identify early molecular events involved in the mechanisms leading to obesity-related complications, before these molecular mechanisms result in clinically identifiable specific diseases.

TOOLS FOR SYSTEMS BIOLOGY

The use of high throughput technologies, such as microarrays (also called DNA chips), creates enormous opportunities but each methodology brings its own specific problems. As tens of thousands of mRNAs can be measured simultaneously, this inevitably leads to large quantities of data. Other approaches such as proteomics or metabolomics also provide huge amounts of data referring to related biological processes. However, the data produced by these techniques are different in nature and, therefore, an important challenge is to integrate these heterogeneous types of data in meaningful metabolic network frames. Therefore, in parallel with the development of these technologies, a variety of new analytical methods are currently being developed to analyze and integrate these heterogeneous datasets. These tools are vital to the extraction of information and interpretation of results in order to reveal the "big picture."

TRANSCRIPTOMICS

Transcriptional profiling can measure the relative abundance of every mRNA in a sample. Simple analysis of these experiments can be used to select candidate genes for further inspection, but analysis of microarray data in the context of other biological knowledge, both from other experiments and from the literature can be used to elucidate the underlying physiological changes and mechanisms. We believe that the incorporation of transcriptomic data with other high throughput techniques will lead to new insights into health and disease.

MICROARRAY BASICS

There can be tens of thousands of spots (or features) on a microarray, each containing probes for a specific nucleotide sequence. There are two principal types of microarray: two-color (spotted) cDNA arrays involve using a robot to spot presynthesized cDNA probes onto precise locations on the array (1). Two different samples, each labeled with a different fluorophore are competitively hybridized to this type of array. A "dye-swap" experiment, where the two samples are labeled with the other fluorophore is performed, so that variability due to differential labeling can be quantified. Oligonucleotide arrays, such as those produced by Affymetrix, are made by synthesizing the oligonucleotides on the array directly, using techniques such as photolithography. Just one sample is hybridized to these arrays. Figure 1 illustrates microarray design and use. Whichever type of array is used, replicate hybridizations are required in order to quantify variability and allow statistical analysis.

Once the labeled RNA sample has been hybridized to the microarray, it is then scanned to measure the fluorescence at each feature, which corresponds to the amount of RNA that has hybridized to the complementary sequence of the probe. For spotted arrays, this will involve measuring the fluorescence in the two channels corresponding to the two samples. The end results from this type of microarray will be the relative abundance of each mRNA across the two samples. As only one sample is applied to oligonucleotide arrays, different arrays are compared in order to describe expression differences between samples.

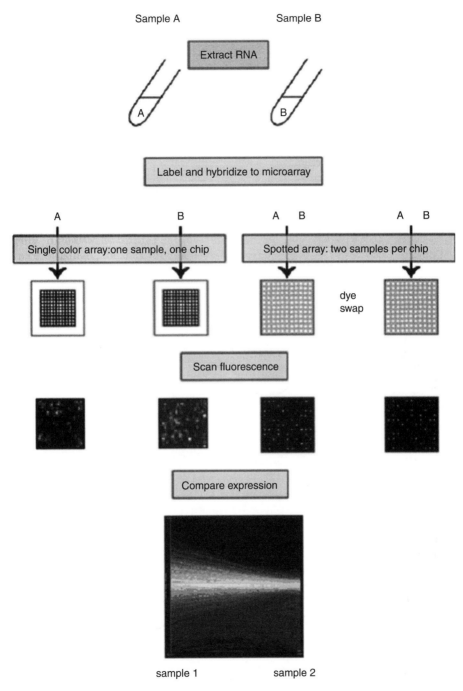

FIGURE 1 The basics of microarrays for transcriptional profiling.

THE BEST RESULTS FROM THE BEST EXPERIMENTAL DESIGNS

Microarray experiments involve comparing one sample to another. The choice of microarray platform is a major factor in experimental design, and careful thought should be given to experimental design (2). This is particularly important where two-color microarrays are used, as decisions have to be made regarding which samples are cohybridized to which chip (Fig. 2). If the aim of the experiment is simply to characterize expression differences between a knockout and a wild type mouse, then this is obvious. However, if there is also a treatment given to the two mice, will the treated knockout sample be hybridized to the untreated knockout, or the wild type treated, or the wild type untreated? One solution is to competitively hybridize each sample using the same reference RNA (3). As the reference RNA contains a known and standard amount, this means that all arrays and all future experiments using the same standards are comparable. This requires more

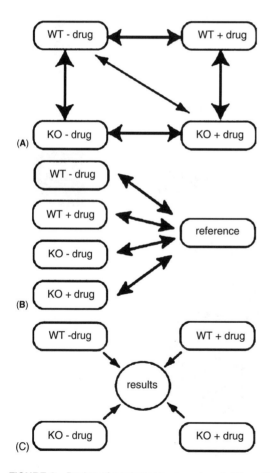

FIGURE 2 Design of a microarray experiment. Alternative hybridization strategies (**A, B**) for two-color microarrays; (**C**) strategy for single sample arrays.

chips, and cost is an important factor in microarray experiment design. Although more expensive than two color, spotted arrays, the commercial, oligonucleotide arrays provide greater flexibility as any array can be compared to any other from the same experiment.

Microarrays are expensive to buy and use. However, many institutions and organizations have access to some kind of spotted array facility (although this may have a limited choice of formats or oligonucleotide sets). A wide variety of commercially produced microarrays is available, including whole-genome arrays for several organisms, focused arrays that just contain probes for a target of interest (such as the insulin signaling pathway), or custom arrays, where the user specifies the probes.

It is becoming standard for journals to require microarray data to be deposited in one of the online microarray databases for publication. The three main databases are ArrayExpress (4) at the European Bioinformatics Institute, Gene Expression Omnibus (GEO) (5) at the NCBI, and the Stanford Microarray Database (6). Data deposited in these databases must comply with the minimum information about a microarray experiment (MIAME) standards (7), providing information to enable interpretation of the results and reproduction of the experiment.

MICROARRAYS: THE GOOD, THE BAD, AND THE FUTURE

Reproducibility of microarray data has been long identified as a problem (8). Technical variability such as preferential labeling, cross-hybridization, inconsistent spotting are problems, which are being and have been addressed, but even if these were all perfected, it will never be possible to eliminate biological variability: not all cells are the same, and certainly not all humans are the same; there will always be some degree of variation between them. In order to obtain statistically significant expression changes, microarray experiments must be repeated several times. Candidate genes obtained from a microarray experiment should be verified using a quantitative method such as real-time RT-PCR (9). It is not unusual to find that the fold change in expression is considerably different between the two platforms, but for a highly expressed gene with a reasonable or large fold change according to the microarray, there is generally a qualitative agreement with RT-PCR. Multiwell PCR microfluidics cards may provide a rapid and cost-effective method of validating a large number of candidates.

Microarrays are only as good as the probes they contain. Currently, whole-genome arrays are available, containing probes for each known or predicted gene. Chromosome or genome tiling arrays are on the way, these will cover the entire genome, with regularly spaced or overlapping probes (10). This will open up systems biology to the effects of exons, microRNA, noncoding or junk DNA, or unpredicted genes (11). The single-nucleotide polymorphism (SNP) arrays contain allele-specific probes and can be used for whole-genome association studies (see Chapter 6.1) (12).

Messenger RNA abundance does not necessarily correlate with protein levels (13–15). The activity of many proteins is also regulated, so it is important to remember that using microarrays will only reveal which genes are transcriptionally regulated. Messenger RNA degradation or stability also affects the abundance, and differences in abundance of splice variant mRNAs cannot always be detected.

ANALYZING THE DATA

So how do you get from a microarray experiment to the promised revelations? Analysis of microarray data is an expanding field. While some stages of data extraction and interpretation are still being debated in the literature, there is nearly consensus on some issues, such as normalization techniques. It is desirable to do some inter- and intra-array normalization in order to minimize the experimental variability between spots and arrays and maintain the biological variability. After this, the user will be left with a large dataset, ready for interpretation. There are several software packages available, both free and commercial, to assist with the analysis and interpretation of microarray data, e.g., Bioconductor (16), GeneSpring (Agilent).

Filtering the Data to Identify Simple Targets

The simplest way to look at microarray data is to make the comparison between two different samples, and produce a list of genes whose expression changes significantly between the different conditions. Annotations for these genes are available online see Ref. (17) for a review, and microarray software packages can assist with annotating simple gene lists, which can then be scanned to look for interesting genes. Examples of this type of simple analysis can be found in Yechoor et al. (18), looking at the effect of the MIRKO mutation in mice (mice deficient for insulin receptor in the muscle), and Horton et al. (19), investigating SREBP transgenic mice. This method is useful for finding simple targets, which tend to be highly expressed genes with large fold changes in expression, and these tend to be well-characterized genes with good annotations. However, inspection of a list of several hundred significantly regulated genes will still leave far more information than can be digested! It is also typical to come across at least one gene with poor or no annotation, especially if an entire genome was represented on the array.

Using Clustering and Patterns to Identify Complex Pathways

Another simple analysis to do is to cluster the data and look for patterns of expression (20). This is more appropriate where several conditions have been profiled, such as a time series or a range of different tissues. Clustering of microarray data is commonly used to classify either genes or samples. As coexpressed genes tend to have similar functions, grouping genes in this way can give an indication of the function of unannotated genes (21). Hierarchical clustering systematically places genes into a "tree"; genes with similar expression patterns are connected by short branches (Fig. 3). Clusters are then defined by slicing the hierarchical tree. Alternatively, using the array data to classify samples is an important diagnostic tool and has been applied to several types of cancer (22–25), in order to identify the subclassification of disease. In future this could be used clinically to optimize or personalize a patient's treatment.

These approaches have several drawbacks. Different distance measures result in different clusters, and should be carefully chosen, according to the purpose of the clustering. Because the distance measures are calculated from the expression data, a repeated experiment would not give precisely the same expression data and would, therefore, not be expected to return exactly the same clusters. Clustering data from whole-genome arrays is possible, but does not

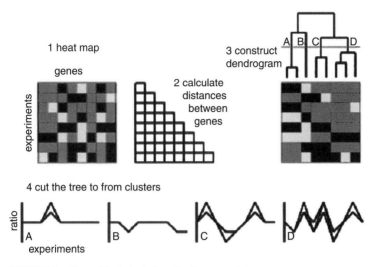

FIGURE 3   Hierarchical clustering of microarray data.

always give conclusive results. However, using clustering can be useful for finding subsets of the data with particular expression patterns that are interesting and merit further investigation.

DIGGING DEEPER: KNOWLEDGE-BASED APPROACHES

The methods described in the section, "Transcriptomics," are designed to analyze microarray data in isolation. Here, we begin to incorporate information from other sources. Published literature and online databases contain a host of information, from protein and DNA sequences, enzyme functions, metabolic pathways, to protein-protein and protein-DNA interactions. This is where the systems biology approach truly begins.

Functional Knowledge

An increasingly common approach to the analysis of microarray data is pathway analysis. There are several different approaches, all aiming to discover biochemical pathways that are activated or inactivated. This is termed enrichment of a pathway or functional annotation within all or a subset of the microarray data. These methods can be used to look for enrichment effects where the fold change in expression of specific genes is small but the global effects in a specific pathway may despite being subtle still have biological relevance. This is particularly relevant to obesity studies where biologically relevant changes in energy balance may only require changes of small magnitude. There are various software packages available that can perform this type of enrichment analysis. Many of these are freely available online to run or download, see Ref. (26) for more information.

There are several sources of this kind of annotation information. KEGG (27), GenMAPP (28), and Biocarta (www.biocarta.com) contain pathways such as metabolic or signaling pathways. In addition, the Gene Ontology project (29) classifies function and location in a hierarchical manner, for example fatty acid biosynthesis is a subset of lipid synthesis, which in turn is part of cellular lipid metabolism.

Gene Set Enrichment Analysis (GSEA)

Gene set enrichment analysis (GSEA) is a novel method that can find pathways that are subtly but consistently affected by a perturbation. It was first presented by Mootha et al. (30) but has been recently revised and updated to address a few problems (31). Tian et al. (32) also describe a related method. The original GSEA paper (30) compared gene expression in muscle from diabetics and controls, but did not find any significantly dysregulated genes. They used GSEA to look for differences between the two groups. This method involves ranking all of the genes on the microarray by some measure, such as expression change; they used signal-to-noise ratio. Proceeding down the ranked list, each gene in turn is compared to a pathway or functional annotation (gene set) of interest. If that gene is found on the pathway, a figure is added to the "enrichment score"; if it is not on the pathway, an amount is subtracted from the score. When all of the genes on the ranked list have been compared to the pathway, the maximum value that the enrichment score reached is defines the "maximum enrichment score" (MES). The greater this score, the greater the enrichment of that pathway. There is a second step to the analysis, which involves making a random pathway and calculating the MES. This is done many times, in order to calculate the random distribution of enrichment scores. The MES for the original pathway is compared to the random distribution in order to give it a *p*-value: if a higher MES is obtained 10 times from a 1000 random pathways, the MES from the real pathway can be assigned a *p*-value of .01 (Fig. 4A). Using this strategy the analysis of diabetic versus control muscle samples was able to show a subtle but significant down regulation of oxidative phosphorylation in the diabetic tissue that was not evident using conventional statistical approaches.

The advantages of GSEA over other methods are that it is applied to a ranked list of all the genes on the microarray, and that it can find subtly regulated pathways. However, it can be problematic where there is more than one micro-array comparison in the experiment, such as a system of four conditions: a knockout versus wild type mouse, with and without some treatment. Perhaps the "interesting" genes are those with expression changes in the knockout compared to the wild type and expression changes in the treated knockout versus untreated. This strategy filters the data and gives a shorter list of the genes of interest. There is a second type of pathway analysis, which may be more appropriate here: a group of methods that use "hit counting."

Hit Counting

These methods use a filtered list of genes from the microarray data and test the hypothesis that the list of genes from the microarray is enriched in genes from the pathway. Depending on the method used, the result may be an enrichment score and a significance measure, e.g., GenMAPP (28), or just the significance value, e.g., Onto-Tools (33). This is calculated from different factors: (a) the number of genes on the microarray, (b) the number of genes on a subset of the microarray (such as 1.5-fold up regulated genes), (c) the number of genes on a pathway of interest, and (d) the number of 1.5-fold up regulated genes that appear on the pathway (the number of "hits"). The methods more commonly used include the hypergeometric

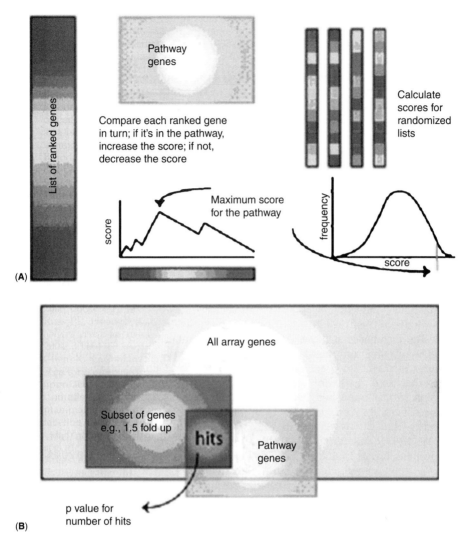

FIGURE 4 Enrichment analysis of microarray data. (**A**) Gene set enrichment analysis and (**B**) hit counting enrichment analysis.

and binomial distributions. These methods provide information regarding the probability of seeing that many hits by chance (Fig. 4B). Results from hit counting methods are generally intuitive and easy to understand. However, as they perform enrichment analysis on data that has been filtered, subjective decisions have to be made a priori regarding the significance and or fold change thresholds and these may bias the results.

Patti et al. (34) used the hit counting algorithm of GenMAPP (28) to find a downregulation of genes involved in oxidative phosphorylation in the muscle of diabetic patients compared to controls. This was in agreement with the GSEA method used by Mootha et al. (30). It is reassuring that the two complementary methods of enrichment pathways analysis came to the same conclusion as this validates both microarrays as a means of measuring gene expression and pathway analysis of the resulting data.

Module Maps

Segal et al. (35) had a related approach to incorporating functional knowledge into microarray data analysis. They applied this to two very large microarray datasets; one where yeast were given different environmental stimuli (36) and a compendium of different cancer array experiments. They compared a collection of pathways and functional annotations (gene sets) to the arrays and used a hit counting method (the hypergeometric distribution) to identify which gene sets were in enriched in each array. Where a cluster of related gene sets have a similar expression pattern, the core genes within these sets were extracted to form a "module." These modules better describe the genes involved in a biological process as it contains genes whose expression corresponds to the expression of the gene sets. After the modules had been extracted, they were used to produce a "module map," describing the processes and functions affected in each type of cancer.

Other Uses of Enrichment Methods to Investigate Obesity-Relevant Genes

There are other gene sets that can be tested for enrichment. These include looking for regulation of parts of the genome by searching for commonly regulated chromosome bands or quantitative trait loci (QTLs). Ghazalpour et al. (37) and Schadt et al. (38) both use microarray data to implicate new genes in susceptibility to obesity. Databases such as TRANSFAC (39) contain information about regulatory elements in promoters, so it is becoming possible to look for enrichment of promoter elements in a set of genes, which indicate the common transcription factors that bind upstream of the genes and regulate their expression. Another option is to use published lists of regulated genes from other experiments and compare them to your data (40). Although there is a considerable amount of microarray data deposited in online databases, it can be time consuming to extract a simple list of regulated genes from a single experiment, never mind from a series of experiments. The LOLA database (41) contains a collection of such lists that can be easily downloaded. However, the number of lists in the database is limited, as is the information provided for each experiment. HomGL (42) enables comparisons to be made across species. Literature searches can be incorporated into enrichment analysis, looking for overrepresentation of a word or annotation in published abstracts (43) or cocitation of genes in abstracts (44).

An important consideration in this type of analysis, and any analysis making multiple comparisons, is to correct for multiple hypothesis testing. Where multiple pathways are compared to the same data, it is likely that some pathways are incorrectly flagged as significantly dysregulated. The false discovery rate is one statistical method that can reduce the number of these false-positive results (45). Multiple testing corrections make use of the assumption that all the pathways being tested are independent of each other. This may not be the case as many pathways overlap and a protein may appear in more than one pathway.

Enrichment analysis is limited by the quality of the pathways or other annotations being tested. Many metabolic or signaling pathways have gaps where a gene has yet to be identified, be it generally or species-specific (46). The majority of genes are not represented on any pathway, and the problem is confounded by the fact that different annotation sources use different types of accession numbers, all of which have to be cross-referenced to the microarray. Other types of gene sets are also incomplete, such as those containing promoter elements: just because a promoter contains a consensus sequence that can bind a particular protein, which does not mean that the gene is regulated by that transcription factor.

Interactome Knowledge

Microarray analysis is expanding to use other information, such as interaction data and networks. This approach is still less widespread than pathway analysis as the tools involved either require considerable bioinformatic expertise or expensive commercial software, although this will probably soon change. Essentially, the idea is to overlay the expression profiling data onto a network of interactions, such as known protein-protein (47), protein-DNA (e.g., transcription factors (39)), or protein-metabolite interactions (e.g., metabolic pathways (27,28)). These types of interactions may be looked at on their own, or together. This will give an indication of which parts of the global network in the cell are affected and may suggest mechanisms or targets.

There are several programs for specifically looking at protein-DNA interactions. These generally query the publicly accessible databases containing information on transcription factor binding sites TRANSFAC (39) or JASPAR (48) and then screen the promoter sequences for overrepresentation of known sites, e.g., Toucan (49). As transcription factors do not act in isolation to regulate gene expression, there are examples of using combinatorial methods to look for pairs or groups of transcription factor binding sites (50–52).

As with pathway analysis, the application of protein-DNA interactions to microarray data analysis requires a good standard of biological knowledge to start with. Often the binding sites or transcription factors binding to DNA are unknown, so the binding site databases are incomplete. Confounding this is that just because the promoter of a gene contains a sequence matching that of a known binding site, it is not necessarily true that a transcription factor binds to it. There is also a certain amount of variation in the DNA sequence that a protein binds to. As the binding sites are short sequences, even allowing for a small number of mismatches from the consensus sequence would be expected to predict several binding sites, many of which will be false positives. Transcription factor binding predictions have to be verified, both to check that a protein binds to the predicted consensus, and that this binding has an effect on gene expression. However, the completion of several genome sequencing projects and high throughput methods of looking for protein-DNA interactions, such as chromatin immunoprecipitation in combination with microarrays, are improving the standard and quantity of information for transcription factor binding sites. The integration of binding data with the context of the binding sites (location relative to other binding sites or the transcriptional start site, orientation, conservation across species) should improve the predictions these methods make.

Calvano et al. (53) used software from Ingenuity called Pathways Analysis in order to relate their array data to the entire "interactome": all known interactions of all types. The interaction data were from the Ingenuity Pathways Knowledge Base, constructed from a comprehensive mining of 200,000 publications. Subjects were given a dose of bacterial endotoxin to activate the innate immune response and microarrays used to measure gene expression in whole blood leukocytes over a 24-hour time course. Using this software, the authors were able to follow the effects of the immune response with time, and observe how different parts of the network responded at different times.

GOING FISHING: LOOKING FOR THE UNKNOWN

The previous section described combining microarray data with biological knowledge. But it can be difficult to find enrichment or patterns if you don't know what you're looking for! Searching for protein-DNA interactions, such as transcription factor binding sites, is a good example of this type of problem. Let us take a group of genes with similar expression patterns that were identified using microarrays. No known regulatory elements were found in the promoters of these genes that could explain their coregulation. There is considerable redundancy and "wobble" in transcription factor binding sites and there are also several orphan nuclear receptors, therefore it is a reasonable hypothesis that there is a novel binding site in the promoters of these genes.

There are several different programs available that can look for overrepresented short sequences (i.e., binding sites) in a given set of input sequences (the promoters of the coexpressed genes), e.g., WeederWeb (54) or BEARR (55). Some of these methods are reviewed by Wasserman (56). Once a candidate binding site has been found, it can be matched against similar sequences in the transcription factor binding site databases to see if there is a for known transcription factors binding to that sequence. This approach was used by Mootha et al. to find the binding sites for estrogen-related receptor alpha (ESRRA) and GA-binding protein transcription factor, alpha subunit 60 kDa (GABPA) and elucidate their role in regulating the expression of oxidative phosphorylation genes (57) in the context of diabetes.

These methods tend to produce many false-positive sequences, and it has been recommended to use several different programs (58,59) and to validate predicted sites experimentally. The number of false-positive results can be improved by masking the parts of the promoter sequence that are repetitive elements (60), and also by finding which parts of the promoters are conserved between similar species (61).

FINAL ANALYSIS: DATA INTEGRATION

The methods we have so far described have involved integrating transcriptomic data with various sources of information. Next we turn to integrating gene expression data with other experimental data from the same system (Fig. 5). This may consist of phenotyping data, biochemical assays, or kinetic measurements. There are several omic approaches that can generate high throughput data, including metabolomics (62–64) (studies of small molecules in cells, tissues, and biofluids; profiling their levels and fluxes), lipidomics (65) (profiling lipids), and proteomics (66) (protein abundances and dynamics). Technical introduction and details are provided in Chapters 10.1 and 10.5.

An Array of Omic Data

Proteomics and metabolomics have emerged as rapidly developing and increasingly utilized technologies for characterization of complex phenotypes found in medical systems biology research (64,67). Each of these technologies offers distinct glimpses of biological phenomena, and the systems approach involves a combined and parallel study across all these levels, using bioinformatics to integrate and interpret the heterogeneous biological information (68,69).

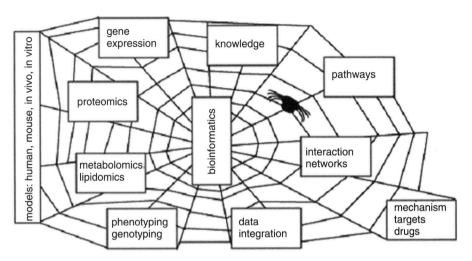

FIGURE 5 Integration of data using a systems biology approach.

Metabolites are known to be important regulators of systems homeostasis. As such, level changes in the abundance of specific groups of metabolites may be descriptive of systems responses to environmental or genetic interventions, and their study may therefore be a powerful tool for characterization of complex phenotypes as well as for development of biomarkers for specific physiological responses. Among the emerging omics technologies, metabolomics has gained the prominence most recently, yet it may also be considered as the oldest of the omics approaches. The pioneering research on use of metabolic fingerprinting to characterize disease phenotypes, with application of multivariate methods to analyze and interpret the data, dates back to the 1970s and 1980s (70–72). With today's advances in analytical technologies and more powerful information technology solutions for handling large volumes of analytical data, the metabolomics approach is becoming more feasible, making it one of the core components of systems biology research.

Lipidomics can be considered as a subfield of metabolomics, which aims to use global lipid profiling approaches to elucidate the biological processes in the context of lipids and their relations to other entities of the biological system. Lipids are known to play an important role as structural components (e.g., cell membranes), energy storage components, and as signaling molecules. For example, changes in lipid function due to peroxidation or imbalanced fatty acid composition may contribute to development of disorders such as atherosclerosis, diabetes, or Alzheimer's disease. With the advances in metabolomics methods, the profiling approaches, including informatics methods applied to other *omics* platforms, are increasingly being applied to the study of lipids. There have been significant developments both on the analytical and data processing side toward the mature platforms for lipid analyses (73–76); also the related bioinformatics is benefiting from the recent work of the LIPIDMAPS consortium funded by NIH (http://www.lipidmaps.org), which has been developing new lipid nomenclature (77) and will greatly facilitate the computational approaches to lipidomics and their applications in biomedical and more generally life science research.

High dimensionality of molecular profile data is posing new challenges for data analysis and interpretation. Univariate statistics approaches are generally not appropriate due to the complex correlation structure of profile data. In the case of multivariate analyses, special caution is necessary due to inherent nonlinearity of biological phenomena as reflected in molecular profiles, as well as due to the noise that can be attributed either to the systematic error specific to experimental platform, or to inherently biological factors and therefore of relevance to the study. An outline of a typical metabolomics platform is illustrated in Figure 6.

The first pass step in handling complex molecular profile data is data processing, where the raw data from the experimental platform is converted into a format that can be handled by numerical analyses. As discussed in Chapter 10.1, in case of mass spectrometry applications commonly utilized in metabolomics and proteomics, this includes spectral filtering, peak detection, aligning of multiple samples, as well as normalization that aims to reduce the systematic error by adjusting the intensities within each sample run (78). Following the processing, the data are ready for statistical analyses. Exploratory analysis is an essential next step to detect trends in the data and elucidate what are the main phenotypes within the monitored groups.

Integrated Analyses

New computational approaches are being developed to integrate the data across different *omics* levels. Some of these methods involve looking for signatures, patterns, or correlations between mRNA, proteins, metabolites, or other measured variable. However, it is important to remember that correlation does not prove mechanism. Although sometimes a correlation may represent a direct

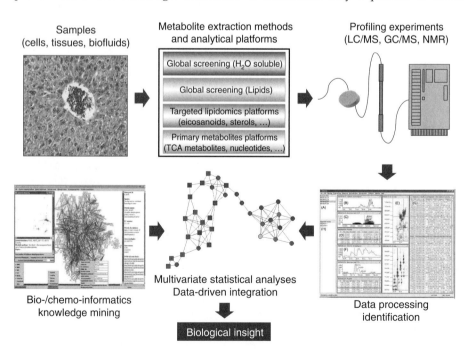

FIGURE 6 (*See color insert.*) Schematic of metabolomics and lipidomics.

cause and effect relationship, it may also be the result of indirect or down-stream effects of other changes. Messenger RNA and protein abundance do not necessarily correlate; for a review of integration of proteomic and transcriptomic data (13,79).

There are several examples of integrated analyses across metabolome, proteome, and transcriptome levels. For example, Orešič et al. utilized the nuclear magnetic resonance (NMR)–based metabolomics, liquid chromotography/mass spectrometry (LC/MS)–based lipidomics, LC/MS–based proteomics, as well as transcriptomic analyses to characterize the ApoE3 transgenic mouse model of atherosclerosis prior to disease onset (69,80,81). Correlation network analyses based on kernel approaches were utilized to integrate across multiple *omic* levels.

Li and Chan studied hepatocytes cultured in high or low insulin concentrations (82). Gene expression was measured using microarrays, and metabolites using high-performance liquid chromatography (HPLC) and biochemical assays. A combination of partial least squares analysis and a genetic algorithm was used to find a subset of genes that could predict function based on their expression. They then incorporated biological knowledge of the genes in order to piece together their roles in the metabolic network.

Griffin et al. investigated orotic acid–induced fatty liver in two different rat strains (83). They measured gene expression using microarrays, metabolites using NMR, and profiled lipids using gas chromatography. The metabolite and transcriptomic data were analyzed separately and then integrated using a supervised partial least squares multivariate analysis. Analysis of correlated metabolites and mRNAs using bootstrapping found the most positively and negatively correlated metabolite-messenger pairs. This revealed relationships between nucleotide, fatty acid, glycerolipid, and cholesteryl ester biosynthesis. Development of fatty liver was associated with accumulation of unsaturated fatty acids yet there was decreased transcription of stearoyl CoA desaturase, an important enzyme in their synthesis.

A different analytical approach was used by Hirai et al. in their investigation of nutritional stress in *Arabidopsis* (84). They used cDNA macroarrays to profile gene expression and HPLC and mass spectrometry to measure metabolites in root and leaf tissue. Principal components analysis showed that the effects of long-term sulfur deficiency are different from those of short-term. A self-organizing map approach suggested that genes involved in glucosinolate metabolism are transcriptionally regulated; glucosinolates can be used to store sulfur and their accumulation in nutrient starved roots protects the plant against pathogens.

These methods use experiments to provide the data to make or test models, which can be further refined in vitro or in silico. These models may be mathematical or kinetic representations, or simple hypotheses of potential mechanisms. The more detailed models can be constructed in several ways. Kinetic parameters and concentrations can give a model of a metabolic pathway, such as glycolysis (85), and the control and regulation of a system can be described using metabolic control analysis (86,87). Control analysis was applied to microarray data to distinguish between direct and indirect expression changes (88).

The complementary approach is to start with as complete a representation of biological knowledge as possible (the model), use one or more high throughput profiling techniques and observe the effects on the network or system as a whole. This is becoming possible, due to large databases detailing the different types of interactions (protein-protein, enzyme-metabolite, etc.). Because metabolite, protein, and mRNA abundance are regulated by metabolite, protein, and mRNA abundance, using all types of interaction data will give a better description of the perturbation than looking at one type of interaction in isolation. Gopalacharyulu et al. (89) have such an system. Calvano et al. (53) used the Ingenuity Pathways Knowledge Base database (www.ingenuity.com) to analyze their microarray data. The most ambitious aim of systems biology is the "computation of life," the goal of the Silicon Cell project (90), which hopes to integrate "genomic, transcriptomic, proteomic, metabolomics and cell-physiomic information" to produce a complete description of the cell. It remains to be seen if such a bottom-up approach is practically applicable to the computational modeling at the level of integrative physiology.

USING SYSTEMS BIOLOGY TO SEE THE BIG PICTURE OF OBESITY

As indicated in the introduction of this chapter and clearly shown in other chapters of this book, obesity is a complex syndrome. Current research in obesity focuses on questions related to the factors involved in energy balance and complications derived from its deviations. As varied as the questions are the experimental approaches. Among them high throughput techniques and systems biology approaches are progressively being incorporated to the experimental design applied to studies in humans, to in vitro tissue culture and genetically manipulated mouse models (91).

Investigation of the whole human would be the most physiologically relevant, but there is limited capacity to study manipulations in humans, other than drug responses or genetic variants. The natural variability from human to human allows the study of SNP and QTLs, but complicates the identification of markers of disease or response to therapeutics. The success of a system biology strategy applied to human obesity requires exquisite genetic and phenotypic characterization of the individuals to identify homogeneous experimental groups for environmental or therapeutic trials. However, when the biological material analyzed is of high quality, a powerful systems biology approach may lead to important new concepts such as the involvement of mitochondrial defects in the development of diabetes (30,34).

For our strategy of research, we consider that use of animal models have some advantages particularly when the genetic background is homogeneous and the conditions for the environmental challenges (e.g., diet, drugs, exercise to be investigated) well controlled. In fact, our strategy takes advantage of the homogeneity of genetically modified mouse models to identify relevant molecular mechanisms to be subsequently evaluated in humans. In our opinion this strategy allows a subsequent focused candidate approach to validate the relevance of specific hypothesis in humans. We also apply a systems biology approach to in vitro models relevant to obesity. In fact, before moving to in vivo models we applied this approach to relatively simple in vitro systems to validate the approach (92). However, we are becoming sceptical about the translatability of some of the data produced in vitro to in vivo, particularly in aspects related to adipogenesis (93). For instance we have identified similar disagreement when comparing the potential of differentiation in vitro or in vivo of preadipocytes genetically modified to lack PPARG2 expression (94). The reason may be related to factors operating exclusively in vivo, such as nutritional pressure and/or effects secondary to compensatory responses and modulatory signals generated in other organs. In our experience applying a systems biology approach in vitro may be useful to distinguish primary from secondary and compensatory effects induced in vivo (95).

Publications on the systems biology of obesity are still sparse. There are multiple papers describing transcriptional profiling in several tissues in metabolically relevant tissues (e.g., adipose tissue (96), brown fat (97), skeletal muscle (30,34), liver (92), beta cells (98), or heart (99)). Interestingly, very little has been published looking at microarrays of the brain or specific nuclei despite its relevance controlling energy homeostasis. Similarly papers combining transcriptomics, proteomics, and metabolomics are still scarce. However, these complex approaches are feasible. A good example of this approach is the recent paper from Hackl et al. (100) using spotted arrays to profile the differentiation of a preadipocyte cell line. This was followed by an in-depth bioinformatic analysis of 780 differentially expressed genes, including mapping of functions, pathways, and cellular localization. Further analysis revealed few shared transcription factor binding sites, and no clustering to chromosomal location.

The current limitations of the use of a systems biology approach to obesity are not different from other diseases. First of all it requires a multidisciplinary collaborative effort involving experts in very different areas including biology, informatics, physics, mathematics, and medicine. Secondly, each one of the components requires constant refinement and integration. For instance one big challenge facing systems biology is the refinement of current biological knowledge into compartments. The pathway and interaction data that are available online do not make any allowance for differences in tissue specificity. One of the gene ontology annotations (101) is cellular location and there are data published detailing mRNA abundance in many different human and mouse tissues (102,103), but this information has yet to be incorporated into pathway and other annotation data.

CONCLUSION

The completion of genome sequencing projects has allowed the development of microarrays containing probes for thousands, or even all genes in an organism. In addition, other high throughput technologies have advanced, and with the large volume of biological information available online, systems biology projects are now possible. Integration of all these data sources can generate hypotheses, propose targets and narrow down possible mechanisms within cells or systems, suggest how this goes wrong in disease, and offer therapeutic targets.

Systems biology is a promising tool to unravel complex systems. From this point of view, it seems ideal for understanding the interactions between the different components of energy homeostasis and its deviations from normality toward pathological states such as obesity or leanness. Therefore systems biology appears as an excellent platform to attain the final goal: understanding the "big picture" of obesity and related complications.

REFERENCES

1. DeRisi JL, Iyer VR, Brown PO. Exploring the metabolic and genetic control of gene expression on a genomic scale. Science 1997; 278:680–6.
2. Churchill GA. Using ANOVA to analyze microarray data. Biotechniques 2004; 37: 173–5,177.
3. Baker SC, Bauer SR, Beyer RP, et al. The external RNA controls consortium: a progress report. Nat Methods 2005; 2:731–4.

4. Parkinson H, Sarkans U, Shojatalab M, et al. ArrayExpress—a public repository for microarray gene expression data at the EBI. Nucleic Acids Res 2005; 33:D553–5.
5. Barrett T, Suzek TO, Troup DB, et al. NCBI GEO: mining millions of expression profiles—database and tools. Nucleic Acids Res 2005; 33:D562–6.
6. Sherlock G, Hernandez-Boussard T, Kasarskis A, et al. The Stanford microarray database. Nucleic Acids Res 2001; 29:152–5.
7. Brazma A, Hingamp P, Quackenbush J, et al. Minimum information about a micro-array experiment (MIAME)-toward standards for microarray data. Nat Genet 2001; 29:365–71.
8. Lee ML, Kuo FC, Whitmore GA, et al. Importance of replication in microarray gene expression studies: statistical methods and evidence from repetitive cDNA hybridizations. Proc Natl Acad Sci USA 2000; 97:9834–9.
9. Bustin SA, Benes V, Nolan T, et al. Quantitative real-time RT-PCR—a perspective. J Mol Endocrinol 2005; 34:597–601.
10. Mockler TC, Chan S, Sundaresan A, et al. Applications of DNA tiling arrays for whole-genome analysis. Genomics 2005; 85:1–15.
11. Frey BJ, Mohammad N, Morris QD, et al. Genome-wide analysis of mouse transcripts using exon microarrays and factor graphs. Nat Genet 2005; 37:991–6.
12. Syvanen AC. Toward genome-wide SNP genotyping. Nat Genet 2005; 37(Suppl): S5–10.
13. Greenbaum D, Colangelo C, Williams K, et al. Comparing protein abundance and mRNA expression levels on a genomic scale. Genome Biol 2003; 4:117.
14. Gygi SP, Rochon Y, Franza BR, et al. Correlation between protein and mRNA abundance in yeast. Mol Cell Biol 1999; 19:1720–30.
15. Tian Q, Stepaniants SB, Mao M, et al. Integrated genomic and proteomic analyses of gene expression in mammalian cells. Mol Cell Proteomics 2004; 3:960–9.
16. Gentleman RC, Carey VJ, Bates DM, et al. Bioconductor: open software development for computational biology and bioinformatics. Genome Biol 2004; 5:R80.
17. Guffanti A, Reid JF, Alcalay M, et al. The meaning of it all: web-based resources for large-scale functional annotation and visualization of DNA microarray data. Trends Genet 2002; 18:589–92.
18. Yechoor VK, Patti ME, Ueki K, et al. Distinct pathways of insulin-regulated versus diabetes-regulated gene expression: an in vivo analysis in MIRKO mice. Proc Natl Acad Sci USA 2004; 101:16525–30.
19. Horton JD, Shah NA, Warrington JA, et al. Combined analysis of oligonucleotide microarray data from transgenic and knockout mice identifies direct SREBP target genes. Proc Natl Acad Sci USA 2003; 100:12027–32.
20. Eisen MB, Spellman PT, Brown PO, et al. Cluster analysis and display of genome-wide expression patterns. Proc Natl Acad Sci USA 1998; 95:14863–8.
21. Hughes JD, Estep PW, Tavazoie S, et al. Computational identification of cis-regulatory elements associated with groups of functionally related genes in *Saccharomyces cerevisiae*. J Mol Biol 2000; 296:1205–14.
22. Alizadeh AA, Eisen MB, Davis RE, et al. Distinct types of diffuse large B-cell lymphoma identified by gene expression profiling. Nature 2000; 403:503–11.
23. Chen X, Cheung ST, So S, et al. Gene expression patterns in human liver cancers. Mol Biol Cell 2002; 13:1929–39.
24. Ross DT, Scherf U, Eisen MB, et al. Systematic variation in gene expression patterns in human cancer cell lines. Nat Genet 2000; 24:227–35.
25. van't Veer LJ, Dai H, van de Vijver MJ, et al. Gene expression profiling predicts clinical outcome of breast cancer. Nature 2002; 415:530–6.
26. Curtis RK, Orešič M, Vidal-Puig A. Pathways to the analysis of microarray data. Trends Biotechnol 2005; 23:429–35.
27. Kanehisa M, Goto S, Kawashima S, et al. The KEGG resource for deciphering the genome. Nucleic Acids Res 2004; 32:D277–80 [database issue].
28. Doniger SW, Salomonis N, Dahlquist KD, et al. MAPPFinder: using Gene Ontology and GenMAPP to create a global gene-expression profile from microarray data. Genome Biol 2003; 4:R7.

29. Harris MA, Clark J, Ireland A, et al. The Gene Ontology (GO) database and informatics resource. Nucleic Acids Res 2004; 32:D258–61 [database issue].

30. Mootha VK, Lindgren CM, Eriksson KF, et al. PGC-1alpha-responsive genes involved in oxidative phosphorylation are coordinately downregulated in human diabetes. Nat Genet 2003; 34:267–73.

31. Subramanian A, Tamayo P, Mootha VK, et al. Gene set enrichment analysis: a knowledge-based approach for interpreting genome-wide expression profiles. Proc Natl Acad Sci USA 2005; 102:15545–50.

32. Tian L, Greenberg SA, Kong SW, et al. Discovering statistically significant pathways in expression profiling studies. Proc Natl Acad Sci USA 2005; 102:13544–9.

33. Draghici S, Khatri P, Bhavsar P, et al. Onto-Tools, the toolkit of the modern biologist: Onto-Express, Onto-Compare, Onto-Design and Onto-Translate. Nucleic Acids Res 2003; 31:3775–81.

34. Patti ME, Butte AJ, Crunkhorn S, et al. Coordinated reduction of genes of oxidative metabolism in humans with insulin resistance and diabetes: potential role of PGC1 and NRF1. Proc Natl Acad Sci USA 2003; 100:8466–71.

35. Segal E, Shapira M, Regev A, et al. Module networks: identifying regulatory modules and their condition-specific regulators from gene expression data. Nat Genet 2003; 34:166–76.

36. Gasch AP, Spellman PT, Kao CM, et al. Genomic expression programs in the response of yeast cells to environmental changes. Mol Biol Cell 2000; 11:4241–57.

37. Ghazalpour A, Doss S, Sheth SS, et al. Genomic analysis of metabolic pathway gene expression in mice. Genome Biol 2005; 6:R59.

38. Schadt EE, Lamb J, Yang X, et al. An integrative genomics approach to infer causal associations between gene expression and disease. Nat Genet 2005; 37:710–7.

39. Matys V, Fricke E, Geffers R, et al. TRANSFAC: transcriptional regulation, from patterns to profiles. Nucleic Acids Res 2003; 31:374–8.

40. Newman JC, Weiner AM. L2L: a simple tool for discovering the hidden significance in microarray expression data. Genome Biol 2005; 6:R81.

41. Cahan P, Ahmad AM, Burke H, et al. List of lists-annotated (LOLA): a database for annotation and comparison of published microarray gene lists. Gene 2005; 360:78–82.

42. Bluthgen N, Kielbasa SM, Cajavec B, et al. HOMGL-comparing genelists across species and with different accession numbers. Bioinformatics 2004; 20:125–6.

43. Matsunaga T, Muramatsu MA. Knowledge-based computational search for genes associated with the metabolic syndrome. Bioinformatics 2005; 21:3146–54.

44. Jensen LJ, Knudsen S. Automatic discovery of regulatory patterns in promoter regions based on whole cell expression data and functional annotation. Bioinformatics 2000; 16:326–33.

45. Storey JD, Tibshirani R. Statistical significance for genomewide studies. Proc Natl Acad Sci USA 2003; 100:9440–5.

46. Cary MP, Bader GD, Sander C. Pathway information for systems biology. FEBS Lett 2005; 579:1815–20.

47. Stelzl U, Worm U, Lalowski M, et al. A human protein–protein interaction network: a resource for annotating the proteome. Cell 2005; 122:957–68.

48. Sandelin A, Alkema W, Engstrom P, et al. JASPAR: an open-access database for eukaryotic transcription factor binding profiles. Nucleic Acids Res 2004; 32:D91–4.

49. Aerts S, Thijs G, Coessens B, et al. Toucan: deciphering the cis-regulatory logic of coregulated genes. Nucleic Acids Res 2003; 31:1753–64.

50. Frith MC, Li MC, Weng Z. Cluster-buster: finding dense clusters of motifs in DNA sequences. Nucleic Acids Res 2003; 31:3666–8.

51. Pilpel Y, Sudarsanam P, Church GM. Identifying regulatory networks by combinatorial analysis of promoter elements. Nat Genet 2001; 29:153–9.

52. Sharan R, Ben-Hur A, Loots GG, et al. CREME: cis-regulatory module explorer for the human genome. Nucleic Acids Res 2004; 32:W253–6.

53. Calvano SE, Xiao W, Richards DR, et al. A network-based analysis of systemic inflammation in humans. Nature 2005; 437:1032–7.

54. Pavesi G, Mereghetti P, Mauri G, et al. Weeder Web: discovery of transcription factor binding sites in a set of sequences from co-regulated genes. Nucleic Acids Res 2004; 32:W199–203.

55. Vega VB, Bangarusamy DK, Miller LD, et al. BEARR: batch extraction and analysis of cis-regulatory regions. Nucleic Acids Res 2004; 32:W257–60.

56. Wasserman WW, Sandelin A. Applied bioinformatics for the identification of regulatory elements. Nat Rev Genet 2004; 5:276–87.

57. Mootha VK, Handschin C, Arlow D, et al. Erralpha and Gabpa/b specify PGC-1alpha-dependent oxidative phosphorylation gene expression that is altered in diabetic muscle. Proc Natl Acad Sci USA 2004; 101:6570–5.

58. Osada R, Zaslavsky E, Singh M. Comparative analysis of methods for representing and searching for transcription factor binding sites. Bioinformatics 2004; 20:3516–25.

59. Tompa M, Li N, Bailey TL, et al. Assessing computational tools for the discovery of transcription factor binding sites. Nat Biotechnol 2005; 23:137–44.

60. Stepanova M, Tiazhelova T, Skoblov M, et al. A comparative analysis of relative occurrence of transcription factor binding sites in vertebrate genomes and gene promoter areas. Bioinformatics 2005; 21:1789–96.

61. Suzuki Y, Yamashita R, Shirota M, et al. Sequence comparison of human and mouse genes reveals a homologous block structure in the promoter regions. Genome Res 2004; 14:1711–8.

62. Fiehn O. Metabolomics—the link between genotypes and phenotypes. Plant Mol Biol 2002; 48:155–71.

63. Fiehn O, Weckwerth W. Deciphering metabolic networks. Eur J Biochem 2003; 270:579–88.

64. van der Greef J, Davidov E, Verheij E, et al. The role of metabolomics in systems biology: a new vision for drug discovery and development. In: Harrigan GG, Goodacre R, eds. Metabolic Profiling: Its Role in Biomarker Discovery and Gene Function Analysis. Boston, MA: Kluwer Academic Publishers, 2003:171–98.

65. Wenk MR. The emerging field of lipidomics. Nat Rev Drug Discov 2005; 4:594–610.

66. Patterson SD, Aebersold RH. Proteomics: the first decade and beyond. Nat Genet 2003; 33(Suppl):311–23.

67. van der Greef J, Stroobant P, van der Heijden R. The role of analytical sciences in medical systems biology. Curr Opin Chem Biol 2004; 8:559–65.

68. Nicholson JK, Holmes E, Lindon JC, et al. The challenges of modeling mammalian biocomplexity. Nat Biotechnol 2004; 22:1268–74.

69. Orešič M, Clish CB, Davidov EJ, et al. Phenotype characterisation using integrated gene transcript, protein and metabolite profiling. Appl Bioinformatics 2004; 3:205–17.

70. Pauling L, Robinson AB, Teranishi R, et al. Quantitative analysis of urine vapor and breath by gas–liquid partition chromatography. Proc Natl Acad Sci USA 1971; 68:2374–6.

71. Tas AC, van der Greef J, de Waart J, et al. Comparison of direct chemical ionization and direct probe electron impact/chemical ionization pyrolysis for characterization of Pseudomonas and Serratia bacteria. J Anal Appl Pyrolysis 1985; 7:249–55.

72. Windig W, Meuzelaar HL. Nonsupervised numerical component extraction from pyrolysis mass spectra of complex mixtures. Anal Chem 1984; 56:2297–303.

73. Ekroos K, Chernushevich IV, Simons K, et al. Quantitative profiling of phospholipids by multiple precursor ion scanning on a hybrid quadrupole time-of-flight mass spectrometer. Anal Chem 2002; 74:941–9.

74. Han X, Gross RW. Global analyses of cellular lipidomes directly from crude extracts of biological samples by ESI mass spectrometry: a bridge to lipidomics. J Lipid Res 2003; 44:1071–9.

75. Koivusalo M, Haimi P, Heikinheimo L, et al. Quantitative determination of phospholipid compositions by ESI-MS: effects of acyl chain length, unsaturation, and lipid concentration on instrument response. J Lipid Res 2001; 42:663–72.

76. Orešič M, Katajamaa M, Seppänen-Laakso T. Lipidomics as a tool for characterization of biological systems. Lipid Technol 2005; 17:59–63.

77. Fahy E, Subramaniam S, Brown HA, et al. A comprehensive classification system for lipids. J Lipid Res 2005; 46:839–61.
78. Katajamaa M, Orešič M. Processing methods for differential analysis of LC/MS profile data. BMC Bioinformatics 2005; 6:179.
79. Hegde PS, White IR, Debouck C. Interplay of transcriptomics and proteomics. Curr Opin Biotechnol 2003; 14:647–51.
80. Clish CB, Davidov E, Orešič M, et al. Integrative biological analysis of the APOE*3-leiden transgenic mouse. Omics 2004; 8:3–13.
81. Davidov E, Clish CB, Orešič M, et al. Methods for the differential integrative omic analysis of plasma from a transgenic disease animal model. Omics 2004; 8:267–88.
82. Li Z, Chan C. Integrating gene expression and metabolic profiles. J Biol Chem 2004; 279:27124–37.
83. Griffin JL, Bonney SA, Mann C, et al. An integrated reverse functional genomic and metabolic approach to understanding orotic acid-induced fatty liver. Physiol Genomics 2004; 17:140–9.
84. Hirai MY, Yano M, Goodenowe DB, et al. Integration of transcriptomics and metabolomics for understanding of global responses to nutritional stresses in *Arabidopsis thaliana*. Proc Natl Acad Sci USA 2004; 101:10205–10.
85. Olivier BG, Snoep JL. Web-based kinetic modelling using JWS online. Bioinformatics 2004; 20:2143–4.
86. Fell D. Understanding the Control of Metabolism. London, UK: Portland Press, 1997.
87. Kacser H, Burns JA. The control of flux. Biochem Soc Trans 1995; 23:341–66.
88. Curtis RK, Brand MD. Analysing microarray data using modular regulation analysis. Bioinformatics 2004; 20:1272–84.
89. Gopalacharyulu PV, Lindfors E, Bounsaythip C, et al. Data integration and visualization system for enabling conceptual biology. Bioinformatics 2005; 21(Suppl 1):i177–85.
90. Snoep JL. The Silicon Cell initiative: working towards a detailed kinetic description at the cellular level. Curr Opin Biotechnol 2005; 16:336–43.
91. van der Greef J, McBurney RN. Innovation: rescuing drug discovery: in vivo systems pathology and systems pharmacology. Nat Rev Drug Discov 2005; 4:961–7.
92. Lelliott CJ, Lopez M, Curtis RK, et al. Transcript and metabolite analysis of the effects of tamoxifen in rat liver reveals inhibition of fatty acid synthesis in the presence of hepatic steatosis. FASEB J 2005; 19:1108–19.
93. Soukas A, Socci ND, Saatkamp BD, et al. Distinct transcriptional profiles of adipogenesis in vivo and in vitro. J Biol Chem 2001; 276:34167–74.
94. Medina-Gomez G, Virtue S, Lelliott C, et al. The link between nutritional status and insulin sensitivity is dependent on the adipocyte-specific peroxisome proliferator-activated receptor-gamma2 isoform. Diabetes 2005; 54:1706–16.
95. Lelliot CJ, Lopez M, Curtis RK, et al. Transcript and metabolite analysis of the effects of tamoxifen in rat liver reveals inhibition of fatty acid synthesis in the presence of hepatic steatosis. FASEB J 2005; 19:1108–19.
96. Hackl H, Buckard TR, Sturn A, et al. Molecular processes during fat cell development revealed by gene expression profiling and functional annotation. Genome Biol 2005; 6: R108.
97. Tseng YH, Butte AJ, Kokkotou E, et al. Prediction of preadipocyte differentiation by gene expression reveals role of insulin receptor substrates and necdin. Nat Cell Biol 2005; 7:601–11.
98. Scearce LM, Brestelli JE, McWeeney SK, et al. Functional genomics of the endocrine pancreas: the pancreas clone set and PancChip, new resources for diabetes research. Diabetes 2002; 51:1997–2004.
99. Castro-Chavez F, Yechoor VK, Saha PK, et al. Coordinated upregulation of oxidative pathways and downregulation of lipid biosynthesis underlie obesity resistance in perilipin knockout mice: a microarray gene expression profile. Diabetes 2003; 52:2666–74.
100. Hackl H, Buckard TR, Sturn A, et al. Molecular processes during fat cell development revealed by gene expression profiling and functional annotation. Genome Biol 1995; 6: R108.

101. Ashburner M, Ball CA, Blake JA, et al. Gene ontology: tool for the unification of biology. The Gene Ontology Consortium. Nat Genet 2000; 25:25–9.
102. Su AI, Wiltshire T, Batalov S, et al. A gene atlas of the mouse and human protein-encoding transcriptomes. Proc Natl Acad Sci USA 2004; 101:6062–7.
103. Zhang W, Morris QD, Chang R, et al. The functional landscape of mouse gene expression. J Biol 2004; 3:21.

Frédéric Capel and Dominique Langin

INSERM, U858, Laboratoire de Recherches sur les Obésités, Institut de Médecine Moléculaire de Rangueil, Institut Louis Bugnard IFR 31, Université Paul Sabatier, and Centre Hospitalier, Universitaire de Toulouse, Toulouse, France

Hubert Vidal

INSERM UMR870, INRA U-1235, and Human Nutrition Research Centre, Laennec Medical Faculty, Lyon 1 University, Lyon, France

Karine Clément

INSERM, U872, Nutriomique, Centre de Recherche des Cordeliers, Université Pierre et Marie Curie-Paris6, UMRS 872, Université Paris Descartes, Assistance Publique Hôpitaux de Paris, AP-HP, and Department of Endocrinology and Nutrition, Pitié-Salpêtrière Hospital, Paris, France

The molecular pathogenic mechanisms for obesity and related disorders are still largely unknown. The identification of physiological and biological factors underlying the metabolic disturbances observed in obesity is a key step in developing better therapeutic outcomes. Obesity is a complex phenomenon characterized by an increased fat mass in different anatomical sites. In addition, each stage in the development of obesity, weight gain, weight maintenance, and variable response to treatment, could probably be associated with different molecular mechanisms. Adipose tissue present, we do not know for example of any biological markers or molecular predictors of passing from one stage to the other (1). For a better understanding of the development of obesity, in vitro and in vivo studies of adipocyte differentiation, differences between each type of fat depot and the development of related disorders are essential to identify the key gene involved in these phenomena.

The use of DNA microarrays and related "omics" techniques that allow the comparison of global expression changes in thousands of genes between different conditions appears as a useful tool to advance research in identifying master genes involved in human obesities.

In this chapter, we focus on how transcriptomic technology is being used to study the molecular determinants of obesity and its complications. Particularly, we are giving some examples of how applications of microarray technique on adipose tissue refine our understanding of adipocyte differentiation and the particularities of subcutaneous and visceral adipose tissue biology. We show how microarray technology provided new insights for the comprehension of the transcriptional regulation of genes encoding currently known molecules as well as novel biomolecules, which are involved in energy homeostasis and in other pathways. Many gene expression regulations were investigated to understand changes in body fat mass content that occurred during obesity development and energy restriction-induced weight loss. Inflammation is one of the pathways that are profoundly affected by obesity and was then regularly found to be modulated adipose tissue the transcriptional level when microarray technology was used. A more complete view of the biological events leading to obesity or weight loss should be obtained with data-gathering of genetic, transcriptomic, and other "omics" studies. It could then lead to a better understanding of energy homeostasis and to discovery of robust biomarkers.

TRANSCRIPTOMICS: DNA CHIP TECHNOLOGY AND GOALS

Technical details regarding microarray approach and methods of analysis are provided in Chapters 10.1 and 10.2. Briefly microarray technology is based on the reverse concept of dot blot and Northern blot analysis. The DNA is attached to the solid phase (probe), whereas labeled cDNA (or RNA) is in solution (target). Large numbers of cDNA sequences or synthetic DNA oligomers can be fixed onto a glass slide (or other substrate like filters) in known locations on a grid. Arrays with thousands of spotted DNA have been developed by academic consortium or companies (see Chapter 10.1). Different kinds of microarrays are available, allowing the study of constitutive genes of a whole genome of an organism or a specific metabolic pathway or cellular process. Each RNA sample is transcribed into cDNA and labeled with different fluorophores (typically Cy3 and Cy5). The measured amount of target bound to each probe reflects the level of expression of the gene. This measurement is frequently performed by simultaneous competitive hybridization of two labeled cDNA. While initially used for simple organisms, this approach now indexes thousands of known and newly discovered genes into various large groups defined by expression similarities in terms of physiological pathways, for example respiration, cell division, and response to chemical or thermal stress. For this purpose, several bioinformatic tools have been developed (see Chapter 10.2). Starting from a list of several hundreds of genes, it is possible to identify a biological process or sets of coregulated functions that can be affected by a dietary intervention, a drug treatment, or a pathological state. This kind of screening is now applied for the understanding of complex human diseases including cancer, aging and more recently metabolic diseases, including diabetes and obesity. For example, it was observed that oxidative phosphorylation genes regulated by the peroxisome proliferator-activated receptor gamma (PPARG), coactivator 1 alpha (PGC1A) are globally downregulated in skeletal muscle of type-2 diabetic patients (2,3). The key objective is to dissect and characterize the regulatory pathways and networks involved in energy balance and to define the resulting signaling patterns in gene expression. Among the goals of future projects that could be achieved is the identification of clusters of genes that are recruited or modified by given nutritional conditions, their links in terms of biological function, their coregulation in different tissues, the gene markers specific for some nutrients, differences/similarities in different models of obesity, and eventually the patterns of tissue expression in individuals with different polymorphisms in these genes. Studies of the gene expression profiling in adipose tissue could help to understand what happens during weight changes and what supports the improvement of obesity complications. As enough subcutaneous adipose tissue can be obtained by simple needle-biopsy aspiration, gene expression measurements in this tissue may provide a suitable tool to a better individual characterization of obese patients.

Studies of Adipocyte Differentiation

Adipose mass increases in part through the recruitment and differentiation of existing pools of preadipocytes into adipocytes. DNA microarrays enable the examination of gene expression profiles of cells across differentiation and should allow the discovery of novel adipogenic mediators and biomarkers of adipogenesis.

Microarray studies have been performed using 3T3L1 murine cells, the most widely used model for adipocyte differentiation studies in vitro. A large number of genes encoding transcription factors and coregulators, and signaling molecules are positively (such as PPARG, CEBPA, signal transducer and activator of transcription 1, STAT1, or iron responsive element binding protein) or negatively (Jun/Fos family members) regulated throughout differentiation (4). This study revealed a differential expression kinetic between genes encoding key transcription factors and target genes characteristic of the adipocyte phenotype such as the phosphoenolpyruvate carboxykinase gene. Cell cycle and cytoskeletal-related genes were also downregulated by differentiation. After 24 hours, 4 days, and 1 week of differentiation into adipocytes, expression of genes encoding proteins involved in lipid metabolism, such as stearoyl-CoA desaturase increased regularly, whereas genes encoding components of acute-phase inflammatory response [serum amyloid 3 (SAA3), haptoglobin, (HP)] are similarly expressed throughout differentiation (5,6). Comparing in vivo human mature adipocytes and preadipocytes, two distinct gene expression profiles were found. As compared to preadipocytes, overexpression of several genes involved in lipid metabolism was confirmed in human adipocytes. Additionally, the genes encoding E2F transcription factor 5, p130-binding (E2F5), a transcription factor involved in cell cycle control and SMARC (SWI/SNF related, matrix associated, actin-dependent regulator of chromatin, subfamily), a protein possessing helicase and ATPase activities, were identified to be more expressed in adipocytes. The preadipocytes predominantly expressed genes encoding extracellular matrix components, such as fibronectin, osteonectin, matrix metalloproteins, and novel proteins such as lysyl oxidase (7). Recently, it was found that differentiation of human fibroblasts toward adipocytes in vivo was associated with increased expression of genes encoding factors involved in cell motility and chemotaxis (8). Microarray studies comparing gene expression of in vitro preadipocytes and adipocytes to their in vivo counterparts revealed that preadipocytes and adipocytes in vivo display a particular phenotype that is not entirely mimicked by preadipocytes and adipocytes in vitro (4), confirming the importance of in vivo studies. For example, metabolic enzymes and leptin are predominantly expressed in vivo.

DEVELOPMENT OF OBESITY AND ASSOCIATED COMPLICATIONS

The molecular links between expanded adipose tissue and obesity complications are still to be discovered. Animal models of obesity such as the diet-induced obesity in rodents represent useful models for human obesity and have sometimes provided candidates. Indeed, a high-fat intake is well known to promote fat mass development. In mouse adipose tissue, a large number of genes, including genes encoding enzymes of the lipid metabolism or markers of adipocyte differentiation and genes related to detoxification were down regulated by diet-induced obesity (9). Similar observations and a down regulation of SREBP1-regulated genes were made in the leptin-deficient mice suggesting that adipocytes from enlarged adipose tissue exhibit reduced lipogenic skills (10,11). Other genes displayed increased expression both in diet-induced obesity and ob/ob mice, such as those encoding inflammatory markers, and cytoskeletal and extracellular matrix proteins (12,13).

The comparison between obese and lean subjects has confirmed this observation. Pangenomic analysis showed that genes involved in inflammation are overexpressed in subcutaneous and omental adipose tissues of obese subjects when compared with nonobese subjects (14,15). The regulation of inflammatory pathways will be developed in a following section. In conclusion, obesity affects strongly the expression profile in adipose tissue of genes involved in inflammatory process, metabolism, cytoskeleton, and extracellular matrix.

GENE EXPRESSION IN SUBCUTANEOUS AND VISCERAL ADIPOSE TISSUES

The anatomical distribution of adipose tissue is a key indicator of metabolic alterations and cardiovascular diseases. The excess of fat mass in the upper part of the body constitutes a classical risk factor for diabetes and cardiovascular diseases (16,17). There are marked differences between subcutaneous and visceral adipose tissues in the expression and secretion of key adipose genes such as leptin (18) and adiponectin (19) as well as proinflammatory factors like plasminogen activator inhibitor 1, which has been related to the pathogenic effects of visceral fat (20). The large-scale screening of genes differentially expressed in human or animal subcutaneous and visceral adipose depots allowed the identification of biomarkers of visceral obesity that may represent the mediators of metabolic alterations. The new adipose tissue-secreted protein visfatin alters glucose homeostasis and is highly expressed in visceral fat (21) where it is overexpressed in severe obese subjects as compared to lean controls (22). Genes related to immune process were also found to be strongly expressed in visceral adipose tissue (23,24). Pangenomic approach allowed the identification of 44 putatively differentially expressed genes in subcutaneous and omental fat tissues in men with severe abdominal obesity. Differential expression of genes involved in immune response such as calcyclin but also in lipid turnover regulation in human fat cells was observed (25). In other studies, carboxypeptidase E (*CPE*), thrombospondin-1 (*THBS1*), and some complement components were overexpressed in visceral adipose tissue (26,27). Additionally, visceral and subcutaneous adipose tissues exhibited differential expression levels of genes, which are involved in lipid metabolism and turnover. Following energy restriction, increased expression of hormone-sensitive lipase (*HSL*), uncoupling protein (*UCP2*), and adrenergic beta receptors (*ADRBs*) was reported only in visceral fat of obese rat, although the gene encoding fatty acid synthase was selectively downregulated in subcutaneous adipose tissue (28). Gene-encoding complement factor D (adipsin, CFD), a protein involved in fat cell's lipid turnover is more expressed in subcutaneous than in human omental adipose tissue, although the overexpression of phospholipid transfer protein, which could be related to insulin resistance and alterations in high-density lipoprotein metabolism was observed in omental adipose tissue (25). These studies have also led to the identification of a large number of genes expressed in adipose tissue whose function is still unknown. Subcutaneous and visceral adipose tissues harbor marked differences in gene expression profiles, in particular concerning inflammatory and lipid metabolism pathways. More studies are required to identify the determinants of the differences between the two fat depots.

OBESITY-RELATED INFLAMMATION

Inflammation is now widely recognized to be associated with the development of obesity and insulin resistance. Transcriptomic analyses contributed to the recognition of these associations and provided new insights for a better understanding of the relationship between obesity and the inflammatory state. We mentioned in a previous section some studies in rodents and humans using microarrays, which have shown an obesity-induced overexpression of genes related to inflammatory pathways. The mRNA levels of a hundredth of genes involved in inflammation are increased in subcutaneous adipose tissue of obese subjects comparatively to nonobese subjects (14). Differences have also been observed in omental adipose tissue; e.g., the gene encoding the receptors of Fc fragment (known to mediate antibody-dependent inflammatory response) of immunoglobulin (IgG) and other genes implicated in immunity processes are up regulated in obese subjects (15). These results suggest a possible link between adipose tissue and immunity as previously suggested in another gene expression study (24). Changes in gene expression profiles in subcutaneous adipose tissue from obese subjects after 4 weeks of very low-caloric restriction diet confirmed the importance of the function related to inflammation (14). In adipose tissue of obese individuals, the very low-caloric restriction diet led to a decrease of the gene expression level of these factors to the level observed in nonobese subjects (Fig. 1). It was also observed that weight loss decreased the expression of gene-encoding acute phase reactant such as serum amyloid A1 and A2 (SAA1, SAA2) (29,30). SAA is involved in AA amyloidosis, which is a complication of many inflammatory conditions (31,32).

An important question was the site of expression of inflammatory genes. The animal and human studies previously cited (12–14) indicated that overexpressed genes related to inflammation might be produced by infiltrating macrophages. Recent studies confirmed the role of macrophage infiltration in the expression of inflammatory markers in adipose tissue. The positive correlation between macrophage number in the stroma vascular fraction of human adipose tissue and body mass index supports this hypothesis (14). Moreover, pangenomic analysis showed that, compared to adipocytes, the stroma vascular fraction of subcutaneous adipose tissue (containing macrophages) exhibited an overexpression of genes related to defense, immune, and inflammatory responses (30). Elsewhere, it was

Obese (day 28) Non-obese Obese (day 0)

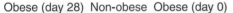
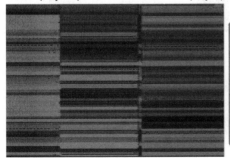

Haptoglobin
β2microglobulin
α2macroglobulin
Serum amyloides
TNF factor families
Interleukin 1

FIGURE 1 (*See color insert.*) Cluster of inflammatory-related gene expression in adipose tissue of non-obese subjects and obese patients before and after VLCD. Each row represents one gene and each column represents one clinical situation or nutritional condition. The intensity of colors of each gene represents the mean in $\log_2$ of gene expression ratios of 7 non-obese subjects and 10 obese subjects before and after VLCD. Green, red, and black colors represent, respectively, the genes downregulated, upregulated, and equal to median. Examples of inflammatory genes are given beside the cluster. *Abbreviation*: VLCD, very low-calorie diet.

found that chemokine (C–C motif) receptor 2 (CCR2), a receptor of monocyte chemoattractant proteins (MCPs) is required to induce macrophage-related gene expression in obese mice and contributes to the inhibition of the expression of metabolism-related genes, such as *PPARG* or fatty acid-binding protein 4 (FABP4) (33). Concomitantly with reduced macrophage number, expression of chemokine (C–C motif) ligand 2 (CCL2 or) MCP1 and other genes involved in macrophage attraction is strongly inhibited by weight loss in human adipose tissue (Fig. 2) (30). In energy-restricted rats, gene expression of this factor was decreased in visceral fat. In addition, the development of diabetes was reversed and expression level of genes involved in lipid metabolism and cellular signaling was modulated in several tissue involved in energy homeostasis (34). These studies show that the beneficial effect of weight loss on obesity-related complications may be associated with the modification of the inflammatory profile in adipose tissue, probably due to a decrease in the macrophage content in the stroma vascular fraction but also a change in the phenotype of macrophages (14). Indeed, the increased expression of macrophagic anti-inflammatory genes such as interleukin-10 and interleukin-1 receptor antagonist during weight loss suggests a modification of macrophage properties. The way is paved to future clinical and cellular studies that aim adipose tissue determining the impact of these molecular adaptations on the development of obesity and associated insulin resistance.

TWO NOVEL BIOMARKERS ASSOCIATED WITH OBESITY

We and others have observed the decreased expression of a gene encoding the acute phase reactant serum amyloid A after weight loss (14,35–37). The SAA are apolipoprotein A, usually known to be synthesized by the liver and to be involved in cholesterol transport and in early response to injury. We have shown that *SAA*

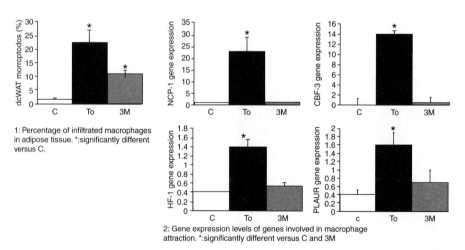

FIGURE 2 Reduction of macrophage number and gene expression in subcutaneous adipose tissue by weight loss. Percentage of infiltrated macrophages in adipose tissue and expression level of four genes involved in macrophage attraction were determined in lean subjects (C) and morbid obese subjects before (T0) and three months after weight loss surgery (3M). *Abbreviations:* MCP1, monocyte chemotactic protein-1; CSF3, colony-stimulating factor 3; HIF-1, hypoxia-inducible factor 1 alpha; PLAUR, plasminogen activator urokinase receptor.

gene expression is increased in adipose tissue of obese subjects and significantly correlates with adipocyte size and inflammatory biomarkers. This finding was confirmed by immunohistochemistry analysis of adipose tissue showing mainly staining in adipocytes in contrast to many inflammatory-related proteins. The production of SAA by human adipose tissue has been confirmed by several independent teams and correlates with adipocyte size (29,36,37). SAA could play a local role in the adipose tissue, for example, in enhancing the synthesis of inflammatory protein by the macrophage and the free fatty acid release from adipose cells. Although no obvious evidence of a relationship between insulin sensitivity surrogates and SAA was observed in morbidly obese subjects (38), improvement of insulin sensitivity using thiazolinediones showed a decrease of SAA in adipose tissue and in the serum of less severely obese subjects (36). It was then suggested that this inflammatory adipokine could link obesity with its metabolic and vascular complications (39). In agreement, with this hypothesis, studies in obese subjects revealed significant associations between adipose tissue and plasma levels of SAA and surrogates of sleep apnea, a condition frequently linked with cardiovascular diseases (40).

The second biomarker identified in human adipose tissue by large-scale analysis was cathepsin S (CTSS) (41). CTSS is a cysteine protease known to degrade several components of the extracellular matrix in atherosclerotic plaques and to be involved in immunity processes notably the antigen presentation. Several studies showed that various models of atherosclerosis-prone mice had higher CTSS levels in their atherosclerosis lesions compared with their lean counterparts (42). Human investigations showed abnormal presence of CTSS in atherosclerotic lesions whereas no expression of CTSS was detected in normal arteries (43). The role of CTSS in atherogenesis has been established in transgenic mice model, atheroma-prone (low-density lipoprotein receptor-deficient mice) crossed with CTSS −/− mice, subjected to high-cholesterol diet, which showed significant reductions in atheroma lesions (44,45). A recent study performed on a large cohort of patients not selected on body mass index, showed that serum CTSS levels were increased in patients with atherosclerotic stenosis (46). Specialists of the cardiovascular field thus suggest that elevated levels of CTSS in vascular wall promote atherosclerosis. Using pangenomic arrays and real-time PCR combined with bioinformatics treatment of the data, we have shown in independent groups of individuals that CTSS is produced by human adipose cells, increased in obesity and decreased with weight loss both in adipose tissue and in serum (47). CTSS secretion in adipose tissue explants is enhanced by inflammatory markers (48). Extracellular matrix remodeling is a key process associated with adipogenesis and CTSS a potent elastolytic protein. These properties prompted us to assess the potential role of CTSS in adipocyte differentiation. A set of experiments analyzing fibronectin cleavage using both a specific inhibitor and a recombinant protein showed that CTSS facilitates adipogenesis adipose tissue at least in part by degrading fibronectin in the early steps of differentiation (48). Other cathepsins such as cathepsin K (CTSK) may also be involved in the facilitation of adipose differentiation (49). Taken together, these results indicate that CTSS and eventually other members of the cathepsin family, released locally by preadipocytes promotes adipogenesis, suggesting a possible contribution of this protease to fat mass expansion in obesity. In addition, given the potential deleterious effect of CTSS on the arterial wall, this protease represents a plausible molecular link between enlarged fat mass and developing atherosclerosis.

Biomarkers of Nutritional Status and Predictors of Weight Changes

Microarray studies could help in characterizing the molecular response of obese patients to a nutritional intervention or a treatment. As it is not well established how the macronutrient composition of the diet could modulate the response to a hypocaloric diet, microarrays represent then a potential diagnostic tool to determine the most appropriate diet for each patient. Little is known about the effect of energy restriction and macronutrients on the regulation of adipose tissue gene expression. The recent multicentric European study on the effects of low-fat and moderate-fat, 10-week low-calorie diets NUGENOB (nutrient-gene interactions in obesity: NUGENOB www.nugenob.org) (50) showed that, as observed for anthropometric parameters, energy restriction, rather than the fat/carbohydrate ratio is of importance to modify the transcriptional program in human adipose tissue (51,52). Up to now, no difference in adipose tissue gene expression was observed between the two diets using a candidate gene expression approach. Energy restriction induced a decrease in key genes involved in lipid metabolism (fatty acid synthase, stearoyl CoA desaturase) and an increase in the expression of *PGC1A*. Therefore, the identification of molecular biomarkers of the nutritional status (e.g., the level of fat in the diet) requires an investigation on a large number of subjects and genes. Such a study is ongoing in our laboratories. Further works are necessary for a better understanding of weight variations and changes in nutritional status. In particular, food with a low glycemic index and proteins may help in weight control, in part because of improving satiety feeling. Few and inconclusive data are available about these hypotheses. The European program DIOGENES (diet, obesity, and genes, www.diogenes-eu.org) is intended to assess the effect of diets differing in their glycemic index and protein content for preventing weight regain during a 6 month weight maintenance period, after several weeks of caloric restriction. Molecular biomarker of the nutritional status will be identified to determine how these diets could modulate the expression of specific genes in adipose tissue. Both the NUGENOB and DIOGENES programs offer the opportunity to characterize molecular predictors of weight changes based on mRNA profiling. Different algorithms applied to clinical data and plasma parameters reveal poor prediction of weight loss suggesting that other data such as gene expression profiles may be of interest alone or in combination to build good predictive models (see Chapter 10.4). The predictors may be single genes or combinations of several genes that best predict weight loss. The reduction in size of the data may constitute a key point in setting up a reliable method of prediction.

LIMITATIONS OF MICROARRAY USE

Although information and resources are growing, it should be kept in mind that there are still many difficulties and pitfalls in the interpretation of microarray data. Details have been given in Chapters 10.1 and 10.2. Some practical examples regarding human investigation are provided as below. One issue constantly faced in research using human tissues is the small number of samples studied related to the potential huge number of genes that can be evaluated adipose tissue the same time. The cost of these techniques is limiting and there is also limited availability of human tissues that are less accessible to biopsy such as heart, skeletal muscle, or liver (and obviously brain). However, this later hurdle can be overcome as improvement in mRNA amplification and microarray signal sensitivity allow the use of minute quantities of tissues. For example, the hormonal control of skeletal muscle gene expression (53,54) and the distinctive patterns of expression induced by obesity and hypertension in the heart (55) have been described. It is critical to obtain adipose tissue some stages an integrated view of gene signatures in different tissues under different conditions (see Chapter 10.2). The development of large human tissue banks appears to be necessary. Furthermore in the perspective of finding gene predictors of clinical changes after environmental modifications, experiments are mandatory to get enough power in data analysis that is now the objective of the NUGENOB and DIOGENES programs funded by the European Union. The tremendous source of variability adipose tissue different levels by using these techniques needs to be mentioned. mRNA measurements are inherently highly variable (biological variability). The variability also depends on the level of expression of the gene with increased variability for lowly expressed genes. The methods by themselves induce variability: mRNA extraction, probe labeling, hybridization, scanning, and image analysis. In addition, conventional statistical analysis of thousand of values in parallel will reveal differences that are only attributable to the random normal distribution of the data, thus adequate procedures for multiple testing have to be applied. Thus, validation of a candidate gene is systematically performed by RT-qPCR. Another aspect is related to the standardization procedures not only due to experimental variations but to the reported gene information (Table 1). As mentioned in Chapter 10.2, this aspect is currently improving. However, an assessment of the current DNA microarray available literature shows that there is little standardization in the field with regard to the methods, analysis and controls used, as well as with data validation (Table 1). For example, most functional gene annotations in many publications are made manually, enabling bias in interpretation and limiting the possibility of comparing information among different independent studies (Table 1). The examples of transcriptomic approaches described above already emphasize the need for standardization. Working groups have proposed different procedures recommended for the representation of microarray information. The exchange of information between different data systems and research groups for further integrative approach is mandatory. By using microarray techniques, one should always keep in mind that the resulting gene expression does not necessarily reflect the proteins that serve as the functional effectors of cellular processes detailed in Chapters 10.4 and 10.5.

COMBINING "OMIC" APPROACHES

Since the physiopathology of obesity is complex, it becomes apparent that a multidisciplinary research effort, involving the combination of various fields (i.e., clinical, biochemical, genetic, transcriptomic, proteomic, and metabolomic) is necessary with the aim of increasing our knowledge of the complexity of biological traits and processes of the disease. The use of other "omics" technologies such as proteomic and metabolomic, which assess the protein and metabolites products offers additional and complementary opportunities (Fig. 3). In the complex picture of the physiopathology of obesity adipose tissue its different stages of evolution, studies of genes, proteins, and metabolites may contribute to revealing the role of certain signals and then could provide better understanding of the mechanisms of energy homeostasis. For example, the DIOGENES program will allow a concomitant analysis of genetic background (based on candidate genes associated with obesity), gene expression, peptides and proteins analyses during different weight loss and weight maintenance programs in obese subjects from several European countries (see above). Relevant markers of the nutritional status or the capacity to lose or

TABLE 1 Examples of Limitations in the Microarray Data Analysis Performed on Animal and Human Adipose Tissues

Reference number	Type of study	Number of genes on microarrays	% of differentially expressed genes	Validation	Multiple testing	Annotation
Rodent studies						
(10)	Obesity	11,000	10%	No	No	Manual
(11)	Obesity	6500	25%	Yes ($n=20$)	No	Manual
(58)	High-fat diet	12,500	15%	Yes ($n=3$)	No	Manual
(9)	High-fat diet	12,488	6%	Yes ($n=6$)	No	Manual
(59)	Obesity	12,000	0.1%	No	No	No
(60)	High-fat diet	76	~30%	Yes ($n=23$)	No	Manual
Human studies						
(24)	Subcutaneous/visceral fat	Affymetrix U95A human genome	N/A	No	No	Manual
(14)	Caloric restriction	40,000	~5%	Yes ($n=10$)	Yes	Manual
(25)	Subcutaneous/visceral fat	44	36%	No	No	Manual
(15)	Visceral obesity	1152	13%	Yes ($n=6$)	No	Manual
(7)	Preadipocyte/adipocyte	~9000	~1%	Yes ($n=5$)	Yes	Gene ontology tree machine
(35)	Obesity	40,000	~2%	Yes	Yes	Manual
(51)	Caloric restriction	8793	~1%	Yes ($n=7$)	No	Gene ontology

Note: Number of genes on microarrays represents the number of cDNA or genes spotted on arrays. % mobilized genes means % of genes that were significantly selected under the tested condition. Validation of microarray data was performed using quantitative RT-PCR or Northern blot analyses. Multiple testing controls for genes selected by chance when a large number of genes is analyzed in parallel. Annotation assigns genes into functional classes.

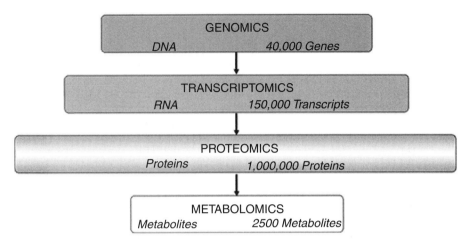

FIGURE 3 Information stored in omics-derived components. In agreement with current molecular biology dogma, DNA is transcribed into RNA, which is translated in proteins. The metabolome appears to be the smallest compartment.

maintain body weight should be then identified. The combination of all these techniques requires the development of data mining tools to fully exploit various data. One of the future challenges is to process the mass of information generated from diverse phenotypic and genotypic characteristics as well as different nutritional conditions. The advances in technology now allow for combining the search for gene variation/mutation and the gene expression profiling on a genome-wide basis. Thus, the overlap between gene profiling studies, the whole genome scan and the candidate genes map available in humans and rodents will constitute important steps in combining information. A proof-of-concept of this new approach was provided by a study in which gene expression data and genome-wide scan were combined in standard inbred mice strains (56). The strains were crossed together and the F2 generation was fed with a high-fat diet for 4 months. Phenotypes were obtained with regard to obesity-related traits and metabolic parameters. Gene expression levels in the liver were compared in obese and lean animals and molecular signatures of the lean and the obese states were identified. A second step aimed adipose tissue identifying genes or chromosomal regions linked to obesity phenotype was achieved by using genome-wide scans. The variation of liver gene expression in the animal strains was used as a quantitative trait loci (eQTL). mRNA levels proved to be a highly valuable trait that gave stronger association with chromosomal loci than usual endophenotypes parameters. The linkage study not only identified chromosomal regions involved in the control of adiposity, but also in the control of the liver gene expression. Recently, another study using the same approach combining gene expression profiling in fat and kidney with linkage analysis was used to identify genes involved in the metabolic syndrome (57).

CONCLUSION

The choice of a candidate gene in obesity research is based on several arguments including the physiological role of its encoded protein in the development and complications of obesity, its chromosomal location in a region linked to obesity in human or animal models, the phenotypic consequences of its genetic manipulation in gene knockout or transgenic mouse models and eventually the in vitro functional characteristics of gene mutations or variations studied. The pattern of expression of the gene transcripts in key tissues for weight control, or even its modification of expression in response to the environment can be used. All criteria are rarely taken into account. The future will tell us whether they are good targets for intervention. Among the limitations to this integrated approach, one can cite the difficulty of having large enough samples as well as biocomputing tools that are still in their infancy for accessing the question of multiple interactions with no "a priori hypotheses." This picture will probably change rapidly in the future thanks to developing technologies.

REFERENCES

1. Mercer JG, O'Reilly LM, Morgan PJ. Increasing the impact of European obesity research in preparation for the European research area: a report on the 2003 European Commission Obesity Workshop. Obes Rev 2004; 5:79–85.
2. Mootha VK, Lindgren CM, Eriksson KF, et al. PGC-1alpha-responsive genes involved in oxidative phosphorylation are coordinately downregulated in human diabetes. Nat Genet 2003; 34:267–73.
3. Patti ME, Butte AJ, Crunkhorn S, et al. Coordinated reduction of genes of oxidative metabolism in humans with insulin resistance and diabetes: Potential role of PGC1 and NRF1. Proc Natl Acad Sci USA 2003; 100:8466–71.
4. Soukas A, Socci ND, Saatkamp BD, et al. Distinct transcriptional profiles of adipogenesis in vivo and in vitro. J Biol Chem 2001; 276:34167–74.
5. Jessen BA, Stevens GJ. Expression profiling during adipocyte differentiation of 3T3-L1 fibroblasts. Gene 2002; 299:95–100.
6. Burton GR, Nagarajan R, Peterson CA, et al. Microarray analysis of differentiation-specific gene expression during 3T3-L1 adipogenesis. Gene 2004; 329:167–85.
7. Urs S, Smith C, Campbell B, et al. Gene expression profiling in human preadipocytes and adipocytes by microarray analysis. J Nutr 2004; 134:762–70.
8. Hong KM, Burdick MD, Phillips RJ, et al. Characterization of human fibrocytes as circulating adipocyte progenitors and the formation of human adipose tissue in SCID mice. FASEB J 2005; 19:2029–31.
9. Moraes RC, Blondet A, Birkenkamp-Demtroeder K, et al. Study of the alteration of gene expression in adipose tissue of diet-induced obese mice by microarray and reverse transcription-polymerase chain reaction analyses. Endocrinology 2003; 144: 4773–82.
10. Nadler ST, Stoehr JP, Schueler KL, et al. The expression of adipogenic genes is decreased in obesity and diabetes mellitus. Proc Natl Acad Sci USA 2000; 97:11371–6.
11. Soukas A, Cohen P, Socci ND, et al. Leptin-specific patterns of gene expression in white adipose tissue. Genes Dev 2000; 14:963–80.
12. Weisberg SP, McCann D, Desai M, et al. Obesity is associated with macrophage accumulation in adipose tissue. J Clin Invest 2003; 112:1796–808.
13. Xu H, Barnes GT, Yang Q, et al. Chronic inflammation in fat plays a crucial role in the development of obesity-related insulin resistance. J Clin Invest 2003; 112:1821–30.
14. Clement K, Viguerie N, Poitou C, et al. Weight loss regulates inflammation-related genes in white adipose tissue of obese subjects. FASEB J 2004; 18:1657–69.
15. Gomez-Ambrosi J, Catalan V, Diez-Caballero A, et al. Gene expression profile of omental adipose tissue in human obesity. FASEB J 2004; 18:215–7.
16. Donahue RP, Abbott RD. Central obesity and coronary heart disease in men. Lancet 1987; 2:1215.
17. Ducimetiere P, Richard JL. The relationship between subsets of anthropometric upper versus lower body measurements and coronary heart disease risk in middle-aged men. The Paris Prospective Study. I. Int J Obes 1989; 13:111–21.

18. van Harmelen V, Reynisdottir S, Eriksson P, et al. Leptin secretion from subcutaneous and visceral adipose tissue in women. Diabetes 1998; 47:913–7.
19. Motoshima H, Wu X, Sinha MK, et al. Differential regulation of adiponectin secretion from cultured human omental and subcutaneous adipocytes: effects of insulin and rosiglitazone. J Clin Endocrinol Metab 2002; 87:5662–7.
20. Bastelica D, Morange P, Berthet B, et al. Stromal cells are the main plasminogen activator inhibitor-1-producing cells in human fat: evidence of differences between visceral and subcutaneous deposits. Arterioscler Thromb Vasc Biol 2002; 22:173–8.
21. Fukuhara A, Matsuda M, Nishizawa M, et al. Visfatin: a protein secreted by visceral fat that mimics the effects of insulin. Science 2005; 307:426–30.
22. Pagano C, Pilon C, Olivieri M, et al. Reduced plasma visfatin/pre-B cell colony-enhancing factor in obesity is not related to insulin resistance in humans. J Clin Endocrinol Metab 2006; 91:3165–70.
23. Yang YS, Song HD, Li RY, et al. The gene expression profiling of human visceral adipose tissue and its secretory functions. Biochem Biophys Res Commun 2003; 300:839–46.
24. Gabrielsson BG, Johansson JM, Lonn M, et al. High expression of complement components in omental adipose tissue in obese men. Obes Res 2003; 11:699–708.
25. Linder K, Arner P, Flores-Morales A, et al. Differentially expressed genes in visceral or subcutaneous adipose tissue of obese men and women. J Lipid Res 2004; 45:148–54.
26. Gabrielsson BL, Carlsson B, Carlsson LM. Partial genome scale analysis of gene expression in human adipose tissue using DNA array. Obes Res 2000; 8:374–84.
27. Ramis JM, Franssen-van Hal NL, Kramer E, et al. Carboxypeptidase E and thrombospondin-1 are differently expressed in subcutaneous and visceral fat of obese subjects. Cell Mol Life Sci 2002; 59:1960–71.
28. Li Y, Bujo H, Takahashi K, et al. Visceral fat: higher responsiveness of fat mass and gene expression to calorie restriction than subcutaneous fat. Exp Biol Med 2003; 228(10):1118–23.
29. Sjoholm K, Palming J, Olofsson LE, et al. A microarray search for genes predominantly expressed in human omental adipocytes: adipose tissue as a major production site of serum amyloid A. J Clin Endocrinol Metab 2005; 90:2233–9.
30. Cancello R, Henegar C, Viguerie N, et al. Reduction of macrophage infiltration and chemoattractant gene expression changes in white adipose tissue of morbidly obese subjects after surgery-induced weight loss. Diabetes 2005; 54:2277–86.
31. Urieli-Shoval S, Linke RP, Matzner Y. Expression and function of serum amyloid A, a major acute-phase protein, in normal and disease states. Curr Opin Hematol 2000; 7:64–9.
32. Merlini G, Bellotti V. Molecular mechanisms of amyloidosis. N Engl J Med 2003; 349:583–96.
33. Weisberg SP, Hunter D, Huber R, et al. CCR2 modulates inflammatory and metabolic effects of high-fat feeding. J Clin Invest 2006; 116:115–24.
34. Colombo M, Kruhoeffer M, Gregersen S, et al. Energy restriction prevents the development of type 2 diabetes in Zucker diabetic fatty rats: coordinated patterns of gene expression for energy metabolism in insulin-sensitive tissues and pancreatic islets determined by oligonucleotide microarray analysis. Metabolism 2006; 55:43–52.
35. Poitou C, Viguerie N, Cancello R, et al. Serum amyloid A: production by human white adipocyte and regulation by obesity and nutrition. Diabetologia 2005; 48:519–28.
36. Yang RZ, Lee MJ, Hu H, et al. Acute-phase serum amyloid A: an inflammatory adipokine and potential link between obesity and its metabolic complications. PLoS Med 2006; 3:e287.
37. Jernas M, Palming J, Sjoholm K, et al. Separation of human adipocytes by size: hypertrophic fat cells display distinct gene expression. FASEB J 2006; 20:1540–2.
38. Poitou C, Coussieu C, Rouault C, et al. Serum amyloid A: a marker of adiposity-induced low-grade inflammation but not of metabolic status. Obesity (Silver Spring) 2006; 14:309–18.
39. O'Brien KD, Chait A. Serum amyloid A: the other inflammatory protein. Curr Atheroscler Rep 2006; 8:62–8.

40. Poitou C, Coupaye M, Laaban JP, et al. Serum amyloid A and obstructive sleep apnea syndrome before and after surgically-induced weight loss in morbidly obese subjects. Obes Surg 2006; 16:1475–81.
41. Taleb S, Lacasa D, Bastard JP, et al. Cathepsin S, a novel biomarker of adiposity: relevance to atherogenesis. FASEB J 2005; 19:1540–2.
42. Jormsjo S, Wuttge DM, Sirsjo A, et al. Differential expression of cysteine and aspartic proteases during progression of atherosclerosis in apolipoprotein E-deficient mice. Am J Pathol 2002; 161:939–45.
43. Sukhova GK, Shi GP, Simon DI, et al. Expression of the elastolytic cathepsins S and K in human atheroma and regulation of their production in smooth muscle cells. J Clin Invest 1998; 102:576–83.
44. Shi GP, Sukhova GK, Kuzuya M, et al. Deficiency of the cysteine protease cathepsin S impairs microvessel growth. Circ Res 2003; 92:493–500.
45. Sukhova GK, Zhang Y, Pan JH, et al. Deficiency of cathepsin S reduces atherosclerosis in LDL receptor-deficient mice. J Clin Invest 2003; 111:897–906.
46. Liu J, Ma L, Yang J, et al. Increased serum cathepsin S in patients with atherosclerosis and diabetes. Atherosclerosis 2006; 186:411–9.
47. Taleb S, Cancello R, Poitou C, et al. Weight loss reduces adipose tissue cathepsin S and its circulating levels in morbidly obese women. J Clin Endocrinol Metab 2006; 91:1042–7.
48. Taleb S, Cancello R, Clement K, et al. Cathepsin s promotes human preadipocyte differentiation: possible involvement of fibronectin degradation. Endocrinology 2006; 147:4950–9.
49. Xiao Y, Junfeng H, Tianhong L, et al. Cathepsin K in adipocyte differentiation and its potential role in the pathogenesis of obesity. J Clin Endocrinol Metab 2006; 91:4520–7.
50. Petersen M, Taylor MA, Saris WH, et al. Randomized, multi-center trial of two hypo-energetic diets in obese subjects: high- versus low-fat content. Int J Obes (Lond) 2006; 30:552–60.
51. Viguerie N, Vidal H, Arner P, et al. Adipose tissue gene expression in obese subjects during low-fat and high-fat hypocaloric diets. Diabetologia 2005; 48:123–31.
52. Dahlman I, Linder K, Arvidsson Nordstrom E, et al. Changes in adipose tissue gene expression with energy-restricted diets in obese women. Am J Clin Nutr 2005; 81:1275–85.
53. Clement K, Viguerie N, Diehn M, et al. In vivo regulation of human skeletal muscle gene expression by thyroid hormone. Genome Res 2002; 12:281–91.
54. Viguerie N, Clement K, Barbe P, et al. In vivo epinephrine-mediated regulation of gene expression in human skeletal muscle. J Clin Endocrinol Metab 2004; 89:2000–14.
55. Philip-Couderc P, Pathak A, Smih F, et al. Uncomplicated human obesity is associated with a specific cardiac transcriptome: involvement of the Wnt pathway. FASEB J 2004; 18:1539–40.
56. Schadt EE, Monks SA, Drake TA, et al. Genetics of gene expression surveyed in maize, mouse and man. Nature 2003; 422:297–302.
57. Hubner N, Wallace CA, Zimdahl H, et al. Integrated transcriptional profiling and linkage analysis for identification of genes underlying disease. Nat Genet 2005; 37:243–53.
58. Lopez IP, Marti A, Milagro FI, et al. DNA microarray analysis of genes differentially expressed in diet-induced (cafeteria) obese rats. Obes Res 2003; 11:188–94.
59. Takahashi K, Mizuarai S, Araki H, et al. Adiposity elevates plasma MCP-1 levels leading to the increased CD11b-positive monocytes in mice. J Biol Chem 2003; 278:46654–60.
60. Lopez IP, Milagro FI, Marti A, et al. High-fat feeding period affects gene expression in rat white adipose tissue. Mol Cell Biochem 2005; 275:109–15.

Proteomics and Metabonomics Routes Toward Obesity

Martin Kussmann and Michael Affolter

Functional Genomics Group, Bioanalytical Science Department, Nestlé Research Center, Lausanne, Switzerland

Obesity is a condition resulting from a chronic imbalance between energy intake and energy expenditure (1,2). Behind this simple observation there is a complex disease involving genetic, environmental, and behavioural factors (3,4). Obesity is strongly correlated with type 2 diabetes mellitus, a common disorder of glucose and lipid metabolism: it often causes insulin resistance, a decline in the ability of insulin to stimulate glucose uptake in the body, which leads to compensatory oversecretion of this hormone by the pancreatic beta-cells and, eventually, to beta-cell exhaustion and development of type 2 diabetes mellitus (2,5). Overconsumption of energy (6), types of fats, proteins, and carbohydrates absorbed (7) and micronutrient deficiencies (8) have been associated with obesity and type 2 diabetes.

Roughly a hundred genes are reported to date to be potentially involved in obesity and about 20 of them, most of them apolipoproteins, have been studied in diet response or association studies (9). Early (even prenatal) nutritional (metabolic) imprinting seems to play an important role for later susceptibility to obesity (10).

Proteomics is well-established in the pharmaceutical industry mainly for biomarker and drug target discovery. The potential of proteomics for diabetes and obesity (diabesity) research is now increasingly being recognized. Metabonomics has been employed in (pre-) clinical research, in environmental and biomedical applications and in toxicology (11). More recently, it has gained a strong impact in nutritional research (12) and is nowadays more and more integrated into biomarker discovery for diabesity. Hence, protein and metabolite profiling will increasingly complement the more established transcriptomic platforms in diabesity biomarker and target identification. This chapter summarizes applications of proteomics, metabonomics, and transcriptomics to both obesity and diabetes.

OMICS APPLIED TO OBESITY
Omics in Animal Models for Obesity

Several research groups investigated gene expression differences between lean and obese animal models: Carre et al. looked at differential expression and genetic variation of hepatic messenger RNAs from genetically lean and fat chickens (13). Stricker-Krongrad et al. studied the central and peripheral deregulation of melanin-concentrating hormone in obese Zucker rats (14).

Microarray profiling was conducted in studies of mouse genetic models for obesity: Nadler et al. for example used DNA microarrays to identify differences in gene expression in adipose tissue from lean, obese, and obese-diabetic mice (15). They showed that a decrease in expression of genes normally involved in adipogenesis is associated with obesity, and identified genes important for subsequent development of type 2 diabetes.

More recently, Zucker obese rats were compared to normal animals by metabonomic means. Granger and Plumb employed ultraperformance liquid chromatography [(UPLC), providing separation power superior to conventional high-performance liquid chromatography (HPLC)] and time-of-flight mass spectrometry (ToF-MS) to distinguish obese and normal rats based on their urinary metabolite profile (16,17). With the same objective in mind, Williams et al. undertook a combined approach consisting of ^{1}H-NMR spectroscopy and HPLC-MS (18).

Proteomics of Adipose Tissue

Adipose tissue has been recognized not only as a fat and energy depot but also as an endocrine organ (19) secreting a number of hormones. This tissue has therefore been analyzed in terms of possible links between obesity and insulin resistance (20). Proteins secreted by fat cells (adipocytes) encompass adiponectin, angiotensinogen, adipsin, acylation-stimulating protein, tumor necrosis factor, interleukin-6 and plasminogen activator inhibitor 1 (21). These proteins regulate lipid metabolism, inflammation, cardiovascular functions, vascular haemostasis, and immunity. The adipocyte transcriptome, its changes during differentiation and its regulation by growth factors and pathological conditions have been examined by microarray-based studies (22–24, and see Chapter 10.3).

Apart from being subjected to microarrays, adipose tissue has become an interesting object for studying proteomic patterns related to obesity. The Swiss 2D-PAGE database provides two-dimensional gel electrophoretic protein maps of white and brown adipose tissue (25,26). Protein recovery from adipose tissue is a challenge though because of the high fat content of the sample. Corton et al. developed a sample preparation particularly adapted to solubilization and isoelectric focusing of AT-recovered proteins submitted to 2DE analysis (27). They compared protein profiles of the intra-abdominal adipose tissue of morbidly obese women with and without polycystic ovary syndrome. Kratchmarova et al. embarked on a proteomic route toward the identification of secreted factors during the differentiation of preadipocytes to adipocytes in vitro (28).

Proteomics and Metabonomics of PPARs

Peroxisome proliferator-activated receptors (PPARs) have become important "Omic objects" in diabesity research. The PPAR transcription factors are fatty acid–activated receptors, which regulate genes involved in lipid metabolism and homeostasis (29–31). PPARs can be interpreted as sensors of intracellular lipid and fatty acid concentrations (32,33). PPARα is preferentially expressed in the liver, while PPARγ is predominantly found in adipose tissue (34). Activation of PPARα leads to peroxisome proliferation and increased beta-oxidation of fatty acids. PPARγ activation results in adipocyte differentiation as well as improved insulin signaling of mature adipocytes.

The insulin sensitizer drug rosiglitazone has been shown to bind and activate PPARγ1 in adipocytes and PPARγ2 in hepatocytes. The identification of new molecular targets associated with fatty acid oxidation and PPARγ nuclear receptor regulation in insulin resistance tissues is a key research goal. Sanchez et al. employed a proteomic approach to identify such targets (35). Lean and obese C57 Bl/6J leptin-deficient mice were given rosiglitazone. The drug impaired glucose tolerance and dyslipidemia in these mice but had no significant effect in the lean mice. Liver, white and brown adipose tissue, and muscle proteins were analyzed by 2DE-MS/MS. Thirty-four polypeptides were differentially expressed between lep^{ob}/lep^{ob} and lean mice and 11 were significantly modulated by rosiglitazone treatment of the obese mice. None of the proteins was modulated by rosiglitazone treatment of the lean mice. The identity of these differentially expressed proteins revealed components of fatty acid and carbohydrate metabolism as well as proteins with unknown function.

Also the lipid metabonome-wide effects of rosiglitazone were investigated in a type 2 diabetes mouse model (36). While dietary supplementation with the drug-suppressed type 2 diabetes in obese male mice, chronic treatment with rosiglitazone exacerbated hepatic steatosis. Metabonomic assessment showed that the drug induced hypolipidemia and de novo fatty acid synthesis, decreased intraperoxisome lipid biosynthesis, altered free fatty acid, and cardiolipin metabolism in heart and resulted in an abnormal accumulation of polyunsaturated fatty acids in adipose tissue. Since many rosiglitazone effects on tissue metabolism were reflected in the plasma lipid profile, metabonomics bears great potential for developing clinical assessments of metabolic response to drug therapy.

The effects of a therapeutic dose of a PPARα agonist (Wy 14,643) in the leptin-deficient mouse were investigated by proteomic means (2DE-MS/MS approach). The agonist showed upregulation of 16 liver proteins, 14 of which are implied in peroxisomal fatty acid metabolism (37). In a related study, Chu et al. concluded that livers with Wy 14,643-mediated activation are transcriptionally geared toward fatty acid combustion (38). Edvardsson et al. extended their classical 2DE-based proteomic investigations by a comparison of hepatic protein expression of lean and obese mice to obese mice treated with PPARα and PPARγ agonists (39). Livers from obese mice displayed higher levels of enzymes involved in fatty acid oxidation and lipogenesis compared to lean mice and these differences were further amplified by treatment with PPARα and γ activators.

Mitochondrial Proteomics

Mitochondria are the "power houses" of the cells and essential organelles for cellular homeostasis. They are predominantly known for their oxidative phosphorylation machinery and for containing enzymes for free fatty acid metabolism and the Kreb's cycle. Other functions with mitochondrial contribution are heme biosynthesis, ketone body generation, generation of and self-protection against reactive oxygen species (ROS), cellular calcium signaling, and programmed cell death. It is therefore not surprising that the energy-metabolism-linked pathologies diabetes and obesity can be associated with mitochondrial dysfunction (40).

As a consequence, mapping of mitochondrial components is of interest to gain further insight in such disorders. Proteomic approaches to mitochondrial (dys-)function have been developed and recently reviewed (41). In this context, an integrated analysis of protein composition, tissue diversity, and gene regulation in mouse mitochondria was presented combining proteomics with transcriptomics (42). Comparisons to other species and 2DE studies of isolated mammalian mitochondria (43,44) suggest a proteome complexity of approximately 1200 polypeptides, with currently only 600 to 700 proteins being identified through proteomic and genetic approaches (45–48).

Gene and Metabolite Markers for Susceptibility and Treatment of Obesity and Insulin Resistance

Several strategies have been employed to identify susceptibility genes for obesity and insulin resistance such as positional cloning, microarray-based transcriptomic profiling, and a combination of the latter with gene linkage analysis (2). Two transcriptomic studies in humans were conducted to reveal potential candidate genes for insulin resistance: one investigation dealt with gene expression profiling of skeletal muscle tissues from equally obese, nondiabetic insulin-sensitive and insulin-resistant Pima Indians (49); the other looked at the gene expression profile in the skeletal muscle of type 2 diabetes patients and the effect of insulin treatment (50). Two more recent investigations focused on potential gene regulators showing a coordinated differential expression in subjects with insulin resistance and/or diabetes (51,52). Tobe et al., employing a mouse model, reported on increased expression of the *Srebp1* gene in mice with the insulin receptor substrate 2 deficiency in the liver (53). Regrettably, to date complementary proteomic cohort studies with the objective of identifying protein biomarkers for obesity/diabetes susceptibility are largely missing.

Several authors proposed microarray-derived candidate target genes for the treatment of obesity and related disorders: Kaszubska et al. found that protein tyrosine phosphatase 1B negatively regulates leptin signaling in a hypothalamic cell line; Matsuzaka et al. cloned and characterized a mammalian fatty acyl-CoA elongase as a lipogenic enzyme regulated by SREBPs; and Sone et al. discovered that acetyl-coenzyme A synthetase is a lipogenic enzyme controlled by SREBP1 and energy status (54–56).

Proteomics and Metabonomics in Diabetes Mechanisms and Diagnostics

A mouse Swiss 2D-PAGE database has been established for type 2 diabetes (57). These 2DE reference maps are annotated with protein identifications and were generated from mouse white and brown adipose tissue, pancreatic islets, liver, and skeletal muscle. They can be accessed through http://www.expasy.org/ch2d/.

Finding new molecular targets associated both with islet cell dysfunction and protection is an important objective in diabetes research. In a ground-laying study, glucose-responsive proteins in pancreatic islets from rats were separated and visualized by 2DE (58). More recently, the effect of the drug rosiglitazone on differential expression of diabetes-related proteins in pancreatic islets of obese mice was examined following a 2DE-based proteomic strategy (35). This paper is discussed in more detail in the previous paragraphs on PPARs. A global protein analysis of normal mouse pancreatic islets revealed proteins previously found implicated in Alzheimer's disease to be highly expressed (59), a finding, which triggered speculations about potential parallel pathophysiologies between Alzheimer's disease and type 2 diabetes.

A series of diabetes-related proteomic studies aimed at the identification of possibly deleterious or protective proteins in the initial cytokine-induced beta-cell damage in type-1 diabetes (60–62). The complexity of IL-1 beta effects on islet protein expression supports the hypothesis that in type-1 diabetes development is the result of a collective, dynamic instability, rather than the outcome of a single factor (63).

In order to elucidate molecular alterations associated with insulin resistance in muscle tissue, human skeletal muscle biopsies from patients with type 2 diabetes were compared to healthy controls at 2DE level and eight potential markers were identified (64).

Complementary to the search of candidate marker genes, metabolic profiling has been more recently applied to find surrogate markers of type 2 diabetes (65).

The discrimination of type 2 diabetes patients from healthy controls was achieved by metabonomic profiling of serum fatty acids (66) and plasma phospholipids (67). Genetically modified mouse models for disorders of fatty acid metabolism were employed to pursue a nutrigenomics approach to insulin resistance and type 2 diabetes (68).

Omics-Driven Obesity Research Networks

The European-funded 5th framework program "NUGENOB" (www.nugenob.org) stands for "Nutrition, Genes, and Obesity." The main objectives of this research consortium were to (*i*) identify and characterize novel nutrient-sensitive candidate genes for obesity; (*ii*) analyse differential gene expression in adipose tissue in relation to the acute intake of a high-fat meal as well as long term intake of a hypocaloric diet with either a high or a low fat content; (*iii*) assess effects of functional variants of the candidate genes on physiological responses in obese subjects to a high-fat test meal: appetite, energy expenditure, partitioning, and circulating obesity-related hormones and metabolites; and (*iv*) identify on this basis predictors of changes in body weight and composition during dietary intervention, including changes in fat intake. The paper by Arvidsson et al. (69) showed the effects of the different diets on the protein secretion from AT obtained during the NUGENOB programme.

The main objectives of the 6th European framework program "DIOGENES" (for "Diet, Obesity, and Genes") programme will be achieved in a long-term 6 to 12 months dietary intervention study, using a novel factorial design to investigate the potential benefit of a high protein diet or a diet with low glycemic index. In proteomic terms, the principal objective is the identification of plasma biomarkers for nutritional status and weight change. This will be done by monitoring concentration changes of 20 plasma peptides known to be correlated with nutritional status and body composition (cytokines, adipokines, and satiety peptides) using innovative antibody arrays and multiplex antibody-based technologies. Differential peptide display will be employed as a powerful tool for differential profiling of small proteins and peptides and is based on an efficient generation and fractionation of a low-molecular-weight protein complement and its multidimensional quantitative display by mass spectrometry and proprietary software (70).

CONCLUSIONS

Efforts undertaken to date to "shed Omics-emitted light" on the molecular mechanisms of diabetes and obesity can be summarized as follows: (a) proteomic and genomic inventories of diabesity-related organs and organelles in different species (e.g., pancreatic islets, adipose tissue, mitochondria); (b) elucidation of the crucial link between obesity and diabetes, which appears to be insulin resistance; (c) search for transcriptomic, proteomic, and metabonomic biomarkers, which may indicate disposition, onset, development, and success of treatment of these diseases (Omics for prediction, diagnostics, and monitoring); (d) focus on targets of treatment like PPARs; and (e) large-scale dietary intervention studies combined with Omics-driven biomarker discovery for energy metabolism.

While transcriptomics represents an established technology platform for marker and target discovery in the context of diabesity, proteomics increasingly adds to the picture and the contribution of metabonomics is emerging.

ACKNOWLEDGMENT

Dr. Laurent-Bernard Fay, head of Bioanalytical Sciences, NRC and Dr. Katherine Macé, group leader Energy and Metabolic Health, NRC are thankfully acknowledged for scientific advice and critical reading.

REFERENCES

1. Tataranni PA, Ravussin E. Energy metabolism and obesity. In: Wadden TA, Stunkard AJ, eds. Handbook of Obesity Treatment. New York: Guilford Press, 2002:42.
2. Permana PA, DelParigi A, Tataranni PA. Microarray gene expression profiling in obesity and insulin resistance. Nutrition 2004; 20:134–8.
3. Bouchard C, Perusse L. Heredity and body fat. Ann Rev Nutr 1988; 8:259.
4. World Health Organization. Preventing and managing the global epidemic. In: Obesity. Geneva: World Health Organization, 1997.
5. Tataranni PA, Borgadus C. Obesity and diabetes mellitus. In Porte DJ, Sherwin RS, Baron A, eds. Diabetes Mellitus. 6th ed. New York: McGraw-Hill, 2003:401.
6. Willett W. Isocaloric diets are of primary interest in experimental and epidemiological studies. Int J Epidemiol 2002; 31:694–5.
7. Jenkins DJ, Kendall CW, Augustin LS, et al. Glycemic index: overview of implications in health and disease. Am J Clin Nutr 2002; 76:266S–73.
8. Fairfield KM, Fletcher RH. Vitamins for chronic disease prevention in adults: scientific review. JAMA 2002; 287:3116–26.
9. Kaput J. Diet-disease gene interactions. Nutrition 2004; 20:26–31.
10. Waterland RA, Jirtle RL. Early nutrition, epigenetic changes at transposons and imprinted genes, and enhanced susceptibility to adult chronic disease. Nutrition 2004; 20:63–8.
11. Robertson DG. Metabonomics in toxicology: a review. Toxicol Sci 2005; 85:809–22.
12. Whitfield PD, German AJ, Noble PJ. Metabonomics: an emerging post-genomic tool for nutrition. Br J Nutr 2004; 92:549–55.
13. Carre W, Bourneuf E, Douaire M, et al. Differential expression and genetic variation of hepatic messenger RNAs from genetically lean and fat chickens. Gene 2002; 299:235–43.
14. Stricker-Krongrad A, Dimitrov T, Beck B. Central and peripheral dysregulation of melanin-concentrating hormone in obese Zucker rats. Brain Res Mol Brain Res 2001; 92:43–8.
15. Nadler ST, Stoehr JP, Schueler KL. The expression of adipogenic genes is decreased in obesity and diabetes mellitus. Proc Natl Acad Sci USA 2000; 97:11371.
16. Plumb RS, Granger JH, Stumpf CL, et al. A rapid screening approach to metabonomics using UPLC and oa-TOF mass spectrometry: application to age, gender and diurnal variation in normal/Zucker obese rats and black, white and nude mice. Analyst 2005; 130:844–9.
17. Granger J, Plumb R, Castro-Perez J, et al. Metabonomic studies comparing capillary and conventional HPLC-oa-TOF MS for the analysis of urine from Zucker obese rats. Chromatographia 2005; 61:375–80.
18. Williams RE, Lenz EM, Evans JA, et al. A combined (1)H NMR and HPLC-MS-based metabonomic study of urine from obese (fa/fa) Zucker and normal Wistar-derived rats. J Pharm Biomed Anal 2005; 38:465–71.
19. Kim S, Moustaid-Moussa N. Secretory, endocrine and autocrine/paracrine function of the adipocyte. J Nutr 2000; 130:3110S.
20. Mohamed-Ali V, Pinkney JH, Coppack SW. Adipose tissue as an endocrine and paracrine organ. Int J Obes Relat Metab Disord 1998; 22:1145.
21. Moustaid-Moussa N, Urs S, Campbell B, et al. Gene expression profiling in adipose tissue. In: Berdanier CD, Moustaid-Moussa N, eds. Genomics and Proteomics in Nutrition. New York: Marcel Dekker, 2004:257–80.

22. Maeda K, Okubo K, Shimomura I, et al. Analysis of an expression profile of genes in the human adipose tissue. Gene 1997; 190:227–35.

23. Yang YS, Song HD, Li RY, et al. The gene expression profiling of human visceral adipose tissue and its secretory functions. Biochem Biophys Res Commun 2003; 300:839–46.

24. Nadler ST, Attie AD. Please pass the chips: genomic insights into obesity and diabetes. J Nutr 2001; 131:2078–81.

25. Sanchez JC, Chiappe D, Converset V, et al. The mouse SWISS-2D PAGE database: a tool for proteomics study of diabetes and obesity. Proteomics 2001; 1:136–63.

26. Lanne B, Potthast F, Hoglund A, et al. Thiourea enhances mapping of the proteome from murine white adipose tissue. Proteomics 2001; 1:819–28.

27. Corton M, Villuendas G, Botella JI, et al. Improved resolution of the human adipose tissue proteome at alkaline and wide range pH by the addition of hydroxyethyl disulfide. Proteomics 2004; 4:438–41.

28. Kratchmarova I, Kalume DE, Blagoev B. A proteomic approach for identification of secreted proteins during the differentiation of 3T3-L1 pre-adipocytes to adipocytes. Mol Cell Proteomics 2002; 1(3):213–22.

29. Spiegelman BM. PPAR-gamma: adipogenic regulator and thiazolidinedione receptor. Diabetes 1998; 47:507–14.

30. Wahli W, Braissant O, Desvergne B. Peroxisome proliferator activated receptors: transcriptional regulators of adipogenesis, lipid metabolism and more. Chem Biol 1995; 2:261–6.

31. Schoonjans K, Staels B, Auwerx J. Role of the peroxisome proliferator-activated receptor (PPAR) in mediating the effects of fibrates and fatty acids on gene expression. J Lipid Res 1996; 37:907–25.

32. Wahli W, Braissant O, Desvergne B. Peroxisome proliferator activated receptors: transcriptional regulators of adipogenesis, lipid metabolism and more. Chem Biol 1995; 2:261–6.

33. Schoonjans K, Staels B, Auwerx J. Role of the peroxisome proliferator-activated receptor (PPAR) in mediating the effects of fibrates and fatty acids on gene expression. J Lipid Res 1996; 37:907–25.

34. Wahli W, Braissant O, Desvergne B. Peroxisome proliferator activated receptors: transcriptional regulators of adipogenesis, lipid metabolism and more. Chem Biol 1995; 2:261–6.

35. Sanchez JC, Converset V, Nolan A, et al. Effect of rosiglitazone on the differential expression of obesity and insulin resistance associated proteins in lep/lep mice. Proteomics 2003; 3:1500–20.

36. Watkins SM, Reifsnyder PR, Pan HJ, et al. Lipid metabonome-wide effects of the PPARgamma agonist rosiglitazone. J Lipid Res 2002; 43:1809–17.

37. Edvardsson U, Alexandersson M, Brockenhuus-von-Lowenhielm H, et al. A proteome analysis of livers from obese (ob/ob) mice treated with the peroxisome proliferator WY14,643. Electrophoresis 1999; 20:935–42.

38. Chu R, Lim H, Brumfield L, et al. Protein profiling of mouse livers with peroxisome proliferator-activated receptor alpha activation. Mol Cell Biol 2004; 24:6288–97.

39. Edvardsson U, von Lowenhielm HB, Panfilov O, et al. Hepatic protein expression of lean mice and obese diabetic mice treated with peroxisome proliferator-activated receptor activators. Proteomics 2003; 3:468–78.

40. Wallace DC. Mitochondrial diseases in man and mouse. Science 1999; 283:1482–8.

41. Da Cruz S, Parone PA, Martinou JC. Building the mitochondrial proteome. Expert Rev Proteom 2005; 2:541–51.

42. Mootha VK, Bunkenborg J, Olsen JV, et al. Integrated analysis of protein composition, tissue diversity, and gene regulation in mouse mitochondria. Cell 2003; 115:629–40.

43. Lopez MF, Kristal BS, Chernokalskaya E, et al. High-throughput profiling of the mitochondrial proteome using affinity fractionation and automation. Electrophoresis 2000; 21:3427–40.

44. Rabilloud T, Kieffer S, Procaccio V, et al. Two-dimensional electrophoresis of human placental mitochondria and protein identification by mass spectrometry: toward a human mitochondrial proteome. Electrophoresis 1998; 19:1006–14.

45. Da Cruz S, Xenarios I, Langridge J, et al. Proteomic analysis of the mouse liver mitochondrial inner membrane. J Biol Chem 2003; 278:41566–71.

46. Ozawa T, Sako Y, Sato M, et al. A genetic approach to identifying mitochondrial proteins. Nat Biotechnol 2003; 21:287–93.

47. Taylor SW, Fahy E, Zhang B, et al. Characterization of the human heart mitochondrial proteome. Nat Biotechnol 2003; 21:281–6.

48. Westermann B, Neupert W. `Omics' of the mitochondrion. Nat Biotechnol 2003; 21:239–40.

49. Yang X, Pratley RE, Tokraks S, et al. Microarray profiling of skeletal muscle tissues from equally obese, non-diabetic insulin-sensitive and insulin-resistant Pima Indians. Diabetologia 2002; 45:1584–93.

50. Sreekumar R, Halvatsiotis P, Schimke JC, et al. Gene expression profile in skeletal muscle of type 2 diabetes and the effect of insulin treatment. Diabetes 2002; 51:1913.

51. Mootha VK, Lindgren CM, Eriksson KF. PGC-1 alpha-responsive genes involved in oxidative phosphorylation are coordinately down-regulated in human diabetes. Nat Genetics 2003; 34:267.

52. Patti ME, Butte AJ, Crunkhorn S. Coordinated reduction of genes of oxidative metabolism in humans with insulin resistance and diabetes: potential role of PGC1 and NRF1. Proc Natl Acad Sci USA 2003; 100:8466.

53. Tobe K, Suzuki R, Aoyama M, et al. Increased expression of the sterol regulatory element-binding protein-1 gene in insulin receptor substrate-2(-/-) mouse liver. J Biol Chem 2001; 276:38337–40.

54. Sone H, Shimano H, Sakakura Y, et al. Acetyl-coenzyme A synthetase is a lipogenic enzyme controlled by SREBP-1 and energy status. Am J Physiol Endocrinol Metab 2002; 282:E222–30.

55. Kaszubska W, Falls HD, Schaefer VG, et al. Protein tyrosine phosphatase 1B negatively regulates leptin signaling in a hypothalamic cell line. Mol Cell Endocrinol 2002; 195:109–18.

56. Matsuzaka T, Shimano H, Yahagi N, et al. Cloning and characterization of a mammalian fatty acyl-CoA elongase as a lipogenic enzyme regulated by SREBPs. J Lipid Res 2002; 43:911–20.

57. Sanchez JC, Chiappe D, Converset V, et al. The mouse SWISS-2D PAGE database: a tool for proteomics study of diabetes and obesity. Proteomics 2001; 1:136–63.

58. Collins H, Najafi H, Buettger C. Identification of glucose response proteins in two biological models of β-cell adaptation to chronic high-glucose exposure. J Biol Chem 1992; 267(2):1357–66.

59. Nicolls MR, D'Antonio JM, Hutton JC. Proteomics as a tool for discovery: proteins implicated in Alzheimer's disease are highly expressed in normal pancreatic islets. J Proteome Res 2003; 2(5):199–205.

60. Sparre T, Bergholdt R, Nerup J, et al. Application of genomics and proteomics in Type 1 diabetes pathogenesis research. Expert Rev Mol Diagn 2003; 3:743–57.

61. Larsen PM, Fey SJ, Larsen MR, et al. Proteome analysis of interleukin-1beta-induced changes in protein expression in rat islets of Langerhans. Diabetes 2001; 50:1056–63.

62. Sparre T, Christensen UB, Mose LP, et al. IL-1beta induced protein changes in diabetes prone BB rat islets of Langerhans identified by proteome analysis. Diabetologia 2002; 45:1550–61.

63. Freiesleben DB, Bak P, Pociot F, et al. Onset of type 1 diabetes: a dynamical instability. Diabetes 1999; 48:1677–85.

64. Hojlund K, Wrzesinski K, Mose-Larsen P. Proteome analysis reveals phosphorylation of Aor synthase β-subunit in human skeletal muscle and proteins with potential roles in Type-2 Diabetes. J Biol Chem 2003; 278(12):10436–42.

65. Whitfield PD, German AJ, Noble PJ. Metabonomics: an emerging post-genomic tool for nutrition. Br J Nutr 2004; 92:549–55.

66. Yang J, Xu G, Hong Q, et al. Discrimination of Type 2 diabetic patients from healthy controls by using metabonomics method based on their serum fatty acid profiles. J Chromatogr B Analyt Technol Biomed Life Sci 2004; 813:53–8.

67. Wang C, Kong H, Guan Y, et al. Plasma phospholipid metabolic profiling and biomarkers of type 2 diabetes mellitus based on high-performance liquid chromatography/electrospray mass spectrometry and multivariate statistical analysis. Anal Chem 2005; 77:4108–16.

68. Wood PA. Genetically modified mouse models for disorders of fatty acid metabolism: pursuing the nutrigenomics of insulin resistance and type 2 diabetes. Nutrition 2004; 20:121–6.
69. Arvidsson E, Viguerie N, Andersson I, et al. Effects of different hypocaloric diets on protein secretion from adipose tissue of obese women. Diabetes 2004; 53:1966–71.
70. Jurgens M, Schrader M. Peptidomic approaches in proteomic research. Curr Opin Mol Ther 2002; 4:236–41.

Quantitative Proteomics for Analysis of Adipocyte Development and Function

Ariane Minet and Karsten Kristiansen
Eukaryotic Gene Expression and Differentiation Group, Department of Biochemistry and Molecular Biology, University of Southern Denmark, Odense, Denmark

Irina Kratchmarova
Center for Experimental Bioinformatics, Department of Biochemistry and Molecular Biology, University of Southern Denmark, Odense, Denmark

In the recent years after the complete sequencing of the human genome there has been an increased focus on the investigation of the products of the genes, namely the proteins. Up to date around 22,000 protein-coding genes have been predicted in the human genome and comprehensive studies of these encompass new challenges and prospects (1). In general, proteomics can be defined as large-scale studies of the proteome that combine investigation of protein structure, function, and expression. Proteomics also includes studies of protein folding, localization, interaction, and posttranslational modifications. Lately, the term systems biology was introduced to denote comprehensive studies aiming at delineating the complex interplay of molecular processes controlling whole body homeostasis. Integral part of this approach includes the study of dynamic networks of interacting molecules, the determination of changes in protein profiles in response to environmental changes, and the determination of the combined actions of diverse signaling networks that lead to a differential outcome for the organism. Obtaining and combining information about such networks is of particular importance considering the main processes occurring in the cells: proliferation, differentiation, survival, and apoptosis.

Differentiation of mammalian cells is a dynamic process that involves dramatic changes in the cellular machinery. The conversion from one cell type to another is triggered in response to external stimuli such as alterations in the cellular environment, communication between different cell types and overall physiological changes. The differentiation process can be divided into three stages—each stage being represented by a specific phenotype and gene expression profile. Under the influence of the surroundings a stem cell gives rise to precursor cells that in turn can become terminally differentiated to a defined cell type. It is of great importance to study the mechanisms of cell differentiation and commitment in order to understand and eventually modulate or influence critical points during the conversion. The use of hormones, particular compounds, or drug treatments to influence the conversion process is only possible if the critical time nodes and switches are well known. Proteomics and in particular mass spectrometry (MS)-based quantitative proteomics have proven successful in investigating changes that occur during differentiation. Here we focus on the latest advances in MS-based quantitative proteomics applied to the study of adipocyte development and function.

QUANTITATIVE MASS SPECTROMETRY-BASED PROTEOMICS—APPLICATIONS

Obtaining quantitative information about the changes that occur during the differentiation process is an essential step in understanding adipocyte biology. For a period of more than 30 years, especially after the establishment of model cell culture systems, a tremendous amount of research has been concentrated on the investigation of adipocytes and the possible links between obesity and obesity-associated complications such as type 2 diabetes, cardiovascular diseases, and atherosclerosis. Some of the widely utilized methods for analysis of protein profiles and changes in expression levels include metabolic ^{35}S-labeling, ^{125}I-labeling, measurement of enzyme activities, immunotitration and immunoblotting (2–5). In this way, by comparing changes in the expression of specific proteins a variety of adipose conversion markers have been identified, ranging from transcription factors, enzymes, membrane proteins to secreted molecules. Recently, advances in the technologies and applications in the field of MS-based quantitative proteomics have allowed large scale in-depth analysis of the adipocyte proteome including investigation of changes that occur during the differentiation process. In addition these advances permitted direct comparison of the levels of specific proteins in adipose tissue samples. The existing methods developed for quantitative proteomics using a mass spectrometer as a read out can be divided into two main groups based on the usage or not of a stable isotope for the quantitation of protein changes (6).

Quantitation Without Stable Isotopes

Quantitation without stable isotopes encompasses gel electrophoresis and chromatography-based approaches. In the first case, one- or two-dimensional gel electrophoresis is used as a mean to resolve proteins followed by visualization of the protein bands or spots using different types of stains or fluorescent dyes. Typically, protein samples originating from different stages are separated on a gel and then the bands or spots that show differential expression are excised, digested with protease and identified by MS (Fig. 1A). In the second case, the two protein samples are digested, the resulting mixtures of peptides separated by chromatography and the signal intensity from one peptide originating from one sample is compared to the signal intensity from the same peptide originating from another sample. In this approach the extracted ion chromatogram originates from the liquid chromatography profile of the sample during the mass spectrometric analysis.

The gel electrophoresis approach has been extensively applied to study a variety of changes that occur during adipocyte conversion. In general, samples are collected during differentiation and following separation and staining they are compared either visually or using sophisticated scanners and software to identify up- or downregulated proteins. Using cell culture models, such semiquantitative analyses have been performed on fibroblasts or preadipocytes and differentiated adipocytes. Comparison of crude cell lysates using mainly two-dimensional electrophoresis followed by identification by MALDI-MS has led to a substantial accumulation of data detailing changes in protein expression during adipocyte conversion (7,8). In one of these studies, changes during adipocyte differentiation in response to either a combined treatment with dexamethasone, isobutyl methyl xanthine and insulin or treatment with the Peroxisome proliferator-activated receptor gamma (PPARg) agonist (glitazone) were compared. Over 2000

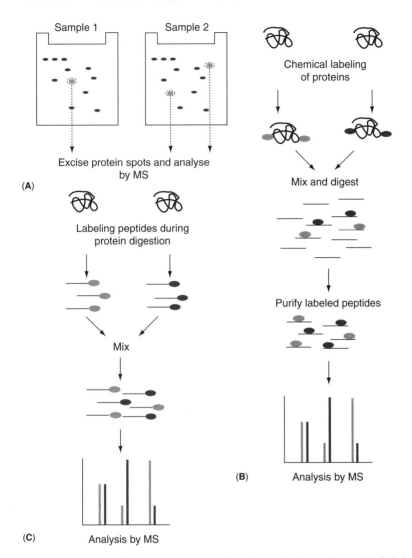

FIGURE 1 Methods for mass spectrometry-based quantitation analyses. (**A**) Gel electrophoresis–based approach. Protein mixtures are resolved by two dimensional polyacrylamide gel electrophoresis (2D-PAGE) and stained. Protein spot patterns are compared, and differentially appearing spots are excised, proteolytically digested, and identified by MS. (**B**) Chemical labeling strategy. Protein samples are labeled using isotopically labeled tags, mixed, and digested. Labeled peptides are desalted, affinity purified, and analyzed. (**C**) Enzymatic labeling. During proteolytic digest the enzyme catalyzes $^{16}O/^{18}O$ exchange, resulting in differential labeling of two samples. Peptide mixtures are combined and analyzed by MS. *Abbreviation*: MS, mass spectrometry.

alterations in the protein profiles during the differentiation process were found using two-dimensional electrophoresis and 300 proteins were identified by MS analysis (7). Using a similar approach, changes in protein expression during adipocyte differentiation and changes following starvation of mature adipocytes were identified (9). In addition, the effect of tumor necrosis factor alpha (TNFa) on the background of caloric restriction/starvation was investigated. Interestingly, treatment with TNFA resulted in pronounced protein changes toward the preadipocyte-like expression pattern. It was also demonstrated that the remodeling of the cytoskeleton that occurred during this dedifferentiation did not impair lipolysis, and furthermore, it was shown that the glycolysis/gluconeogenic pathways were differentially regulated during differentiation and starvation (9). Proteomic analysis of primary cultures of human adipose-derived stem cells resulted in the identification of over 40 upregulated and 13 downregulated proteins (10).

A major disadvantage of these types of investigations is the limitation imposed by the low dynamic range and inefficient recovery of high or loss of very low-molecular-weight proteins in two-dimensional gel electrophoresis resulting in the identification of mainly high abundant molecules such as cytoskeletal proteins and highly expressed metabolic enzymes (11). Reducing complexity of the sample, for example subcellular fractionation, can at least partially overcome these limitations.

In a study of changes in mitochondrial biogenesis during adipogenesis, a crude mitochondrial fraction was isolated using velocity gradient centrifugation and separated on one-dimensional gels. This approach resulted in identification of numerous mitochondrial proteins, which expression of which increased 20- to 30-fold during adipocyte differentiation. In addition, the effect of the antidiabetic drug rosiglitazone on the mitochondrial protein composition in mature adipocytes was investigated (12). In another proteomic study the changes in the protein profiles of factors secreted by preadipocytes or terminally differentiated adipocytes were studied by collecting media containing the secreted molecules, resolving the proteins on a one-dimensional gel, excising the bands that were distinct and analyzing them using liquid chromatography-MS. Fibronectin (FN1) and serpin peptidase inhibitor, clade F, member 1 (SERPINF1 or PEDF) were found to be specific for the undifferentiated state whereas 20 secreted proteins were upregulated in adipocytes. Using this strategy several proteins not previously known to be secreted by adipocytes were identified (13). A number of adipokines were also identified using the combination of two-dimensional electrophoresis and MS. In this study, brefeldin A or low temperatures were used to inhibit endoplasmic reticulum/Golgi dependent and independent secretory pathways, respectively. Based on the obtained protein profiles it was suggested that mature adipocytes possess an additional unique secretory pathway (14).

Another line of research includes identification of the proteins associated with cell organelles, surrounding lipid droplets or associated with particular membrane structures. In one such study it was revealed how hormonal stimulation of lipolysis altered the composition of the proteins associated with the lipid droplets (15). This study was complemented by an investigation providing the first map of the mouse adipose lipolytic proteome, which was shown to comprise all known intracellular lipases (16). Major peripheral proteins associated with the cytosolic surface of the caveolae in human adipocytes have been revealed by vectorial analyses of the protein domains that were exposed to the opposite membrane sides of proteins by proteolysis and MS (17). The composition and changes in the complement of mitochondrial proteins have been investigated in adipose tissue during the development of obesity, in the obese state, and after treatment with the antidiabetic drug rosiglitazone. The results obtained in this study interestingly suggested that thiazolidinediones besides the well-characterized PPARg-dependent insulin-sensitizing effects also work via changes in the composition of mitochondrial proteins (18).

The gel electrophoresis-based approach for identification and quantitation has been applied to create tissue-specific expression profiles as well. The proteome of the white adipose tissue from epididymal fat pads was mapped resulting in the identification of 140 protein spots (19). The importance of insulin signaling was examined in a study that compared the proteome of adipocytes in mice with a fat-specific knockout of the insulin receptor mice with wild-type mice. The adipocytes were separated according to size followed by fractionation into cytosolic and membrane subfractions. The proteins were resolved by gel electrophoresis and identified by MS. This approach revealed 27 changes in protein expression influencing key steps in lipid and energy metabolism depending on the presence or absence of the insulin receptor. Intriguingly, approximately half of the changes were not detectable at the mRNA level emphasizing the importance of the acquisition of proteomic data (20).

The effect of high-fat diet has been investigated by comparison of the expression of proteins in muscle, liver, and white and brown adipose tissues from mice. Fifty differentially expressed proteins were found comparing lean and obese mice. Strikingly, the majority of these differences were detected in the brown adipose tissue reflecting the important role of this tissue in diet-induced thermogenesis (21).

In summary, the combination of gel electrophoresis with MS has yielded a substantial amount of information on the proteome of adipocytes, but has its limitations in the lack of producing accurate quantitative data. The chromatography-based approach for protein quantitation relies on the fact that the peak area obtained from liquid chromatography-MS correlates with the concentration of the protein/peptide (6,22). Hence, it is possible to obtain semiquantitative data even in complex mixtures such as human sera (23). The extraction ion chromatogram can be easily applied to study adipose conversion and to follow changes during the differentiation process at a subcellular level. A major advantage of the extraction ion chromatogram-based quantitation is that it is label free thus it can be applied to any sample. A disadvantage is that it is only partially quantitative and requires highly reliable and reproducible analysis of the samples.

Quantitation with Stable Isotopes

In the recent years a tremendous amount of research and efforts have been concentrated on the development of technologies that result in accurate and confident quantitation of proteins in complex protein mixtures containing hundreds or even thousands of proteins. Such methods are MS-based and generally employ the use of stable isotopes like ^{2}H, ^{13}C, ^{18}O, and ^{15}N. Based on the method of incorporation of the isotopes, the quantitation approaches can be divided into two major groups: chemical and metabolic ones.

Chemical and Enzyme Catalyzed Labeling Strategies: ICAT, iTRAQ, Hys-tag, and $^{16/18}$O-Labeling

The prototype and mostly utilized of the chemical modification-based methodologies for protein quantitation is the isotope-coded affinity tag—ICAT (24). It depends on the use of two isotopically labeled tags that contain eight ^{1}H or ^{2}H atoms—light and heavy tag, respectively. When comparing two different samples, one sample is reacted with the light tag, one with the heavy tag. The tags bind specifically to cysteine residues. The peptides originating from proteolytic digest of either of the samples can easily be distinguished based on the mass difference of the tags resulting in a characteristic mass shift of the modified peptides. The presence of a biotin group in the light and heavy tags allows selective enrichment of the labeled peptides using avidin affinity chromatography, thus, reducing greatly the complexity of the mixture (Fig. 1B).

ICAT has been applied to a variety of cell culture and tissue samples and has proven to be a reliable and relatively easy applicable method to perform quantitative proteomics. The protocol has been used to create differential expression profiles of microsomal proteins from native and in vitro-differentiated human myeloid leukemia cells, to investigate secreted proteins during osteoclast differentiation, to follow dynamic changes of transcription factors during erythroid differentiation as well as to compare protein changes in livers of mice treated for different periods of time with three PPAR agonists (25–28). Disadvantages of ICAT are the targeting of only cysteine-containing peptides, the altered retention times of the light compared to the heavy form during chromatographic separation and the insufficient elution of the peptides from the beads. To overcome some of these problems a cleavable ^{12}C and ^{13}C-based reagent, cICAT was developed. These tags exhibit improved coelution profiles during liquid chromatography separation and increased recovery after enrichment of the labeled peptides (29).

Additional reagents that target cysteine residues have been developed including the HysTag peptide. The HysTag contains an affinity ligand (His(6)-tag) enabling robust purification and flexibility. It was successfully used for quantitative proteomic analyses of proteins from enriched plasma membrane preparations from mouse fore- and hindbrain (30). This type of studies may prove to be of value for investigation of brain tissue samples originating form normal, obese, and diabetic mouse models, studies justified by connection between increased body mass and brain physiology (31). Quantitative analysis has also been performed using an isobaric tag for relative and absolute quantitation (iTRAQ). This reagent attaches to lysine residues and give rise to the generation of reporter ions in the mass spectrometer that are used for quantitation (32). A major disadvantage is that this approach requires access to an advanced mass spectrometer since obtaining quantitative information is entirely dependent on the ability of the instrument to detect the reporter group in the low mass region. To the best of our knowledge the chemical labeling strategies mentioned above have not so far been applied directly to investigate adipocyte biology, but they clearly have the potential to be utilized in future comparative studies on both cell lines and tissue samples and to track changes in protein expression levels occurring as a result of the differentiation process per se or as a result of dietary or other physiological changes.

A different quantitative proteomic method applying stable isotopes has been used to study secretory proteins from rat adipose cells (33). In this strategy two samples (conditions) are compared and the isotopic label is introduced during the proteolytic digestion of the samples (Fig. 1C). One sample is digested in $H_2^{16}O$ and the other in $H_2^{18}O$, resulting in incorporation of one or two ^{18}O atoms into the carboxylic groups created by the proteolytic cleavage of the proteins. The samples are then combined and analyzed by MS. This labeling method was applied to identify and quantify changes in the secretion profiles of rat adipocytes treated or not with insulin. It resulted in the identification of a total of 84 secreted factors and the quantitation of the changes that occurred in response to insulin (33).

In summary, the chemical- and enzyme-catalyzed labeling strategies can be applied to a variety of different samples, tissues, and protein mixtures enabling the generation of quantitative protein expression data that provide better understanding of the biological systems and function. These methods depend on the efficient chemistry, and a major disadvantage of these is that the label is introduced in late stages of the work flow. Sample preparation usually includes isolation, fractionation, and protein purification prior to the labeling step, thus, increasing the probability for introduction of errors in the quantitative analysis. This can be minimized by carefully reproducing the experimental conditions and applying statistical methods for evaluation of the data.

Metabolic Labeling Strategies: ^{15}N-Labeling and Stable Isotope Labeling by Amino Acids in Cell Culture (SILAC)

The metabolic labeling strategies rely on the introduction of a stable isotope into the proteins while they are being de novo synthesized in the cell. In contrast to the standard radioactivity-based pulse-chase assays, the stable isotope is fully incorporated into the whole proteome. There are two means of introducing the stable isotope—using either media containing ^{15}N-labeled ammonium sulfate or media supplemented with a stable isotope-labeled amino acid. ^{15}N labeling strategies have been used for quantitative analysis of yeast phosphopeptides and a mouse melanoma cell line (34,35). Additionally, several organisms have been metabolically labeled using ^{15}N as a label such as bacteria (*E. coli* and Deinococcus), *C. elegans*, *D. melanogaster*, and rat (34,36,37).

SILAC is an increasingly popular method for quantitative MS-based proteomics (38,39). The principles of SILAC are fairly simple and this method can be applied to study various of biological processes. SILAC uses the incorporation of a stable isotope-labeled amino acid into the proteins in such way that the entire proteome of a given cellular population becomes encoded either with the light or heavier version of the same amino acid (Fig. 2). This is achieved by growing and expanding the cells in labeling media for a number of population doublings. Generally, after five population doublings the entire proteome of the cells is labeled close to 100%. After complete labeling is accomplished the cells are pooled together or lyzed and then the protein extracts are combined in a 1:1 ratio according to their protein concentration. The protein mixture is then purified or fractionated, optionally separated on a one-dimensional gel, proteolytically digested, and analyzed using MS. Using the SILAC protocol, the cells can be induced to differentiate after labeling or be treated with different growth factors, hormones, or inhibitors. It is also a very powerful approach for the investigation of posttranslational modifications such as methylation, phosphorylation, ubiquitnation, sumoylation, and nitrosylation.

The SILAC methodology has been proven to be successful in studying signal transduction cascades initiated by growth factors. A long-standing problem when performing classical interaction studies is the question of how to distinguish true interaction partners from the background binding proteins. This issue has been addressed by applying SILAC to investigate functional protein-protein interactions in epidermal growth factor (EGF) signaling. Using the SH2 domain of the protein Grb2 228 (an adapter protein in the Ras pathway) was identified, of which 28 were found to be selectively enriched upon EGF stimulation (40). In a similar way SILAC can be applied not only to study protein-protein and specific-domain protein interactions but also defined peptide-motive interactions (41). The protein interaction networks are not simple static systems but highly dynamic and obtaining information about the changes that occur not only in space but also in time is of critical importance for the understanding of any biological process that takes place in the cell. Recently, temporal analysis of signaling events induced by EGF led to the generation of dynamic

Medium with "light"   Medium with "heavy"
amino acid   amino acid

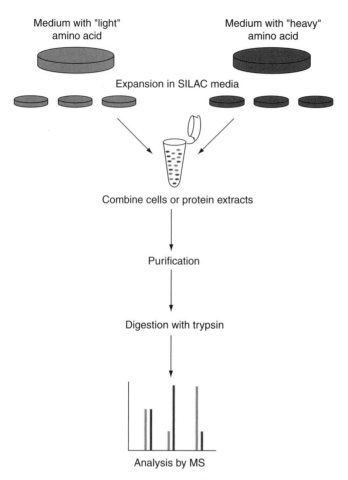

Expansion in SILAC media

Combine cells or protein extracts

Purification

Digestion with trypsin

Analysis by MS

FIGURE 2 Schematic representation of the SILAC method. Cells are grown and expanded in SILAC medium containing "light" or "heavy" amino acid. After complete incorporation of the respective amino acid in the proteome, cells or protein extracts are combined and subjected to protein purification procedures. Proteins are proteolytically digested and analyzed by liquid chromatography tandem mass spectrometry. *Abbreviations*: MS, mass spectrometry; SILAC, stable isotope labeling by amino acids in cell culture.

phosphorylation profiles in the early stage after growth factor stimulation (42,43). Additionally, quantitative analysis of the human nucleoli proteome revealed the dynamics of the nucleolar proteins and characterized the protein flux through the cellular organelles over time, providing a global synopsis of the organelle changes in response to different metabolic states (44). SILAC is also used to compare entire signaling networks that can lead to the discovery of control points in the differentiation process. The differentiation of the mesenchymal stem cells into osteoblasts was found to be stimulated by EGF but not by platelet-derived growth factor (PDGF). Using SILAC the EGF and PDGF-induced tyrosine phosphoproteomes were compared resulting in determination of the common and differentially utilized signaling molecules. The phosphatidylinositol 3-kinase (PI3K) pathway was exclusively activated by PDGF and chemical inhibition of it led to enhanced differentiation in the presence of PDGF (45). Application of similar strategies will enable the in-depth investigation of critical nodes and complexes involved in insulin signaling. Insulin binds to the insulin receptor and initiates series of phosphotyrosine-dependent signaling events. The adipocyte function and metabolism is dependent on an efficient response to insulin and any malfunction in the signaling cascade can have serious consequences for the whole organism. In addition, delineating insulin signaling and the changes that occur in the development of insulin resistance are key issues in understanding the pathology of type 2 diabetes. The SILAC protocol has already been applied to study tyrosine kinase substrates in the insulin signaling pathway in adipocytes. Labeling the adipocytes either with a light or heavy form of tyrosine enabled the identification of nine tyrosine phosphorylated effectors after treatment with insulin (46). In another study proteins that specifically interact with the insulin-regulated glucose transporter (GLUT4 or SLC2A4) in an insulin-dependent manner were identified in myotubes. Using GLUT4 as bait, 36 proteins were found to change their interaction with the transporter in response to insulin, among these several cytoskeleton-related proteins. In particular, alpha-actinin-4 was shown to associate with GLUT4 in order to facilitate its routing to the plasma membrane (47). Recently, it was demonstrated that SILAC can be applied to study tissue samples as well. Using cell culture–derived isotope tags as an internal standard more than 1000 proteins from mouse whole brain samples and Neuro2A cells were identified and quantified (48). The SILAC method represents a reliable and easily applicable method for quantitative protein analysis and can be used to elucidate a variety of pathways, metabolic changes, and treatment conditions. A disadvantage is the requirement for the cells to be expanded in labeling media for a number of population doublings, and thus SILAC can not be used in a straightforward fashion to study changes in tissue samples.

CONCLUSION

Systematic and comprehensive analyses of adipocyte development and function can be achieved only when combining genomic, proteomic, and metabolomic analysis. The advances of MS-based quantitative proteomics and the large variety of existing methods will lead to a rapid accumulation of comprehensive data set representing the adipocyte proteome. In addition, the application of different labeling strategies to study adipocyte and adipose tissue will enable targeted quantitative and in-depth investigation of signaling pathways and crosstalk between cascades, generation of transcriptome and secretome profiles, changes in the composition of mitochondria and other organelles in response to differential treatment, utilization of nutrients and drugs. The accumulation of such quantitative data will ultimately lead to better understanding of the process of adipose conversion and discover possible novel drug targets that can be used for treatment of diseases associated with increased adipose mass.

ACKNOWLEDGMENT

We would like to thank Dr. Blagoev for critically reading the manuscript. Work in the authors' laboratory has been supported by The Danish Biotechnology Program, The Danish Natural Science Research Council, The Danish National Research Foundation and the European Community (contract QLK1-CT-2001-00183).

REFERENCES

1. Rual JF, Venkatesan K, Hao T, et al. Towards a proteome-scale map of the human protein–protein interaction network. Nature 2005; 437:1173–8.
2. Mackall JC, Student AK, Polakis SE, et al. Induction of lipogenesis during differentiation in a "preadipocyte" cell line. J Biol Chem 1976; 251:6462–4.
3. Spiegelman BM, Green H. Control of specific protein biosynthesis during the adipose conversion of 3T3 cells. J Biol Chem 1980; 255:8811–8.
4. Rubin CS, Hirsch A, Fung C, et al. Development of hormone receptors and hormonal responsiveness in vitro. Insulin receptors and insulin sensitivity in the preadipocyte and adipocyte forms of 3T3-L1 cells. J Biol Chem 1978; 253:7570–8.
5. Sidhu RS. Two-dimensional electrophoretic analyses of proteins synthesized during differentiation of 3T3-L1 preadipocytes. J Biol Chem 1979; 254:11111–8.
6. Ong SE, Mann M. Mass spectrometry-based proteomics turns quantitative. Nat Chem Biol 2005; 1:252–62.
7. Welsh GI, Griffiths MR, Webster KJ, et al. Proteome analysis of adipogenesis. Proteomics 2004; 4:1042–51.
8. Choi KL, Wang Y, Tse CA, et al. Proteomic analysis of adipocyte differentiation: Evidence that alpha2 macroglobulin is involved in the adipose conversion of 3T3 L1 preadipocytes. Proteomics 2004; 4:1840–8.
9. Renes J, Bouwman F, Noben JP, et al. Protein profiling of 3T3-L1 adipocyte differentiation and (tumor necrosis factor alpha-mediated) starvation. Cell Mol Life Sci 2005; 62:492–503.
10. DeLany JP, Floyd ZE, Zvonic S, et al. Proteomic analysis of primary cultures of human adipose-derived stem cells: modulation by adipogenesis. Mol Cell Proteomics 2005; 4:731–40.
11. Gygi SP, Corthals GL, Zhang Y, et al. Evaluation of two-dimensional gel electrophoresis-based proteome analysis technology. Proc Natl Acad Sci USA 2000; 97:9390–5.
12. Wilson-Fritch L, Burkart A, Bell G, et al. Mitochondrial biogenesis and remodeling during adipogenesis and in response to the insulin sensitizer rosiglitazone. Mol Cell Biol 2003; 23:1085–94.
13. Kratchmarova I, Kalume DE, Blagoev B, et al. A proteomic approach for identification of secreted proteins during the differentiation of 3T3-L1 preadipocytes to adipocytes. Mol Cell Proteomics 2002; 1:213–22.
14. Wang P, Mariman E, Keijer J, et al. Profiling of the secreted proteins during 3T3-L1 adipocyte differentiation leads to the identification of novel adipokines. Cell Mol Life Sci 2004; 61:2405–17.
15. Brasaemle DL, Dolios G, Shapiro L, et al. Proteomic analysis of proteins associated with lipid droplets of basal and lipolytically stimulated 3T3-L1 adipocytes. J Biol Chem 2004; 279:46835–42.
16. Birner-Gruenberger R, Susani-Etzerodt H, Waldhuber M, et al. The lipolytic proteome of mouse adipose tissue. Mol Cell Proteomics 2005; 4:1710–7.
17. Aboulaich N, Vainonen JP, Stralfors P, et al. Vectorial proteomics reveal targeting, phosphorylation and specific fragmentation of polymerase I and transcript release factor (PTRF) at the surface of caveolae in human adipocytes. Biochem J 2004; 383(Pt 2):237–48.
18. Wilson-Fritch L, Nicoloro S, Chouinard M, et al. Mitochondrial remodeling in adipose tissue associated with obesity and treatment with rosiglitazone. J Clin Invest 2004; 114:1281–9.
19. Lanne B, Potthast F, Hoglund A, et al. Thiourea enhances mapping of the proteome from murine white adipose tissue. Proteomics 2001; 1:819–28.
20. Bluher M, Wilson-Fritch L, Leszyk J, et al. Role of insulin action and cell size on protein expression patterns in adipocytes. J Biol Chem 2004; 279:31902–9.
21. Schmid GM, Converset V, Walter N, et al. Effect of high-fat diet on the expression of proteins in muscle, adipose tissues, and liver of C57BL/6 mice. Proteomics 2004; 4:2270–82.
22. Andersen JS, Wilkinson CJ, Mayor T, et al. Proteomic characterization of the human centrosome by protein correlation profiling. Nature 2003; 426:570–4.

23. Chelius D, Bondarenko PV. Quantitative profiling of proteins in complex mixtures using liquid chromatography and mass spectrometry. J Proteome Res 2002; 1:317–23.
24. Gygi SP, Rist B, Gerber SA, et al. Quantitative analysis of complex protein mixtures using isotope-coded affinity tags. Nat Biotechnol 1999; 17:994–9.
25. Han DK, Eng J, Zhou H, et al. Quantitative profiling of differentiation-induced microsomal proteins using isotope-coded affinity tags and mass spectrometry. Nat Biotechnol 2001; 19:946–51.
26. Kubota K, Wakabayashi K, Matsuoka T. Proteome analysis of secreted proteins during osteoclast differentiation using two different methods: two-dimensional electrophoresis and isotope-coded affinity tags analysis with two-dimensional chromatography. Proteomics 2003; 3:616–26.
27. Brand M, Ranish JA, Kummer NT, et al. Dynamic changes in transcription factor complexes during erythroid differentiation revealed by quantitative proteomics. Nat Struct Mol Biol 2004; 11:73–80.
28. Tian Q, Stepaniants SB, Mao M, et al. Integrated genomic and proteomic analyses of gene expression in mammalian cells. Mol Cell Proteomics 2004; 3:960–9.
29. Yi EC, Li XJ, Cooke K, et al. Increased quantitative proteome coverage with (13)C/(12)C-based, acid-cleavable isotope-coded affinity tag reagent and modified data acquisition scheme. Proteomics 2005; 5:380–7.
30. Olsen JV, Andersen JR, Nielsen PA, et al. HysTag—a novel proteomic quantification tool applied to differential display analysis of membrane proteins from distinct areas of mouse brain. Mol Cell Proteomics 2004; 3:82–92.
31. Prodi E, Obici S. The brain as a molecular target for diabetic therapy. Endocrinology 2006; 2664–9.
32. Ross PL, Huang YN, Marchese JN, et al. Multiplexed protein quantitation in *Saccharomyces cerevisiae* using amine-reactive isobaric tagging reagents. Mol Cell Proteomics 2004; 3:1154–69.
33. Chen X, Cushman SW, Pannell LK, et al. Quantitative proteomic analysis of the secretory proteins from rat adipose cells using a 2D liquid chromatography-MS/MS approach. J Proteome Res 2005; 4:570–7.
34. Conrads TP, Alving K, Veenstra TD, et al. Quantitative analysis of bacterial and mammalian proteomes using a combination of cysteine affinity tags and ^{15}N-metabolic labeling. Anal Chem 2001; 73:2132–9.
35. Oda Y, Huang K, Cross FR, et al. Accurate quantitation of protein expression and site-specific phosphorylation. Proc Natl Acad Sci USA 1999; 96:6591–6.
36. Krijgsveld J, Ketting RF, Mahmoudi T, et al. Metabolic labeling of *C. elegans* and *D. melanogaster* for quantitative proteomics. Nat Biotechnol 2003; 21:927–31.
37. Wu CC, MacCoss MJ, Howell KE, et al. Metabolic labeling of mammalian organisms with stable isotopes for quantitative proteomic analysis. Anal Chem 2004; 76:4951–9.
38. Ong SE, Blagoev B, Kratchmarova I, et al. Stable isotope labeling by amino acids in cell culture, SILAC, as a simple and accurate approach to expression proteomics. Mol Cell Proteomics 2002; 1:376–86.
39. Ong SE, Kratchmarova I, Mann M. Properties of ^{13}C-substituted arginine in stable isotope labeling by amino acids in cell culture (SILAC). J Proteome Res 2003; 2:173–81.
40. Blagoev B, Kratchmarova I, Ong SE, et al. A proteomics strategy to elucidate functional protein–protein interactions applied to EGF signaling. Nat Biotechnol 2003; 21:315–8.
41. Schulze WX, Mann M. A novel proteomic screen for peptide–protein interactions. J Biol Chem 2004; 279:10756–64.
42. Blagoev B, Ong SE, Kratchmarova I, et al. Temporal analysis of phosphotyrosine-dependent signaling networks by quantitative proteomics. Nat Biotechnol 2004; 22:1139–45.
43. Olsen JV, Blagoev B, Gnad F, et al. Global, in vivo, and site-specific phosphorylation dynamics in signaling networks. Cell 2006; 127:635–48.
44. Andersen JS, Lam YW, Leung AK, et al. Nucleolar proteome dynamics. Nature 2005; 433:77–83.
45. Kratchmarova I, Blagoev B, Haack-Sorensen M, et al. Mechanism of divergent growth factor effects in mesenchymal stem cell differentiation. Science 2005; 308:1472–7.

46. Ibarrola N, Molina H, Iwahori A, et al. A novel proteomic approach for specific identification of tyrosine kinase substrates using [^{13}C]tyrosine. J Biol Chem 2004; 279:15805–13.
47. Foster LJ, Rudich A, Talior I, et al. Insulin-dependent interactions of proteins with GLUT4 revealed through stable isotope labeling by amino acids in cell culture (SILAC). J Proteome Res 2006; 5:64–75.
48. Ishihama Y, Sato T, Tabata T, et al. Quantitative mouse brain proteomics using culture-derived isotope tags as internal standards. Nat Biotechnol 2005; 23:617–21.

Section 11: Conclusion

11.1 Exciting Advances and New Opportunities

Claude Bouchard and Tuomo Rankinen

Human Genomics Laboratory, Pennington Biomedical Research Center, Baton Rouge, Louisiana, U.S.A.

Genetic epidemiology has been helpful in defining the magnitude of the familial risk and the genetic contribution to obesity in a population perspective. The level of heritability has been considered in a large number of twin, adoption and family studies, and the estimates vary considerably. However, serious doubts have been raised in many quarters concerning not only high heritability values for obesity phenotypes but even moderate levels, for instance in the range of 30% to 60%, in light of the recent dramatic increase in the prevalence of excess weight around the world. It should be by now clear that the debate has shifted from the population estimates of the genetic risks to the actual genes and mutations predisposing or causing obesity and related diseases. This does not mean that research on population genetic issues pertaining to obesity should not be encouraged. We still have a lot more to learn in these areas. But the field needs to move on to more sophisticated designs and to research paradigms that have the statistical power to address fundamental population genetic questions.

One example is that of assortative mating studies. A few papers have recently revealed that such studies could provide new insights not only into the genetics of obesity but also on the dynamics of the ongoing prevalence increase in a given population (1–3). In a Canadian study, it was observed that spousal correlations were stronger in parents of lean offspring as well as in parents of obese children but lower in parents of children with average adiposity (3). More recently in a study based on three cohorts from Sweden, it was found that spouse concordance for obesity was associated with a 20-fold higher obesity risk in biological offspring compared to children of parents who were not concordant for obesity (2). These observations suggest that much remains to be learned by mining parents and offspring databases.

HYPOTHESES ABOUT THE CAUSES

The rapid increase in prevalence and the fact that the obese are becoming more severely obese need to be taken into account in any attempt to understand the causes of what has become arguably the most pressing public health problem of the 21st century. However, there are few certainties concerning the true causes of the phenomenon. An important fact to keep in mind when approaching the study of the causes of the obesity epidemic is that it is driven by pervasive positive energy balance. This appears to be simple and straightforward. But it is not. Numerous factors can influence how much energy is consumed and how much is expended over long periods of time. In addition, a number of physiological and metabolic properties affect energy processing, storage and mobilization in a variety of states.

The numerous causes of the epidemic can be grouped under four major headings: physical and built environment, social environment, behavior and biology.

These four categories of potential affectors encompass agents that participate in the modulation of energy balance in any given individual (Fig. 1).

The list of attributes of the physical and built environment contributing to the obesity epidemic includes: suburban sprawl, absence of sidewalks, reliance on the automobile, public and corporate building design, environmental pollutants, and undoubtedly others. Many components of the social milieu can also be seen as potential effectors of body weight status: pressure to consume, recreational eating, powerful and constant advertising, pressure to be sedentary, etc. They are just as complex as the factors of the physical environment and interact in many intricate ways with each other.

The importance of behavior favoring positive energy balance is supported by a large number of studies. These behaviors include excess caloric intake from the consumption of high caloric density foods, high fat diets, high sugar intake, low calcium intake, low protein intake, etc. However, there is no convincing evidence that diets rich or poor in any of the macronutrients have a significant effect on body weight if they are compared to one another at isocaloric levels. One other lifestyle component that has received much attention is the time spent in a sedentary state. There is some evidence that the greater the time spent watching TV, playing video games, working at the computer, etc, the higher the risk level for gaining weight and becoming obese. People who are very active are generally not overweight and seldom obese. It is important to recognize that some of the inconsistencies observed among behavioral studies are not due to the intrinsic properties of the diet or physical activity regimen being tested. They are rather simply the result of the poor compliance of participants to the prescribed experimental interventions.

Finally, biology needs to be taken into account when defining the causes of obesity. A large number of factors have been implicated in animal and human studies. Among the most frequently, although not always consistently, reported

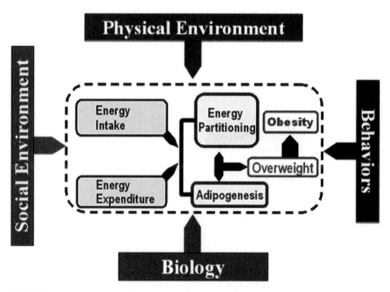

FIGURE 1 A network of factors that modulate the various components of the energy balance equation.

biological predictors of weight gain or obesity, one finds a low resting metabolic rate, a low thermic effect of food, a low lipid oxidation rate, high levels of adipose tissue lipoprotein lipase activity and low levels of lipid mobilization rates, abnormal biology of leptin and other hormones, poor regulation of appetite and satiety, low skeletal muscle oxidative potential, etc. Moreover, many genetic studies have concluded that there is in our genome a latent predisposition to be in or to achieve positive energy balance for long periods of time.

IS THERE A BIOLOGICAL PREDISPOSITION?

There is a synergistic relationship between genes and environment: in the presence of a genetic predisposition to obesity, the severity of the disease is largely determined by lifestyle and environmental conditions. When individuals living in a "restrictive" environment evolve towards an "obesogenic" environment, such as that found in industrialized countries, most are likely to gain weight. However, those with a high genetic predisposition for obesity will gain the most weight, whereas those resistant to obesity will gain little, if any, weight. We reviewed the evidence for such a gene-environment interaction effect with a focus on experimental studies based on pairs of identical twins in a previous chapter of this book (see Chapters 2.3 and 2.4). Another example of this gene-environment interaction effect can be found in a population apparently predisposed to obesity and type 2 diabetes, such as the Pima Indians. Pima Indians living in the restrictive environment of the remote Mexican Sierra Madre mountains have a lower prevalence of obesity and type 2 diabetes mellitus than those living in the obesogenic environment of Arizona, in the Southwestern United States (4).

These suggestive observations on Pima Indians are reinforced by the results of three experimental studies conducted with pairs of identical twins, one positive (5) and two negative (6,7) energy balance with highly standardized protocols. These experiments confirm that the magnitude of a subject's response to changes in lifestyle or environmental conditions (from rather restrictive to more obesogenic or vice versa) depends on a predisposition thought to be largely inherited.

The model suggested by these empirical observations is depicted in Figure 2. The "obesogenic environment" favors obesogenic behavior. The net effect of an obesogenic behavior profile is determined by the biological terrain. In some cases,

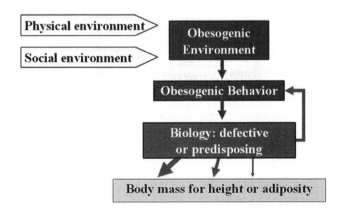

FIGURE 2 Relationships between an obesogenic environment favoring obesogenic behavior.

the biology is truly defective and obesity is then almost inevitable. In most cases, however, one's biology translates into a highly heterogeneous biological predisposition to obesity. A biological susceptibility to obesity can also manifest itself by favoring the adoption of obesogenic behavior.

WHERE DOES THE BIOLOGICAL PREDISPOSITION RESIDE?

It is commonly accepted that evolutionary circumstances have led to the progressive selection of biological traits favoring the conservation of energy, thus allowing survival through the reproductive ages under conditions of limited food availability or even prolonged periods of food deprivation. All populations of the world have experienced, at one time or another, periods of food shortages that may have had consequences on the demographics of these populations. It is not unrealistic to speculate that those who were metabolically more energy efficient may have been selected for under these circumstances.

Five Genetic Hypotheses

It is quite common to invoke the paper published in 1962 by James V. Neel (8) as the key reference for the "thrifty genotype" hypothesis whose overall purpose was to provide an explanation for the current increase in the prevalence of excess weight in human populations. Unfortunately, the reliance on this 1962 paper is a case of bad citation. What Neel was describing in 1962 under the label of a thrifty genotype was essentially a suggestion that a basic defect in diabetes mellitus could be a quick insulin response to food, which would have served to minimize the renal loss of glucose in a feast or famine environment. For decades, obesity researchers and others alike have wrongly cited this paper in support of an energy balance–related thrifty genotype. It was only in more recent times, i.e., more than 35 years later, that Neel revisited the concept and broadened it to include obesity (9–11).

For a long time, scientists have entertained the view that the ability to increase metabolic rate in response to dietary and other challenges was potentially an important mechanism to prevent weight gain. This has proven to be exceedingly difficult to demonstrate in humans. Adaptive thermogenesis can theoretically occur by two mechanisms: by increasing ATP utilization or by uncoupling of fuel oxidation from ATP generation or work (12). ATP utilization is increased by physical activity, by diet-induced thermogenesis, by operation of so-called futile cycles, or by growth. On the other hand, uncoupling fuel oxidation from the production of ATP occurs in all cells to some extent but particularly in brown adipose tissue where it is regulated. Pathways that may contribute to adaptive thermogenesis typically require an activation of the sympathetic nervous system and include leptin, melanocortin, UCPs pathways, and adrenergic receptor mediated pathways. However, even though the hypothesis is highly attractive, these thermogenic mechanisms have a limited capacity to buffer large and sustained energy imbalance. Indeed, the current obesity epidemic would seem to be a striking demonstration of the fact that adaptive thermogenic capacity in humans is limited and that the contribution of a thrifty genotype, if any, is quite small.

Even though a thrifty genotype hypothesis deserves to be further investigated, it is by no means the only potential explanation for the apparent genetic vulnerability that modern homo sapiens seems to exhibit in an obesogenic environment. We believe that at least four other hypotheses should be examined in future genetic studies (Fig. 3). For instance, while we have strong mechanisms to defend body weight against starvation, it appears that a large number of people are poor regulators of energy intake. Family and twin studies have revealed that there is a significant heritability component to energy and nutrient intake. The preponderance of the evidence suggests that carriers of genetic traits favoring hyperphagia are quite prevalent (hyperphagic genotype). For instance, at normal leptin levels for fat mass, energy intake is in balance with energy expenditure while at low leptin levels for fat mass, energy intake is poorly regulated and tends to exceed energy expenditure (13).

One re-interpretation of the thrifty genotype hypothesis can also be proposed. It requires a distinction between the energy expenditure of physical activity versus the energy expenditure associated with an efficient or thrifty metabolism. Indeed, one way to conserve energy under caloric deprivation is to reduce the energy expenditure for physical activity to a minimum. Individual differences were undoubtedly present in this regard throughout evolution. Those who were most able to keep the wastage of energy for activity to a minimum were likely to derive survival and reproductive advantages. The conservation of energy through sedentary time may have been an important survival element in a harsh environment. However, it has become a liability in our obesogenic environment (sedentary genotype). In support of this hypothesis, there are family and twin studies that have identified a significant component to the level of physical activity. There are also family lines for a couch potato lifestyle. Candidate gene studies have identified a few markers of activity level or sedentarism. A recent genomic scan has uncovered three quantitative trait loci (QTLs) for inactivity and several more for differences in physical activity level (see Chapter 8.2) (14).

A fourth hypothesis has to do with human variation in rates of substrates oxidation. There is robust evidence to the effect that high rates of lipid oxidation in the normal weight are desirable and could protect against excessive weight gain. For instance, a high respiratory exchange ratio or respiratory quotient indicative of a higher relative rate of carbohydrate oxidation, or alternatively a low lipid oxidation rate (low lipid oxidation genotype), has been associated with weight gain over time in Pima Indians (15), in men of the Baltimore Longitudinal Study on Aging (13), and in a group of nonobese women gaining more than 3 kg over 3 years (16). However, these findings could not be replicated in the Quebec Family Study over a 5.5-year follow-up period (12).

The fifth hypothesis can be labeled the "adipogenesis genotype." The most severe forms of obesity appear to be characterized by large fat cells and a higher than normal number of adipose cells. The ability to maximize fat storage during periods of caloric abundance may have served a useful purpose during much of

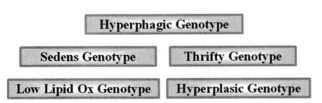

FIGURE 3 Five genetic hypotheses for the latent predisposition to obesity.

our evolutionary history but may be associated with greater amounts of weight gain in our current obesogenic environment.

Single Genes Causing Obesity

The identification of genes and mutations causing obesity in a small number of cases can illuminate the biology of candidate pathways involved in the pathophysiology of the more common forms of obesity. At present, only a few hundred human obesity cases caused by single-gene mutations have been described. However, the number of such cases is likely to increase substantially as we begin to understand which genes to target and where to look in the human genome. Eleven genes have been implicated thus far in these single-gene cases: *CRHR1, CRHR2, GPR24, LEP, LEPR, MC3R, MC4R, NTRK2, POMC, PSCK1,* and *SIM1* (see http://www.gene.ucl.ac.uk/cgi-bin/nomenclature/searchgenes.pl for full names). Until now, genetic screening for obesity has concentrated on the identification of mutations in specific genes in persons who were severely obese, with the greatest success rates being recorded in cases with an early age of onset. Additionally, almost 50 loci known to be related to Mendelian syndromes exhibiting human obesity as one of the clinical manifestations have been mapped to a specific region, and the causal genes or strong candidates have been identified for most of them. Overall, these single-gene disruptions already account for about 5% of the obesity cases, and their importance is likely to grow with better screening programs. However, these single gene cases cannot account for the latent genetic predisposition that is revealed only upon exposure to an obesogenic environment. Interestingly none of these genes appear to have their primary deleterious effects through metabolic rate or energy expenditure.

Genes and More Common Forms of Obesity

In most cases, obesity is a complex multifactorial phenotype; inter-individual variation in such phenotypes is thought to result from the action of multiple genes and environmental factors. These genes tend to have small effects but the variant allele(s) is typically quite common in the population. Figure 4 depicts the contrast between the genes with very large effects and those of interest in this section. A recent review of the literature performed in the context of the latest update of the Human Obesity Gene Map (17) revealed that positive associations with obesity phenotypes have been reported with more than 127 candidate genes. Among these genes, 22 are supported by at least five positive studies: *ACE, ADIPOQ, ADRB2, ADRB3, DRD2, GNB3, HTR2C, IL6, INS, LDLR, LEP, LEPR, LIPE, MC4R, NR3C1, PPARG, RETN, TNFA, UCP1, UCP2, UCP3, VDR.* Overall, the results of these association studies are quite heterogeneous and at times inconsistent. Even for these 22 genes, there are a large number of negative studies. Nonetheless, several of these genes may turn out to be small but significant predictors of the obesity risk.

A careful analysis of the nature of these 22 candidate genes reveals that most of them relate to three of the five genotypes theorized in the previous section. Table 1 provides the distribution of these 22 candidate genes among five genetic hypotheses. The majority of these genes relate to the thrifty, hyperphagic, and low-lipid-oxidation-rate genotypes. At this time, few of these genes relate to the sedentary and adipose tissue hyperplasic genotypes but they have been less frequently the focus of relevant genetic studies.

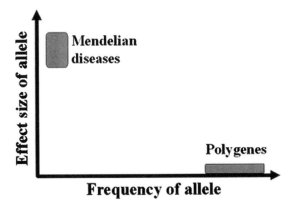

FIGURE 4 Frequency and effect size of alleles at genes causing obesity or genes that are part of more complex genotypes associated with a predisposition to obesity. *Source*: From Ref. 41.

OTHER POTENTIAL CONTRIBUTORS

A biological predisposition to excessive weight gain may lie in our genetic diversity but it may also be associated with events that are not the direct consequence of our genetic heritage. Among these other factors, we would like to emphasize in utero environment, lactation, epigenetic events and the potential role of viruses.

In utero environment

The topic of the fetal origin of adult risk factor profile and diseases has received considerable attention over the last two decades. In the case of obesity, it has been hypothesized that a low birth weight, taken as a marker of maternal nutritional deficiencies, was associated with childhood and adulthood obesity (18). However, the evidence in support of this hypothesis is mixed. There are studies on both sides of the issue. High birth weight is also associated with a higher risk of obesity later in life. Most of us are certainly prepared to accept that maternal nutrition has consequences for the fetus, and some of these effects are likely to translate into individual differences in disease risk later in life. This has, however, proven to be difficult to demonstrate in the case of human obesity. In fact, one could conclude that, at present, the evidence for a role of maternal nutrition, fetal nutritional status, and infant nutrition is stronger for adulthood metabolic and endocrine anomalies than obesity (18,19). There is, however, a body of animal data suggesting that maternal nutrition

TABLE 1 Distribution of Candidate Genes with Five or More Replications Across the Genetic Hypotheses

Genotype	Gene(s)
Thrifty	*ADRB2, ADRB3, UCP1, UCP2, UCP3*
Hyperphagic	*DRD2, HTR2C, LEP, LEPR, MC4R, NR3C1*
Sedens	*DRD2, MC4R*
Low lipid oxidation	*ACE, AD1POQ, GNB3, IL6, INS, LDLR, LIPE, RTN, TNFA*
Hyperplasic	*PPARG, VDR*

before and during pregnancy contributes to the risk of excess weight and adiposity in the offspring from a number of genetic backgrounds (20–24). Interestingly, a recent study has shown that Wistar rat offspring of mothers who were undernourished during pregnancy had a diminished locomotor activity level shortly after birth and subsequently later in life (14 months) compared to rats born from mothers who were fed ad libitum during pregnancy (25).

Lactation

Health authorities generally recommend that the newborn be exclusively breast fed for the first six months of life if the mother can do so adequately. However, a sizable fraction of mothers in the developed countries use infant formulas or rely on breast feeding for only a few weeks. Even though infant formulas are thought to be nutritionally adequate, breast milk contains some unique nutrients. Several studies have suggested that breast feeding is protective against childhood and adolescent overweight. In one particular study, duration of breastfeeding was associated with significantly reduced risk of being overweight at adolescence, particularly when the duration of breastfeeding extended beyond nine months (26). However, there are several studies that did not observe a relationship between the duration of breastfeeding and the risk of overweight.

Some experimental evidence indicates that polyunsaturated fatty acids of the omega-6 series are more potent promoters of adipogenesis in vitro and of adipose tissue expansion during pregnancy and the lactation period, compared to polyunsaturated fatty acids of the omega-3 series (27). It has been proposed that the content of n-6 polyunsaturated fatty acids in the breast milk of American women has increased substantially over the last 50 years while that of the n-3 polyunsaturated fatty acids has remained constant. This phenomenon has not been seen in European women. Ailhaud and Guesnet have proposed that the polyunsaturated fatty acids composition of breast milk and of dietary fats in general may favor the continuous development of adipose tissue during the pregnancy, lactation, and infancy period, thus setting the stage for an enhanced predisposition to obesity. This is obviously a controversial issue that requires a great deal of research.

Epigenetic Events

The two preceding sections suggest that epigenetic events may be implicated in creating susceptibility over and above that inscribed in the DNA sequence of genes. The nature of epigenetic modifications of DNA and histones as well as their potential relevance to the risk of obesity was discussed in a previous chapter. This is a new research path that may help us understand some of the variance unaccounted for in more classical genetic studies.

Viruses

The role of infections in the etiology of obesity has not been studied to a significant extent. However, Dhurandhar began in the early 90s probing the hypothesis that a viral infection may be involved in the etiology of obesity. To date, seven pathogens have been associated with obesity in animal models but their role in human obesity remains unclear (28). The adenovirus type 36 (Ad-36) antibody is found six times more frequently in the serum of human obese individuals (30%) than in the normal weight subjects (5%) (29). Ad-36 is the first human virus to be implicated in obesity. However, a cause-and-effect relationship has not been proposed yet, and potential mechanisms for the association remain unclear.

NEW AND MORE POWERFUL TOOLS

Advances of the last few years in genomics, mouse genetics, knockout and transgenic models, RNAi technologies, bioinformatics and computational biology (see some aspects developed in section 10) to name but a few are having a strong impact on our ability to understand the genetic architecture of the causes or the predisposition to obesity. It is not possible to highlight all the developments that are likely to influence human genetic studies of obesity in the years to come. However, we have chosen to mention three tools that became recently available which have the potential to make a difference in our research paradigms. These are referred to as the HapMap resource, the ability to perform genome-wide association studies, and the option to combine expression studies with exploration of single nucleotide polymorphisms (SNPs).

Hapmap

In 2005, The International HapMap Consortium published the first detailed haplotype map of the human genome (30). We are likely to see further refinement of the HapMap in the coming years. But already we have a tool that should improve our ability to identify the genotypes that contribute to the predisposition to common diseases (31). Even though we need more data regarding the applicability of the HapMap in a variety of ethnic groups, there is no doubt that it represents an important advance that can contribute to the understanding of the underlying biology of obesity.

Genome-Wide Association

Introduction of microarray-based SNP genotyping methods has drastically increased the throughput and reduced the cost of SNP genotyping. Ability to assay hundreds of thousands of DNA sequence variants in a single experiment has also made genome-wide association studies a reality, and the first such study was published in 2005 (32). Of considerable interest to the obesity research community was the series of genome-wide association reports focusing on Type 2 diabetes (33–37). Table 2 provides an overview of the genetic loci identified in at least one of these studies with a comparison across five cohorts. It was particularly striking that TCF7L2 was replicated across all five studies and that HHEX and SLC30A8 were also quite consistently replicated across the studies.

In the Wellcome case control study, SNPs in the FTO gene region on chromosome 16 were strongly associated with type 2 diabetes, but the association was abolished by adjustment for BMI (38). This led to the notion that the FTO gene was a strong candidate for the predisposition to human obesity, a hypothesis that was tested in 13 cohorts with 38,759 participants. The 16% of adults who were homozygotes for the risk allele at SNP rs9939609 weighed 3 kg more and had a 1.7-fold increased risk of obesity when compared to those without the risk allele (38).

Thus, it has become quite clear that from now on genome-wide association scans will be an essential part of the efforts to identify genetic loci and SNPs predisposing to human obesity. However, a genome-wide association study remains a major intellectual and financial undertaking, and several questions need

TABLE 2 Results from T2DM Genome-wide Association Studies

Chr	Gene	Map	Wellcome (35)	Broad (34)	Fusion (36)	DeCode (37)	French (33)
1	PKN2	88,855,326	No	Yes	Yes	No	No
3	PPARG	12,368,125	Yes	Partly	Yes	No	No
3	IGF2BP2	186,994,389	Yes	Yes	Yes	No	No
3	IGF2BP2	187,011,782		Yes		No	No
4	FLJ39370	113,152,901	No	Yes	No	No	No
6	CDKAL1	20,769,013	Yes	Yes	Yes		No
6	CDKAL1	20,787,688				Yes	No
8	SLC30A8	118,253,964	Yes	Not quite	Yes	Yes	Yes
9	(CDKN2B)	22,019,547	Yes	No	Partly	No	Yes
9	(CDKN2B)	22,124,094	Yes	Yes	Yes	No	Yes
10	HHEX	94,452,862	Partly	Yes	Partly	Yes	Yes
10	HHEX	94,455,539	Yes				
10	TCF7L2	114,744,078	Yes	Yes	Yes	Yes	Yes
11	KCNJ11	17,365,206	Yes	Yes	Yes	No	No
11		41,871,942	No	No	Yes	No	Partly
16	FTO	52,373,776	Yes	No	Partly	No	No

Source: From Refs. 33–37.

to be addressed to optimize the benefits from such an investment. These include the optimal number of SNPs, the optimal sample size and study design, the optimal statistical methods for a given study design, the control of multiple testing bias, and others. All these questions are topics of lively discussion and detailed research in the genetic community around the world.

Expression Studies with SNPs

The field is known as "genetical genomics." It combines the power of RNA microarray technologies with the advantages of classic mapping techniques by using gene expression levels as quantitative traits that are mapped to quantitative trait loci (examples are provided in Section 10). Even though it has not been widely applied to humans yet, the approach offers too much not to be taken seriously. It should make it possible to define the nature of the sequence variation that contributes to complex phenotype or disease traits from the point of view of the system or pathways that can be captured in the expression studies. The method could be applied to the biology of the adipose tissue and skeletal muscle in relevant experimental or observational designs for obesity (39).

CONCLUSION

The obesity epidemic we are facing today began manifesting itself only over the past three or four decades and can clearly not be explained by changes in our genome. The rapid weight gain in the population is more likely due to a changing environment that encourages consumption and discourages expenditure of energy, behaviors that are poorly compatible with our preagricultural hunter-gatherer genes. Therefore, most obesity cases are caused by maladaptive behaviors nurtured by an obesogenic environment.

However, there are biological determinants of the predisposition to become obese. We are proposing that the "thrifty genotype" is not the only, and probably not the best, genetic hypothesis to account for the apparent vulnerability that some people exhibit in the presence of an obesogenic environment. We believe that the "hyperphagic genotype" and the "sedentary genotype" have even more to contribute to our understanding of the highly complex concept of the "predisposition" to obesity.

Even though the genetic information is still scanty, we speculate that one can recognize four levels of genetic contributions to the risk of obesity. When obesity is caused by an invalidated gene resulting in the lack of a competent protein affecting a pathway impacting on the regulation of energy balance, then obesity is a disorder with a genetic origin. In such cases, the environment has only a permissive role in the severity of the phenotype. It is difficult to conclude firmly about the prevalence of cases of genetic obesity, as there remain undoubtedly a large number of genes to be evaluated in this regard. Based on the body of data accumulated to date, it would seem that cases of genetic obesity could represent up to 5% of the obesity cases and a larger percentage of the severely obese.

For the more common forms of obesity, we propose dividing them into those with a strong genetic predisposition and those with a slight genetic susceptibility. In contrast with the first category (genetic obesity), those with a strong genetic predisposition are not characterized by a clearly defective biology that can be reduced to a gene and a mutation or some other abnormalities. The strong predisposition results from susceptibility alleles at a number of loci. In an environment that does not favor obesity, these individuals would likely be overweight. They become obese and potentially severely obese in an obesogenic environment. One could hypothesize that a large fraction of the 62 million obese adult Americans are characterized by such a strong genetic predisposition.

A third group is arbitrarily defined as having inherited a slight genetic predisposition to obesity. Here again, one could hypothesize that most of the 68 million overweight adult Americans are representative of this level of susceptibility. In a restrictive environment, they may be normal weight or slightly overweight. An obesogenic environment will result in a large fraction of them becoming obese.

Finally, a fourth group includes those who are genetically resistant to obesity. They remain normal weight or almost normal weight in a wide range of obesogenic conditions. One could speculate that the 67 million normal weight adult Americans include a substantial portion who are resistant to obesity. These four types are depicted with respect to differences in obesogenic conditions in Figure 5.

An important question is whether genetic tests can be developed for population screening in order to predict the level of risk for the common polygenic forms of obesity. The practical usefulness of genetic testing for complex multifactorial diseases has been questioned (40). This skepticism stems from limitations associated with incomplete penetrance, variable expressivity within and across populations, and the low magnitude of risks typically associated with a defective genotype in the population. Despite the fact that many "obesity genes" have been mapped, high-penetrant high-risk genotypes have not been consistently found for the most common forms of obesity. Therefore, the contribution of a given "obesity gene" to the development of common obesity will be difficult to quantify and is likely to be low. The prediction of risk may improve by considering multiple genes simultaneously. However, the usefulness of predictive testing for the common forms of obesity remains to be fully understood.

Major behavioral changes would be needed on the part of large segments of the population of industrialized societies to curb the current increase in the

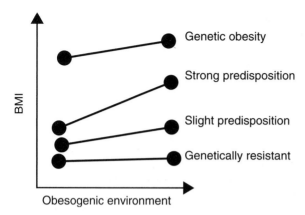

FIGURE 5 Four levels of genetic susceptibility to obesity in relation to differences in obesogenic conditions. *Source*: From Ref. 35.

prevalence of excess weight. However, we have learned over the past two decades or so that while behavior can be modified in the short term, most people revert back to familiar patterns after a few months or years. There are considerable environmental and societal forces that make it difficult for most people with a predisposition to obesity to adopt a preventive lifestyle that would allow them to achieve and maintain a normal body weight. Without major environmental and societal changes, it is almost certain that the obesity epidemic will continue to spread around the world as recent decades have revealed that human beings are biologically vulnerable in the presence of circumstances favoring positive energy balance.

REFERENCES

1. Hebebrand J, Wulftange H, Goerg T, et al. Epidemic obesity: are genetic factors involved via increased rates of assortative mating? Int J Obes Relat Metab Disord 2000; 24(3):345–53.
2. Jacobson P, Torgerson J, Sjostrom L, et al. Spouse resemblance in body mass index—effects on adult obesity prevalence in the offspring generation. Am J Epidemiol 2007; 165(1):101–8.
3. Katzmarzyk PT, Hebebrand J, Bouchard C. Spousal resemblance in the Canadian population: implications for the obesity epidemic. Int J Obes Relat Metab Disord 2002; 26(2):241–6.
4. Ravussin E, Valencia ME, Esparza J, et al. Effects of a traditional lifestyle on obesity in Pima Indians. Diabetes Care 1994; 17(9):1067–74.
5. Bouchard C, Tremblay A, Despres JP, et al. The response to long-term overfeeding in identical twins. N Engl J Med 1990; 322(21):1477–82.
6. Bouchard C, Tremblay A, Despres JP, et al. The response to exercise with constant energy intake in identical twins. Obes Res 1994; 2:400–10.
7. Hainer V, Stunkard AJ, Kunesova M, et al. Intrapair resemblance in very low calorie diet-induced weight loss in female obese identical twins. Int J Obes Relat Metab Disord 2000; 24(8):1051–7.
8. Neel J. Diabetes mellitus: a "thrifty" genotype rendered detrimental by "progress"? Am J Hum Genet 1962; 14:353–62.
9. Neel JV, Weder AB, Julius S. Type II diabetes, essential hypertension, and obesity as "syndromes of impaired genetic homeostasis": the "thrifty genotype" hypothesis enters the 21st century. Perspect Biol Med 1998; 42 (1):44–74.

10. Neel JV. When some fine old genes meet a 'new' environment. World Rev Nutr Diet 1999; 84:1–18.

11. Neel JV. The "thrifty genotype" in 1998. Nutr Rev 1999; 57(5 Pt 2):S2–9.

12. Katzmarzyk PT, Perusse L, Tremblay A, et al. No association between resting metabolic rate or respiratory exchange ratio and subsequent changes in body mass and fatness: 5-1/2 year follow-up of the Quebec family study. Eur J Clin Nutr 2000; 54(8):610–4.

13. Seidell JC, Muller DC, Sorkin JD, et al. Fasting respiratory exchange ratio and resting metabolic rate as predictors of weight gain: the Baltimore Longitudinal Study on Aging. Int J Obes Relat Metab Disord 1992; 16:667–74.

14. Simonen RL, Rankinen T, Perusse L, et al. Genome-wide linkage scan for physical activity levels in the Quebec Family study. Med Sci Sports Exerc 2003; 35(8):1355–9.

15. Zurlo F, Lillioja S, Esposito-Del Puente A, et al. Low ratio of fat to carbohydrate oxidation as predictor of weight gain: study of 24-h RQ. Am J Physiol 1990; 2591(5): E650–7.

16. Marra M, Scalfi L, Covino A, et al. Fasting respiratory quotient as a predictor of weight changes in nonobese women. Int J Obes Relat Metab Disord 1988; 22:601–3.

17. Rankinen T, Zuberi A, Chagnon Y, et al. The Human Obesity Gene Map: The 2005 Update. Obesity 2006; 14(4):529–644.

18. Barker D. Fetal origins of obesity. In: Bray GA, Bouchard C, eds. Handbook of Obesity. New York: Marcel Dekker, 2004; 109–16.

19. Adair LS, Prentice AM. A critical evaluation of the fetal origins hypothesis and its implications for developing countries. J Nutr 2004; 134(1):191–3.

20. Lim K, Shimomura Y, Suzuki M. Effect of high-fat diet feeding over generations on body fat accumulation. In: Romos DR, et al., eds. Obesity: Dietary Factors and Control. Tokyo/S. Karger, Basel: Japan Science Society, 1991; 181–90.

21. Wu Q, Mizushima Y, Komiya M, et al. The effects of high-fat diet feedling over generations on body fat accumulation associated with lipoprotein lipase and leptin in rat adipose tissues. Asia Pacific J Clin Nutr 1999; 8(1):46–52.

22. Wu Q, Mizushima Y, Komiya M, et al. Body fat accumulation in the male offspring of rats fed high-fat diet. J Clin Biochem Nutr 1998; 25:71–9.

23. Levin BE, Dunn-Meynell AA. Maternal obesity alters adiposity and monoamine function in genetically predisposed offspring. Am J Physiol Regul Integr Comp Physiol 2002; 283(5):R1087–93.

24. Levin BE, Govek E. Gestational obesity accentuates obesity in obesity-prone progeny. Am J Physiol 1998; 275(4 Pt 2):R1374–9.

25. Vickers MH, Breier BH, McCarthy D, et al. Sedentary behavior during postnatal life is determined by the prenatal environment and exacerbated by postnatal hypercaloric nutrition. Am J Physiol Regul Integr Comp Physiol 2003; 285(1):R271–3.

26. Gillman MW, Rifas-Shiman SL, Camargo CA, et al. Risk of overweight among adolescents who were breastfed as infants. JAMA 2001; 285(19):2461–7.

27. Ailhaud G, Guesnet P. Fatty acid composition of fats is an early determinant of childhood obesity: a short review and an opinion. Obes Rev 2004; 5:21–6.

28. Dhurandhar N. The viral hypothesis: one new potential pathway to obesity. In: Medeiros-Neto G, Halpern A, Bouchard C, eds. Progress in Obesity Research: 9. Montrouge, France: John Libbey Eurotext, 2003.

29. Atkinson R, Dhurandhar N, Allison DB, et al. Evidence for an association of an obesity virus with human obesity at three sites in the United States. Int J Obesity 1998; 22: S1–314.

30. Altshuler D, Brooks LD, Chakravarti A, et al. A haplotype map of the human genome. Nature 2005; 437(7063):1299–320.

31. Phimister EG. Genomic cartography—presenting the HapMap. N Engl J Med 2005; 353(17):1766–8.

32. Klein RJ, Zeiss C, Chew EY, et al. Complement factor H polymorphism in age-related macular degeneration. Science 2005; 308(5720):385–9.

33. Sladek R, Rocheleau G, Rung J, et al. A genome-wide association study identifies novel risk loci for type 2 diabetes. Nature 2007; 445(7130):881–5.

34. Diabetes Genetics Initiative of Broad Institute of Harvard and MIT, Lund University, and Novartis Institutes of BioMedical Research, Saxena R, Voight BF, et al. Genome-wide association analysis identifies loci for type 2 diabetes and triglyceride levels. Science 2007; 316(5829):1331–6.

35. Zeggini E, Weedon MN, Lindgren CM, et al. Replication of genome-wide association signals in UK samples reveals risk loci for type 2 diabetes. Science 2007; 316(5829): 1336–41.

36. Scott LJ, Mohlke KL, Bonnycastle LL, et al. A genome-wide association study of type 2 diabetes in Finns detects multiple susceptibility variants. Science 2007; 316(5829): 1341–45.

37. Steinthorsdottir V, Thorleifsson G, Reynisdottir I, et al. A variant in CDKAL1 influences insulin response and risk of type 2 diabetes. Nat Genet 2007; 39(6):770–5.

38. Frayling TM, Timpson NJ, Weedon MN, et al. A common variant in the FTO gene is associated with body mass index and predisposes to childhood and adult obesity. Science 2007; 316(5826):889–94.

39. Secko D. Genetics embraces expression. Scientist 2005; 19:26–9.

40. Holtzman NA, Marteau TM. Will genetics revolutionize medicine? N Engl J Med 2000; 343(2):141.

41. Loos RJ, Bouchard C. Obesity—is it a genetic disorder? J Intern Med 2003; 254(5): 401–25.

Index